Diagnostic and Operative Arthroscopy

James R. Andrews, M.D.

Medical Director, American Sports Medicine Institute
Orthopaedic Surgeon
Alabama Sports Medicine & Orthopaedic Center
Birmingham, Alabama

Laura A. Timmerman, M.D.

Associate Clinical Professor
Department of Orthopaedic Surgery
University of California, Davis
Sacramento, California
Private Practice
Oakland, California

W.B. Saunders Company

A Division of Harcourt Brace & Company

Philadelphia   London   Toronto   Montreal   Sydney   Tokyo

W.B. SAUNDERS COMPANY
A Division of Harcourt Brace & Company

The Curtis Center
Independence Square West
Philadelphia, Pennsylvania 19106

Library of Congress Cataloging-in-Publication Data

Diagnostic and operative arthroscopy / [edited by] James R. Andrews,
Laura A. Timmerman.—1st ed.

    p.   cm.

   ISBN 0–7216–5690–0

    1. Joints—Endoscopic surgery. 2. Arthroscopy. I. Andrews,
James R. (James Rheuben). II. Timmerman, Laura A.
   [DNLM: 1. Arthroscopy—methods. 2. Surgery, Endoscopic—methods.
WE 304 D536 1997]

  RD686.D53 1997   617.4′72059—dc20

  DNLM/DLC   96–26906

DIAGNOSTIC AND OPERATIVE ARTHROSCOPY   ISBN 0–7216–5690–0

Printed in the United States of America.

Last digit is the print number: 9   8   7   6   5   4   3   2   1

Dedication

This work is dedicated to:

The Orthopaedic and Primary Care Fellows who have challenged us over the years. Their dedication to their work with us has inspired us beyond our own limitations, and through them we have learned the true meaning of a team approach to accomplishing our goals.

Our mentors, Jack C. Hughston, M.D.; Frank C. McCue, M.D.; and Albert Trillat, M.D., who freely gave us so much of their knowledge and wisdom and made us what we are.

Lanny Johnson, M.D., who pioneered modern arthroscopic techniques, freely sharing his expertise and knowledge with us all.

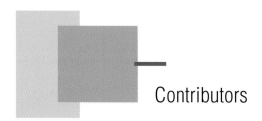

Contributors

GARY ANDERSON, M.D. Orthopaedic Surgeon, Orthopaedic Associates, Oklahoma City, Oklahoma. *Degenerative Arthritis of the Shoulder*.

JAMES R. ANDREWS, M.D. Clinical Professor of Orthopaedics and Sports Medicine, University of Virginia Medical School, Charlottesville, Virginia; Medical Director, American Sports Medicine Institute, Birmingham, Alabama; Orthopaedic Surgeon, Alabama Sports Medicine and Orthopaedic Center, Birmingham, Alabama. *Arthroscopic Surgical Techniques*; *Normal and Pathologic Arthroscopic Anatomy of the Shoulder*; *Degenerative Arthritis of the Shoulder*; *Diagnostic Arthroscopy of the Knee*; *Normal and Pathologic Arthroscopic Anatomy of the Knee*; *Synovial Lesions of the Knee*.

FREDERICK M. AZAR, M.D. Clinical Instructor, University of Tennessee, Memphis, Tennessee; Active Staff, The Campbell Clinic, Inc. *Diagnostic Arthroscopy of the Knee*.

J. W. THOMAS BYRD, M.D. Assistant Clinical Professor, Vanderbilt University School of Medicine, Department of Orthopaedics and Rehabilitation, Nashville, Tennessee; Orthopaedic Surgeon, Southern Sports Medicine and Orthopaedic Center, Nashville, Tennessee. *Diagnostic and Operative Arthroscopy of the Hip*.

WILLIAM G. CLANCY Jr, M.D. Clinical Professor of Orthopaedics and Sports Medicine, University of Virginia Medical School, Charlottesville, Virginia; Orthopaedic Surgeon, Alabama Sports Medicine and Orthopaedic Center, Birmingham, Alabama. *Meniscus Tears/Repair*; *Posterior Cruciate Ligament*.

KEVIN M. DUKES, M.D. Clinical Instructor, University of Oklahoma College of Medicine, Orthopaedic Surgeon, Tulsa Orthopaedics and Sports Medicine Center, Tulsa, Oklahoma. *Operating Room Environment*.

JAN P. ERTL, M.D. Assistant Clinical Professor of Orthopaedics, University of California, Davis; Chief of Trauma Service, Kaiser Permanente, Kaiser Permanente Medical Center, Sacramento, California. *Arthroscopic Techniques of Fracture Fixation of the Knee*.

RICHARD D. FERKEL, M.D. Clinical Instructor of Orthopaedic Surgery, University of California, Los Angeles; Attending Surgeon and Director of Sports Medicine Fellowship, Southern California Orthopaedic Institute, Van Nuys, California. *Operative Arthroscopy of the Ankle*; *Subtalar Arthroscopy: Diagnostic and Operative Techniques*.

GREGORY M. FOX, M.D. Orthopaedic and Sports Medicine Physician, Bloomington Bone and Joint Clinic, Bloomington, Indiana. *Normal and Pathologic Arthroscopic Anatomy of the Shoulder*.

WILLIAM P. GARTH, Jr, M.D. Associate Professor of Orthopaedics, University of Alabama, Birmingham, Alabama; Medical Director of University of Alabama Sports Medicine, The Childrens Hospital of Alabama. *Patellofemoral Joint*.

SCOTT D. GILLOGLY, M.D. Clinical Assistant Professor, Department of Surgery, Uniformed Services University of Health Sciences; Director of Sports Medicine, Georgia Baptist Orthopaedic Residency Program; Orthopaedic Surgeon, Atlanta Knee and Shoulder Clinic, Atlanta, Georgia. *Complications of Shoulder Arthroscopy*.

STEPHANIE L. GLAZE, R.N. HealthSouth Medical Center, Birmingham, Alabama. *Arthroscopic Surgical Techniques*.

GORDON I. GROH, M.D. Director of Shoulder and Elbow Surgery, University of Colorado; Orthopaedics, Mission Memorial Hospital, Asheville, North Carolina; St. Joseph's Hospital, Asheville, North Carolina. *Arthroscopic Acromioplasty*.

JAMES J. GUERRA, M.D. Head, Section of Sports Medicine, Cleveland Clinic Florida, Fort Lauderdale, Florida. *Normal and Pathologic Arthroscopic Anatomy of the Shoulder*.

JAMES F. GUHL, M.D. Clinical Professor of Orthopaedic Surgery, Medical College of Wisconsin, Milwaukee, Wisconsin. *Diagnostic Arthroscopy of the Ankle*.

JOHN GUIDO, Jr, P.T., C.S.C.S. Physical Therapist, Berushone Institute of Orthopedic and Sports Physical Therapy, Wyomissing, Pennsylvania. *Adhesive Capsulitis*.

MICHAEL M. HECKMAN, M.D. University of Texas Health Science Center, Department of Orthopaedics, Assistant Clinical Professor, University of Texas Medical School, San Antonio, Texas; Private Practice Orthopaedics, Corpus Christi, Texas. *Arthroscopic Acromioplasty*.

MARY LLOYD IRELAND, M.D. Assistant Professor, Department of Surgery (Orthopaedics), College of Medicine, University of Kentucky, Lexington, Kentucky; Orthopaedic Surgeon, Kentucky Sports Medicine, Lexington, Kentucky. *Degenerative Arthritis of the Knee*.

ROBERT W. JACKSON, M.D. Clinical Professor, Department of Orthopaedics, University of Texas, Southwestern, Dallas, Texas; Chief, Department of Orthopaedics, Baylor University Medical Center, Dallas, Texas. *History of Arthroscopy*.

MICHAEL E. JOYCE, M.D. Clinical Assistant Professor, Department of Orthopaedic Surgery, University of Connecticut School of Medicine, Farmington, Connecticut; Orthopaedic Surgeon, Connecticut Sports Medicine and Orthopaedic Center, Team Orthopaedic Surgeon at

University of Connecticut and Eastern Connecticut State University. *Normal and Pathologic Arthroscopic Anatomy of the Knee.*

STEPHEN L. KOLLIAS, M.D. Assistant Professor, Sports Medicine and Shoulder Surgery, Department of Orthopaedic Surgery, Indiana University Medical Center, Indianapolis, Indiana. *Labral Tears.*

SCOTT D. KUIPER, M.D. Orthopaedic Surgeon, Louisville Orthopaedic Clinic, Louisville, Kentucky. *Posterior Cruciate Ligament.*

LAWRENCE J. LEMAK, M.D. Clinical Assistant Professor of Orthopaedics and Rehabilitation, University of Virginia Medical School, Charlottesville, Virginia; Orthopaedic Surgeon, Alabama Sports Medicine and Orthopaedic Center, Birmingham, Alabama. *Treatment of Articular Cartilage.*

MEHRDAD M. MALEK, M.D. Director, Washington Orthopaedics and Knee Clinic, Oxen Hill, Maryland. *Complications of Knee Arthroscopy.*

RICHARD A. MARDER, M.D. Associate Professor of Orthopaedic Surgery; Chief, Sports Medicine Service, University of California, Davis, Medical Center, Sacramento, California. *Arthroscopic Techniques of Fracture Fixation of the Knee.*

SCOTT DAVID MARTIN, M.D. Orthopaedic Attending, Brigham and Women's Hospital, Boston, Massachusetts; Clinical Instructor, Harvard Medical School, Boston, Massachusetts. *Arthroscopic Resection of the Acromioclavicular Joint.*

MICHAEL M. MARUSHACK, M.D. Orthopaedic Surgeon, Orthopaedic Surgeons East, Birmingham, Alabama. *Treatment of Articular Cartilage.*

DANIEL G. McBRIDE, M.D. Orthopaedic Surgeon, Hampshire Orthopaedics, Northampton, Massachusetts. *Meniscus Tears/Repair.*

KEITH MEISTER, M.D. Assistant Professor of Orthopaedics, Division of Sports Medicine, University of Florida, Shands Hospital, University of Florida, Shands Clinic at Hampton Oaks, Gainesville, Florida; Team Physician, University of Florida, Gainesville, Florida. *Diagnostic Arthroscopy of the Shoulder.*

BARRY PHILLIPS, M.D. Associate Professor of Orthopaedic Surgery, University of Tennessee, Memphis, Tennessee; Active Staff, Campbell Clinic, Germantown, Tennessee. *Anterior Cruciate Ligament Injuries.*

GARY G. POEHLING, M.D. Professor and Chairman, Bowman Gray School of Medicine, Winston-Salem, North Carolina. *Diagnostic Arthroscopy of the Wrist; Operative Arthroscopy of the Wrist.*

DAVID S. RUCH, M.D. Assistant Professor of Orthopaedic Surgery, Bowman Gray School of Medicine, Winston-Salem, North Carolina; Assistant Professor, Hand and Microsurgery, Trauma and Reconstructive Surgery, Bowman Gray School of Medicine, Winston-Salem, North Carolina. *Diagnostic Arthroscopy of the Wrist; Operative Arthroscopy of the Wrist.*

CHARLES M. RULAND, M.D. Orthopaedic Surgeon, Anne Arundel Orthopaedic Surgeons, Annapolis, Maryland. *Operative Arthroscopy of the Ankle.*

YVONNE E. SATTERWHITE, M.D., C.S.C.S. Team Physician Berea College, Sue Bennett College, Lindsey Wilson College; Assistant Team Physician, Eastern Kentucky University; Orthopaedic Surgeon, Kentucky Sports Medicine Clinic, Lexington, Kentucky. *Shoulder Instability.*

KURT C. SCHLUNTZ, M.D. Orthopaedic and Sports Medicine Physician, Physicians Plaza, Oak Ridge, Tennessee. *Synovial Lesions of the Knee.*

NEAL C. SMALL, M.D. Clinical Assistant Professor, Department of Orthopaedic Surgery, University of Texas, Southwestern Medical School, Dallas, Texas; Medical Director, Associated Arthroscopic Institute, Plano, Texas. *Complications of Knee Arthroscopy.*

STEPHEN J. SNYDER, M.D. Orthopaedic Surgeon, Southern California Orthopedic Institute, Van Nuys, California. *Labral Tears.*

STEPHEN R. SOFFER, M.D. Director, Eastern Sports Medicine and Orthopedic Institute, Berkshire Orthopedic Associates, Wyomissing, Pennsylvania. *Adhesive Capsulitis; Diagnostic Arthroscopy of the Elbow.*

JAMES W. STONE, M.D. Assistant Clinical Professor, Medical College of Wisconsin; Orthopaedic Physician, Milwaukee, Wisconsin. *Diagnostic Arthroscopy of the Ankle.*

KURT T. STROEBEL, M.D. Orthopaedic and Sports Medicine Physician, Palmetto Orthopaedic and Sports Medicine Center, Sumter, South Carolina. *Patellofemoral Joint.*

TIMOTHY B. SUTHERLAND, M.D. Instructor, Department of Orthopaedic Surgery, University of California, Davis, Sacramento, California; Desert Orthopaedic Center, Las Vegas, Nevada. *Rotator Cuff Tears.*

LAURA A. TIMMERMAN, M.D. Associate Clinical Professor, Department of Orthopaedic Surgery, University of California, Davis; Team Physician, University of California, Berkeley; Chief of Orthopaedics, Merrithew Hospital, Martinez, California; Private Practice, Oakland, California. *Throwing Shoulder; Operative Arthroscopy of the Elbow.*

MARK M. WILLIAMS, M.D. Attending Physician, Florida Sports Medicine and Orthopaedic Center, Panama City, Florida. *Subtalar Arthroscopy: Diagnostic and Operative Techniques.*

RICHARD I. WILLIAMS, M.D. Orthopaedic Surgeon, Upper Cumberland Orthopaedic Surgery, Cookeville, Tennessee. *Degenerative Arthritis of the Knee.*

Preface

The purpose of this book is to provide a comprehensive guide to arthroscopic surgery—from the basic diagnostic level to advanced operative procedures. We understand there are several ways to achieve the same outcome and have attempted to present a variety of techniques for different procedures. Preparation, equipment, and set-up are critical in arthroscopy, and we have spent time on these areas. Our goal is to provide one reference source with a "how-to-do" orientation for all levels of surgeons, from orthopaedic residents to arthroscopic subspecialists.

James R. Andrews, M.D.
Medical Director
American Sports Medicine Institute
Birmingham, Alabama

Laura A. Timmerman, M.D.
Oakland, California

Acknowledgments

We want to thank all the members of the American Sports Medicine Fellowship Society. It is the contribution of the Fellows, both during and after their training, that provided the inspiration and energy for this project. In addition, we appreciate the time and effort of the contributing authors and understand the commitment involved in seeing a chapter to completion. We also want to thank the American Sports Medicine Institute, especially Mrs. Jerry Conner and Mr. Dale Baker; Dan Nichols, Medical Illustrator in Atlanta, Georgia; and the excellent editors at W.B. Saunders Co. for their hard work in the preparation of this book.

James R. Andrews, M.D.
Medical Director
American Sports Medicine Institute
Birmingham, Alabama

Laura A. Timmerman, M.D.
Oakland, California

Notice

Medicine is an ever-changing field. Standard safety precautions must be followed, but as new research and clinical experience broaden our knowledge, changes in treatment and drug therapy become necessary or appropriate. Readers are advised to check the product information currently provided by the manufacturer of each drug to be administered to verify the recommended dose, the method and duration of administration, and contraindications. It is the responsibility of the treating physician relying on experience and knowledge of the patient to determine dosages and the best treatment for the patient. Neither the Publisher nor the editor assumes any responsibility for any injury and/or damage to persons or property.

The Publisher

Contents

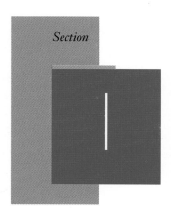

Basic Principles

History of Arthroscopy

Robert W. Jackson

The science of endoscopy has made great strides since Phillip Bozzini (1773–1809) presented his Lichtleiter to the Joseph Academy of Medical Surgery in Vienna in 1806. This instrument for looking into the bladder was not well received and was regarded as a mere toy. Almost 50 years later, in 1853, A.J. Desormeaux (1815–1882) introduced the gastrogen endoscope, which used a light source provided by the combustion of a mixture of turpentine and gasoline, with mirrors to transmit the light into the bladder.[1] In 1876, following the introduction of electricity, Max Nitze (1848–1906) used an electrically heated platinum wire glowing white-hot, encased in a water-cooled goose quill, to provide the first light source from within the bladder.[1] The next major advance occurred when Thomas Edison (1847–1931) developed the incandescent lamp in 1880, which solved most of the previous problems of illumination and allowed cystoscopy to flourish.[1]

THE PIONEERS OF ARTHROSCOPY

Professor Kenji Takagi (1888–1963) of Tokyo University is generally given credit for being the first to successfully apply the principles of endoscopy to a knee joint.[2–5] In 1918, he viewed the interior of a cadaver knee using a cystoscope. His hope was that, by means of endoscopy of the knee, he would be able to diagnose and treat tuberculosis in its early stages and thus avoid the physical and psychologic problems that were created in the Japanese population by a stiff knee. He developed endoscopic instruments specifically for this purpose, and on July 6, 1932, he gave the first report of endoscopy of the knee to the Japanese Orthopaedic Association.[6] This report was illustrated with black-and-white pictures taken through the cystoscope. By 1936, he was successful in obtaining color pictures and movie film of the interior of a knee joint. Working closely with him during this developmental phase was Dr. Saburo Iino, who was the first to describe and name the various plicae, or folds, of synovium within the knee joint.[7]

As so often happens in science, another investigator was also exploring the use of endoscopy in the knee joint. In 1919, Dr. Eugen Bircher (1882–1956), using a Jacobeus laparoscope developed by the Georg Wolf Company, examined the knees of a small number of patients[8] and, in 1922, published the results of his investigation of 21 patients with osteoarthritis.[9] These were the first publications on arthroscopy; Bircher called the technique arthroendoscopy.

In 1925, Phillip Kreuscher (1884–1943) published in the *Illinois Medical Journal* a plea for the early diagnosis of semilunar cartilage disease by use of an arthroscope.[10] Unfortunately the instrument that he developed and used has been lost. He was, however, an original thinker and must be given credit for the first publication in English on this topic. A year later, E.W. Geist published a "preliminary report" on arthroscopy in the journal *Lancet*.[11]

In 1930, Dr. Michael Burman (1901–1975) spent a fellowship year in Berlin studying endoscopic techniques. On his return to New York, he published several classic articles on this new method of examining joints, along with his associates at the Hospital for Joint Diseases, Drs. Finkelstein, Mayer, and Sutro.[12–15] However, problems with the technology of the time led to frequent breakage of the equipment, and his pioneering foresight was met with skepticism and derision from many of his colleagues.

European pioneers in the 1930s included Drs. Sommer (1937),[16] Vaubel (1938),[17] and Wilke (1939),[18] who published in the German literature their early experiences with arthroscopy.

THE REAWAKENING

World War II interrupted the further development of arthroscopy. After the war, the concept was once again explored, and the technique slowly gained momentum. In Japan, Dr. Masaki Watanabe (1921–1994), who had been a student of Prof. Takagi, continued Takagi's work. The Japanese in the postwar era developed extensive expertise

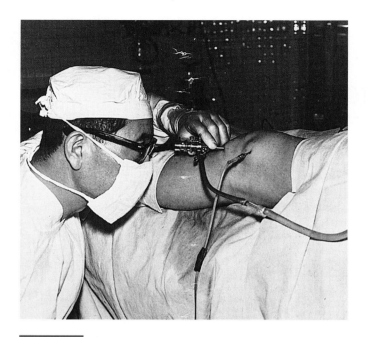

Figure 1–1 • Dr. Masaki Watanabe performs arthroscopy at the Tokyo Teishin Hospital in 1964.

in electronics and optics, and Dr. Watanabe, working with several companies, developed new and better arthroscopes and numbered them successively.[3] In 1958, he produced the Watanabe 21, which proved to be the first truly successful arthroscope (Fig. 1–1).[19] The Watanabe 21 had a magnificent lens with an angle of vision of 102 degrees in saline solution. It also had a depth of focus from 0.5 mm to infinity. Fiber light was the next major advance and was a feature of the Watanabe 22 arthroscope. The Watanabe 24 arthroscope was 1.7 mm in diameter, used a single glass (Selfoc) fiber, and was designed for use in small joints.

Dr. Watanabe also performed the first recorded surgical procedures under arthroscopic control. In 1955, he removed a xanthomatous giant cell tumor from the suprapatellar pouch of a patient. He also performed a partial meniscectomy under arthroscopic control in 1962.[4] His colleagues, Dr. Hiroshi Ikeuchi and Dr. Sakae Takeda, also deserve much credit as they played significant roles in the early development of the techniques of operative arthroscopy. In 1957, Dr. Watanabe published the first edition of his *Atlas of Arthroscopy*, with Takeda and Ikeuchi as coauthors.[20] The atlas was illustrated by S. Fujihashi and was revised for a second edition in 1969 with photographs of pathologic conditions of joints.[21]

In somewhat parallel development, publications appeared in the French literature by Drs. Hurter in 1955[22] and Imbert in 1956.[23] Several rheumatologists, including Drs. Jayson and Dixon in England[24] and Drs. Robles-Gil, Katona, and Barroso in Mexico,[25] were using the arthroscope on joints in the early 1960s.

In 1964, Dr. Robert Jackson went to Tokyo on a research scholarship to work at Tokyo University. He was introduced to the work of Dr. Watanabe by Dr. Isao Abe.

He attended Dr. Watanabe's operating sessions at the Tokyo Teishin Hospital on every possible occasion.[26] Dr. Watanabe taught Dr. Jackson his techniques in exchange for English lessons. Dr. Jackson returned to the University of Toronto in 1965 and was joined a year later by Dr. Abe. Together they further refined and promoted the technique of arthroscopy and published their early experience in the *Journal of Bone and Joint Surgery* in 1972.[27] Dr. Jackson's first major presentation on the subject of arthroscopy in North America was at the inaugural meeting of the Association of Academic Surgeons in Toronto in 1967. He also gave the first instructional course on the subject at the annual meeting of the American Academy of Orthopaedic Surgeons in 1968 and did so yearly until 1974. In the late 1960s and early 1970s, numerous visitors came to Toronto to learn the technique. These early pioneers included Drs. John Joyce III (1914–1991), Ward Casscells (1915–1996),[28] John McGinty, David Drez, and Kenneth DeHaven.

In 1969, Dr. Richard O'Connor (1933–1980) visited Dr. Watanabe in Tokyo and soon was expounding on the benefits of partial meniscectomy. In the early 1970s, Dr. Lanny Johnson began his work with a modified Watanabe 24, called the Needle Scope, and he soon became known for his teaching and technical innovations.

Meanwhile, in Europe, Dr. Harold Eikelaar defended his thesis on arthroscopy in 1973 and received the highest possible degree in surgery from the University of Groningen in Holland.[29] Dr. Henri Dorfmann in France, Drs. Jan Gillquist and Ejnar Eriksson in Sweden, Mr. Adrian Henry in England, Dr. Hans Rudolph Henche in Switzerland, Drs. John Ohnsorge and Werner Glinz in Germany, and Dr. O. Wruhs in Austria also played significant roles in the teaching and development of new techniques in arthroscopy during those early days.

THE RAPID GROWTH

The 1970s were years of rapid progress. In 1974, Mr. David Dandy of Cambridge, England, took a fellowship year in Toronto and coauthored with Dr. Jackson the first English monograph on the subject of arthroscopy, published in 1976.[5] Also in 1974, the International Arthroscopy Association (IAA) was founded in Philadelphia, and Dr. Watanabe was honored as the first president. The stated purpose of the IAA was to educate orthopaedic surgeons in the value of the technique and to spread awareness of arthroscopy through IAA chapters throughout the world. The first formal course in arthroscopy was given in 1973 at the University of Pennsylvania under the chairmanship of Dr. Joyce. During the next few years numerous courses were given by the IAA and by other academic institutions. Excellent courses were organized annually by Drs. Richard O'Connor, Robert Metcalf, John McGinty, Ejnar Eriksson, Theo VanRens, and many others.

In 1981, the North American chapter of the IAA became the Arthroscopy Association of North America (AANA). Other arthroscopy associations were soon established in Brazil, India, Mexico, Argentina, and Germany.

THE SHIFT TO SURGERY

Although arthroscopy started as an aid to diagnosis, events in the 1980s produced a major shift in attitudes. First, it became generally accepted that arthroscopy provided a diagnostic accuracy that was far greater than that which could be produced by clinical examination and any other diagnostic modality. Second, the ability to see pathologic conditions, coupled with the desire to treat them under arthroscopic control, with minimal morbidity and fewer complications, led to the revolutionary concept of minimally invasive surgery. This desire spawned the development of new instruments and new techniques specifically designed to treat a large variety of conditions. Dr. Johnson developed the first powered tools, such as the shaver and the bur. Dr. O'Connor was central in developing the operating arthroscope; use of the arthroscope has since given way to the technique of triangulation. Numerous other individuals developed specific instruments for use in operations, such as the suction punch developed by Dr. T. Whipple, and the graspers and cutting tools developed by Drs. O'Connor, Dandy, and Jackson. Techniques for the knee joint developed rapidly, including meniscus repair and transplantation, pioneered by individuals such as Drs. Robert Stone, Charles Henning, Dilworth Cannon, Russell Warren, and Gregory Keene. Anterior cruciate ligament reconstruction was pioneered by Drs. David Drez, Douglas Jackson, Donald Shelbourne, and many others. Examination of the shoulder, ankle, and elbow, and techniques related to those joints, were pioneered by Drs. James Andrews, Steven Snyder, Harvard Ellman, Richard Caspari, and James Guhl. The symptomatic treatment of osteoarthritis was popularized by Drs. Robert Jackson, Lanny Johnson, Whit Ewing, Jerome Jennings, and others. It is now being recognized by rheumatologists as superior to the use of anti-inflammatory medication. Teaching was enhanced by anatomic models such as those developed by Drs. Robert Eilert and Howard Sweeney, only recently giving way to cadaver parts for teaching purposes. Many books have been written, and videotapes have been prepared to aid in the teaching of arthroscopy. The establishment of *Arthroscopy, The Journal of Arthroscopic and Related Surgery* in 1985 was a major step forward. The Orthopaedic Learning Center opened in Chicago in 1994; together with the American Academy of Orthopaedic Surgeons, they teach arthroscopic and other surgical techniques.

Arthroscopic surgery has been a true revolution and perhaps the most important event in orthopaedics in this century.

In perspective, the momentum has slowed slightly. The basic instrumentation is fairly uniform, visualization with television is routine, and standard techniques are commonly employed throughout the world. However, progress is still evolving in the application of these techniques to problems that afflict other joints, such as the ankle, the wrist, the shoulder, the elbow, and the lumbar spine. Where this surgical revolution will end is hard to predict. The application of new energy sources such as the laser, now being explored as a reparative tool rather than a resecting tool, is noted. Resurfacing of arthritic joints under arthroscopic control might also be a possibility in the near future.

Without doubt, arthroscopy is an exciting and developing field with a constantly evolving history. It has played a leading role in the new concept of minimally invasive surgery and has stimulated the spread of this concept to most of the other surgical disciplines.

Finally, it is fascinating to reflect on how much progress has been made in the treatment of joint problems since the first recorded surgery for meniscal disease in 1885.[30] It is even more remarkable, when one reflects on the last three decades, how medicine has moved rapidly from the scalpel to the scope in the treatment of joint problems.

References

1. From Lichtleiter to fiber optics. Catalogue prepared by the staff of the National Museum for the History of Science, Leiden, the Netherlands, on the occasion of the 16th Congress of the International Society for Urology.
2. Joyce JJ: Foreword, symposium on arthroscopy. Orthop Clin North Am 10:3, 1979.
3. Watanabe M: The development and present status of the arthroscope. J Jpn Med Instr 24:11, 1954.
4. Watanabe M, Bechtol RC, Nottage WM, et al.: The history of arthroscopy. In Shahriaree H (ed.): O'Connor's Textbook of Arthroscopic Surgery, 2nd ed. Philadelpha, J.B. Lippincott Co., 1992, pp 213–217.
5. Jackson RW and Dandy DJ: Arthroscopy of the Knee. New York, Grune & Stratton, 1976.
6. Takagi K: Practical experiences using Takagi's arthroscope. Nippon Seikeigeka Gakkai Zasshi 8:132, 1933.
7. Iino S: Normal arthroscopic findings of the knee joint in the adult cadaver. Nippon Seikeigeka Gakkai Zasshi 14:467–523, 1940.
8. Bircher E: Die Arthroendoskopie. Zentralbl Chir 48:1460–1461, 1921.
9. Bircher E: Beitrag zur Pathologie und Diagnose der Meniscus-Verletzung. Bruns Beitr Klin Chir 127:239–250, 1922.
10. Kreuscher PH: Semilunar cartilage disease: a plea for early recognition by means of the arthroscope and early treatment of this condition. Ill Med J 47:290–292, 1925.
11. Geist EW: Arthroscopy: preliminary report. Lancet 46:306–307, 1926.
12. Burman MS: Arthroscopy or direct visualization of joints: an experimental cadaver study. J Bone Joint Surg 13:669–695, 1931.
13. Burman MS, Finkelstein H, and Mayer L: Arthroscopy of the knee joint. J Bone Joint Surg 16:255–268, 1934.
14. Burman MS and Mayer L: Arthroscopic examination of the knee joint. Arch Surg 2:846, 1936.
15. Burman MS and Sutro CJ: Arthroscopy by fluorescence: experimental study. Arch Phys Ther 16:423, 1935.
16. Sommer R: Die Endoskopie des Kniegelenkes. Zentralbl Chir 64:1692–1697, 1937.
17. Vaubel E: Die Endoskopie des Kniegelenkes. Z Rheumaforsch 1:210–213, 1938.
18. Wilke KH: Endoskopie des Kniegelenkes an der Leiche. Bruns Beitr Klin Chir 169:75–83, 1939.
19. Watanabe M and Takeda S: The number 21 arthroscope. Nippon Seikeigeka Gakkai Zasshi 34:1041, 1960.
20. Watanabe M, Takeda S, and Ikeuchi H: Atlas of Arthroscopy. Tokyo, Igaku Shoin Ltd., 1957.
21. Watanabe M, Takeda S, and Ikeuchi H: Atlas of Arthroscopy, 2nd ed. Tokyo, Igaku Shoin Ltd., 1969.
22. Hurter E: L'arthroscopie: nouvelle méthode d'exploration du genou. Rev Chir Orthop 41:763–766, 1955.
23. Imbert R: L'arthroscopie du genou: sa technique. Marseille Chir 8:368–369, 1956.

24. Jayson MI and Dixon ASJ: Arthroscopy of the knee in rheumatic disease. Ann Rheum Dis 27:503–511, 1968.
25. Robles-Gil J, Katona G, and Barroso MR: Arthroscopy as an aid to diagnosis and investigation. Excerpta Med Int Congr Ser 143:16, 1968.
26. Jackson RW: Memories of the early days of arthroscopy: 1965–1975: the formative years. Arthroscopy: 3:1–3, 1987.
27. Jackson RW and Abe I: The role of arthroscopy in the management of disorders of the knee. J Bone Joint Surg Br 52:310–322, 1972.
28. Casscells SW: Arthroscopy of the knee joint. J Bone Joint Surg Am 53:278–298, 1971.
29. Eikelaar HR: Arthroscopy of the knee. Thesis for a doctorate in orthopaedic surgery at the University of Groningen, 1975.
30. Annandale T: An operation for displaced semilunar cartilage. Br Med J 779, 1885.

2 Operating Room Environment

Kevin M. Dukes

Since the introduction of arthroscopy into North America in 1964 by Robert Jackson, the technology has rapidly progressed. Approximately 98% of practicing orthopaedists utilize arthroscopy in their practice.[1] It is believed to be the most common outpatient procedure performed in the United States. There has been an increase in different joints that are treated arthroscopically. The indications and types of procedures have increased as well. Consequently, this has led to an explosion of instrument development. It is beyond the scope of this chapter to discuss all the products available on the market today.

ARTHROSCOPES

There are a variety of sizes and angles of arthroscopes. Arthroscopes vary in diameter, focal length, and lens angles. The diameter of the arthroscope is important in providing the rigidity needed to prevent bending. If the arthroscope is bent, it alters the path of the light beams, which can affect the resolution of the image. Arthroscopes are available in 2.7 mm, 4.0 mm, and 5.0 mm. Generally, larger arthroscopes are used in larger joints that require manipulation within the joint and that provide more space. Smaller-diameter arthroscopes provide greater maneuverability within the joint and are useful in the wrist and ankle. A larger 5.0 mm arthroscope is useful in hip arthroscopy.[2] Important optic properties are focal length, field of vision, and resolution. Focal length is dependent on the length of the arthroscope. A longer focal length produces a smaller depth of field but greater magnification.[3] Larger camera angles provide a wider field of vision, which is the area in which the camera can receive light and see. This angle is measured by the lines from the distal tip of the arthroscope to two points at the extreme of an object (Fig. 2–1). Most arthroscopes used in orthopaedic surgery have angles of 0, 30, and 70 degrees (Fig. 2–2). The cost of a wider-angle arthroscope is increased distortion (Fig. 2–3). Although the 30 degree arthroscope is

often more useful, it has greater distortion than a 0 degree arthroscope. There is approximately 30% distortion in a wide-angle arthroscope of 100 degrees. An advantage of the angle arthroscope is that the field of view can effectively be increased by rotating the arthroscope (Fig. 2–4). The field of view is reduced in aqueous media as compared with air media. The tip must be 40–50% farther from an object in an aqueous media to obtain the same field of view as in air.[4] Unlike endoscopy, in which resolution is limited by the human eye, videoimaging is limited by the video chip or pixel or by the monitor resolution. Scratches, chips, or residue built up on the lens can cause a blurred or unfocused image. There are many sophisticated camera systems that provide excellent images. The light source is also an important component in quality images. Adequate lighting is necessary to safely visualize inside a joint so that inadvertent damage to the articular surface can be avoided. Fiberoptic cables are used to transmit light from the source. The primary determinants of the amount of light provided are the light source intensity and the area of the fiberoptic bundles. Most light sources provide variable intensity, which allows for illumination in dark regions. Intensity may be controlled manually or by an automatic feedback sensor. Large dark areas result from a decrease in the amount of light and indicate broken fibers or poor packing of fibers in the cable.[4] Arthroscopes fit into a cannulated system, which allows the surgeon to place the camera easily into the joint (Fig. 2–5). Blunt and sharp trocars introduce the cannula through the soft tissue into the joint. Caution is needed when placing the sharp trocar tip through the soft tissue to avoid inadvertent damage to the articular surface. Blunt trocars can be used to penetrate the joint capsule. If frequent changes are required, Wiessinger rods or switching sticks are helpful in minimizing soft-tissue trauma on reinsertion of the cannula. If frequent changes in portals are necessary, extra cannulae help minimize soft-tissue injury to the portals from frequent introductions. Cannulae have side portals to allow inflow or outflow of fluid through the arthroscope.

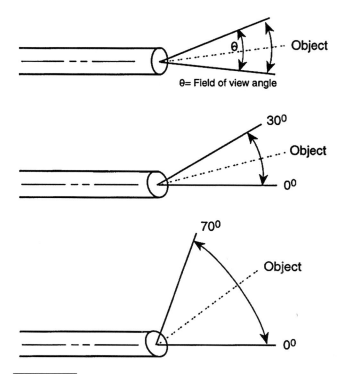

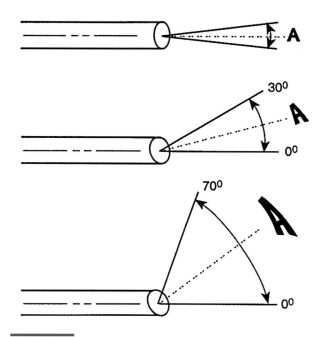

Figure 2–3 • Arthroscopic distortion. As the field of view increases, so does the amount of distortion of the image.

Figure 2–1 • Field of view angle. Wider camera angles provide a larger viewing area.

PREOPERATIVE ANTIBIOTICS

The rate of occurrence of septic arthritis following arthroscopy has been reported to be 0.4–3.4%.[5, 6] This is a serious and potentially disabling complication. D'Angelo and Ogilvie-Harris[7] reported on the cost-effectiveness of prophylactic antibiotics in arthroscopic surgery. Forty-four percent of their infected patients had symptomatic sequelae. They reported few side effects of antibiotics and

relatively low cost. It was concluded that if the incidence of infection is greater than 0.08%, it would be most cost-effective to give prophylactic antibiotics. They were unable to identify any specific risk factors that could be used to predict complications. This is in contrast to the study by Wertheim, Gillespie, and Klaus,[8] who reported an infection rate of 0.07% in a retrospective review of 800 arthroscopic procedures. They concluded that it is justified not to give prophylactic antibiotics. Wieck et al.[9] in a prospective double-blind study of 437 patients reported no significant differences in those receiving preoperative antibiotics and those not given antibiotics. There were no infections in the cefazolin group and one superficial infection in the control group. One allergic reaction occurred in the cefazolin group, which required treatment. Because of potential complications and cost, the researchers found no evidence to support the routine use of prophylactic antibiotics in arthroscopic surgery. If prophylactic antibiotics are given, they should be given approximately 20 minutes before surgery to obtain maximum tissue concentrations.[10] A comprehensive study by Armstrong, Bolding, and Joseph[11] discussed septic arthritis after arthroscopy. They discussed that previous rates of septic arthritis may have been low because the reports involved a method of voluntary reporting. The actual number may have been underreported. In their retrospective study of 4,256 patients they reported a 0.42% infection rate. *Staphylococcus aureus* was the most common infectious agent, followed by coagulase-negative *Staphylococcus*. The primary risk factor was the length of surgery. Prophylactic antibiotics provided a small but not statistically significant protective effect. Seventy percent of patients had symptoms within 3 days, and all had symptoms within 11 days. Débridement and 2 weeks of intravenous antibiotics appeared satisfactory in the treatment. The researcher reported excellent long-term results in 73% of patients.

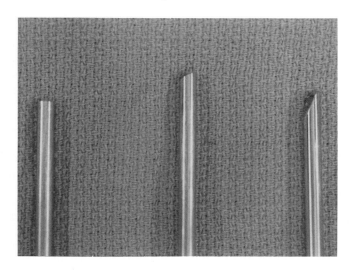

Figure 2–2 • Arthroscopes left to right: 0 degree, 30 degrees, and 70 degrees.

Rotation of Arthroscope 180⁰

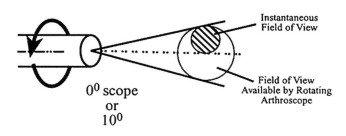

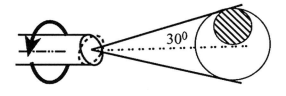

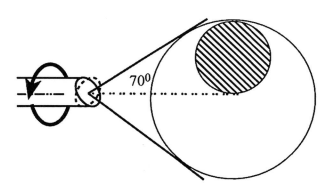

Figure 2–4 • The overall viewing area can be increased by simply rotating the arthroscope.

SET-UP

Patient positioning is important in the preparation of the procedure. It is important to be familiar with all the traction and holding devices as well as with their advantages and potential complications.

Knee arthroscopy can be assisted with use of either a leg holder or a post (Fig. 2–6). The leg holder provides stability needed to stress the medial and lateral compartments. The holder allows the surgeon to manipulate the leg without an assistant.

Neurapraxia to the lateral femoral cutaneous nerve may result if the holder is placed too tight. The side post allows more maneuverability of the leg during the procedure, which may be helpful in repair of a meniscus or reconstruction of the anterior or medial collateral ligaments. Excessive stress on the knee may result in ligament injuries to the knee, most commonly the mid cruciate ligament. When shoulder arthroscopy is performed with the

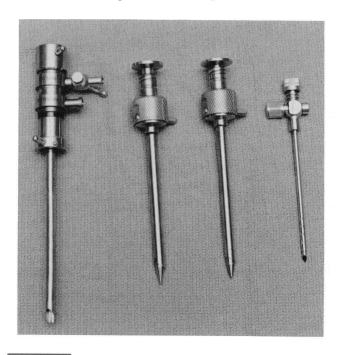

Figure 2–5 • Cannula system left to right: sheath with a bridge for the camera; sheaths with blunt and sharp trocars; egress cannula.

patient in the lateral decubitus position, shoulder suspension can be done with an overhead frame (Fig. 2–7). Andrews, Carson, and Ortega[12, 13] recommended 70 degrees of abduction and 15 degrees of forward flexion with longitudinal traction. Traction of 20 lb or less can be used with minimal risk of neurapraxia. Transient dysesthesias of the radial sensory nerve have been reported with inadequate padding of the wrist.[14] Although permanent neurologic injury has been reported,[15] most injuries are transient. Rodeo, Forster, and Weiland[16] used the beach-chair position, citing lower incidence of brachial plexus strain. However, they cautioned about the position of the head because of reported hypoglossal nerve injury.[17]

Ankle arthroscopy has been performed with and without traction. Invasive and noninvasive devices assist in distraction of the joint. Noninvasive clover-hitch ankle straps are safe and provide satisfactory distraction. Invasive devices utilize cortical pins in the tibia and calcaneus to distract the joint. Guhl[18] cites as advantages of invasive devices that they provide increased room for visualization and manipulation of instruments and allow larger instruments and therefore reduce the risk of breaking instruments within the joint and scuffing the articular surface. Guhl recommended that traction be limited to 30–50 lb of traction. However, there are potential complications of pin breakage, pin tract infections, neurovascular damage, and the creation of stress risers. Ferkel and Scanton[19] did not note an increased rate of complications with invasive devices. Skeletal distraction is contraindicated in the presence of an open physis, reflex sympathetic dystrophy and infection, and severe degenerative joint disease.[18, 19]

Elbow arthroscopy may be performed with the patient in the supine or prone position. The prone position

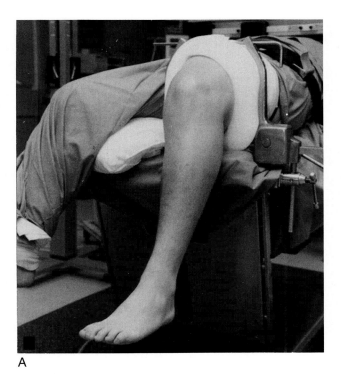

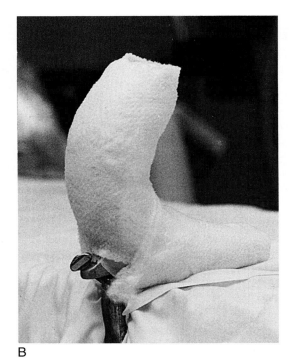

A

B

Figure 2–6 • *A*, Knee holder. *B*, Lateral stress post.

allows for easy range of motion of the arm and good stability of the elbow. Gravity may allow the neurovascular structures to move from the joint capsule. The supine position can be used with an overhead traction device. It may be easier to conceptualize the anatomy; however, some believe that posterior access may be more difficult.[20]

Wrist arthroscopy is commonly performed with the patient's elbow in the supine position, with elbow flexed 90 degrees and the hand suspended overhead by Chinese fingertraps. Digital nerve neurapraxia has been reported, particularly in the presence of distal interphalangeal osteophytes.[21] Traction should be limited to 5–7 lb for a maximum of 2 hours.[22] Mounted traction devices are also available. There have been no reports of compartment syndrome in wrist arthroscopy.

Hip arthroscopy may be used with the patient either in the supine or the lateral position; however, both positions require the use of a fracture table with longitudinal

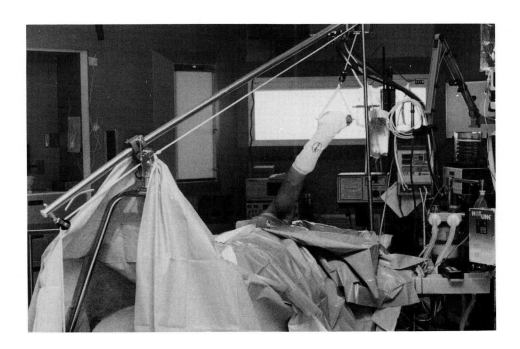

Figure 2–7 • Shoulder suspension device.

traction. This traction is provided on a fracture table with a central perineal post. Longitudinal traction should be limited to 25–50 lb for less than 60 minutes. Approximately 8 mm of distraction can be produced.[22] Excessive traction may lead to pudendal nerve injuries.

Tourniquets allow for clearer visualization of the joint and can be used in elbow, wrist, knee, and ankle arthroscopy. Neurapraxia may be minimized by limiting duration to 2 hours and pressure to 250 mm Hg in the upper extremity and 350 mm Hg in the lower extremity.[16, 22] There is little evidence to support deflating the tourniquet for 10 minutes, then reinflating if a duration of longer than 2 hours is required. The widest cuff that can be used is the most effective. There have been muscle and nerve changes associated with increased tourniquet time.[23–25] This could have important implications in rehabilitation after surgery. Contraindications to use of a tourniquet include ischemia, suspected deep venous thrombosis (DVT), and sickle cell anemia. The extremity should not be exsanguinated if there is potential infection, tumor, or DVT. Complications may occur if excessive pressure or duration occurs. Tourniquet pressure gauges should be standardized on a regular basis to avoid inadvertent excess pressure. Epinephrine has been advocated in shoulder arthroscopy to minimize bleeding and improve visualization. One-half ampule of epinephrine per 3L of irrigation fluid is recommended.[26] Preinjection of the subacromial space may also help reduce bleeding when performing a subacromial decompression. Ideally, if there is a 50 mm Hg gradient between the systolic pressure and pump pressure, bleeding can be minimized and visualization can be improved.

FLUID MANAGEMENT

A considerable number of papers have discussed the merits and problems with various irrigation solutions. Concern about the effects of irrigation fluids on the chondrocytes has led to research on the biochemical and mechanical changes that may occur. Considerable dispute still exists.

Initial reports believed that Ringer solution was more physiologic and supported cartilage metabolic activity.[27] Normal saline solution was shown to inhibit proteoglycan synthesis. Differences were most notable with 8-hour incubation times, with little difference in solutions used for less than 2 hours. A more physiologic solution was recommended for arthroscopic surgery.

Later, Arciero et al.[28] used SO_4 metabolism as a marker for cartilage metabolism and demonstrated no significant differences in irrigation solutions. Constant short-term irrigation with any of the solutions caused little damage to the chondrocyte. They felt that normal saline solution, Ringer lactate solution, and sterile water could be used safely.

Bert et al.[29] were the first to use scanning electron microscopy to evaluate effects of different irrigating fluids on the ultrastructure of the cartilage. They concluded that water caused the most damage, followed by Ringer solution and sodium chloride with little effect by glycine. However, an artifact may have been caused by the biopsy procedure and pre-existing disease of the cartilage.

Because of the lack of controls and questionable experimental technique, there has been some skepticism.

Follow-up studies using scanning electron microscopy were conflicting.[30, 31] Yang and colleagues[30] controlled for the variables missing in the study by Bert et al.[29] Yang and colleagues found that normal saline solution, water, Ringer solution, and sorbitol in irrigation for 1–2 hours caused no detrimental effects. Gradinger, Trager, and Klauser[31] studied effects on ultrastructure using electron microscopy (Fig. 2–8). They believed that the ridges and furrows were deeper in the cartilage that was immersed in Ringer solution for 4 hours. The specimens

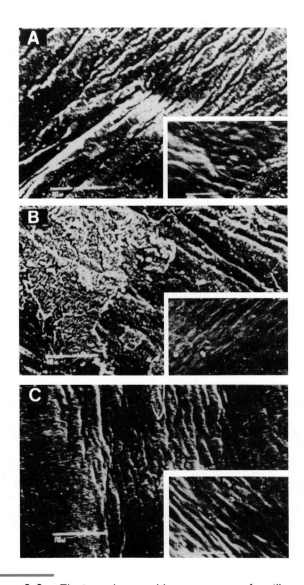

Figure 2–8 • Electronmicrographic appearance of cartilage surface. *A*, Control cartilage fixed without prior incubation of the cartilage. Original magnification ×2400 (inset ×240). *B*, Cartilage incubated in Ringer solution for 4 hours. Original magnification ×2400 (inset ×240). *C*, Cartilage incubated in 10% mannitol for 4 hours. Original magnification ×2400 (inset ×240). (From Gradinger R, Trager J, and Klauser RJ: Influence of various irrigation fluids on articular cartilage. Arthroscopy 11:263–269, 1995.)

using the 10% mannitol more closely resembled the control specimens.

Studies have also tested the effect of various solutions on proteoglycan content. The amount of deformation is highly related to the proteoglycan content of the cartilage. Jurvelin et al.[32] used mechanical properties to test for articular cartilage degeneration. They showed that using Ringer solution resulted in an increased amount of deformity, suggesting degeneration. Nonionic solution retained the biochemical properties better than did Ringer solution. Jurvelin et al. postulated that the changes in the mechanical properties are due to proteoglycan extraction by the Ringer solution. This was supported by Gradinger, Trager, and Klauser.[31] They showed there was greater proteoglycan extraction with Ringer solution and sodium chloride solution (Fig. 2–9 and Table 2–1). The extraction of the proteoglycan appears to be related to ion concentration. However, only the higher 0.9% sodium chloride solution caused significant proteoglycan extraction. It may be possible that high ion concentrations displace the proteoglycans from their binding sites. High carbohydrate solutions seem to spare proteoglycan elution. Ion-free solutions may preserve the biochemical properties of the cartilage better than high ion solutions.

While the debate about the effects of various solutions on the ultrastructure of cartilage continues, there does appear to be some evidence that proteoglycan extraction may occur. It is not certain if this is clinically significant. Further long-term clinical studies may help elucidate the effects of irrigating solutions. The author is unaware of any deleterious effects of normal saline solution. At the author's institution, normal saline is the most economic solution available.

Conductivity of the irrigating media was a previous concern with the use of an electrocautery. The newer Teflon-coated electrocautery minimizes dispersion and allows for use of the electrocautery with normal saline solutions.

The author recommends that irrigation fluids not be placed in a warming chamber before use. Superficial skin burns can occur if fluid is too warm.

Arthroscopy requires a careful understanding of fluid management in order to perform precise and safe surgery.

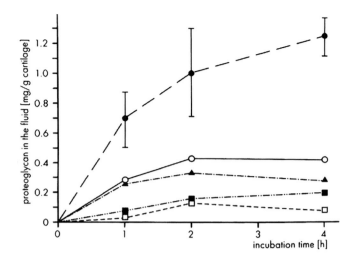

Figure 2–9 • Proteoglycan loss from bovine articular cartilage on incubation in selected aqueous media. Chopped bovine articular cartilage was incubated in Ringer solution (● - - - ●), water (○ - - - ○), 5% sorbitol (▲- . -▲), 2% mannitol (■ - . . - ■), and 10% mannitol (□ - - - □). The proteoglycan content in the fluid was determined after 1, 2, and 4 hours. The bars for the standard deviation are shown for Ringer solution only because of intelligibility of the figure (see Table 2–1). (From Gradinger R, Trager J, and Klauser RJ: Influence of various irrigation fluids on articular cartilage. Arthroscopy 11:263–269, 1995.)

A fluid serves to provide a more effective medium for visualization than either synovial fluid or gas. Irrigation also allows the surgeon to clear debris from the knee as well as to distend the knee to improve visualization. It is important to have clear visual fields in order to avoid inadvertent damage to the articular surface. Equally important is an understanding of flow and pressure in order to avoid serious complications such as compartment syndrome.[16, 33–37] Careful attention is also necessary in using the pump during shoulder arthroscopy. Complete airway obstruction has been reported while using an automated pump. This is extremely important for patients having shoulder arthroscopy with an interscalene block.[38]

		Incubation Time (hours)		
No.	**Medium**	*1*	*2*	*4*
1	Ringer	0.693 ± 0.185	1.01 ± 0.297	1.24 ± 0.121
2	Water	0.274 ± 0.192	0.430 ± 0.199	0.417 ± 0.186
3	Sorbitol 5%	0.271 ± 0.215	0.332 ± 0.240	0.281 ± 0.174
4	Sorbitol 20%	0.143 ± 0.205	0.231 ± 0.197	0.189 ± 0.146
5	Mannitol 2%	0.066 ± 0.074	0.159 ± 0.113	0.201 ± 0.191
6	Mannitol 10%	0.031 ± 0.056	0.145 ± 0.121	0.070 ± 0.070
7	Rheomacrodex G	0.087 ± 0.095	0.184 ± 0.199	0.101 ± 0.100

Table 2–1 Proteoglycan Loss from Bovine Articular Cartilage on Incubation in Selected Aqueous Media

n = 5. Proteoglycan in the medium ± SD (milligrams per gram of cartilage).
From Gradinger R, Trager J, and Klauser RJ: Influence of various irrigation fluids on articular cartilage. Arthroscopy 11:263–269, 1995.

It is thought that a minimum of 28 mm Hg of intra-articular pressure is necessary to perform tamponading of blood vessels within the knee.[39] Pressure of 30–70 mm Hg is believed to be necessary for adequate distention of the knee. However, authors have shown that this pressure is not static and varies with knee position and instrumentation.[39, 40]

Funk et al.[40] reported that pressures of 20 mm Hg increased to 150 mm Hg or higher by flexing the knee 30–80 degrees. They showed that extravasation of fluid occurred at 50 mm Hg. They also believed that scarred or small knees with stiffer capsules would generate greater pressures more quickly. Ewing et al.[39] also studied the effects of knee position as well as the effects of instrumentation. Pressures significantly increased with forced flexion of the knee and the figure-four position (Table 2–2). Extremely high pressure was generated when the portals were closed to form a closed system. They also noted a negative pressure was generated with a suction shaver.

Fluid management is performed either with gravity inflow or with an automated pump. Gravity inflow allows a safe method of irrigation; however, there is little control of flow or pressure. Automated pumps have the advantages of variable flow or pressure, increased pressure capabilities, less bleeding, and decreased need for a tourniquet.

Gravity flow appears to provide satisfactory irrigation.[41, 42] Amount of flow is determined by the pressure gradient created by the height of the bag above the joint and the diameter of the tubing used.

Poiseuille's law

$$\text{Flow} = \frac{\text{pressure gradient} \times \text{diameter}^4}{\text{viscosity} \times \text{length}}$$

Pumps are helpful, particularly if there is a variable intra-articular pressure such as when suction shavers are being used or with increased bleeding such as anterior cruciate ligament surgery. The pump may increase pressure to perform tamponading of vessels or increase flow to clear debris. It is important to avoid increased flow that may lead to turbulence or increased pressure that can cause fluid extravasation and possible compartment syndrome.

Morgan[41] recommended that flow occur through the arthroscope because it avoids flow from being obstructed by knee position and allows for irrigation at the site of visualization. If a pump is to be used, the pressure setting should be slightly above the threshold of bleeding, and the pump should have an automated pressure variable shut-off alarm. A closed system should be avoided at all times.

Bergstrom and Gilquist[43] reported that the maximum pressure that can be generated by gravity is 100 mm Hg versus pressures greater than 200 mm Hg with the pump. This allows for greater flow and distention; however, they noted the warning signs of induration and swelling.

Dolle and Augustini[44] compared three different irrigation systems (Arthropump, 3M pump, SARNS 5500) and noted that although these systems were effective in regulating flow, particularly when suction was used, no system provided protection against high pressures generated by rapid flexion.

INSTRUMENTATION

A large assortment of manually operable instruments is commercially available. The probe is the most commonly used instrument in the examination of the knee. It is used to lift, depress, and pull the meniscus to evaluate for tears and its integrity and stability. The probe is also useful in palpating articular defects and in determining their depth. The probe usually measures 3 mm from inside the angle to the tip and 5 mm from outside the angle to the tip (Fig. 2–10).

Table 2–2	Pressure Changes Versus Knee Position (mm Hg)		
Knee Position	**Mean**	**Standard Deviation**	**Range**
Extension	−11.7	101.6	−107/315
Flexion	78.0	71.6	−75/405
Forced flexion	159.3	101.0	50/393
Internal rotation with forced flexion	155.8	125.5	20/380
Figure four	144.0	103.2	−163/455
Suction shaver insertion	−60.7	30.5	−127/−45
Outflow opening	−91.8	50.8	−460/−25
Outflow closure	72.0	30.4	−58/141

From Ewing JW, Noe DA, Kitaoka HB, et al.: Intra-articular pressures during arthroscopic knee surgery. Arthroscopy 2:264–269, 1986.

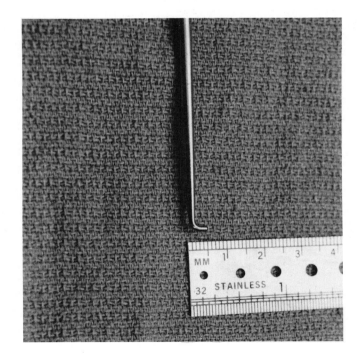

Figure 2–10 • Probe.

Graspers come in two types, one that locks and one that requires continuous pressure. They also vary in the configuration of their teeth. Graspers are essential for grasping tissue within the knee. Pieces of meniscus or loose bodies are removed using this instrument (Fig. 2–11). Suction graspers are also helpful in removing loose bodies.

Basket forceps are used in performing meniscectomies by removing small pieces of tissue. They are available in 2.7 mm sizes for larger working space and more aggressive excision. A smaller 2.1 mm size is available for smaller working areas to decrease the risk of damage to the articular surface. Forceps that angle up and to the right and left are available to access otherwise difficult areas (Figs. 2–12 and 2–13). Suction punches pull tissue into the forceps to assist in tissue resection (Fig. 2–14).

Chondral awls are instruments used in large chondral defects to penetrate the subchondral bone in a controlled fashion in order to establish vascular channels. Various angles are available to reach difficult locations (Fig. 2–15).

Reusable and arthroscopic knives are available in traditional scalpel style as well as back-cutting knives (Fig. 2–16). An underwater electrocautery can be used arthroscopically for hemostasis and tissue-cutting, such as lateral releases (Fig. 2–17).

A variety of specially designed power instruments are available. Variable speed control as well as forward, reverse, and oscillate modes provides versatility with each blade. It is important to be familiar with the types of blades commercially available and the indications for each blade. In general there are soft-tissue resectors and bony resectors in small and large diameters. Typically, soft-tissue resectors are used for débriding synovial, bursal, and

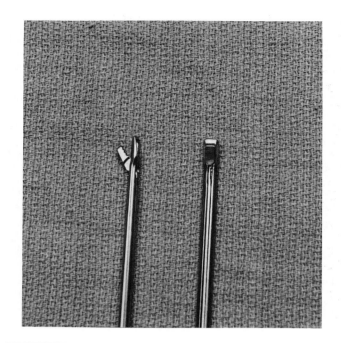

Figure 2–12 • Punch forceps.

meniscal tissue, whereas bone resectors are used for acromioplasty and notchplasty. Newer curved blades are available to assist in getting to hard-to-reach areas (Fig. 2–18). Tissue-cutting rates are affected by the type of tissue being resected. Synovial tissue is more effectively resected in an oscillate mode, whereas bone tissue is more

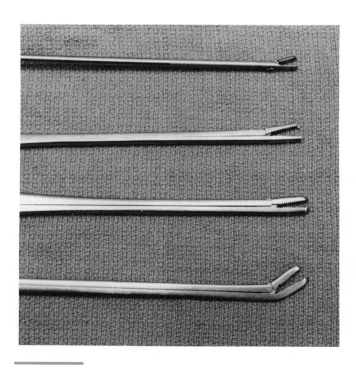

Figure 2–11 • *(Top to bottom),* Small graspers with teeth, needle-nose graspers with teeth, blunt-tip graspers, and angled pituitary graspers.

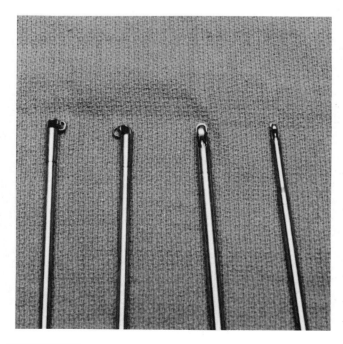

Figure 2–13 • Side-biting punch forceps.

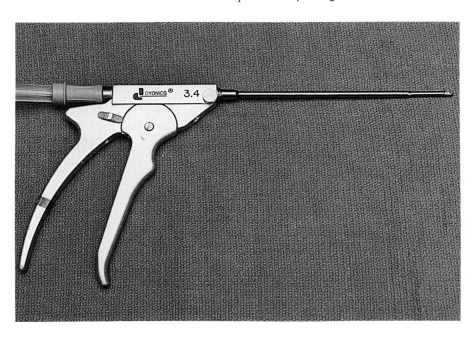

Figure 2–14 • Suction punch forceps.

effectively resected with the forward mode.[45] The reverse mode may be used to polish surfaces (Fig. 2–19).[45]

Suture Anchors

Suture anchors provide a convenient method of attaching soft tissue to bone. It is technically easier to insert suture anchors than to make bone tunnels. Suture anchors have a lower profile than screws and washers. An important feature is the ability to place the soft tissue in an exact location even when there is limited working room. Instrumentation is also available for arthroscopic procedures. Several procedures, such as rotator cuff repairs, Bankart repairs, capsular shifts, biceps tendon repairs, and thumb ulnar collateral ligament repairs have utilized suture anchors.

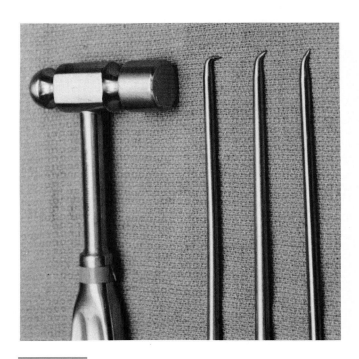

Figure 2–15 • Chondral awls of various angles.

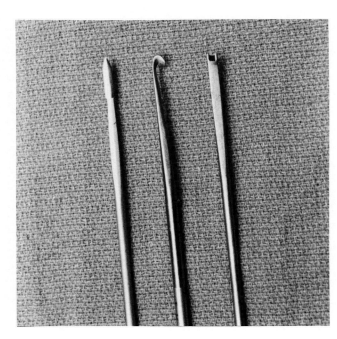

Figure 2–16 • Arthroscopic knives.

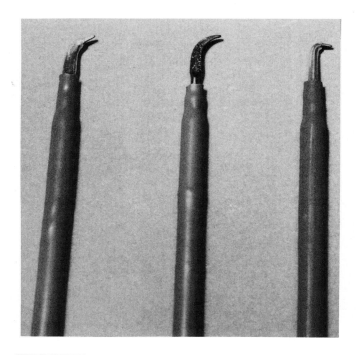

Figure 2–17 • Electrosurgical tips. (From Banas MP: Arthroscopic lateral retinacular release of the patellofemoral joint. Oper Tech Sports Med 2:291–296, 1994.)

There are a variety of designs (Figs. 2–20 to 2–23). These anchors are available in screw and nonscrew designs and in metal, plastic, and bioabsorbable materials in various sizes. This provides the surgeon with several choices. Barber, Herbert, and Click[46] evaluated different suture anchors.

They analyzed the failure mode, pullout strength, and effect of drill-hole size of each anchor in a fresh porcine model. They evaluated design type, anchor size, and composition in diaphyseal and metaphyseal cortex and in cancellous bone trough. Pulling the anchor from the bone was the most common failure, followed by cutout of the suture eyelet. The Statak 5.0 and 5.2 anchors (Zimmer), Revo Screw (Linvatec), and Mitek G4 (Mitek Surgical Products) demonstrated the highest pull-out strength in metaphyseal and cortical bone and cancellous bone. The Mitek G2 was stronger than the Mitek G4 in cancellous trough bone. This phenomenon was thought to be due to the larger entrance hole required for the G4. The highest ultimate strength was that of the Statak anchor; however, the Revo Screw demonstrated the most consistent strength (Figs. 2–24 and 2–25). Larger screws were stronger than small screws in all types of bone; however, the nonscrew type showed less strength in anchors that required larger holes in cancellous bone. In general, the metallic anchors were stronger than the nonmetallic anchors. There was no significant difference among the nonmetallic anchors. Most suture anchors are stronger than the suture that is typically used. An in vivo experiment[47] demonstrated that even anchors with low pullout forces are stronger than No. 2 Ethibond suture within a few weeks.

Nonmetallic anchors have the advantage of not interfering with radiographs and create potentially less complication if they dislodge into the joint. This had led to the development of bioabsorbable suture anchors. Polylactic acid has been used to make plates and screws. Bostman[48] reviewed absorbable implants in the use of fracture treatment. He reported the development of a delayed inflammatory process in absorbable fixation devices, which required surgical drainage of the wound in 7.9%.[49] Elrod

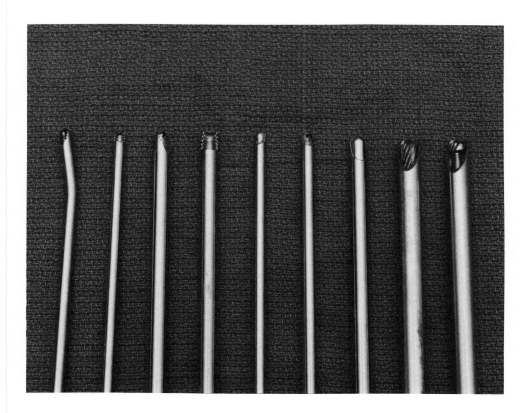

Figure 2–18 • Motorized soft-tissue resectors and burs.

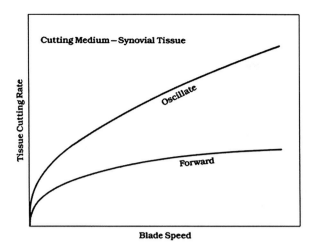

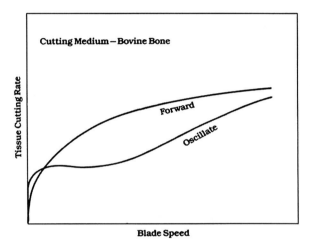

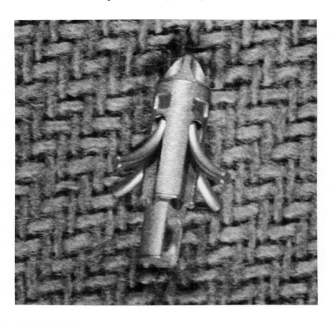

Figure 2–20 • Metal suture anchor.

Figure 2–19 • *(Top)*, Graph demonstrating rate of soft-tissue resection and blade speed and direction. *(Bottom)*, Graph demonstrating rate of bone resection with varying speed and direction. (From Smith & Nephew Dyonics: PS3500EP Arthroscopic Surgical System User's Manual, p 9.)

reported that 10% of the Biotak (Linvatec) tacks used in glenoid labral repairs fragmented and led to synovitis. This could potentially weaken the strength of the anchor and repair. In one study[51] a polylactic acid anchor demonstrated no substantial acute or chronic foreign body reaction. It is uncertain if the presence of a synovial joint may alter the host response.

The orthopaedic surgeon has several suture anchors available, based on design type, composition, size, and ease of insertion. All provide a satisfactory means of reattaching ligaments or tendons to bone.

Figure 2–21 • Threaded anchors. (From Barber FA, Herbert MA, and Click JN: The ultimate strength of suture anchors. Arthroscopy 11:21–28, 1995.)

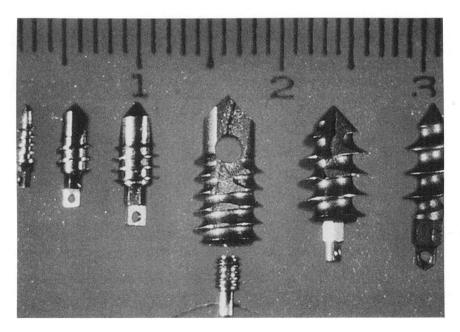

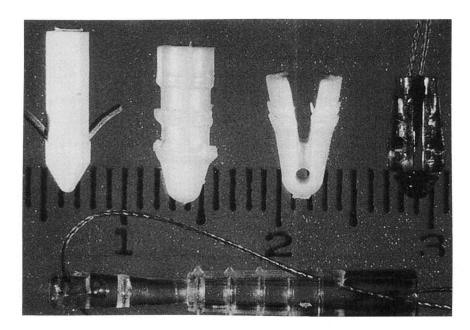

Figure 2–22 • Nonmetallic anchors. (From Barber FA, Hebert MA, and Click JN: The ultimate strength of suture anchors. Arthroscopy 11:21–28, 1995.)

Laser

An increasing interest in laser surgery has led to numerous types of lasers and applications. Lasers (light amplification by stimulated emission of radiation) use electricity to excite a substance to produce photons that are focused and amplified into an energy beam of specific wavelength. Most lasers work in the infrared portion of the spectrum. Much of the medical experience with lasers has been in vascular and general surgery.

There are a variety of lasers. The CO_2 laser was used initially in arthroscopy and orthopedics. It is readily absorbed in water and therefore requires a gas medium to be used. Furthermore, it cannot be transmitted by fiberoptic cables and requires awkward handpieces. The CO_2 laser has a shallow depth of penetration. Char formation has been a problem with CO_2 laser. Carbon remnants may lead to synovitis.[52]

The Nd:YAG laser can be transmitted by fiberoptic cables and can be used in an aqueous medium. The free beam laser cannot be used in arthroscopy because of its large thermal necrosis and depth of penetration. Conductive tips are available to create a tip that is capable of cutting with little collateral injury. However, the use of tips eliminates the ability of the Nd:YAG laser to ablate tissue. These technical problems have precluded its use in arthroscopic surgery.[52] There have been reports of the Nd:YAG laser having a biostimulation effect on tissue.[53, 54] The potassium titanyl phosphate laser is similar to the Nd:YAG laser but has a doubled frequency. It has been approved by

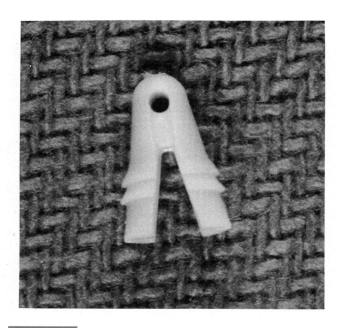

Figure 2–23 • Absorbable anchor.

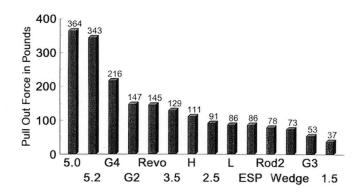

Figure 2–24 • Ultimate pullout strength. *(Left to right)*, Statak 5.0 (Zimmer), Statak 5.2 (Zimmer), Mitek G4 (Miter Surgical), Mitek G2 (Mitek Surgical), Revo Screw (Linvatec), Statak 3.5 (Zimmer), Harpoon (Arthrotek), Statak 2.5 (Zimmer), Arthrotek Lactosorb (Arthrotek), Arthrex ESP (Arthrex), Acufex Tag Rod (Acufex), Acufex Tag Wedge (Acufex), Mitek G3 (Mitek), and Statak 1.5 (Zimmer). (From Barber FA, Herbert MA, and Click JN: The ultimate strength of suture anchors. Arthroscopy 11:21–28, 1995.)

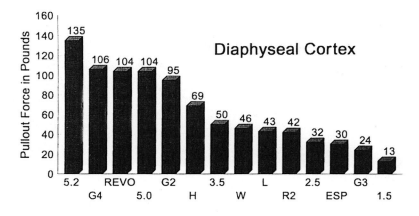

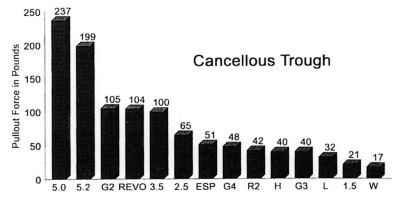

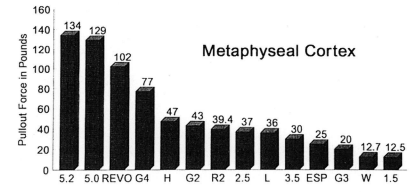

Figure 2–25 • Mean pullout strength. See equipment names in Figure 2–24. (From Barber FA, Herbert MA, and Click JN: The ultimate strength of suture anchors. Arthroscopy 11:21–28, 1995.)

the U.S. Food and Drug Administration for percutaneous diskectomy; however, it has not yet been approved for arthroscopic surgery because of its inefficient power and difficulty with fiber durability.[52]

The Er:YAG laser is precise, but with little tissue penetration, however, it has little hemostasis abilities. Furthermore, it cannot be transmitted through fiberoptic cables. The Er:YAG laser is especially good at bone cutting, which may be more important in osteotomies.[54]

The excimer laser uses various rare gases, such as Xenon, to produce ultraviolet energy beams. It works nonthermally by disrupting molecular bonds.[55] It requires less energy than other lasers. It is precise, with little collateral tissue damage. The main shortcoming is that it is slow and expensive. Unlike the other lasers, which are in the infrared spectrum, the excimer laser is in the ultraviolet spectrum, raising concerns about potential mutigenicity.[54] It is not currently available for arthroscopic surgery.

The most commonly used laser in arthroscopic surgery is the Ho:YAG laser. Dillingham, Fanton, and Thabit[56] have given an excellent overview of this laser. Originally used in vascular surgery, this laser has become the workhorse of lasers in arthroscopic surgery. It is used in an aqueous medium. It is ideal because of its precision, fiberoptic capabilities, and infrared spectrum. It utilizes variable pulse rates, which minimizes tissue damage because of the cooling effect. This allows a delivery of high energy without forming char. It can be used in either a contact (cutting) or near-contact (ablation, coagulation, and shaping) mode.

The applications of lasers can be discussed in terms of those that are clinical and those that are experimental. One of the more common uses is in meniscal surgery. Sherk et al.[55] compared the effects of various lasers on meniscal tissue. The power settings were based on manufacturer recommendations and selected according to those that most

Table 2–3	Adjacent Tissue Damage (Micrometers) Assessed by Light Microscopy of Hematoxylin and Eosin- or Trichrome-Stained Specimens			
	Hematoxylin and Eosin		Trichrome	
Specimen	*Mean*	*Range*	*Mean*	*Range*
Bovie coagulation	250	65–472	478	312–564
Bovie cut	47	16–102	417	205–684
CO_2	54	20–88	447	152–762
Nd:YAG	378	41–715	870	506–1234
YAG contact	60	17–192	191	94–288
Holmium:YAG	82	30–135	552	278–789
Excimer	24	4.5–77	0	

From Sherk HH, Black JD, Prodoehl JA, et al.: The effects of lasers and electrosurgical devices on human meniscal tissue. Clin Orthop 310:14–20, 1995.

closely approximated the speed of the scalpel (Table 2–3). The clinical significance of the amount of thermal damage is not fully understood. Intuitively, it is apparent that collateral tissue damage should be minimized. The electrosurgical devices produced large, irregular surfaces as seen on electron microscopy. There may be areas of necrosis as far as 1,000 μm from the cut surface. Lasers are able to produce a smoother surface.

The Ho:YAG laser was studied in a double-blind prospective study that demonstrated faster resolution of pain and return to normal range of motion in the laser-treated group.[57] Excellent results have also been reported in use for lateral releases. Improved postoperative pain, decreased postoperative effusion, and faster recovery were attributed to the hemostasis achieved with the laser.[58]

Lasers have also been used in shoulder surgery for arthroscopic subacromial decompression to débride synovium, subacromial periosteum, and the vascular coracoacromial ligament. Previous reports of collagen shrinkage in the ophthalmology literature were cited by Hayashi et al.[59] They studied the effects of lasers on joint capsular tissue. They demonstrated that tissue shrinkage correlated with the amount of energy used. In their animal model they concluded that significant tissue shrinkage can be accomplished using a Ho:YAG laser without significantly affecting the viscoelastic properties of the tissue. However, the stiffness of the tissue may be compromised at higher energy. This is important basic science research that provides a foundation for further studies. To date there have not been any clinical studies to demonstrate the efficacy in the treatment of capsular redundancy associated with shoulder instability.

Considerable research has been done to study the use of lasers in the treatment of articular cartilage damage. Vangness and Ghaderi[60] reviewed the literature of lasers and articular cartilage. The excimer laser was used to study its effectiveness in the treatment of stages II and III chondromalacia. They concluded that the excimer laser was superior to traditional instruments in decreasing pain and synovitis. There was no difference in disability, function, rehabilitation, and return to activities. Most of the research has been with the Nd:YAG laser. There have been reports that this laser may stimulate regeneration of carti-

lage defects.[61–66] No studies on Ho:YAG lasers have been done to show any stimulatory effect on articular cartilage. Despite these several studies that suggest that lasers may induce a regenerative effect on articular cartilage, more studies are needed to make these results conclusive. It is important to define which lasers and what parameters should be used. The biological effects on cartilage metabolism need to be further elucidated. The type and quality of cartilage also need to be evaluated.

Another potential use of lasers is tissue repair and tissue welding. Dew et al.[67] reviewed the literature of the basic science and clinical studies. Tissue reaction is affected by the laser energy absorbed, length of exposure, and operating conditions.[68] Tissue response progresses from denaturation to coagulation, ablation, and charring as absorption of energy increases.[69] Initial work in tissue welding was in vascular reanastomosis. Laser welding appears to be a function of protein denaturation. Laser welding of meniscal tissue was studied using an Nd:YAG laser in a pig model. In a comparison of traditional suture repair versus laser-induced tissue welding, it was concluded that laser repair was a time-effective and efficient means of meniscal repair. There was better tissue reapproximation and a less intense inflammatory response. The authors concluded that there were still inconsistencies and, before human clinical trial, certain factors required further study: type of laser, power density, delivering system, animal studies, a reproducible laser, and a method of training.

This author's opinion is that, although there appear to be promising uses of the laser, more basic science research is needed, more cost-effective and reproducible lasers are needed, and more controlled clinical studies need to be performed. Arthroscopic use of lasers should be undertaken only by those who have a clear understanding of the laser, its techniques and indications as well as its potential complications.

Care of Instrumentation

Proper care of arthroscopic equipment is essential to reliable and safe surgery. All arthroscopic instruments should

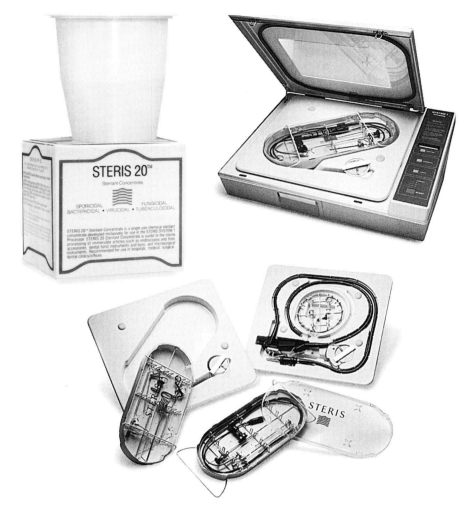

Figure 2–26 • STERIS system (From STERIS Corporation, Mentor, Ohio.)

be properly maintained. The importance of clean and sterile equipment cannot be overemphasized. The complications of infection and potential disease transmission are tragic. It is important to differentiate "clean" and "sterile"; they are not the same. Each instrument should be carefully cleaned before sterilization. Residue may build up, which affects the performance of the arthroscope or the instrument and can also be potentially infectious. Each instrument should be carefully cleaned with water and a mild cleaning substance. There are several methods of sterilization. Instruments may be autoclaved using pressurized steam, or chemically cleaned with either ethylene oxide gas or Cidex (Johnson and Johnson) (which is activated 2% glutaraldehyde), or the STERIS system. Autoclaving is safe and reliable and may be used with most arthroscopy instruments, such as basket forceps, graspers, probes, and

Figure 2–27 • Videoimaging and photos are useful in patient education.

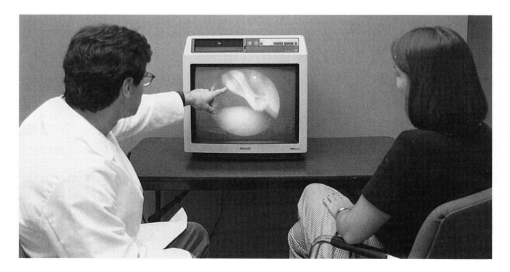

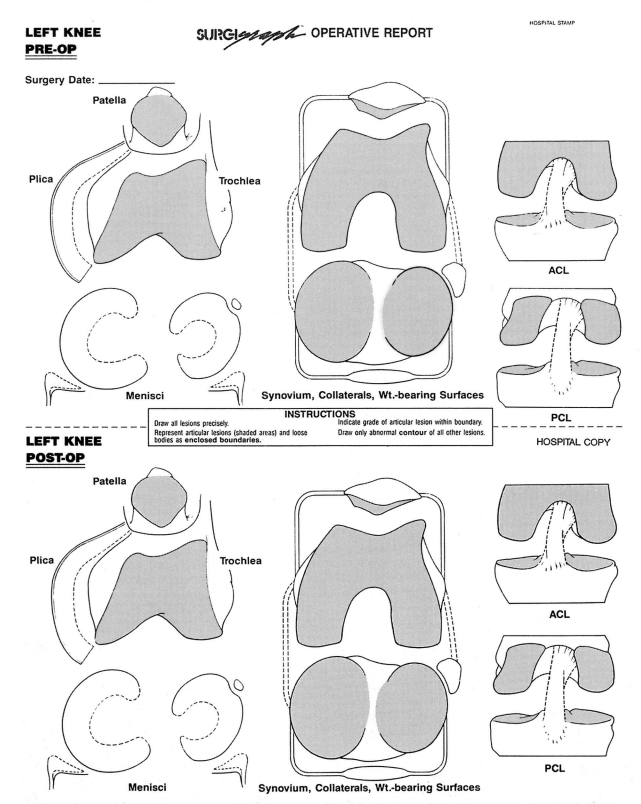

Figure 2–28 • Schematic drawing to record preoperative findings and operative procedures. (From Surgigraph from Terry L. Whipple, M.D.)

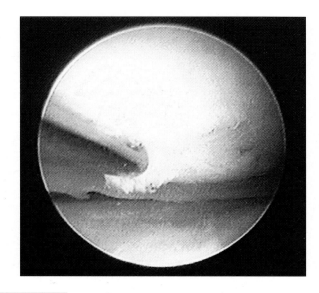

Figure 2–29 • Arthroscopic photograph demonstrating chondral lesion and extent as well as meniscal tear.

cannula systems. It is not safe to autoclave the arthroscopes because it causes deterioration of adhesives between the lenses. Johnson et al.[70] reported on the efficacy of Cidex. They recommended a soak for 15–20 minutes for safe usage. An infection rate of 0.04% was reported. It was noted in their article that Cidex is bactericidal in 10 minutes, killing viruses, *Mycobacterium*, and *Pseudomonas*, but not spores.[71] Two percent glutaraldehyde is not considered to be a sterilizing agent, but it is an acceptable method of disinfection.[72] Ethylene oxide sterilization is another option; however, that requires 12–24 hours, which prohibits timely sterilization. Currently, this author uses the STERIS system (STERIS Corporation), which effectively sterilizes in 20–30 minutes (Fig. 2–26).[73] Its primary active ingredient is peracetic acid, which is buffered to prevent corrosion. A biological control agent is available to monitor the system. Cleaning is still required before using the STERIS system. It is important that, regardless of method of sterilization, a control agent be available to assure safety.

DOCUMENTATION

Increasing sensitivity to medicolegal problems has heightened the role of thorough documentation during arthroscopy. Documentation is also important for making permanent records of the disease at the time of arthroscopy. These records can be used for reference as well as for patient education (Fig. 2–27).

The backbone of documentation is a detailed operative note. The narrative should include both the abnormal findings and the procedures performed and normal findings. A systematic approach is useful so that pertinent normals may not be inadvertently omitted. This author has found schematic drawings to be useful as well (Fig. 2–28).

The art of photography during arthroscopy has been made much simpler. Almost all arthroscopic cameras have systems available for still and video photography. It has been said that a picture is worth a thousand words. This is no more evident than in arthroscopy. Permanent images are able to show location and severity that are not always easily described. People may have different ideas of what "grade II chondromalacia" may mean, but a picture can accurately record the disease (Fig. 2–29).

Still images are useful because they are easily incorporated into the permanent record. Video is more difficult in that it is not an easy reference; however, it does allow for more comprehensive record of the arthroscopy. One difficulty with video is storage for tapes.

References

1. Johnson LL: Arthroscopic Surgery: Principles and Practices, 3rd ed. St. Louis, C.V. Mosby, 1986.
2. Glick JM, Sampson TG, Gordon RB, et al.: Hip arthroscopy by the lateral approach. Arthroscopy 3:4–12, 1987.
3. Kazakakevich Y: Optical specifications used in endoscopy and their definition. Smith and Nephew–Dyonics, 1992.
4. Prescott R: Optical principles of endoscopy. J Med Primatol 5:133–147, 1976.
5. Aritomi H and Yamamoto M: A method of arthroscopic surgery: clinical evaluation of synovectomy with the electric resectoscope and removal of loose bodies in the knee joint. Orthop Clin North Am 10:565–584, 1979.
6. Johnson L, Schneider D, Austin M, et al.: Two percent glutaraldehyde: a disinfectant in arthroscopy and arthroscopic surgery. J Bone Joint Surg 64A:237–239, 1982.
7. D'Angelo GL and Ogilvie-Harris DJ: Septic arthritis following arthroscopy, with cost/benefit analysis of antibiotic prophylaxis. Arthroscopy 4:10–14, 1988.
8. Wertheim SB, Gillespie S, and Klaus R: Role of prophylactic antibiotics in arthroscopic knee surgery. Orthop Trans 4:1101, 1993.
9. Wieck JA, Jackson JK, O'Brien TJ, et al.: A prospective randomized double-blind evaluation of the efficacy of prophylactic antibiotics in arthroscopic surgery. Presented at the Meeting of the Arthroscopy Association of North America, San Francisco, July, 1995.
10. Katz JF and Siffert RS: Tissue antibiotic levels with tourniquet use in orthopedics. Clin Orthop 165:261–264, 1982.
11. Armstrong RW, Bolding F, and Joseph R: Septic arthritis following arthroscopy. Arthroscopy 8:213–223, 1992.
12. Andrews JR and Carson WG: Shoulder joint arthroscopy. Orthopedics 6:1157–1162, 1983.
13. Andrews JR, Carson WG, and Ortega K: Arthroscopy of the shoulder: technique and normal anatomy. Am J Sports Med 12:1–7, 1984.
14. Ellman H: Arthroscopic subacromial decompression: analysis of one to three year results. Arthroscopy 3:173–181, 1987.
15. Matthews LS, Zarins B, Michael RW, et al.: Anterior portal selection for shoulder arthroscopy. Arthroscopy 1:33–39, 1987.
16. Rodeo SA, Forster RA, and Weiland AJ: Current concepts review: neurologic complications due to arthroscopy. J Bone Joint Surg 75A:917–926, 1993.
17. Mullins RC, Dres D, and Cooper J: Hypoglossal nerve palsy after arthroscopy of the shoulder and open operation with the patient in the beach chair position. J Bone Joint Surg 74A:137–139, 1992.
18. Guhl JF: New concepts (distraction) in ankle arthroscopy. Arthroscopy 4:160–167, 1988.
19. Ferkel RD and Scanton PE: Arthroscopy of the foot and ankle. J Bone Joint Surg 75A:1233–1242, 1993.
20. Savoie FH: Presented at Arthroscopy Association of North America Specialty Day, Atlanta, Feb., 1996.
21. Whipple TL: Precautions for arthroscopy of the wrist. Arthroscopy 6:3–4, 1990.
22. Guhl JF, Olsen DW, and Sprague NF: Specific complications: elbow, wrist, hip, and ankle. In Sprague NF (ed.): Complications of Arthroscopy. New York, Raven Press, 1989, pp 199–223.

23. McGinty JB: Ligament, bone and nerve complications. In Sprague NF (ed.): Complications of Arthroscopy. New York, Raven Press, 1989, p 10.
24. Jacobson MD, Pedowitz RA, Oyama BK, et al.: Muscle functional deficits after tourniquet ischemia. Am J Sports Med 22:372–377, 1994.
25. Nitz AJ, Dobner JJ, and Matulionis DH: Pneumatic tourniquet application and nerve integrity: Motor function and physiology. Exp Neurol 94:264–279, 1986.
26. Scarpiento PF, Bramhall JP, and Andrews JR: Arthroscopic management of the throwing athlete's shoulder: indications, techniques, and results. Clin Sports Med 10:913–927, 1991.
27. Reagan B, McInerny VK, Zarins B, et al.: Irrigation solutions for arthroscopy: a metabolic study. J Bone Joint Surg 65A:629–631, 1983
28. Arciero RA, Little JS, Liebenberg SP, et al.: Irrigating solutions used in arthroscopy and their effects on articular cartilage. Orthopedics 9:1511–1515, 1986.
29. Bert JM, Posalaky Z, Snyder S, et al.: Effects of various irrigating fluids on the ultrastructure of articular cartilage. Arthroscopy 6:104–111, 1990.
30. Yang CY, Shun-Chian C, Ching-Liang S, et al.: Effects of irrigation fluids on articular cartilage: a scanning electron microscopy study. Arthroscopy 9:425–430, 1993.
31. Gradinger R, Trager J, and Klauser RJ: Influence of various irrigation fluids on articular cartilage. Arthroscopy 11:263–269, 1995.
32. Jurvelin JS, Jurvelin JA, Kiviranta I, et al.: Effects of different irrigation liquids and times on articular cartilage: an experimental, biochemical study. Arthroscopy 10:667–672, 1994.
33. Bromberg BC: Complications associated with the use of infusion pumps during knee arthroscopy. Arthroscopy 8:224–228, 1992.
34. Noyes FR and Spievak ES: Extra-articular fluid dissection in tissues during arthroscopy. Am J Sports Med 10:346–351, 1982.
35. Fruensgaard S and Holm A: A compartment syndrome complicating arthroscopic surgery. J Bone Joint Surg 70B:146–149, 1988.
36. Ketterl R, Beckurts T, Kovacs J, et al.: Gas-gangrene following arthroscopic surgery. Arthroscopy 5:79–83, 1989.
37. Peek RD and Hayes DW: Compartment syndrome as a complication of arthroscopy. Am J Sports Med 12:464–468, 1984.
38. Hynson JM, Tung A, Guevara JE, et al.: Complete airway obstruction during arthroscopic shoulder surgery. Anesth Analg 76:875–878, 1993.
39. Ewing JW, Noe DA, Kitaoka HB, et al.: Intra-articular pressures during arthroscopic knee surgery. Arthroscopy 2:264–269, 1986.
40. Funk DA, Noyes FR, Grood ES, et al.: The effect of flexion angle on the pressure-volume in the human knee. Arthroscopy 7:86–90, 1991.
41. Morgan CD: Fluid delivery systems for arthroscopy. Arthroscopy 3:288–291, 1987.
42. Oretorp N and Elmersson S: Arthroscopy and irrigation control. Arthroscopy 2:46–50, 1986.
43. Bergstrom R and Gilquist J: The use of infusion pump in arthroscopy. Arthroscopy 2:41–45, 1986.
44. Dolk T and Augustini B: Three irrigation systems for motorized arthroscopic surgery: a comparative experimental and clinical study. Arthroscopy 5:207–314, 1989.
45. Arthroscopic Surgical Systems, User's Manual, Smith & Nephew Endoscopy, 1996.
46. Barber FA, Herbert MA, and Click JN: The ultimate strength of suture anchors. Arthroscopy 11:21–28, 1995.
47. Barber FA, Cawley P, and Prudich JF: Suture anchor failure strength: an in vivo study. Arthroscopy 9:647–652, 1993.
48. Bostman OM: Absorbable implants for the fixation of fractures. J Bone Joint Surg 73A:148–153, 1991.
49. Bostman OM: Intense granulomatous inflammation lesions associated with absorbable internal fixation devices made of polyglycolide in ankle fractures. Clin Orthop 278:193–199, 1992.
50. Elrod BF: Arthroscopic shoulder stabilization with bioabsorbable tack. Arthroscopy Association of North America, April, 1993.
51. Barber FA and Deck MA: The in vivo histology response of an absorbable suture anchor: a preliminary report. Arthroscopy 11:77–81, 1995.
52. Dilingham MG, Price JM, and Fanton GS: Holium laser surgery. Orthopedics 16:563–566, 1993.
53. Spivac J: Metabolic effects of continuous Nd:YAG laser on articular cartilage metabolism. Presented at the Arthroscopy Association of North Carolina, San Diego, April, 1991.
54. Abelow SP: Use of lasers in orthopedic surgery: current concepts. Orthopedics 16:561–566, 1993.
55. Sherk HH, Black JD, Prodoehl JA, et al.: The effects of laser and electrosurgical devices on human meniscal tissue. Clin Orthop 310:14–20, 1995.
56. Dillingham MF, Fanton GS, and Thabit G: Laser-assisted arthroscopic meniscal surgery of the knee. Operative Techniques in Orthopedics 5:39–45, 1995.
57. Dillingham MF and Fanton GS: The use of Ho:YAG laser in operative knee arthroscopy: a double blind prospective study using a new arthroscopically guided laser system. Presented at the Ninth Annual Arthroscopy Association of North America, Orlando, Fla., 1990.
58. Dillingham MF, Fanton GS, and Perkash R: The use of Ho:YAG laser in operative knee arthroscopy: a retrospective study comparing postoperative recovery rates of patients with lateral retinacular release. Presented at the First International Laser in Orthopedics Symposium, San Francisco, 1991.
59. Hayashi K, Markel M, Thabitt, G, et al.: Effects of non-ablative laser energy on joint capsular properties. Am J Sports Med 23:482–487, 1995.
60. Vangness CT and Ghaderi B: A literature review of lasers and articular cartilage. Orthopedics 16:593–598, 1993.
61. Schultz RJ, Krishnamurthy S, Thelmo W, et al.: Effects of laser energy on articular cartilage: a preliminary study. Lasers Surg Med 5:577–588, 1985.
62. Spivak JM, Grande DA, Ben-Yishay A, et al.: The effect of low-level Nd:YAG laser energy on adult articular cartilage in vitro. Arthroscopy 8:36–43, 1992.
63. Herman JH and Khosla RC: In vitro effects of Nd:YAG laser radiation of cartilage metabolism. J Rheumatol 15:1818–1826, 1988.
64. Braderick JP, Eckhausere ML, and Indresaano AT: Morphologic and histologic changes in canine temporomandibular joint tissue following arthroscopically guided Nd:YAG laser exposure. J Oral Maxillofac Surg 47:1177–1181, 1989.
65. Hardi EM, Carlson CS, and Richardson DC: Effect of Nd:YAG laser energy on articular cartilage healing in the dog. Lasers Surg Med 9:595–601, 1989.
66. Kolmer C: Experimental evaluation of stimulatory effects of Nd:YAG laser on canine articular cartilage. In Sherk HH (ed.): Lasers in Orthopedics. Philadelphia, J.B. Lippincott, 1990, pp 140–146.
67. Dew DK, Supik L, Darrow CR, et al.: Tissue repair using lasers: a review. Orthopedics 16:581–587, 1993.
68. Arndt KA, Noe JM, Northham DBC, et al.: Laser therapy: basic concepts of nomenclature. J Am Acad Dermatol 5:649–655, 1981.
69. Hall RR, Beach AD, Baker E, et al.: Incision of tissue by carbon dioxide laser. Nature 232:131–132, 1971.
70. Johnson LL, Schneider DA, Austin MD, et al.: Two percent glutaraldehyde: a disinfectant in arthroscopy and arthroscopic surgery. J Bone Joint Surg 64A:237–239, 1982.
71. Mallison G: The inanimate environment. In Bennet JV and Bracham PS (eds.): Hospital Infections. Boston, Little, Brown, 1979, pp 81–92.
72. Ayliffe GA, Babb JR and Bradley CR: Sterilization of arthroscopes and laparascopes. J Hosp Infect 22:265–269, 199.
73. STERIS operating manual, STERIS Corporation, 1996.
74. Crow S: Practical innovations: protecting patients, personnel, instruments in the OR. AORN J 58:771–774, 1993.

Arthroscopic Surgical Techniques

James R. Andrews • *Stephanie L. Glaze*

GENERAL SURGICAL PRINCIPLES

Basic surgical principles must be appreciated before the arthroscopist attempts arthroscopic surgery. Arthroscopy can become a simple procedure with proper training and patience on the part of the arthroscopist. Nothing related to arthroscopic surgery supersedes experience. The arthroscopist should first attempt small procedures in which an open arthrotomy is anticipated.[1] Surgical time constraints are also to be considered. An arthroscopist should keep in mind the amount of tourniquet time used and the amount of fluid introduced into the joint to prevent fluid extravasation and distortion of the tissue structures for an open procedure. The arthroscopist must understand the equipment being used. The camera and light source are essential to arthroscopy and must be utilized to their full potential. When an arthroscopic pump is utilized, the surgeon must understand all of its technical details to get good visualization and to prevent extravasation of fluid, which could possibly lead to compartment syndrome. It is beneficial for the surgeon to assist in positioning the patient, especially when just beginning to explore arthroscopic surgery. This allows the surgeon to assist the staff in attaining the optimal position of the patient in relation to the positioning device to be used.

THE SURGICAL TEAM

When first exploring arthroscopic surgery, it is good practice to involve the same team to implement the procedures and then begin to train other personnel. The surgeon should act as the leader and take an active role in the training of the arthroscopy team.[1] Consistency of the surgical environment is necessary to achieve optimal results in arthroscopy. Obviously, this consistency begins with the surgical team.

GENERAL ARTHROSCOPIC TECHNIQUES

A novice at arthroscopic surgery should not let frustration interfere with the task at hand. This is all too common an occurrence until the techniques of arthroscopy are mastered. Portal placement for optimal visualization is essential. It is considered good technique to move or redirect the arthroscope when necessary. A methylene-blue pen should be used to outline the bony landmarks of the surgical joint. Entry into the joint is often tricky and can become tedious, especially if scar tissue is present. The great pioneer in arthroscopic surgery, Dr. Lanny Johnson, taught that preparation was 99% of execution (personal communication).

Body Control of the Surgeon

The arthroscopist's hands act like those of an orchestra conductor while working in the joint. Several techniques are described for holding the arthroscope. The authors recommend holding the proximal end of the arthroscope between the thumb and index finger with a firm grasp and a relaxed body posture (Fig. 3–1). The videoarticulated arthroscope should be, therefore, balanced like a paint brush. Control of the arthroscope is maintained by using slow, purposeful motions rather than quick, jerky ones that could cause articular damage. The remaining fingers are used to assist with rotating the direction of the 30 degree angled arthroscope as the joint is scanned. Whether the surgeon is standing or sitting, the table height should be such that the surgeon's arms are at a comfortable level, not strained at any time. The assistant to the surgeon should be placed in the optimal position to assist the surgeon with stabilization of the patient's extremity while remaining out of the view of the monitor. The surgeon's feet should be firmly planted on the ground to secure balance. One foot

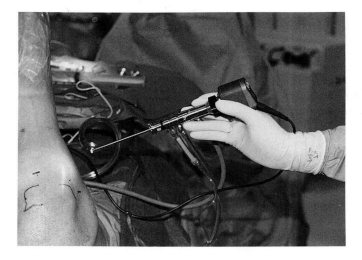

Figure 3–1 • Surgeon holding arthroscope.

maintains balance, and the other foot operates the foot pedals for the shaver or the electrocautery.

Orientation of the arthroscope in the joint is attained much more easily when the surgeon is behind the arthroscope. The television monitor should be placed in front of the surgeon, with nothing obstructing the view. The light cable attached to the arthroscope assists with orientation inside the joint (Fig. 3–2). The monitor shows a mirror image. When an instrument enters the field opposite the arthroscope, a movement of the instrument to the right by the surgeon's hand shows as a movement to the left on the monitor. Orientation to the image on the screen should be attained before attempting the procedure. If an arthroscopic pump is used, the pump should be in clear view of the surgeon. On entering the joint, the arthroscopist must make sure that the pressure and flow measurements are correct and operating normally.

INTRA-ARTICULAR ARTHROSCOPIC TECHNIQUES

Palpation

Palpation of the joint is essential in arthroscopic surgery to facilitate placement of the arthroscope into the joint (Fig. 3–3). With practice and determination, the arthroscopist will become adept at locating bony and soft tissue structures in and around the joint. The arthroscopist should feel around the joint while looking at the structures on the monitor. Palpation of extra-articular soft tissue and bony landmarks, as well as intra-articular ones, takes practice and a special feel for depth perception.

Pistoning

Pistoning of the arthroscope, a push-pull technique, is a useful elementary motion in arthroscopic surgery. Slow, gradual movements should be used to allow the arthroscope to remain in the joint cavity and to allow the surgeon to remain oriented to the objects in view. Pistoning the arthroscope in the joint assists the surgeon in recognizing the size and position of the joint structures in relation to one another. The ability to piston and pull away prevents an elementary problem of "crowding" during any level of arthroscopy.

Scanning

Side-to-side scanning of the joint is a valuable skill that facilitates the arthroscopist's orientation to the joint. Scanning allows the arthroscopist to locate the horizon of the articular surface before moving on to the adjacent structures. When scanning the joint, the surgeon moves from a known to an unknown area in a planned sequence.[1] The arthroscope should be pulled back to a known landmark and the inspection tried again.

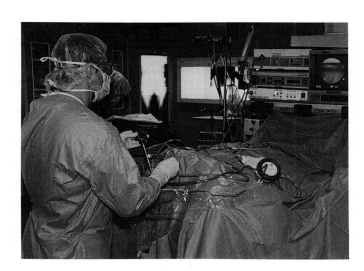

Figure 3–2 • Surgeon facing monitor.

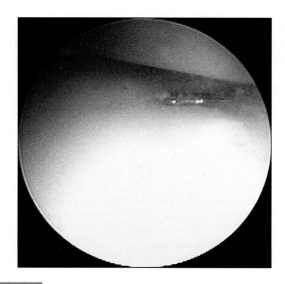

Figure 3–3 • Joint being probed.

Rotation

Rotating the arthroscope in the joint means moving the light cable on the arthroscope. For example, this action rotates the tip of a 30 degree arthroscope enabling a wider view of the area to be inspected. By rotating the arthroscope, the surgeon can view a wider area of the joint without changing his or her position. Utilizing the 0 degree arthroscope does not, of course, change the field of view. The experienced arthroscopist can rotate the arthroscope while holding it in the pencil position and rotating it right to left with the ring and little finger.

Sweeping

Sweeping the arthroscope across the joint requires great care in controlling the movement and angulation of the arthroscope. Quick, jerky movements while practicing could cause damage to the articular surface, the arthroscope, or both. Rotation of the arthroscope is used along with the sweeping motion to explore the joint. Practice is necessary to manage both skills simultaneously.

Many factors should be explored before beginning an arthroscopic procedure. The patient's anatomy is a major factor. The technical ability of the surgeon and the surgical team to complete the procedure should also be noted. The equipment for the procedure should be functioning at optimal levels. There is no room for error in arthroscopic surgery; everyone is looking at the monitor and can see what is occurring in the joint. Great discipline is needed on the part of all members of the team for a successful outcome.

EXTRA-ARTICULAR ARTHROSCOPIC TECHNIQUES

Position of the Arthroscope

Portal selection for arthroscopy is the key to a successful procedure. All too often, the arthroscopist focuses on obtaining entry too quickly to establish a view. A misplaced portal should be either redirected or replaced. An alternate portal may need to be considered if visualization is not optimal or if the instrumentation cannot be used. Often the problem is misdirection of the arthroscope or the instrumentation, and reorientation may be all that is required for proper visualization (Fig. 3–4).

External Manipulation of the Joint

Manipulation of the joint is often overlooked as a functional part of arthroscopy. Rotation of the joint by an assistant allows the surgeon to view the entire joint more effectively (Fig. 3–5). Areas that are difficult to see may come into view after rotation. Distention may also be used to allow better visualization. Distention is achieved by either saline solution injection or by mechanical or physical means. Mechanical distention refers to traction weights, and physical distention refers to an assistant pulling the distraction on the extremity.

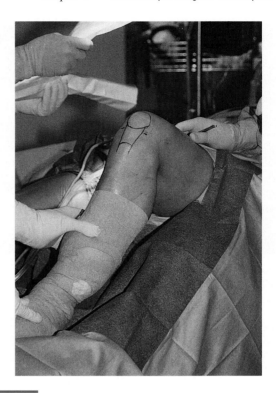

Figure 3–4 • Portal placements and bony anatomy drawn on a patient.

BASIC OPERATING ROOM SET-UP AND EQUIPMENT

Foremost in arthroscopic surgery is the surgeon's confidence in the plan of care. A dedicated operating room (OR) staff, well versed in arthroscopic surgery, is a luxury for some surgeons. The OR set-up is crucial to a successful outcome. According to Gross,[2] an ideal basic set-up is one that is flexible enough to allow the surgeon to flow from one plan to the next with the least disruption. The surgeon's position at the OR table is essential to maintaining orientation in the joint. Patient positioning must be precise in order to maintain useful anatomic orientation. Following is some of Dr. Andrews' preferred patient and surgeon positioning along with a basic OR set-up.

Knee Arthroscopy

Dr. Andrews prefers a technique similar to that of Dr. Lanny Johnson (personal communication). The patient is placed supine on the OR table, and a tourniquet is applied to the operative leg. The surgeon exsanguinates the operative leg and inflates the tourniquet to 300 mm Hg. A padded leg holder is placed on the operative side of the table. The leg is put in the padded leg holder, allowing the knee to extend from the holder four fingerbreadths or approximately 4 in from the superior pole of the patella. This positioning enables use of the femoral condyles as a fulcrum in opening the medial compartment of the knee. Care should be taken not to stress the leg excessively; this

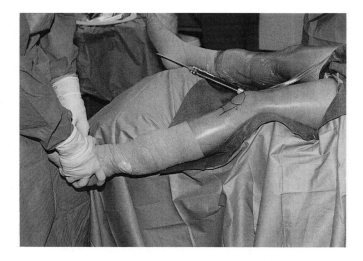

Figure 3–5 • Joint manipulation.

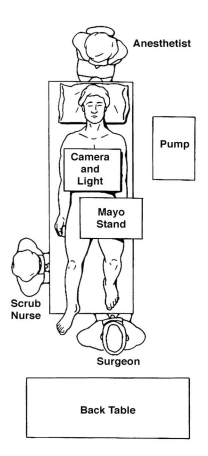

Figure 3–6 • Diagram of knee arthroscopy OR set-up.

could cause damage to the medial collateral ligament. The television monitor is placed directly over the patient's body, with the Mayo stand coming across the patient distal to the monitor. The surgeon stands at the foot of the table in direct line with the monitor for anatomic viewing. An assistant stands beside the surgeon to help manipulate the extremity. The scrub nurse should be positioned behind the Mayo stand within reach of the surgeon. All tubings and cords are draped across the patient superiorly (Fig. 3–6).

Cruciate Ligament Reconstruction

With a cruciate ligament reconstruction, the patient is placed supine on the OR table. A lateral stress post is placed on the lateral side of the table approximately 1 in superior to the femoral condyles. This post is effective in providing lateral countertraction to open the medial compartment during diagnostic arthroscopy. A 10 lb sandbag is placed approximately 3 in from the foot of the table. When the knee is flexed to 90 degrees, the toes should rest on the sandbag. At 45–60 degrees of knee flexion, the heel should rest on the sandbag. This allows for a change of knee-flexion angle during the procedure without the assistant continually holding the leg. All equipment is placed at the head of the table. The television monitor should come across directly over the patient's body. Two Mayo stands are needed for the procedure. The first Mayo stand is placed across the patient's body and should contain all arthroscopic instruments. The second Mayo stand is required for the cruciate ligament repair. The surgeon stands lateral to the operative leg and the assistant is across the table. The scrub nurse stands at the foot of the table. If available, a second scrub nurse could be used to facilitate the arthroscopic instruments (Fig. 3–7).

Sitting Arthroscopy

For some surgeons, sitting on a stool is a more comfortable or natural way to perform arthroscopic knee surgery.

According to Dr. W.G. Clancy, Jr (personal communication, 1996), sitting for arthroscopic surgery allows for the femur to be placed in abduction and internal rotation so that the hip is tight. The anterior hip capsule prevents further internal rotation. The tibia is placed in external rotation, and the heel is placed in the surgeon's groin. Resting the patient's foot against the surgeon's iliac crest maintains the leg in external rotation. The leg is abducted to produce valgus stress and to open the knee medially without the use of a lateral post. The height of the stool the surgeon uses allows the knee to rest in 20 degrees of flexion, increasing the amount of laxity on the medial knee. This position allows the surgeon to view the entire meniscus. Because the surgeon has control over the patient's leg, no assistant is required to hold the leg (personal communication, 1996). Clancy also advocates the use of a 0 degree arthroscope for knee arthroscopy and does not use a tourniquet (Fig. 3–8).

Shoulder Arthroscopy

The authors prefer a lateral decubitus position, as described by Johnson,[1] for shoulder arthroscopy. The patient is placed on the OR table on a bean bag positioner, with the affected arm suspended by overhead traction. The traction apparatus is placed at the foot of the table, with the boom facing the patient's anterior. Ten to fifteen

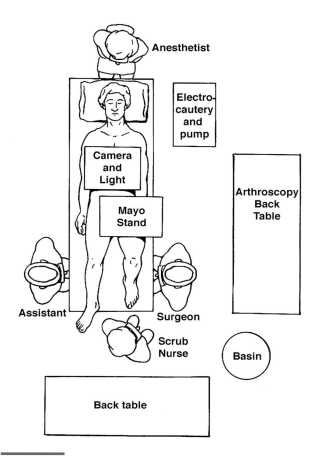

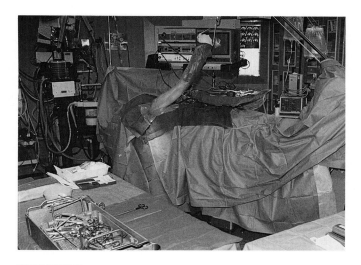

Figure 3–9 • Lateral decubitus position.

Figure 3–7 • Diagram of cruciate ligament OR set-up.

pounds of traction is placed on the pulley system to allow for joint distraction (Fig. 3–9). This position eliminates the need for an assistant to hold traction on the arm while manipulating the joint externally. All equipment should be placed on the side opposite the surgical site. The monitor should be directly across from the surgeon, and the Mayo stand should be across the patient's body. The assistant and the scrub nurse stand beside the surgeon. It is often necessary to angle the table to provide room for the surgical team and the anesthesia team to work (Fig. 3–10).

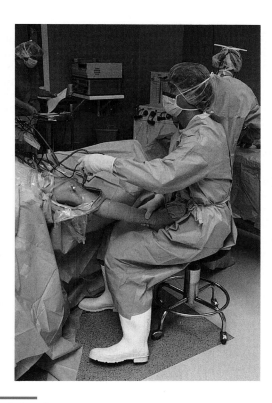

Figure 3–8 • Sitting arthroscopy.

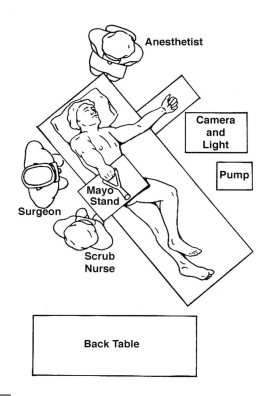

Figure 3–10 • Diagram of shoulder arthroscopy set-up.

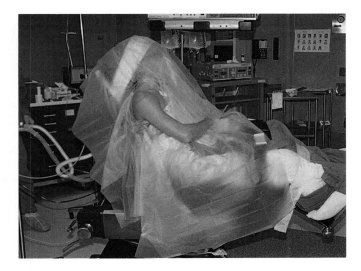

Figure 3–11 • Beach-chair position.

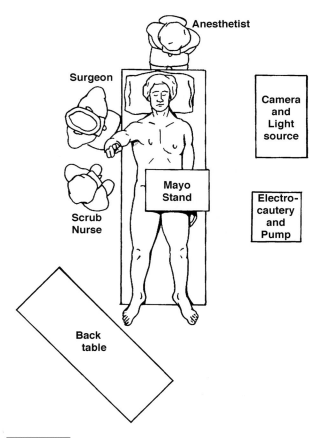

Figure 3–12 • Diagram of elbow arthroscopy repair set-up.

A beach-chair position is the preferred patient position of Skyhar et al.[3] With this position, the advantages include ease of set-up, lack of brachial plexus strain as a result of not using traction, better visualization of all types of arthroscopic shoulder procedures, and easy conversion to an open procedure. With the beach-chair position, the patient is sitting up at approximately 60 degrees of flexion. Care should be taken to flex the knees and to apply proper padding to eliminate stretching the peroneal nerve and artery. Padding the patient's feet is also necessary. A side kidney rest may be used to keep the patient stabilized on the table. The folded sheet should be placed under the scapula to push the joint forward. All equipment is placed just as for the lateral decubitus position (Fig. 3–11).

Elbow Arthroscopy

The patient is placed supine on the OR table. A tourniquet is placed as high on the arm as possible. The patient's forearm is placed in a gauntlet-type holding device and connected to a traction device that hangs overhead. The traction device is placed across the table from the surgical site. The boom arm of the traction device should project superiorly. The gauntlet should be attached to the pulley system on the boom. The arm should hang at 90 degrees of flexion and 90 degrees of abduction. Approximately 5 lb of traction is applied to the pulley system to suspend the arm. The patient should be positioned on the edge of the table to allow the arm to hang free of the table. The surgeon sits directly lateral to the patient. The assistant sits or stands to the side of the surgeon. The Mayo stand is placed over the patient's body, with all cords and tubings running to the side opposite the surgical site. The monitor, pump, and suction are placed opposite the operative site. The arthroscopy pump should always be placed where the surgeon can view the pressures the pump emits (Fig. 3–12). The tourniquet should be inflated 250 mm Hg. Carson, Soffer, and Andrews[4] prefer the tourniquet time be no longer than 90 minutes.

Poehling and Ekman[5] prefer to use a prone position for elbow arthroscopy. According to them, placing the patient prone improves the position of the arthroscope within the joint, facilitates manipulation within the joint, allows for better inspection of the joint, and eliminates the need for overhead traction devices. The OR setup is the same as for a supine patient.

Ankle Arthroscopy

The patient is placed supine on the OR table. A tourniquet is placed around the operative leg. The surgeon exsanguinates the leg and inflates the tourniquet to 300 mm Hg. A leg-holding device is placed on the table as for a knee arthroscopy, with the leg holder angled slightly superior and the patient's leg placed into the holder. The leg holder serves as a stabilizing device, so there is no need to secure the leg as tightly as with a knee arthroscopy. The foot of the bed is then lowered to a 45 degree angle to the table, and the OR table should be elevated to the highest position. The surgeon sits on a stool at the foot of the bed and places the patient's foot on his or her leg for additional stabilization. The monitor is placed directly over the patient's body so that the surgeon is looking in direct line with the patient's body. An assistant is positioned to the side of the surgeon, opposite the extremity prepared for surgery. The Mayo stand with the arthroscopic instruments is positioned over the patient's body. The scrub nurse stands to the side of the patient unless needed as the assistant. When sitting stools are used for an arthroscopic procedure, all suction tubings and pump tubings are best positioned superior and to the side opposite the surgical site. This precaution prevents the surgeon or assistant from rolling over the tubings and disrupting the procedure.

Hip Arthroscopy

The patient is placed supine on the fracture table as described by Byrd.[6] The operative hip is placed in 25 degrees of abduction with neutral rotation and approximately 2 cm of distraction. Usually 25–50 lb of traction is necessary. The opposite leg is placed in a leg holder stirrup and is abducted to allow for fluoroscopy positioning between the legs. A perineal post is placed slightly lateral to the perineal area to assist with hip distraction. A larger perineal post can be used for distraction when shifting the post laterally is not effective. The monitor is placed on the side opposite to the surgical site. All cords and tubings are draped across the patient and rest on the patient's body. The scrub nurse stands behind the surgeon (see Chapter 19). Extra-long instruments and spinal needles are used in hip arthroscopy. With all the equipment needed for hip arthroscopy, a basic set-up drawing placed in the OR assists in facilitating space and use. Glick and colleagues[7] prefer the patient in a lateral decubitus position for hip arthroscopy, citing ease of entry of arthroscopic instruments and the ability to visualize the entire hip joint.

OPERATIVE ARTHROSCOPY

General Techniques

It is best to begin the arthroscopy with a systematic diagnostic arthroscopy. This assessment tells the surgeon where to look, what to expect, and approximately how much time will be needed to accomplish the procedure. Palpation of the joint can be done with a probe, especially in the knee. Use of instrumentation should be understood before attempting arthroscopic surgery. There are several

cutting and grasping tools for removing tissue and loose bodies. Arthroscopic knives are used to cut menisci, labra, and tendons. Basket forceps are used mainly in knee arthroscopy to resect menisci. A Schlesinger grasper is used to grasp tissues and loose bodies. To minimize tissue trauma, a switching stick may be used to transfer the arthroscope to a new portal site.

With the advent of power instruments, arthroscopic surgery is being accomplished with greater success. An arthroscopic shaving system should be available on all procedures. Four basic techniques as described by Johnson[1] are used effectively with an arthroscopic shaving system. First, a shaving action is a back-and-forth movement across the surface. The tissue enters the shaver by means of suction attached to the system. Tissue type will necessitate changing the shaver head. Second, a dabbing or blotting motion is used with the suction action to pull the tissue up into the shaver for cutting. Third, pawing or scratching motion, or a slow motion pulling toward the surgeon, is used on articular cartilage or to smooth meniscus. Each shaving system has an oscillating mode built into it. This oscillating mode helps to facilitate a whittling action used in cutting meniscus and synovial tissue. Fourth, a scooping action can be used to cut irregular or hard tissue. Several shaver tips are available for use.

References

1. Johnson LL: Arthroscopic surgical principles. In Johnson LL: Diagnostic and Surgical Arthroscopy of the Shoulder. St. Louis, Mosby, 1993, pp 115–188.
2. Gross RM: Arthroscopy, basic setup and equipment. Orthop Clin North Am 24:5–18, 1993.
3. Skyhar MJ, Altchek DW, Warren RF, et al.: Shoulder arthroscopy with the patient in the beach chair position. Arthroscopy 4:256–259, 1988.
4. Carson WG, Soffer SR, and Andrews JR: Diagnostic arthroscopy of the elbow. In Andrews JR and Soffer SR (eds.): Elbow Arthroscopy. St. Louis, Mosby, 1994, pp 33–56.
5. Poehling GC and Ekman EF: Arthroscopy of the elbow. In Jackson DW (ed.): Instructional Course Lectures, vol. 44, American Academy of Orthopaedic Surgery, 1995, pp 217–223.
6. Byrd JW: Hip arthroscopy utilizing the supine position. Arthroscopy 10:275–280, 1994.
7. Glick JM, Sampson TG, Gordon RB, et al.: Hip arthroscopy by the lateral approach. Arthroscopy 3:4–12, 1987.

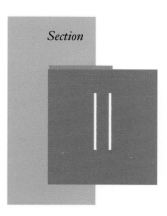

Section

II

The Shoulder

4 Diagnostic Arthroscopy of the Shoulder

Keith Meister

INTRODUCTION

Perhaps the greatest technologic advancement in orthopaedic medicine has been the development of the arthroscope as a viable tool for diagnosis and treatment of intra-articular pathologic problems. The successful use of the arthroscope in orthopaedics has also led to the increasing use of this tool in other medical disciplines. In 1931, Burman[1] examined multiple joints in a cadaver by using a crude arthroscope with poor illumination. He is recognized as the first to visualize the inside of the shoulder. However, the poor technology made it a less than practical instrument for widespread use. Thus, initial interest and experimentation declined.

In the 1950s, Watanabe began developing newer and more practical arthroscopic instrumentation. Newer technology improved visual acuity and expanded the potential for more practical use of the device. The No. 21 arthroscope, developed in 1959 by Watanabe, was a technologic breakthrough that led to the development of routine arthroscopy of the knee in the 1970s.[2, 3]

Development of the use of the arthroscope in the shoulder has lagged behind its application in the knee. As early as 1965, attempts were made to use the arthroscope in the shoulder for treatment of adhesive capsulitis.[4] In 1972, Wiley and Older developed techniques for shoulder arthroscopy while examining cadaveric shoulders.[5] In 1978, Watanabe described the standard anterior and posterior portals.[2] In the early 1980s, Wiley and Older described their clinical applications with techniques developed during their cadaveric experience.[5]

It was during the 1980s that use of arthroscopy in the shoulder not only provided a greater understanding of intra-articular pathology but also became a viable tool for treatment of many common pathologic problems. Initial application was limited to diagnosis, lavage, and removal of loose bodies. During the last decade and a half, application has expanded to treatment of, among others, lesions of instability and the labrum,[6–20] disease of the rotator cuff and biceps tendon,[21–32] acute and chronic injury to the acromioclavicular (AC) joint,[33–35] infection, adhesive capsulitis, osteochondritis dissecans, osteonecrosis, and arthritis.[36–41]

PATIENT SELECTION

Preoperative Evaluation

Arthroscopic surgery is not a substitute for a complete clinical evaluation and assessment of a shoulder problem. The clinician, before use of the arthroscope for evaluation and treatment, needs to have a firm grasp of the skills required for proper preoperative evaluation of the painful shoulder. The current evaluation form and rating system of the American Shoulder and Elbow Society is an accepted outline that is helpful in assisting the clinician in obtaining essential information during evaluation.[41] A brief outline is provided here, and specific, detailed preoperative evaluation of common shoulder problems is discussed in other chapters.

History

Acquiring an adequate history is the essential first step in the diagnosis of any shoulder problem. It is often stated that more than 90% of most orthopaedic diagnoses may be made by obtaining a good history. The timing of onset of symptoms should be questioned: insidious or acute. Pain should be characterized: quality, location, duration, aggravating activities, and alleviating measures. Particularly in overhand athletes, the phase of the throwing cycle in which symptoms are present is often crucial in making a proper diagnosis. The presence or absence of mechanical symptoms, a history of instability, neurologic and vascular complaints, history of neck pain, and prior treatment measures should all be elicited.

Physical Examination

The physical examination should allow for complete evaluation of the upper torso, beginning with the cervical spine. Examination of the cervical spine should note alignment, range of motion, and areas of tenderness.

Examination of the shoulder begins with evaluation for any asymmetry. Palpation of the entire girdle should be accomplished, noting specific common areas of inflammation and tenderness, i.e., rotator cuff, AC joint, coracoid process, and so on. Range of motion should be documented by carefully recording elevation and internal and external rotation at both neutral and 90 degrees of abduction. Stability in the anterior and posterior directions should be assessed by employing the Lachman maneuver of the shoulder, with the arm positioned in the plane of the scapula in neutral rotation. Inferior laxity may be assessed in the sitting position by recording the presence and magnitude of the sulcus. Strength, specifically with notation of magnitude of resistance in abduction and external rotation, is recorded. Specialty maneuvers, such as the impingement tests, clunk test, relocation test, and so on, may be employed depending on the suspected diagnosis and focus of the evaluation. Finally, a neurologic and vascular evaluative examination of the upper extremity should be thorough.

Radiologic Assessment

Standard radiographic profiles are utilized depending on the focus of the evaluation. Evaluation of the painful shoulder utilizes an impingement series, which includes standard anteroposterior views in internal and external rotation, outlet views, and axillary views. Evaluation of the unstable shoulder adds a Stryker notch view to the series. Additional views may be added for assistance in evaluation, depending on the suspected diagnosis. Additional radiologic assessment may include evaluation by arthrography, computed tomography arthrography, ultrasound scan, and magnetic resonance imaging.[42–45] An uncomplicated arthrogram is still the gold standard for quick and inexpensive evaluation of the rotator cuff. Computed tomography arthrography is useful in the evaluation of the rotator cuff, labrum, capsule, and bony architecture. Ultrasonography can also be useful in the evaluation of the rotator cuff, but is highly user-dependent. The indications for and usefulness of magnetic resonance imaging are still being assessed. With better magnets, coils, and computer software, image quality continues to improve, and parameters for the evaluation of soft tissue and bony architecture continue to evolve. The addition of contrast with saline solution or gadolinium can help to highlight the rotator cuff and labrum further, improving the sensitivity of the study.

Adjunctive Testing

Adjunctive testing may include electromyographic analysis, nerve conduction studies, and isokinetic testing of strength. In the general population, isokinetic testing of flexion/extension and internal/external rotation is performed at 60 and 120 degrees/sec. In the overhand athlete, testing of internal/external rotation and abduction/adduction strength is usually performed at higher speeds (180/300 degrees/sec). Videoanalysis of overhand motions can provide additional useful information in the evaluation of shoulder problems in the athletic population.

Indications

Detailed guidelines on indications and technique for the use of the arthroscope in the shoulder for the treatment of common pathologic conditions are covered in other chapters. However, the utility of and indications for when to use the arthroscope in the treatment of common pathologic conditions continue to expand as technology, proficiency, and the understanding of the pathophysiology of many of these conditions grow. It should be a rare instance when the arthroscope is used solely for diagnostic purposes and the clinician enters the joint without clear indications and a specific plan of treatment.

Treatment of problems of the rotator cuff and biceps is commonplace. Arthroscopic subacromial decompression for chronic rotator cuff tendinitis is at least as successful as open techniques.[23, 27, 28] Treatment of partial-thickness tears of the rotator cuff has been successful with arthroscopic débridement.[21, 24] Treatment of small-to-large tears with a closed technique or combined arthroscopic and "mini-open" technique is well established.[22, 26, 29] Treatment of large irreparable tears of the rotator cuff with arthroscopic débridement has been successfully accomplished.[25, 32] Arthroscopic tenodesis of the biceps in cases of chronic bicipital tendinitis can be achieved. Débridement of symptomatic ruptures of the biceps in cases refractory to nonoperative management may be indicated.[46]

Arthroscopic evaluation of the unstable shoulder may provide assistance in planning the proper operative approach. Problems of unidirectional instability, particularly in the anterior direction, with Bankart lesions and little to no underlying capsular laxity may be the clearest indications for arthroscopic stabilization of the shoulder. Multidirectional instability has been treated with arthroscopic techniques, but with clearly less successful outcome. The use of a laser for capsular shrinkage and treatment of some of the more subtle laxity problems is a more recently employed and experimental technique whose efficacy has not yet been determined.[47]

Symptomatic, painful tears of the labrum, unassociated with gross instability, have been treated successfully with arthroscopic débridement.[48, 48a, 49] Tears of the superior labrum from anterior to posterior (SLAP lesions) that occur secondary to acute or repetitive trauma can be treated effectively with débridement or arthroscopic repair.[18, 21, 48–50]

Problems of the AC joint may be addressed with the arthroscope. Isolated degenerative processes may be treated with isolated arthroscopic resection of the distal clavicle by either a subacromial or supraclavicular approach. In cases in which symptoms are secondary to underlying instability, results from resection alone may not be as favorable. Therefore, higher-grade lesions would require a concomitant stabilization of the distal clavicle.[34]

Additional conditions that may be successfully treated with arthroscopic techniques include refractory adhesive capsulitis, removal of loose bodies, sepsis, osteochondritis dissecans, arthritis with synovectomy for rheumatoid disease, and generalized débridement for osteoarthritis.[4, 36, 38–41a]

Contraindications

The numerous neurovascular structures located about the shoulder make it a precarious joint to approach without a thorough knowledge of relational anatomy. Thus, a relative contraindication to the use of arthroscopy in the shoulder lies with the individual who does not have a safe, working knowledge of anatomy and portal access. Additionally, if there is significant distortion of soft tissues or of bony landmarks, a cautious approach to the use of the arthroscope should be taken.

OPERATING ROOM SET-UP

Anesthesia

Two basic anesthetic techniques are now commonly employed in the use of shoulder arthroscopy: general and regional. General anesthesia is the more common technique of the two. The newer short-acting intravenous anesthetic medications routinely employed in the outpatient setting allow for shorter wake-ups and decreased sedation. The primary advantages of a general anesthetic are the lack of experience needed in placing a predictable regional block, less need for patient cooperation, and the ability to use the lateral decubitus position. Additionally, use of a general anesthetic provides the ability to control blood pressure in achieving relative hypotension for hemostasis. This is particularly advantageous in aggressive procedures in the subacromial space.

Regional anesthesia in the form of an interscalene block is becoming more and more popular, particularly as individuals move from the use of a lateral decubitus position to supine beach-chair approaches. For those who use a lateral position for arthroscopy, a regional technique is generally not an alternative because of the difficulty in maintaining an awake patient in this position for a prolonged time.

In a large comparative study involving more than 100 patients,[51] a regional block was found to be safe and effective, with a high degree of patient acceptance. Intraoperatively, it provided excellent analgesia and muscle relaxation. Postoperatively, regional anesthesia was thought to result in fewer side effects, fewer hospital admissions, and a shorter hospital stay than general anesthesia.[51] A long-acting block is also particularly useful in the outpatient setting, providing for long-term anesthesia for control of postoperative pain.

Positioning

There are two basic positioning techniques for use in arthroscopy of the shoulder. The classic position involves placement of the patient in the lateral decubitus position. The second position uses the beach-chair approach.

The lateral position was originally described by Wiley and Older[5] in their early use of the arthroscope in the shoulder. They placed patients in the lateral decubitus position with the flank flexed and the arm draped free. No traction was used. They believed that this position allowed the arm to fall into an adducted and flexed position that facilitated entry into the joint and viewing of the humeral head.

Andrews and Carson[52, 53] later described their technique with the arm held at approximately 70 degrees of abduction and 15 degrees of forward flexion with longitudinal traction. The use of traction facilitated visualization but raised a concern about potential complications to the neurovascular structures as a result of overdistraction.[54–56]

A modification of the lateral position was described by Gross and Fitzgibbons.[57] They changed the direct lateral position to a semilateral position, allowing the patient to roll 30–40 degrees posteriorly to place the glenohumeral joint on a horizontal plane. It was suggested that this variation made the arthroscopy more natural and comfortable, especially when instrumenting from one side of the joint while arthroscoping from the other. Additionally, they applied traction perpendicular to the long axis of the humerus, with the arm in 20 degrees of abduction (Fig. 4–1).

A sitting beach-chair position has been described by Skyhar and colleagues.[58] The patient is placed supine with the torso elevated into the sitting position to at least 60 degrees to the horizontal. The operative side is brought off the edge of the table so that the surgeon can access both sides of the shoulder, and an arm board is placed at the level of the elbow, allowing the arm to hang free. A small bump is placed under the ipsilateral hip to allow better access to the posterior shoulder (Fig. 4–2).

Skyhar and colleagues cited many potential advantages with this position, including ease of set-up, ease in moving to an open procedure, lack of need for a traction set-up, and lack of potential strain to the brachial plexus. Although they have also designed arm holders for use with this technique, this position may still obviate the need for an assistant to manipulate the shoulder. An additional advantage may also be the potential for use of regional anesthesia.

Traction suspension has been carefully evaluated to look at the potential damage to the neurovascular structures with respect to field of visualization, arm position, direction, and amount of applied traction. Pitman et al.[56] used somatosensory evoked potentials (SEPs) to detect neuropraxia during shoulder arthroscopy. SEPs were used to monitor the musculocutaneous, ulnar, and either the median or radial nerves in 20 cases. In 13 patients the arm was placed in 70 degrees of abduction and 15 degrees of forward flexion with 15 lb of traction; in 7 patients the arm was adducted and no more than 5–10 lb of perpendicular traction was applied. In all 20 cases, abnormal SEPs of the

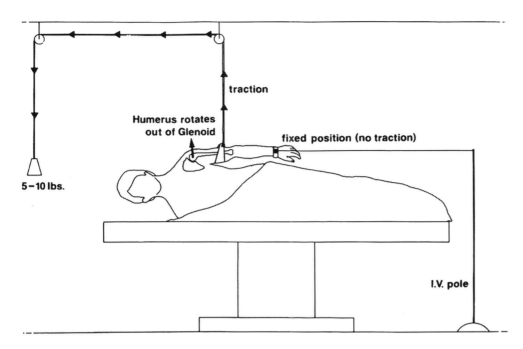

Figure 4–1 • Perpendicular traction applied to the patient in the lateral decubitus position with the shoulder adducted. (From Gross RM: Arthroscopy: basic setup and equipment. Orthop Clin North Am 24:7, 1993.)

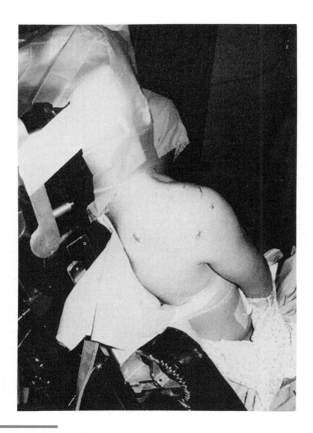

Figure 4–2 • Positioning the patient in the beach-chair position for shoulder arthroscopy. (From Altchek DW, Warren RF, and Skyhar MJ: Shoulder arthroscopy. In Rockwood CA and Matsen FA (eds.): The Shoulder. Philadelphia, W.B. Saunders Co., 1990, p 266.)

musculocutaneous nerve were demonstrated. In 16 cases, they were caused by initial joint distention and in 15 cases by traction; in 11 by longitudinal traction of >12 lb and in 6 by perpendicular traction of >7 lb. In 10 patients there were varying degrees of median, ulnar, and radial nerve entrapment. In spite of these findings, there were only two cases of clinical neuropraxia in this series. Both cases resolved within 48 hours.

Klein and colleagues[55] evaluated the relative strain within the brachial plexus at five selected positions for arthroscopy and correlated each position with viewing capacity. These authors found that the most optimal viewing was achieved with the arm in the classic position of 70 degrees of abduction and 30 degrees of forward flexion, but this position also resulted in the highest rates of strain in the plexus. Increasing the degrees of forward flexion and decreasing the magnitude of abduction generally proved to decrease strain in the plexus. However, a repositioning of the arm resulted in loss of overall visual capacity. These authors, therefore, suggested that multiple arm positions be used during the procedure to maximize viewing and minimize potential injury to the brachial plexus.

Although early authors advocated the use of the lateral decubitus position without traction, most arthroscopists think this is a cumbersome approach. Thus, when traction is used a maximum weight of 10–15 lb in any direction should be utilized. This amount of weight should provide for sufficient visualization with almost any shoulder. Weights should generally be adjusted down in the smaller patient. In the beach-chair position, the weight of the arm alone is said to distract the glenohumeral joint enough to avoid the need for longitudinal traction.[58]

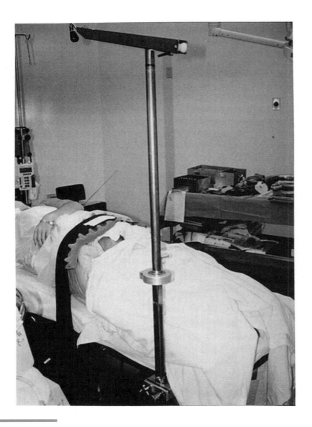

Figure 4–3 • Commercially available shoulder arthroscopy traction for set-up in the lateral decubitus position.

Equipment

A standard operating room table in a dedicated, arthroscopically equipped operating suite should be utilized. The table should be fully adjustable to be able to alter height, tilt in both the long and short planes of the table, and allow flexion/extension of the head, torso, and feet.

In the beach-chair position, no traction is necessary, but an adaptable arm holder off the side of the table may eliminate the need for an assistant to hold the arm during the procedure. Standard arthroscopic shoulder holders may be utilized for the patient in the lateral decubitus position. Longitudinal traction may be applied to the humerus with a commercially available traction arm that allows for adjustment of abduction/adduction and flexion/extension of the arm during the procedure (Fig. 4–3). If perpendicular traction to the humerus is the preferred technique, an intravenous pole may be used at the base of the table and the arm held with this in 20–30 degrees of abduction. Horizontal traction may then be applied with a suspension set-up attached to the ceiling of the operating theater or by a commercially available set-up device that can also attach to the operating table (Fig. 4–4).

Standard equipment for optimal performance of the arthroscopy should include a portable cabinet that is high enough to eliminate the possibility of an obstructed view. The cabinet should house the video monitor, video recorder, and video printer, all for recording normal and pathologic findings (Fig. 4–5).

A standard 4 mm arthroscope is sufficient for use in the shoulder. The smaller-diameter arthroscopes do not really provide any further advantage to warrant their standard use. Both 30 and 70 degree viewing arthroscopes should be available so as to optimize visualization, depending on the portal of use and the complexity of the procedure.

Figure 4–4 • Commercially available device for application of perpendicular traction in the lateral decubitus position.

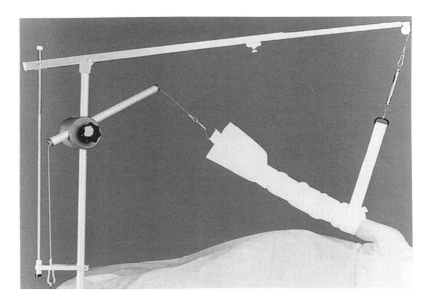

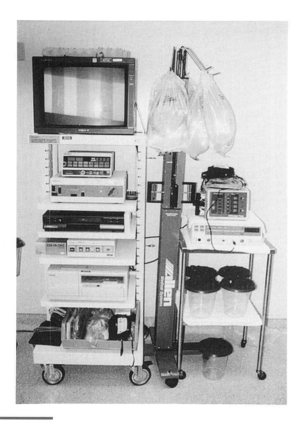

Figure 4–5 • Video cabinet set-up for portability and convenience of use.

Normal saline solution has been shown to be a safe and effective medium for use in the shoulder. Either gravity-assisted flow or a standard arthroscopic pump can be utilized. A pump has the added advantage of allowing for control of flow and pressure, depending on need during the course of the procedure. However, particularly with some of the newer high-flow delivery systems, clinical monitoring of flow to avoid inadvertent extravasation of fluid needs to be emphasized. The systems that measure pressure directly from the scope and not the fluid delivery line may give a more accurate interpretation of actual intra-articular and tissue pressure. These systems may theoretically be safer.

Although hypotensive anesthesia facilitates viewing and the control of active bleeding, particularly in the subacromial space, pressure difference measurements of less than 49 mm Hg between systolic blood pressure and subacromial space pressure should be the goal. These differences have been shown to lead consistently to improved viewing.[59] Additionally, a monopolar arthroscopic cautery and epinephrine added to the saline bags are useful in the control of bleeding during procedures.

A number of different types of cameras are now available for improved viewing capacity. Visual acuity is better achieved with the more advanced and more expensive three-chip, rather than the single-chip, cameras. Most of these cameras allow the surgeon to run both the VCR and the printer with instruments on the hub of the camera. Fogging can be particularly troublesome in the beach-chair position as leaking fluid has a tendency to run down the arthroscope toward the scope camera couple. The direct couple arthroscopes have the advantage of eliminating this problem (Fig. 4–6).

The instrument table should have available multiple cannulas for multiple portal set-up. Additionally, a standard power shaving device with detachable blades and a full complement of hand instruments are needed. Blunted switching sticks are also helpful to have for rapid change of portals when an arthroscope with multiple detachable cannulas is not available (Fig. 4–7).

GENERAL TECHNIQUE

Portals

A number of different portals have been described for the use of the arthroscope in accessing the glenohumeral and AC joints. In the description of each of these portals, it is

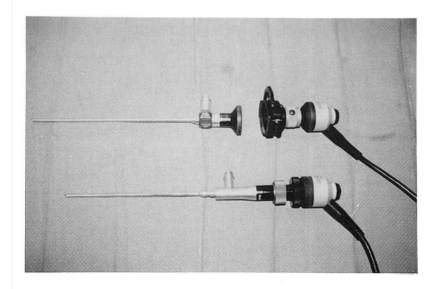

Figure 4–6 • Uncoupled *(top)* and coupled *(bottom)* arthroscopes.

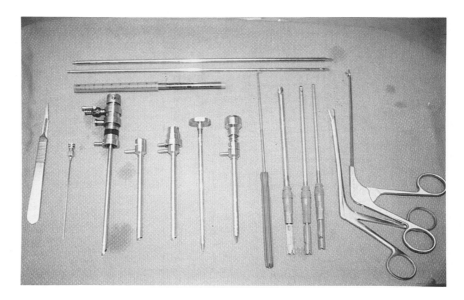

Figure 4–7 • Mayo stand set-up with commonly used instruments for routine arthroscopy.

best to describe and understand them with respect to their general anatomic location. Therefore, we will divide the shoulder into different regions and examine the bony landmarks and relational and arthroscopic anatomy of each of the currently utilized portals. There are now commonly used safe portals in the posterior, anterior, lateral, and superior aspects of the glenohumeral joint and subacromial space, as well as separate portals for access to the AC joint.

Posterior

Wiley and Older[5] are credited with popularizing the posterior approach to instrumentation of the shoulder. During their early cadaveric dissection and use of the Watanabe No. 21 arthroscope, they discovered the utility and ease of access with this approach. The posterior portal is now considered the standard portal for initiation of glenohumeral and subacromial arthroscopy.

The portal as described by Andrews, Carson, and Ortega[52] is located approximately 2 cm inferior and 1 cm medial to the posterolateral tip of the acromion. Although measurements such as these may bring one into the general location for proper portal placement, this point should correspond to the so-called soft spot of the shoulder. This point marks an area overlying the glenohumeral joint at the level of the infraspinatus and teres minor interval. Placement of the portal either too high or too low complicates the procedure either by making instrumentation difficult or by putting the neurovascular structures at risk (Fig. 4–8).

Wolf[60] described an alternative posterior portal that is located slightly inferiorly to this standard placement. His portal is located slightly more medially and inferiorly, lying about 2–3 cm inferior and 1–2 cm medial to the posterolateral tip of the acromion. Placement of the trocar and arthroscope is then along the transverse access of the glenoid, facilitating placement of a lower anterior portal by an inside-out technique.

Placement of a posterior portal at any level first traverses the posterior deltoid. The rotator cuff is then pierced near the infraspinatus and teres minor interval, but usually through the substance of the infraspinatus, to enter into the joint space through the joint capsule at a point just above its equator.

The two primary structures at risk through this posterior portal are the suprascapular nerve medially and the axillary nerve inferiorly. The axillary nerve reaches the undersurface of the deltoid, accompanied by the posterior humeral circumflex artery, at the inferior border of the teres minor. The nerve generally lies 2–4 cm inferior to the classic portal placement. Even a more inferiorly placed portal comes no closer than 1 cm to the nerve (Fig. 4–9).[61–63]

The suprascapular nerve comes at greatest risk at the level of the margin of the posterior glenoid. At that level the nerve lies about 1.8 cm medial at the base of the scapular spine in the spinoglenoid notch. Only a very medially

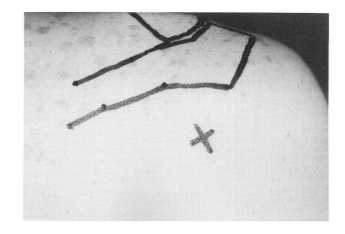

Figure 4–8 • Proper position of the posterior portal.

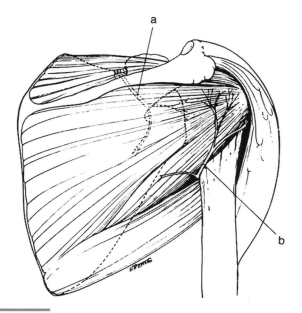

Figure 4–9 • Relational anatomy of the posterior portal. Note the relationship of the suprascapular nerve (a) and the axillary nerve (b) to the posterior aspect of the shoulder. (From O'Brien SJ, Arnoczky SP, Warren RF, et al.: Developmental anatomy of the shoulder and anatomy of the glenohumeral joint. In Rockwood CA and Matsen FA (eds.): The Shoulder. Philadelphia, W.B. Saunders Co., 1990, p 31.)

directed trocar during portal placement should ever come in proximity to this nerve (Fig. 4–10).[64]

Anterior

Anteriorly, an increasing number of safe portals have been described allowing for greater access and instrumentation as more and more technically advanced procedures have been developed. The important bony landmarks include the anterior border of the acromion, the coracoid process, and the AC joint (Fig. 4–11).

A number of authors have described variations of the anterior portals. McIntyre and Caspari[15] and Andrews, Carson, and Ortega[52] have described very similar antero-superior portals. Their portal lies between the coracoid process and acromion, piercing the deltoid and rotator cuff interval just inferior to the biceps. This portal can be established by either an outside-in or inside-out technique.

Matthews et al.[65] described a central or utility anterior portal created in the middle of the space bounded by the humeral head, glenoid, and biceps tendon, remaining above the superior border of the subscapularis and staying lateral to the coracoid process. This portal stays in the middle of the anterior safe intra-articular triangle described that is bounded by the above-mentioned structures.

Any of these superior portals can also be used to access the subacromial space easily by direction of a blunt cannula at the undersurface of the acromion. Particularly in subacromial procedures involving débridement of the distal end of the clavicle, the more superior portals provide a more versatile channel of access.

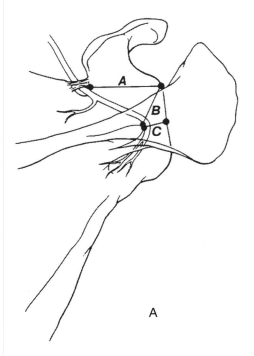

A

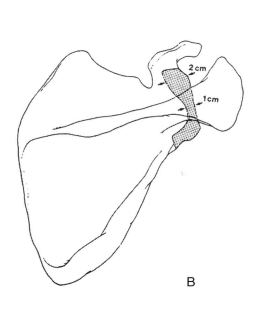

B

Figure 4–10 • *A*, The course of the suprascapular nerve with respect to the posterior glenoid neck (A,B,C). *B*, The safe zone of the posterior glenoid neck. (From Bigliani LU, Dalse RM, McCann PD, et al.: An anatomical study of the suprascapular nerve. Arthroscopy 6:302, 304, 1990.)

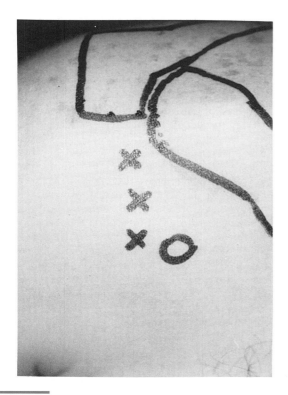

Figure 4–11 • Position of the most commonly used anterior portals.

With respect to the more superiorly located portals, the axillary nerve traverses the underside of the deltoid about 3 cm from the acromial margin. The cephalic vein lies both anterior and lateral to the anterolateral corner of the acromion and is unlikely to be damaged if proper blunt techniques are utilized. Branches of the thoracoacromial artery tend to lie along the medial side of the coracoacromial ligament; therefore, staying lateral to the ligament keeps one in a safe area.[63, 66]

Wolf[60] described what is probably best called a midanterior portal, given references to portals even inferior to this. This portal was developed to obtain more direct access to the lower portion of the anterior glenoid rim for placement of devices during arthroscopic anterior stabilization procedures. An inside-out technique is used to create the portal.

Through the posterior portal, the arthroscope is used to palpate the tip of the coracoid process and allowed to slide off its inferior edge. The arthroscope is then withdrawn from the sheath and the Wissinger rod is passed through the capsule. A cannula is then passed over the exiting rod to create the portal. This portal passes inferior to the tip of the coracoid process at the apex of the angle formed by the conjoined tendon and the pectoralis minor. Wolf claimed that, occasionally, the portal passes through the conjoined tendon.

Wolf found the musculocutaneous nerve to enter the coracobrachialis muscle anywhere from 2 to 8 cm from the tip of the coracoid process, with an average of 5 cm. These measurements were taken with the arm in 30 degrees of abduction, and they increased slightly with further adduc-

tion of the arm. The portal was found to be 1.5–4.0 cm from the musculocutaneous nerve, with an average of 2.9 cm (Fig. 4–12).[60]

Davidson and Tibone[67] have described a true anteroinferior portal with even more direct access to the inferior glenoid. This portal is also established by an inside-out technique. The arthroscope is advanced anterior to the leading edge of the inferior glenohumeral ligament, and a blunt Wissinger rod is used to puncture the capsule and anterior shoulder soft tissues. The importance of placing the arm in maximal adduction, removing lateral traction, and passing the rod as far laterally as possible after piercing the capsule layer was stressed by these authors. The standard 5.5 mm cannula is then passed over the rod and an 8 mm cannula is advanced through the anterior portal in a retrograde fashion.

The relationship of the axillary and musculocutaneous nerves to the portal was measured in nine different positions. There was no statistically significant change in the distance of the relational anatomy for any of the arm positions. The minimum distance from the portal to the axillary nerve was 14 mm, and the average distance was 24.4 mm. The minimum distance from the portal to the musculocutaneous nerve was 12 mm, and the average distance was 22.9 mm.

The portal was also in immediate proximity to the cephalic vein and anterior humeral circumflex artery (<1 cm). After exiting the capsule, the portal passes

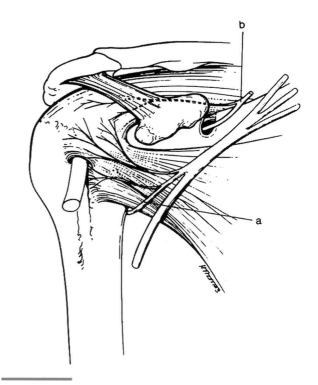

Figure 4–12 • The course of the axillary nerve (a) with respect to the anterior aspect of the shoulder and coracoid; the suprascapular nerve (b). (From O'Brien SJ, Arnoczky SP, Warren RF, et al.: Developmental anatomy of the shoulder and anatomy of the glenohumeral joint. In Rockwood CA and Matsen FA (eds.): The Shoulder. Philadelphia, W.B. Saunders Co., 1990, p 30.)

through the inferior third of the subscapularis, lateral to the conjoined tendon, and within 1 cm of the deltopectoral groove.[67]

The more inferior portals as described by Wolf and Davidson are generally not used as viewing portals. The more superior portals, however, can be used to obtain a better view of the anterior labrum and glenohumeral ligament complex, the posterior undersurface of the rotator cuff, and the posterior glenoid labrum.

Lateral

Multiple portals are described for approach to the lateral aspect of the shoulder with direct access to the subacromial space. Generally, these are not utilized in an approach to the glenohumeral joint except in the event of disruption of the rotator cuff. Because of the normal concavity of the undersurface of the acromion no matter where the portal is placed along the lateral edge of the acromion, it must be at least 2 cm lateral to the edge to allow for access to the entire undersurface of the acromion.

Ellman described both the anterolateral and posterolateral portals. The anterolateral portal was created to allow for access to the anteroinferior surface of the acromion and the coracoacromial ligament. It can also be used to reach over to the AC joint in subacromial procedures requiring access to this articulation. The anterolateral portal is created 2 cm (no greater than 3 cm) lateral to the anterolateral edge of the acromion while viewing from the posterior portal (Fig. 4–13). The posterolateral portal is created 2 cm off of the posterolateral edge of the acromion and was created as an accessory outflow portal by Ellman[23, 24] for subacromial space procedures. This portal is placed about 2 cm off the edge of the posterolateral edge of the acromion with a blunt trocar after an

appropriate skin incision is made (see Fig. 4–13). This portal can also be used for subacromial viewing.

Paulos and Franklin[28] and Paulos and Kody[29] described a central lateral portal for use during instrumentation for subacromial decompression that could be incorporated into an acromial splitting incision for better access to larger tears of the rotator cuff. This portal is located 1 cm lateral to the midpoint of the lateral edge of the acromion (see Fig. 4–13).

A superolateral portal (Fig. 4–14) has been described for additional access to the glenohumeral joint, for viewing during procedures involving the anterior glenoid or for placing anchoring devices in repair of lesions of the superior labrum. Additionally, the posterior capsule and glenoid can be viewed from this portal.

The portal is placed at a position just lateral to the acromion on a line drawn from the acromion to the coracoid process. While viewing the glenohumeral joint from a posterior portal, a needle is placed to enter the joint obliquely, directly above the biceps tendon, piercing the rotator interval. The spinal needle is then replaced with a blunt trocar and arthroscope after skin incision.[48]

The primary structure at risk during use of the lateral portals is the axillary nerve. Injury to this nerve is safely avoided by establishing all portals less than 3 cm lateral to the acromion.

Superior

The supraclavicular fossa portal was first described by Nevaiser[68] for superior access to the glenohumeral joint. The portal is situated in the superior soft spot surrounded by the distal clavicle and the AC joint anteriorly, the acromion laterally, and the spine of the scapula posteriorly (Fig. 4–15).

The portal is established by placing a skin incision 1 cm medial to the medial border of the acromion in the soft spot. A blunt trocar is then directed forward and obliquely through the musculature. Under direct visualization, by aiming laterally and slightly posteriorly the cannula can be advanced into the joint. The cannula passes through the trapezius, a portion of the supraspinatus, and the superior joint capsule, and into the glenohumeral joint.

The structures at greatest risk of damage during use of this portal are the suprascapular nerve and the supraspinatus portion of the rotator cuff. In this region of the shoulder, the suprascapular nerve lies about 3 cm (2.5–3.9 cm) medial to the nerve at the suprascapular notch and about 2.5 cm (1.9–3.2 cm) slightly posterior and medial at the base of the scapular spine.[64]

Souryal and Baker[69] studied the anatomy of the supraclavicular fossa portal. They found that the tendinous portion of the rotator cuff was penetrated in most specimens at any degree of abduction of greater than 60 degrees. No penetration of the musculotendinous portion of the cuff occurred when the arm was at 30 degrees or less of abduction. To avoid the tendinous portion of the cuff, their recommendation for placement of the trocar aiming laterally about 30 degrees and slightly posteriorly should be used.

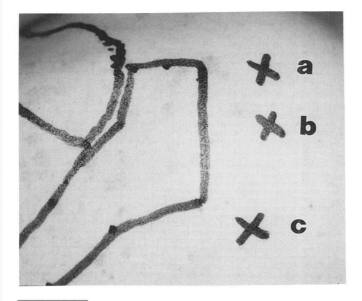

Figure 4–13 • Position of the (a) anterolateral, (b) midlateral, and (c) posterolateral portals.

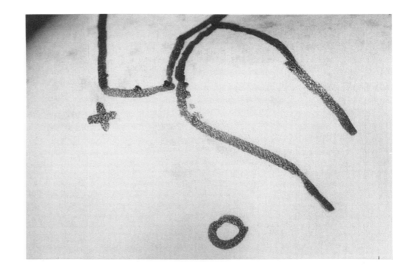

Figure 4–14 • Position of the superolateral portal.

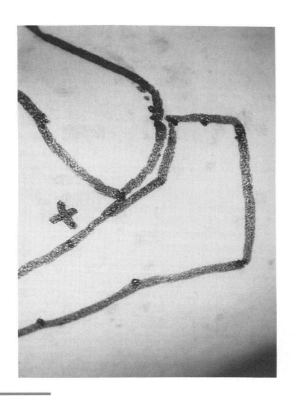

Figure 4–15 • The Nevaiser portal.

Two additional superior portals have been described for use in arthroscopy of isolated disease of the AC joint (Fig. 4–16).[34] The anterosuperior portal is placed in line with the AC joint and 0.75 cm anterior to it. The posterosuperior portal is placed in line with the joint and 0.75 cm posterior to it. Each portal is created with a puncture hole through the skin by a No. 11 scalpel blade, which is carried deeper to pierce the capsule of the AC joint. If the portals are properly placed, which should not be difficult because of the subcutaneous position of the AC joint, there are nei-

ther neurovascular structures at risk nor significant muscles or tendons violated during portal placement.

ARTHROSCOPIC ANATOMY

Biceps/Superior Labrum Complex

The initial view from the posterior portal allows for visualization of the biceps and its attachment to the superior labrum. The biceps is the most distinct structure visualized on entering the joint through the posterior portal (Fig. 4–17). Significant variation can occur in the attachment of the biceps to the superior labrum, as evidenced in the cadaveric study of Vangsness et al.[70] They noted four different types of normal attachment of the biceps to the labrum. In 50% of the biceps, attachment arose from the supraglenoid tubercle. In the other 50%, the biceps arose

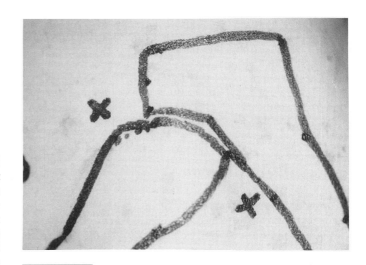

Figure 4–16 • The anterior and posterior portals for access to the acromioclavicular joint.

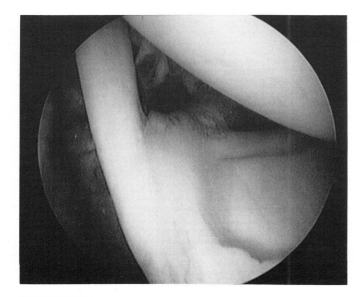

Figure 4–17 • View of the biceps tendon and its origin as seen from the posterior portal.

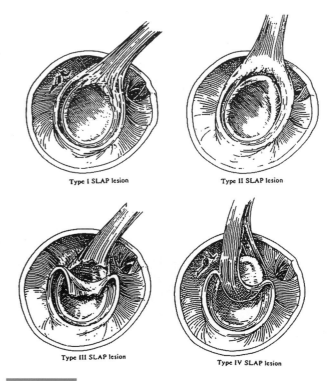

Figure 4–18 • Snyder classification of tears of the superior labrum. (From Snyder SJ, Karzel RP, Del Pizzo, et al.: SLAP lesions of the shoulder. Arthroscopy 6:276–277, 1990.)

directly from the superior labrum. The main labral origin was posterior in more than half. Additional variations described range from complete absence of the tendon to duplicate structures.

Snyder et al.[50] first classified disorders of the superior labrum complex as SLAP (superior labrum from anterior to posterior) lesions, and they characterized four different types. Type I lesions have fraying of the superior labrum with no tears and an intact biceps. Type II lesions, the most common, have stripping of the superior labrum attachment of the biceps off the underlying glenoid. Type III lesions are bucket-handle tears of the superior labrum displaced into the superior aspect of the glenohumeral joint. Type IV lesions are bucket-handle tears of the superior labrum with varying degrees of extension and involvement into the biceps tendon (Fig. 4–18). After reviewing their personal experience, Maffet, Gartsman, and Moseley[71] added three types of lesions to the original categorization that were unclassifiable.

Additional abnormalities in the biceps include isolated lesions, ranging from fraying to frank tearing with complete disruption, and dislocation of the tendon secondary to rupture of the transverse humeral ligament. Complete tears can be associated with type II SLAP lesions.[72]

Rotator Cuff

From a point at the base of the biceps, rotating the arthroscope superiorly allows for visualization of the rotator cuff. The biceps tendon marks the posterior extent of the rotator interval. Posterior to this is the supraspinatus. Proper manipulation of the arthroscope and combined rotation of the humeral head allow for visualization of the infraspinatus and teres minor posteriorly. The undersurface of the rotator cuff is normally covered by a thin layer of syn-

ovium that attaches at the superior margin of the humeral head. In the normal shoulder, the appearance is usually smooth (Fig. 4–19). Burkhart, Esch, and Jolson[73] also described the rotator cable–crescent complex. The rotator crescent is a term used to describe the thin, crescent-shaped sheet of rotator cuff comprising the distal portion:

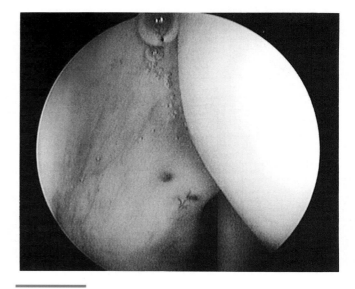

Figure 4–19 • Normal appearance of the undersurface of the rotator cuff as viewed from the posterior portal.

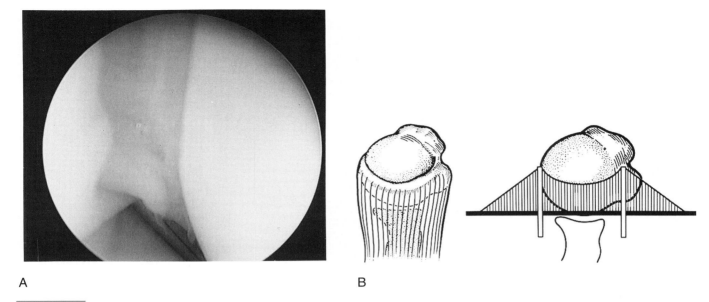

A   B

Figure 4–20 • *A*, The cable-crescent complex in the normal rotator cuff as viewed from the posterior portal. *B*, Schematic of the "suspension bridge" concept of Burkhart. (*B* from Burkhart SS, Esch JC, and Jolson RS: The rotator crescent and rotator cable: an anatomic description of the shoulder's "suspension bridge." Arthroscopy 9:612, 1993.)

of the supraspinatus and infraspinatus insertions. The cable is a thickening of the rotator cuff proximal to the crescent. The cable is important in the transfer of stress by the rotator cuff in support of the "suspension bridge" model of the rotator cuff (Fig. 4–20).

One should take note of the anterior soft spot of the shoulder anterior to the biceps. This is a safe area for placement of the anterior portals. This triangle is bounded by the biceps superiorly, the superior border of the subscapularis inferiorly, and the anterior rim of the glenoid and its labrum medially (Fig. 4–21). The subscapularis lies anterior to the middle glenohumeral ligaments. Rarely, a large portion of the subscapularis tendon can be seen exposing its musculotendinous zone.

Abnormalities of the rotator cuff as viewed from the posterior portal include partial tears of the undersurface of the superior-posterior aspects of the cuff; these tears are noted as fraying of portions of the supraspinatus and infraspinatus (Fig. 4–22). This is often associated with fraying of the posterior labrum as part of the undersurface

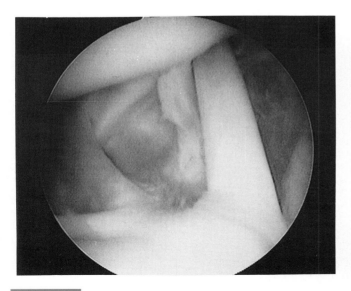

Figure 4–21 • The anterior triangle of the shoulder as viewed from the posterior portal. Note the biceps, superior edge of the subscapularis, and glenoid medially, forming the boundaries of the triangle.

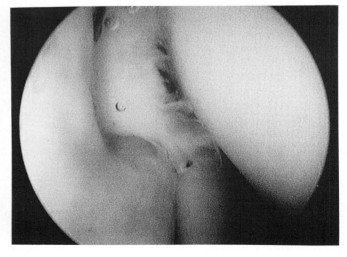

Figure 4–22 • An undersurface tear of the rotator cuff in a young, symptomatic, overhand athlete as viewed from the posterior portal.

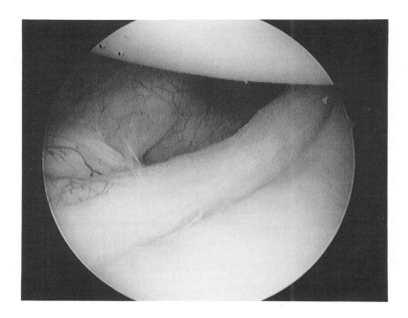

Figure 4–23 • The anterior glenohumeral complex as viewed from the posterior portal with a 30 degree arthroscope.

impingement process in overhand athletes.[30] Complete, full-thickness tears of the rotator cuff can be seen ranging in size from small to massive. Involvement of only the supraspinatus or the entire rotator cuff may be encountered.

Anteriorly, abnormalities of the subscapularis can include rupture and tearing of the upper portion of the subscapularis tendon. Such lesions can occur as isolated entities or in association with other lesions of the cuff and capsule.

Glenoid Labrum

From a point at the anterosuperior margin of the glenoid, directing the arthroscope for an inferior view allows for examination of the anterior glenohumeral complex (Fig. 4–23). In a tighter shoulder, this view may not be easily obtainable and can often be best achieved by utilizing a 70 degree arthroscope from a posterior portal or a standard 30 degree arthroscope from a high anterior portal (Fig. 4–24).

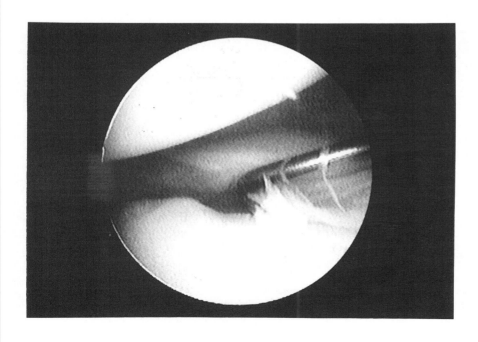

Figure 4–24 • A chronic detachment of the anterior labrum as viewed from the anterior portal.

There can be considerable variation in the size and attachments of the labrum. This is a triangular fibrous structure surrounding and contiguous with the glenoid articular surface. The labrum consists of the same fibrous material as that of the capsule. Its function is to provide attachment of the synovial and capsular structures, primarily the glenohumeral ligaments. The labrum has two attachment points to the glenoid, one directly to the glenoid rim and the other to the periosteum of the scapular neck and the fibrous capsule. The labrum's marginal attachment can vary, with slightly recessed attachments being confused with partial detachments of the labral complex. Appreciation of the articular surface often up and over the edge of the glenoid face can eliminate this misdiagnosis.

Abnormalities of the labrum can include varying degrees of disease, from fraying to detachment. Lesions of the superior labrum have already been discussed. Anterior detachments, or Bankart lesions, are usually associated with patterns of anterior instability (see Fig. 4–24). Although much rarer, similar lesions can be found on the posterior side of the joint in association with varying degrees and patterns of posterior instability. Fraying of either the anterior or posterior labrum should sometimes provide a clue to the examiner to appreciate subtle degrees of instability leading to abnormal translation of the humeral head and disruption of the labral margin. Associated fraying of the posterior superior labrum with undersurface tears of the rotator cuff is now commonly recognized as a source of pain in the overhand athlete (Fig. 4–25).[30]

Glenohumeral Ligament Complex

As with the labrum, there can be considerable variation in size and attachments of the glenohumeral ligaments. The superior, middle, and inferior ligaments are thickened areas of the shoulder capsule. Each is named for its attachment on the humeral head at the anatomic neck rather than on the scapula.

The superior glenohumeral ligament attaches near the top of the lesser tuberosity and inserts into the superior glenoid tubercle at or near the base of the biceps. Arthroscopically, it is often poorly seen because of its subsynovial and anterior position. It has been noted to be an important stabilizer in the prevention of posterior and inferior instability of the shoulder. It additionally contributes to anterior stabilization with the shoulder in external rotation and abduction at less than 90 degrees.[74]

The middle glenohumeral ligament originates from the midportion of the anatomic neck and lesser tuberosity, crosses the subscapularis, and inserts at the midportion of the anterior labrum. At times, the ligament appears cord-like, as noted by Morgan, Rames, and Snyder.[75] An additional normal variation was described by Williams, Snyder, and Buford[76] and termed the Buford complex, in which a cord-like middle glenohumeral ligament is contiguous with the anterosuperior labrum, attaching at the base of the biceps. No other labral tissue is in this area, giving the appearance of a large sublabral hole (Fig. 4–26).

The inferior glenohumeral ligament originates from the inferior portion of the humeral neck; sweeping upward and medially, it attaches at the middle of the glenoid labrum. The ligament is routinely larger than the superior two. A separate thickened band along its superior border can often be seen. A normal inferior glenohumeral ligament is essential for anterior stability of the shoulder.

Abnormal findings in the glenohumeral ligament complex usually involve loss of integrity by disruption at the labral side. However, detachment of the capsular ligaments at the humeral side following episodes of anterior dislocation has been described.[7]

Recesses

Advancement of the arthroscope into the anterior triangle with a view directed inferiorly allows for visualization of the synovial space underlying the subscapularis: the subscapularis recess (Fig. 4–27). This is a frequent spot for loose bodies. The coracoid process can be palpated subcu-

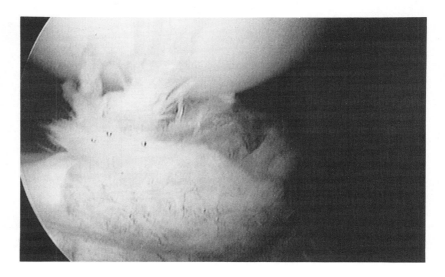

Figure 4–25 • Fraying of the posterior labrum in an overhand athlete with undersurface rotator cuff impingement.

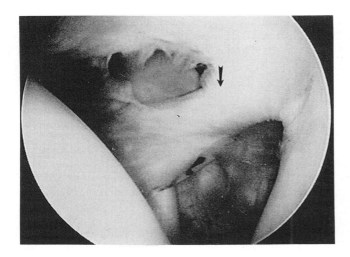

Figure 4–26 • Normal variant of the glenoid attachment of the middle glenohumeral ligament *(arrow)* referred to as the Buford complex. (From Nottage WM: Arthroscopic portals: anatomy at risk. Orthop Clin North Am 24:29, 1993.)

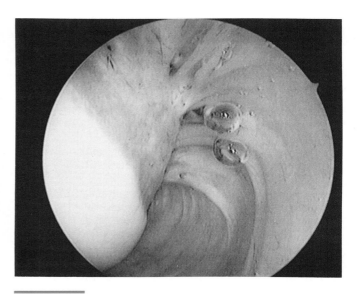

Figure 4–28 • The inferior recess as viewed from the posterior portal. Note the attachment of the capsule at the inferior neck.

taneously, and its base can often be seen anteriorly just superior to the subscapularis tendon. Anterior recesses also include areas above and below the middle glenohumeral ligament. These folds vary in frequency and degree.[75]

The inferior recess can be fully viewed for its contents with the arthroscope slipped inferiorly after anterior viewing. This pocket is the inferior reflection of the capsule and synovial lining at the inferior neck of the humerus. An appreciation of the origins of the capsule should be made while viewing in this region (Fig. 4–28).

The posterior recess is contiguous with the inferior recess and can best be visualized by slightly withdrawing

and rotating the arthroscope to look into the area posterior and medial to the posterior labrum. In most individuals with a well-placed posterior portal, this view is easily achieved. The posterior recess is particularly well viewed in those individuals with a capacious posterior capsule (Fig. 4–29).

Humeral Head and Glenoid

The humeral head and glenoid face are both well visualized from the posterior portal (Fig. 4–30). After leaving the inferior recess and following the margin of the inferior capsule posteriorly, the "bare area" of the head can be seen

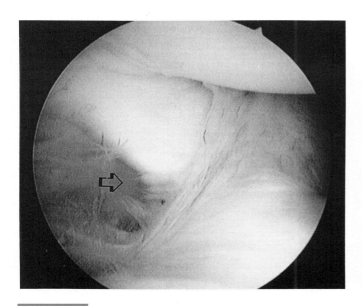

Figure 4–27 • View from the posterior portal of the position of the subscapularis recess *(arrow)*.

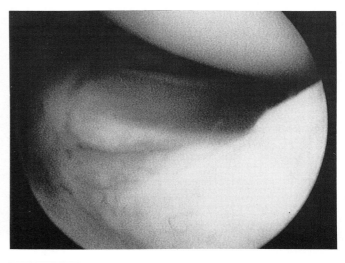

Figure 4–29 • Posterior portal view of the posterior recess.

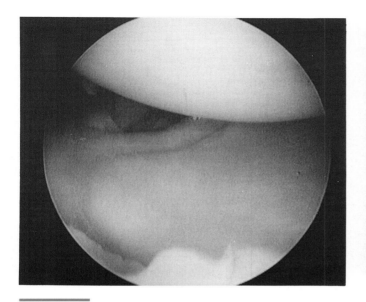

Figure 4–30 • Articulation of the glenoid and humeral head as viewed from the posterior portal.

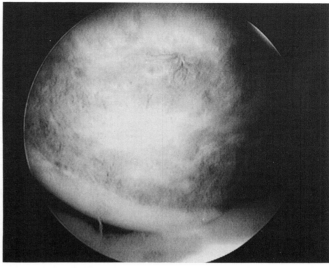

Figure 4–32 • A large Hill-Sachs lesion in an individual with recurrent unidirectional anterior instability.

(Fig. 4–31). This bony region on the posteroinferior aspect of the head is void of articular cartilage and is not to be mistaken for an abnormal finding. This region lies between the attachment of the posterior capsule and the articular surface. Often, small fenestrations can be observed on this bony surface that are representative of several intraosseous vessels. There is no functional significance to this zone except that it is often confused with a small Hill-Sachs lesion.

The Hill-Sachs lesion is a compression fracture of the humeral head resulting from an anterior dislocation and impaction on the anterior glenoid (Fig. 4–32). This lesion distinguishes itself by being located posterosuperiorly

without the normal fenestrations seen on the normal bare area. More centrally located lesions representative of osteochondritis have been described.[38] Rotating the humeral head while viewing from the posterior portal gives an almost complete look at the articular surface.

The glenoid is covered with articular cartilage that typically thins centrally. Slight distraction of the joint allows for a complete view of the articular surface. Chondral or even bony fractures of the edges can represent bony Bankart lesions indicative of prior or recurrent episodes of instability (Fig. 4–33).

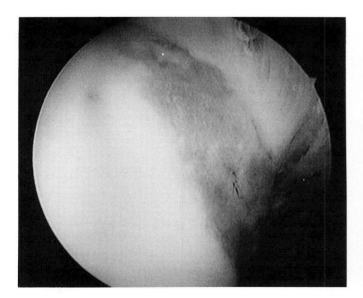

Figure 4–31 • The normal bare area of the posterior aspect of the humeral head.

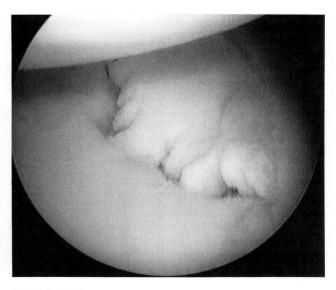

Figure 4–33 • A chondral fracture of the posterior glenoid associated with chronic pain in the dominant shoulder of this pitcher.

Subacromial Space

The subacromial space can be accessed by redirecting the arthroscope through the same posterior portal (Fig. 4–34) by repiercing the posterior deltoid. The usual obstacle to clear viewing in this compartment is the bursa. Often, particularly in an individual with chronic subacromial disease, clearing some of this hypertrophied and inflamed tissue is necessary before adequate visualization. A cleared bursal space allows for complete visualization of the superior surface of the rotator cuff to a point well lateral and distal to the greater tuberosity and medial to the AC joint. The distal portion of the supraspinatus, from its musculotendinous junction to its bony insertion, can be viewed as well as at least the upper 20% of the subscapularis and anterior 20% of the infraspinatus to their respective bony margins (see Fig. 4–34).[77]

Abnormalities of the cuff (specifically, tears) vary considerably with respect to size and involvement of the tendons. Certain partial-thickness tears may be viewed only from the superior surface. Calcification of the tendons may also be seen.

The acromion forms the central and posterior portions of the roof of this space. Its undersurface is usually covered by a thick periosteal layer. Its lateral margin is the insertion point for a major portion of the deltoid fibers. The anterior portion of the acromion serves as the attachment site of the coracoacromial ligament. In many individuals with chronic problems involving the rotator cuff, the anterior portion of the acromion may appear to have a hook or large osteophyte. Recognition of this and débridement during acromioplasty are important factors in successful treatment of the impingement process.

The coracoacromial ligament forms the anterior roof of the acromial arch by attaching under the anterior edge. It is probably a vestigial ligament that may have some biomechanical constraint to superior migration of the humeral head (Fig. 4–35). With the arm in an increasingly elevated position, the rotator cuff comes in direct contact with the ligament and anterior acromion, causing the impingement syndrome. In patients with chronic problems of the rotator cuff, the ligament can become thickened or even calcified. The AC joint lies at the anteromedial corner of the acromion, with the anterior edge of the distal clavicle almost paralleling the anterior margin of the acromion. The distal end of the clavicle is covered partially by the coracoacromial ligament and enclosed by the fibrous capsule of the joint. Often osteophytes off the inferior distal surface of the clavicle are present in the shoulder with pathologic conditions. The osteophytes as well as the AC joint can be débrided from access through the subacromial space.

SURGICAL PROCEDURE

A number of different routines may be utilized in routine arthroscopy of the shoulder, incorporating any of a number of combinations of types of anesthesia, patient positioning, traction set-up, and portal placements. Most important of all, it is necessary for the surgeon to develop a routine that accommodates his or her level of expertise, comfort, and equipment limitations.

Author's Preferred Technique

The patient is first brought into the operating room and placed in the supine position on the operating table. A general anesthetic is preferred to allow for a relaxed examination of the shoulder under anesthesia and lateral decubitus positioning. Following induction of anesthesia, a complete examination is performed with documentation of bilateral range of motion, including elevation, internal and external rotation at 90 degrees of abduction, and external rotation at 0 degrees. A stability examination is then performed and documented in the anterior, posterior, and inferior directions and graded; 1+, humeral head to the glenoid rim; 2+, humeral over the glenoid rim but with spontaneous reduction of the humeral head; and 3+, fixed dislocation of the humeral head. Inferior laxity corresponds to a slightly different scale with 1+ referring to a sulcus of 1 cm, 2+ to 2 cm, and 3+ to 3 cm.

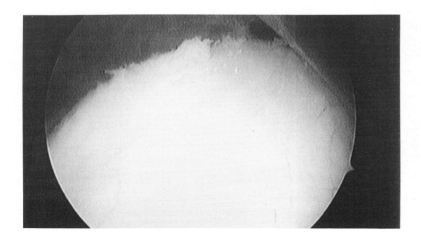

Figure 4–34 • Subacromial view of the superior surface of the rotator cuff.

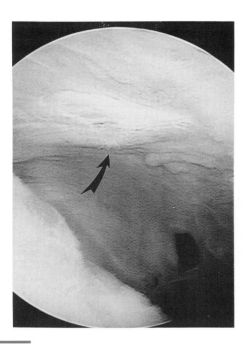

Figure 4–35 • The undersurface of the acromion with the coracoacromial ligament draped across its anterior edge *(arrow)*.

The patient is placed into the lateral decubitus position with an axillary roll made out of a 1 L intravenous bag that is padded with a sheet. A bean bag is used to hold the position of the patient rolled back semilaterally about 30–40 degrees (Fig. 4–36). This places the glenoid face parallel to the floor, allowing for easier orientation of the arthroscope and access to the anterior aspect of the shoulder. The lower legs are flexed, with padding placed under the down leg to protect the peroneal nerve at the lateral aspect of the knee and the bony prominences of the foot and ankle. A pillow is placed between the legs.

A plastic U-drape is applied to the axilla and hemithorax, and an additional plastic drape is placed across the neck to seal off the head and neck from the surgical field. These drapes also provide a barrier to the preparation and arthroscopic fluids used during the procedure. Preparation is preferably done with a Hibistat solution.

Draping follows in a routine fashion. Four sterile towels are placed first: one across the axilla, followed by one anterior and one posterior to the shoulder, with the final towel placed across the base of the neck. These are held with nonpenetrating clamps. A half sheet is placed to cover the remainder of the torso and lower extremities.

The arm is suspended using a commercially available sterile skin traction set-up. This employs a stockinette with a loop at the hand to attach to the traction device. The stockinette is rolled to a point to just above the level of the elbow and held in place with a Coban wrap. Anywhere from 7 to 15 lb is used, but the author finds it rarely necessary to suspend the extremity with greater than 12 lb. The shoulder is positioned in about 45 degrees of abduction and 15 degrees of forward flexion. In the author's experience, this has routinely allowed for complete visualization of the glenohumeral space while putting the neurologic structures on stretch at minimal risk. Draping is completed with a U-drape placed into the axilla and a barrier drape placed across the base of the neck.

The video cabinet is moved level with the head and torso of the patient, providing for an unobstructed view. Suction and electrocautery are placed above the cabinet, and the pump and fluid set-up are below the cabinet in full view of the surgeon (Fig. 4–37).

The surgeon is positioned level at the head of the patient, and a Mayo stand with the standard equipment is brought to the level of the patient's buttock. The pump control is placed within easy reach of the surgeon and parallel to the patient's axilla. The arthroscope is brought posterior to the patient's shoulder, and the shaver set-up is anterior to the patient's shoulder, with the suction brought off the head of the table.

Figure 4–36 • Proper positioning of the patient in the lateral decubitus position with the bean bag.

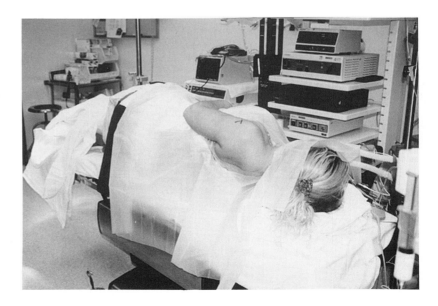

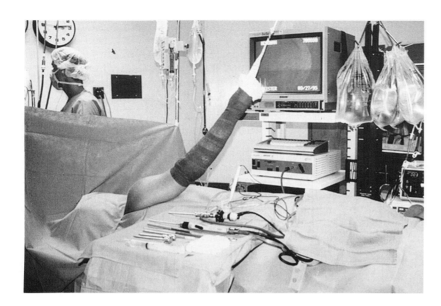

Figure 4-37 • Completed set-up of the patient in the lateral decubitus position for shoulder arthroscopy.

Recommended Procedure

Before proceeding with the case, all bony landmarks—the acromion, scapular spine, distal clavicle, and tip of the coracoid process—are outlined with a surgical pen. A posterior portal site is selected overlying the soft spot of the shoulder usually 2–3 cm inferior and 1 cm medial to the posterolateral edge of the acromion. An anterior portal site is selected lateral to the coracoid process and midway between the coracoid process and acromion, closest to the portal described by Andrews, Carson, and Ortega.[52] A lateral portal is selected 2 cm lateral to the anterolateral edge of the acromion (Fig. 4–38). All three portals are then infiltrated with a total of 10 mL of 1% lidocaine with epinephrine primarily for the control of local bleeding.

A posterior portal is established first. The author has not found it essential to first insufflate the joint before introduction of the trocar. A stab wound incision is made through the skin only with a No. 11 scalpel blade. A blunt trocar and sheath are then pushed through the incision and posterior deltoid while aiming for the tip of the coracoid process marked by a finger of the opposite hand (Fig. 4–39).

Once the rotator cuff is reached with the trocar, the blunt trocar tip can be used to palpate and roll over the posterior rim of the glenoid. After this landmark is appreciated, entry of the trocar into the glenohumeral space is easily achieved. A "pop" should be felt as the posterior capsule is pierced. The arthroscope can then be traded out with the blunt trocar and placed into the sheath (Fig.

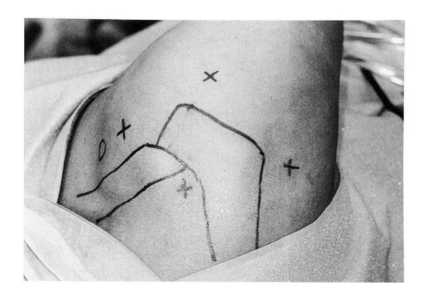

Figure 4-38 • External markings for positioning of the common portals before infiltration.

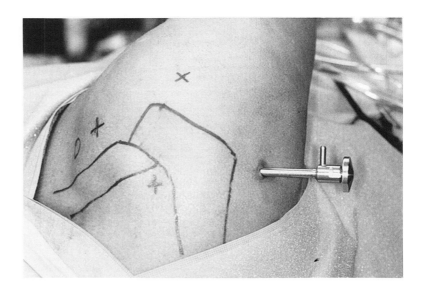

Figure 4–39 • Blunt trocar placement for establishing the posterior portal.

4–40). Before turning on the pump for insufflation, intra-articular placement of the cannula should be appreciated by a dry view of the joint.

The joint is insufflated with the pump, with standard pump settings on 40 mm Hg of pressure and a medium flow rate. In the author's set-up, the joint pressure is sensed directly off the sheath, at the point of outflow, so as to give the most accurate measure of intra-articular flow and pressure. The view of the joint is oriented anatomically, placing the glenoid face in the inferior portion of the view and parallel to the floor. Routine examination of the glenohumeral joint begins at the base of the biceps, appropriately referred to as the nose of the shoulder, and follows a circular, circumferential pattern allowing for evaluation of the entire contents of the glenohumeral complex.

From the biceps attachment site, the arthroscope is rotated clockwise to examine the remainder of its intra-articular portion as well as the undersurface of the supraspinatus. The view is then reoriented to look toward the anterior safe triangle. At this point an anterior portal is established by an outside-in technique.

At the external point marked anteriorly at the initiation of the procedure, a spinal needle can be passed from outside through the anterior triangle in front of the biceps tendon (Fig. 4–41). Once the path of the portal has been established, a No. 11 scalpel blade can be used to pierce the skin, and an additional disposable cannula can be inserted bluntly into the joint. A probe can now be used through the anterior cannula for palpation of the structures of the joint.

Figure 4–40 • Exchange of the blunt trocar for the arthroscope for viewing.

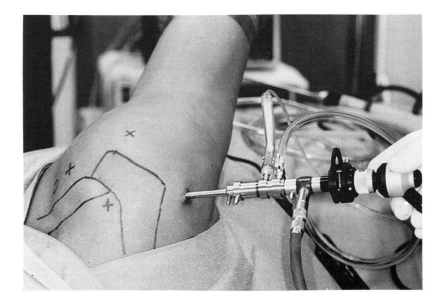

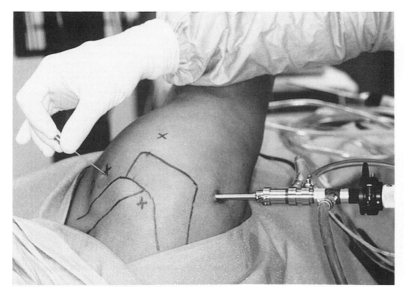

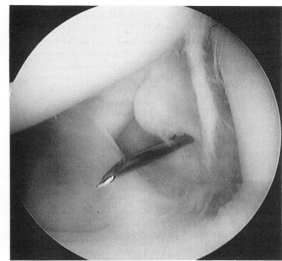

A   B

Figure 4–41 • Safe establishment of the anterior portal under direct visualization with an outside-in technique using a spinal needle. *A,* External view. *B,* Arthroscopic view of the needle piercing the anterior triangle.

Arthroscopic Evaluation

Advancement of the arthroscope anteriorly allows for evaluation of the subscapularis recess and anterior glenohumeral complex. If a better view is desired, either a 70 degree arthroscope can be inserted or, after viewing through the posterior portal is completed, the arthroscope can be placed through the anterior portal.

If the arthroscope cannot be easily manipulated inferiorly from a position over the anterior edge of the glenoid, then it should be retracted and placed into the inferior recess. Here the inferior capsular reflection can be viewed. Retracting the arthroscope slightly and redirecting the view slightly superiorly allow for visualization of the bare area and posterior aspect of the humeral head. Directing the arthroscope further superiorly should allow for additional viewing of the posterior reflection of the capsule and rotator cuff at the humeral head. The remainder of the humeral head can be examined by gentle internal and external rotation of the humerus. The glenoid face should be examined for any defects.

Finally, with further retraction of the arthroscope and redirecting of the viewing, the posterior labrum and posterior recess should be evaluated. Additional procedures may need to be performed and alternative portals established; this depends on the type of pathologic condition being addressed. Information on many of these procedures can be obtained in detail in other chapters.

If an improved view of either the anterior or posterior structures is still desired, the anterior portal is utilized. Under direct visualization, an interchangeable cannula is placed with a blunt trocar through the established anterior portal. The cannula should be left in place posteriorly after withdrawal of the arthroscope for additional instrumentation or probing if desired. The arthroscope is then placed anteriorly; through this portal, an excellent view of the anterior structures, superoposterior rotator cuff, posterior recess, and posterior labrum can be obtained.

After completion of the glenohumeral examination, the joint is evacuated of fluid, and all instruments are withdrawn. The arthroscopic cannula is again loaded with the blunt trocar; by using the previously established posterior portal site, the subacromial space is accessed. With a slightly superior aim, the blunt trocar is pushed through the posterior deltoid. With the tip of the trocar, the posterior edge of the acromion can be palpated and, from here, pushed underneath the posterior edge into the subacromial space. Carefully moving the trocar back and forth underneath the acromion helps to clear the space for better initial viewing.

The arthroscope is introduced, and the pump is restarted. If the disease has been anticipated to be in the subacromial space, then limited viewing is usually available because of the thickened bursal contents. Some clearing of these contents is necessary before adequate viewing.

Under direct visualization, at the point previously marked on the skin, a spinal needle can be used to establish the direction of the anterolateral portal (Fig. 4–42). A No. 11 scalpel blade, longitudinally oriented, is used to establish the portal. The motorized shaver can be introduced with a 4 or 5 mm resector blade to provide an initial clearing of the bursa for viewing of the subacromial contents. An additional cannula is sometimes placed through the previously established anterior portal into the subacromial space for fluid evacuation. The undersurface of the acromion, the coracoacromial ligament, the AC joint and

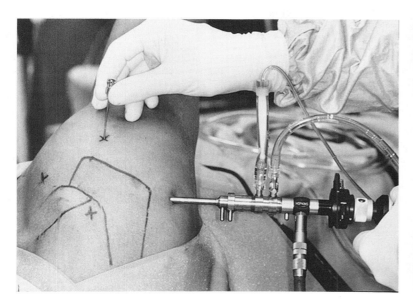

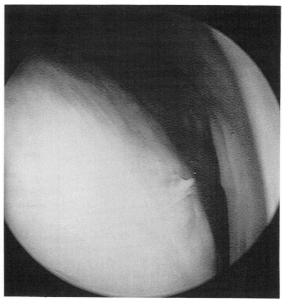

A   B

Figure 4–42 • *A*, External view of establishment of a lateral portal with a spinal needle using an outside-in technique. *B*, Arthroscopic view of the proper placement of the lateral portal with a spinal needle in the subacromial space.

distal clavicle, and the superior surface of the rotator cuff are examined. Detailed instructions on the completion of further surgery in the subacromial space contents can be found in other chapters.

After completion of the procedure, wounds are closed with a simple subcuticular 4-0 Vicryl stitch and covered with Steri-Strips and a dry sterile dressing. A sling is placed on the affected shoulder.

Postoperative Care

Following a routine diagnostic arthroscopic procedure, the patient is encouraged to come out of the sling immediately after the surgery to begin range-of-motion exercises for the elbow, wrist, and shoulder. The patient may begin with pendulum exercises and may progress rapidly to active assisted motion. The sling is usually discarded completely within a few days following surgery. Once full motion and strength are restored, functional activities are reinstituted and a return to full activities is encouraged. More complicated rehabilitation protocols exist for more involved procedures and are not discussed here.

SUMMARY

Arthroscopy of the shoulder has advanced considerably since the mid-1980s, which has allowed the use of the arthroscope in treating many of the problems that had

once required routine open techniques. With a proper understanding of relational anatomy and proper portal placement, the surgeon can continue to employ the arthroscope in the treatment of many of the more complicated shoulder disorders routinely encountered. Understanding one's limitations is essential to performing safe and effective arthroscopic surgery.

References

1. Burman MS: Arthroscopy on the direct visualization of joints: an experimental cadaver study. J Bone Joint Surg 8:669, 1931.
2. Watanabe M: Arthroscopy: the present state. Orthop Clin North Am 10:505, 1979.
3. Watanabe M: The development and present status of the arthroscope. J Jpn Med Inst 25:11, 1954.
4. Andren L and Lundberg BJ: Treatment of rigid shoulders by joint distension during arthroscopy. Acta Orthop Scand 36:45, 1965.
5. Wiley AM and Older MW: Shoulder arthroscopy: investigations with a fiberoptic instrument. Am J Sports Med 8:31, 1980.
6. Altchek DW, Skyhar MJ, and Warren RF: Shoulder arthroscopy for shoulder instability. Instr Course Lect 38:187, 1989.
7. Arciero RA, Taylor DC, Snyder RJ, et al.: Arthroscopic bioabsorbable tack stabilization of initial anterior shoulder dislocations: a preliminary report. Arthroscopy 11:410, 1995.
8. Coughlin L, Rubinovich M, Johansson J, et al.: Arthroscopic staple capsulorrhaphy for anterior shoulder instability. Am J Sports Med 20:253, 1992.
9. Detrisac DA and Johnson LL: Arthroscopic shoulder capsulorrhaphy using metal staples. Orthop Clin North Am 24:71, 1993.
10. Grana WA, Buckley PD, and Yates CK: Arthroscopic Bankart suture repair. Am J Sports Med 21:348, 1993.
11. Green MR and Christensen KP: Arthroscopic Bankart procedure:

two- to five-year followup with clinical correlation to severity of glenoid lesion. Am J Sports Med 23:276, 1995.

12. Green MR and Christensen KP: Arthroscopic versus open Bankart procedures: a comparison of early morbidity and complications. Arthroscopy 9:371, 1993.

13. Hurley JA and Anderson TE: Shoulder arthroscopy: its role in evaluating shoulder disorders in the athlete. Am J Sports Med 18:480, 1990.

14. Lane JG, Sachs RA, and Riehl B: Arthroscopic staple capsulorrhaphy: a long-term follow-up. Arthroscopy 9:190, 1993.

15. McIntyre LF and Caspari RB: The rationale and technique for arthroscopic reconstruction of anterior shoulder instability using multiple sutures. Orthop Clin North Am 24:55, 1993.

16. Pagnani MJ, Speer KP, Altchek DW, et al.: Arthroscopic fixation of superior labral lesions using a biodegradable implant: a preliminary report. Arthroscopy 11:194, 1995.

17. Terry GC, Friedman SJ, and Uhl TL: Arthroscopically treated tears of the glenoid labrum: factors influencing outcome. Am J Sports Med 22:504, 1994.

18. Warner JJP, Kann S, and Marks P: Arthroscopic repair of combined Bankart and superior labral detachment anterior and posterior lesions: technique and preliminary results. Arthroscopy 10:383, 1994.

19. Wolf EM: Arthroscopic capsulolabral repair using suture anchors. Orthop Clin North Am 24:59, 1993.

20. Yoneda M, Hirooka A, Saito S, et al.: Arthroscopic stapling for detached superior glenoid labrum. J Bone Joint Surg Br 73:746, 1991.

21. Andrews JR, Broussard TS, and Carson WG: Arthroscopy of the shoulder in the management of partial tears of the rotator cuff: a preliminary report. Arthroscopy 1:117, 1985.

22. Baker CL and Liu SH: Comparison of open and arthroscopically assisted rotator cuff repairs. Am J Sports Med 23:99, 1995.

23. Ellman H: Arthroscopic subacromial decompression: analysis of one- to three-year results. Arthroscopy 3:173, 1987.

24. Ellman H: Diagnosis and treatment of incomplete rotator cuff tears. Clin Orthop 254:64, 1990.

25. Levy HJ, Gardner RD, and Lemak LJ: Arthroscopic subacromial decompression in the treatment of full-thickness rotator cuff tears. Arthroscopy 7:8, 1991.

26. Levy HJ, Uribe JW, and Delaney LG: Arthroscopic assisted rotator cuff repair: preliminary results. Arthroscopy 6:55, 1990.

27. Olsewiski JM and Depew AD: Arthroscopic subacromial decompression and rotator cuff débridement for stage II and stage III impingement. Arthroscopy 10:61, 1994.

28. Paulos LE and Franklin JL: Arthroscopic shoulder decompression development and application. Am J Sports Med 18:235, 1990.

29. Paulos LE and Kody MH: Arthroscopically enhanced "miniapproach" to rotator cuff repair. Am J Sports Med 22:19, 1994.

30. Walch G, Boileau P, Noel E, et al.: Impingement of the deep surface of the supraspinatus tendon on the posterosuperior glenoid rim: an arthroscopic study. J Shoulder Elbow Surg 1:238, 1992.

31. Warner JJP, Kann S, and Maddox LM: The "arthroscopic impingement test." Arthroscopy 10:224, 1994.

32. Zvijac JE, Levy HJ, and Lemak LJ: Arthroscopic subacromial decompression in the treatment of full thickness rotator cuff tears: a 3 to 6 year follow-up. Arthroscopy 10:518, 1994.

33. Bigliani LU, Nicholson GP, and Flatow EL: Arthroscopic resection of the distal clavicle. Orthop Clin North Am 24:133, 1993.

34. Flatow EL, Duralde XA, Nicholson GP, et al.: Arthroscopic resection of the distal clavicle with a superior approach. J Shoulder Elbow Surg 4:41, 1995.

35. Tolin BS and Snyder SJ: Our technique for the arthroscopic Mumford procedure. Orthop Clin North Am 24:143, 1993.

36. Ellman H, Harris E, and Kay SP: Early degenerative joint disease simulating impingement syndrome: arthroscopic findings. Arthroscopy 8:482, 1992.

37. Ferrari JD, Ferrari DA, Coumas J, et al.: Posterior ossification of the shoulder: the Bennett lesion. Am J Sports Med 22:171, 1994.

38. Hamada S, Hamada M, Nishiue S, et al.: Osteochondritis dissecans of the humeral head. Arthroscopy 8:132, 1992.

39. Hayes JM: Arthroscopic treatment of steroid-induced osteonecrosis of the humeral head. Arthroscopy 5:218, 1989.

40. Wiley AM: Arthroscopic appearance of frozen shoulder. Arthroscopy 7:138, 1991.

41. Hawkins RJ and Bokor DJ: Clinical evaluation of shoulder problems. In Rockwood CA and Matsen FA (eds.): The Shoulder. Philadelphia, W.B. Saunders Co., 1990, pp 149–177.

41a. Matthews LS, LaBudde JK: Arthroscopic treatment of synovial diseases of the shoulder. Orthop Clin North Am 24:101, 1993.

42. Green MR and Christensen KP: Magnetic resonance imaging of the glenoid labrum in anterior shoulder instability. Am J Sports Med 22:493, 1994.

43. Tirman PF, Bost FW, Garcin GJ, et al.: Posterosuperior glenoid impingement of the shoulder: findings at MR imaging and MR arthrography with arthroscopic correlation. Radiology 193:431, 1994.

44. Tuite MJ, Yandow DR, DeSmet AA, et al.: Diagnosis of partial and complete rotator cuff tears using combined gradient echo and spin echo imaging. Skeletal Radiol 23:541, 1994.

45. Wilson AJ: Computed arthrotomography of glenohumeral instability. Top Magn Reson Imaging 6:139, 1994.

46. Curtis AS and Snyder SJ: Evaluation and treatment of biceps tendon pathology. Orthop Clin North Am 24:33, 1993.

47. Thabit G III: Personal communication, 1995.

48. Laurencin CT, Deutsch A, O'Brien SJ, et al.: The superolateral portal for arthroscopy of the shoulder. Arthroscopy 10:255, 1994.

48a. Altchek DW, Warren RF, Wickiewicz TL, et al.: Arthroscopic labral débridement: a three-year follow-up study. Am J Sports Med 20:702, 1992.

49. Martin DR and Garth WP: Results of arthroscopic débridement of glenoid labral tears. Am J Sports Med 23:447, 1995.

50. Snyder SJ, Karzel RP, Del Pizzo W, et al.: SLAP lesions of the shoulder. Arthroscopy 6:274, 1990.

51. Brown AR, Weiss R, Greenberg C, et al.: Interscalene block for shoulder arthroscopy: comparison with general anesthesia. Arthroscopy 9:295, 1993.

52. Andrews JR, Carson WG, and Ortega K: Arthroscopy of the shoulder: technique and normal anatomy. Am J Sports Med 12:1, 1984.

53. Andrews JR and Gidumal RH: Shoulder arthroscopy in the throwing athlete: perspectives and prognosis. Clin Sports Med 6:565, 1987.

54. Burkhart SS: Deep venous thrombosis after shoulder arthroscopy. Arthroscopy 6:61, 1990.

55. Klein AH, France JC, Mutschler TA, et al.: Measurement of brachial plexus strain in arthroscopy of the shoulder. Arthroscopy 3:45, 1987.

56. Pitman MI, Nainzadeh N, Ergas E, et al.: The use of somatosensory evoked potentials for detection of neuropraxia during shoulder arthroscopy. Arthroscopy 4:250, 1988.

57. Gross RM and Fitzgibbons TC: Shoulder arthroscopy: a modified approach. Arthroscopy 3:156, 1985.

58. Skyhar MJ, Altchek DW, Warren RF, et al.: Shoulder arthroscopy with the patient in the beach-chair position. Arthroscopy 4:256, 1988.

59. Morrison DS, Schafer RK, and Friedman RL: The relationship between subacromial space pressure, blood pressure, and visual clarity during arthroscopic subacromial decompression. Arthroscopy 11:557, 1995.

60. Wolf EM: Anterior portals in shoulder arthroscopy. Arthroscopy 5:201, 1989.

61. Blachut PA and Day B: Arthroscopic anatomy of the shoulder. Arthroscopy 5:10, 1989.

62. Matthews LS, Terry G, and Vetter WL: Shoulder anatomy for the arthroscopist. Arthroscopy 1:83, 1985.

63. Nottage WM: Arthroscopic portals: anatomy at risk. Orthop Clin North Am 24:19, 1993.

64. Bigliani LU, Dalse RM, McCann PD, et al.: An anatomical study of the suprascapular nerve. Arthroscopy 6:301, 1990.

65. Matthews LS, Zarins B, Michael RH, et al.: Anterior portal selection for shoulder arthroscopy. Arthroscopy 1:33, 1985.

66. Bryan WJ, Schauder K, and Tullos HS: The axillary nerve and its relationship to common sports medicine procedures. Am J Sports Med 14:113, 1986.

67. Davidson PA and Tibone JE: Anterior-inferior portal for shoulder arthroscopy. Arthroscopy 11:519, 1995.

68. Nevaiser TJ: Arthroscopy of the shoulder. Orthop Clin North Am 18:361, 1987.

69. Souryal TO and Baker CL: Anatomy of the supraclavicular fossa portal in shoulder arthroscopy. Arthroscopy 6:297, 1990.

70. Vangsness CT, Jorgenson SS, Watson T, et al.: The origin of the long head of the biceps from the scapula and glenoid labrum: an anatomical study of 100 shoulders. J Bone Joint Surg Br 76:951, 1994.

71. Maffet MW, Gartsman GM, and Moseley B: Superior labrum–biceps tendon complex lesions of the shoulder. Am J Sports Med 23:93, 1995.

72. Burkhart SS and Fox DL: SLAP lesions in association with complete tears of the long head of the biceps tendon: a report of 2 cases. Arthroscopy 8:31, 1992.

73. Burkhart SS, Esch JC, and Jolson RS: The rotator crescent and rotator cable: an anatomic description of the shoulder's "suspension bridge." Arthroscopy 9:611, 1993.

74. Warner JJP, Deng XH, Warren RF, et al.: Static capsuloligamentous restraints to posterior-inferior translation of the glenohumeral joint. Am J Sports Med 20:675, 1992.

75. Morgan C, Rames RD, and Snyder SJ: Anatomical variations of the glenohumeral ligaments. Presented at the Annual Meeting of the American Academy of Orthopedic Surgeons, Anaheim, Calif., 1991.

76. Williams MM, Snyder SJ, and Buford D Jr: The Buford complex—the "cord-like" middle glenohumeral ligament and absent anterosuperior labrum complex: a normal anatomic capsulolabral variant. Arthroscopy 10:241, 1994.

77. Matthews LS and Fadale PD: Subacromial anatomy for the arthroscopist. Arthroscopy 5:36, 1989.

5

Normal and Pathologic Arthroscopic Anatomy of the Shoulder

James R. Andrews • *James J. Guerra* • *Gregory M. Fox*

INTRODUCTION

Although initially described by Burman[1] in cadaveric joints nearly three-quarters of a century ago, shoulder arthroscopy has only in the last 10–15 years become recognized and accepted as a safe and effective technique in the evaluation and treatment of shoulder disease. Major technologic advancements in fiber optics, video output, and arthroscopic instrumentation, combined with sound knowledge of safe anatomic portals, have resulted in an evolution in shoulder arthroscopy from a diagnostic technique to a more treatment-oriented modality.[2-16] A thorough appreciation of the normal intra-articular anatomy and of the normal variants that may be encountered is an essential prerequisite for orthopaedists performing shoulder arthroscopy. This chapter focuses on the normal as well as the pathologic arthroscopic anatomy of the shoulder. Much like that of the knee, the arthroscopic evaluation of the shoulder should proceed in an organized, structured fashion to ensure complete assessment of the entire intra-articular extent of the joint. The authors' goals are to present an organized and reproducible approach to the arthroscopic examination of the shoulder and to build a general knowledge base of the normal, variant, and pathologic intra-articular anatomy of the shoulder.

As described in Chapter 4, we prefer performing shoulder arthroscopy with the patient in the lateral decubitus position with the shoulder superior. Ten to fifteen pounds of traction is applied to the arm, which is abducted approximately 70 degrees and flexed forward 15 degrees (Fig. 5–1). The posterior portal, located in the "soft spot" between the infraspinatus and teres minor, is the viewing portal of choice for diagnostic arthroscopy. Most of the figures in this chapter are oriented in this fashion (Fig. 5–2).

GLENOHUMERAL JOINT

Biceps Tendon

As one enters the shoulder through the posterior portal, the biceps tendon is generally the first structure identified and is the key anatomic landmark for maintaining proper orientation during arthroscopy of the glenohumeral joint (Fig. 5–3). The long head of the biceps and the popliteus tendons are the only two intra-articular tendons in the body. With the patient in the lateral decubitus position, the biceps tendon is oriented 10–15 degrees inferior to an imaginary vertical line. As the biceps tendon is followed to its proximal attachment, it courses posteriorly across the joint to the supraglenoid tubercle. Generally, it does not attach directly to bone. It appears more typically to be continuous with the posterosuperior glenoid labrum and constitutes a part of or sends fibers to both the anterior and posterior superior labra. This labral attachment of the biceps tendon has been implicated in the development of SLAP (superior labrum from anterior to posterior) lesions in the throwing athlete.[17, 18]

By rotating the arm externally, the biceps tendon can be followed anteriorly to where it exits the joint in the bicipital groove. Visualization may be further facilitated by flexing the elbow. The point of exit of the tendon is an important anatomic landmark. It denotes the normal rotator interval between the subscapularis and the supraspinatus tendons. Normally, the biceps tendon appears glistening and smooth and free of adhesions, fraying, synovitis, or partial tearing. Vincula of the biceps tendon have been described, which are fibrovascular bands that course from the undersurface of the rotator cuff to the bicipital groove, where they attach to the biceps tendon. These structures, which occur in 25% of patients, are thought to be analo-

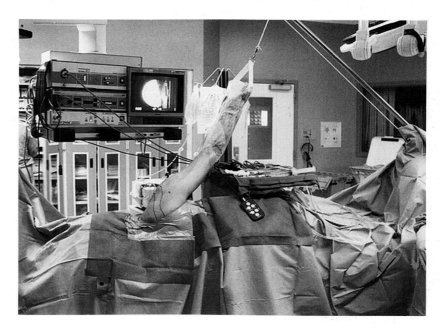

Figure 5–1 • Patient in left lateral decubitus position for right shoulder arthroscopy.

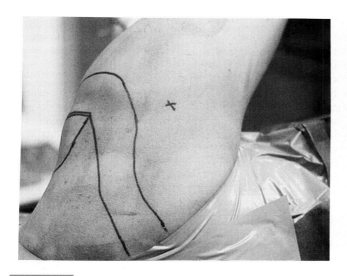

Figure 5–2 • Posterior portal "X" for right shoulder arthroscopy.

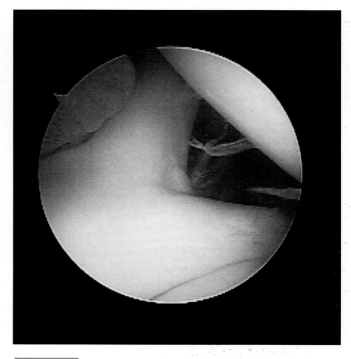

Figure 5–3 • Biceps tendon, right shoulder, arising from superior labrum.

gous to the vincula of the finger flexor tendons and to provide a vascular supply to the biceps tendon.[19]

Pathologic Anatomy

Abnormalities of the biceps tendon are easily identifiable. Hypervascularity at the base of the biceps tendon is commonly associated with rotator cuff tears (Fig. 5–4). Ero-

sion-type tearing of the biceps tendon may occur with the impingement syndrome. In the throwing athlete, a spectrum of injuries may occur, ranging from partial tears and attenuation to complete tears with only a bulbous stump remaining (Fig. 5–5). A concomitant avulsion of the superior glenoid labrum may occur in association with biceps tendon tearing.[17, 18] This is discussed in further detail in the section on the glenoid labrum.

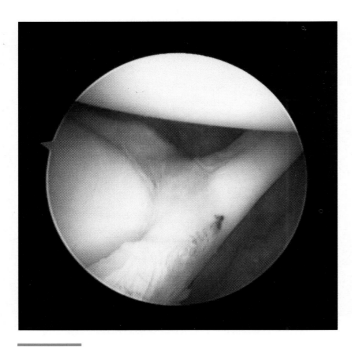

Figure 5–4 • Increased vascularity at base of biceps tendon in left shoulder of a professional baseball pitcher with a rotator cuff tear.

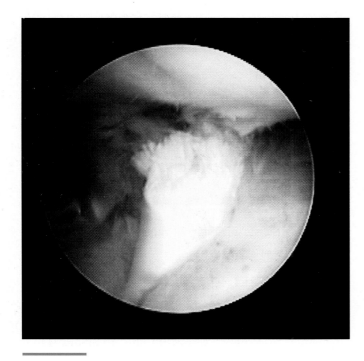

Figure 5–5 • Bulbous stump of ruptured biceps tendon, right shoulder.

Humeral Head and Glenoid

After inspection of the biceps tendon has been completed and proper orientation has been established, the articular surfaces of the humeral head and glenoid may be examined. Both surfaces should appear smooth and are covered by hyaline cartilage (Fig. 5–6). With the patient in the lateral decubitus position, approximately one-third of the articular surface of the humeral head can be viewed through the posterior portal. Visualization of the entire extent of the articular surface of the humeral head can be facilitated by orienting the arthroscope laterally and moving the humerus into internal and external rotation. Anteriorly, the articular hyaline cartilage extends all the way to the synovial reflection at the level of the humeral neck near the insertion of the subscapularis. However, posteriorly, the synovial reflection and rotator cuff attach laterally to the extent of the articular margin, creating a requisite "bare area." This is a normal finding and represents only the nonarticulating intra-articular portion of the humeral head. The size and location of the bare area can vary somewhat, but for the most part the bare area is located directly posteriorly. Characteristically, the bare area can be identified by the small punctate holes, or pits, that house blood vessels (Fig. 5–7).

The glenoid appears as a bean- or pear-shaped tabletop on which the humeral head sits. Its surface is longer in the superior-to-inferior dimension than in the anterior-to-posterior dimension and constitutes a cavity approximately one-fourth the size of the humeral head. The articular cartilage is thickest in the periphery and is most attenuated centrally. After the second decade of life, it is not uncommon to see thinning and fibrillation of the center and lower half of the glenoid. This should not be misinterpreted as a pathologic entity denoting degenerative arthritis or glenohumeral subluxation. A depression, or sulcus, is often present in the middle of the anterior bony glenoid near the attachment of the labrum (Fig. 5–8). This glenoid sulcus may vary in prominence and, similarly, does not denote a pathologic situation.

Pathologic Anatomy

The Hill-Sachs lesion is the most common bony abnormality seen in shoulder arthroscopy (Fig. 5–9). It represents a compression fracture of the posterior humeral head following an anterior glenohumeral dislocation. It must be differentiated from the normally appearing juxta-articular bare area of the humeral head. Confusion arises because both occur posteriorly, and the depth, size, and location of the compression fracture of the Hill-Sachs lesion vary. The bare area can usually be distinguished from a Hill-Sachs lesion by the presence of the small punctate blood vessel holes that are normally present. Similarly, a reverse Hill-Sachs lesion, or a McLaughlin lesion, may be seen on the anterior humeral head following a posterior dislocation.

Avascular necrosis of the humeral head may also be occasionally encountered. This condition is most commonly associated with excessive alcohol intake and sys-

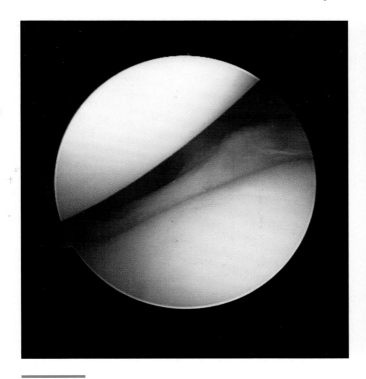

Figure 5–6 • Articular surfaces of glenoid (*bottom*) and humeral head (*top*), left shoulder.

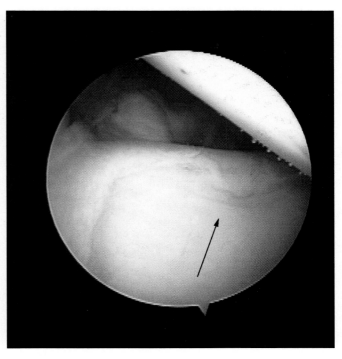

Figure 5–8 • Glenoid sulcus (*arrow*), right shoulder.

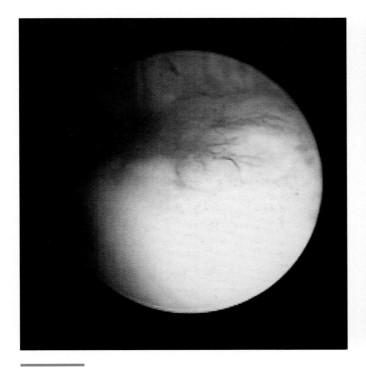

Figure 5–7 • Bare area of humeral head, left shoulder.

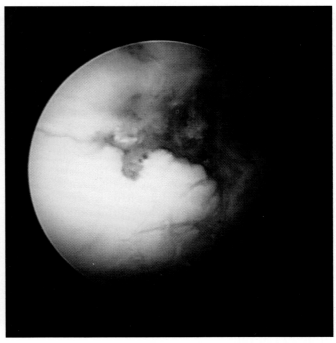

Figure 5–9 • Hill-Sachs lesion, right shoulder.

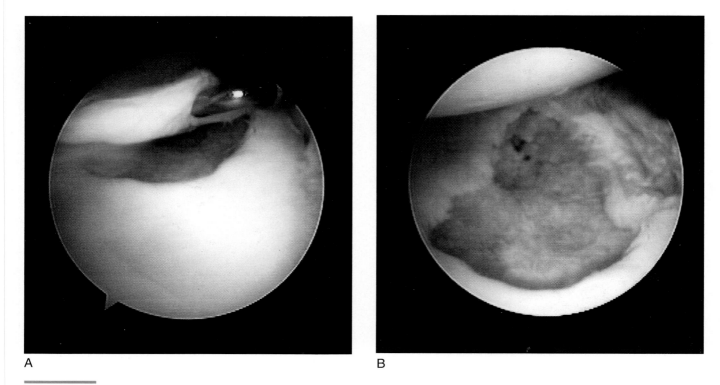

A   B

Figure 5–10 • *A,* Osteochondritis dissecans of the glenoid, right shoulder, in a 20 year old right-handed pitcher. *B,* Defect remaining in inferior glenoid after removal of the loose fragment.

temic steroid use.[20] This lesion may shed cartilaginous fragments, which may be a source of loose bodies. Presently, this lesion is generally not amenable to arthroscopic treatment except for very small lesions that may occasionally benefit from an arthroscopic débridement. In the throwing athlete, osteochondritis dissecans of the glenoid is a rare condition that has been reported[21] (Fig. 5–10).

The most common intra-articular fracture involving the glenoid also accompanies anterior glenohumeral dislocations. With an anterior dislocation or subluxation, the glenohumeral ligaments and labrum may avulse a bony fragment of the anterior glenoid, the so-called bony Bankart lesion (Fig. 5–11). This avulsion fracture may be evaluated arthroscopically, and it is controversial whether it can be managed by arthroscopic means alone.[22–24]

Degenerative osteoarthritic changes are frequently encountered in older patients when performing a diagnostic arthroscopy to evaluate the rotator cuff before a subacromial decompression. Early changes include fibrillation and fragmentation of the articular surfaces and labrum (Fig. 5–12). Later, posterior glenoid wear and inferior osteophyte formation of the humeral head are commonly encountered.

Glenoid Labrum

The glenoid labrum is an ovoid, wedge-shaped fibrocartilaginous rim that circumferentially borders the glenoid. It typically measures 3–4 mm in height, and it deepens the glenoid concavity. In keeping with Bankart's initial description,[25] its primary function is to increase the inherent stability of the glenohumeral joint by restricting anterior and posterior excursion of the humeral head. The addition of the labrum increases the diameter of the glenoid surface to 75% of the humeral head size vertically and to 57% in the transverse direction.[26] Histologic examination has revealed that the labrum is composed of hyaline cartilage, fibrocartilage, and fibrous tissue in a teleologic arrangement. The glenoid surface of the labrum is continuous with the hyaline cartilage of the articular surface of the glenoid, whereas the capsular surface blends with the fibrous tissue of the joint capsule and glenohumeral ligaments. In the middle between the two surfaces is a small transitional zone that is composed of fibrocartilage.[27, 28]

The entire glenoid labrum can be inspected arthroscopically. Beginning superiorly, the labrum is contiguous with the insertion of the biceps tendon into the supraglenoid tubercle. It should appear smooth without fraying, partial or complete tearing, or evidence of hypermobility (Fig. 5–13). Minimal posterior superior detachment of the labrum in the region of the biceps tendon is a normal anatomic variant or result of the aging process and should not be interpreted as a pathologic condition. As the arthroscope is directed further anteriorly, the normal relationship of the labrum to the anterior joint capsule and the glenohumeral ligaments can be confirmed. Additional traction is then placed on the arm, and the arthroscope is directed inferiorly to visualize the inferior labrum. The

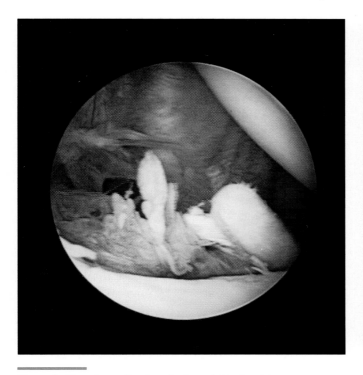

Figure 5–11 • Bony Bankart lesion, right shoulder.

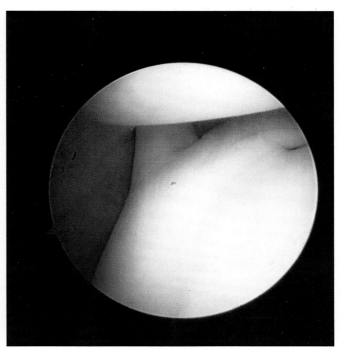

Figure 5–13 • Superior labrum and biceps tendon, right shoulder.

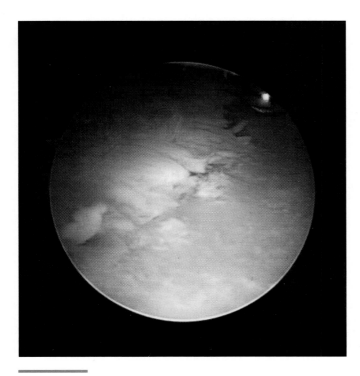

Figure 5–12 • Fragmentation and loss of articular cartilage of the glenoid, right shoulder.

arthroscope is then withdrawn slowly and oriented posteriorly, and the posterior labral rim is inspected. If complete visualization of the posterior rim cannot be obtained, the arthroscope may be placed through the anterior portal to facilitate visualization (Fig. 5–14).

Considerable variation in the size and mobility of the labrum can be encountered. Classifications of the anatomic variations have been variously described. Detrisac and Johnson,[10] in their original description, classified labral variations into five types: superior wedge; anterior wedge; posterior wedge; anterior superior wedge; and, when the entire labrum is enlarged, meniscal. Each type was associated with a pattern of possible normal separation from the underlying bony glenoid. Detrisac later revised his classification to just two basic types.[29] In the first type, most of the labrum, except for the superior aspect, is attached both centrally and peripherally. The superior labrum is attached peripherally but detached centrally. In the second type, the entire labrum is attached both centrally and peripherally.

Pathologic Anatomy

The labrum not only increases the depth of the glenoid fossa but also functions as a load-sharing structure and point of attachment of the glenohumeral ligaments and biceps tendon. Therefore, the labrum may be damaged by

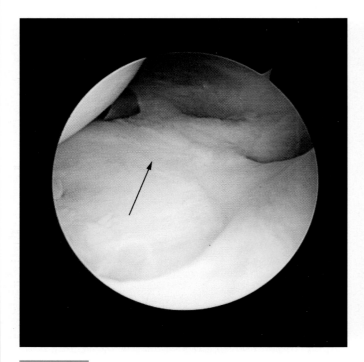

Figure 5–14 • Posterior labrum (*arrow*), right shoulder, viewed from anterior portal.

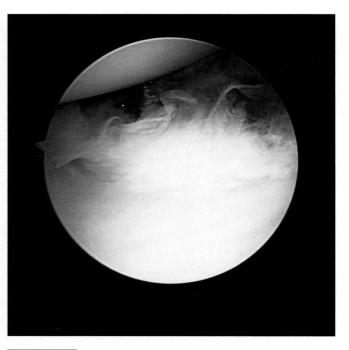

Figure 5–16 • Degenerative tear of anterior labrum, left shoulder.

a variety of potential mechanisms of injury. Included are shear, avulsion or traction, and chronic degeneration. The area of involvement is generally classified in one of the six labral areas[10] (Fig. 5–15). As for meniscal tears, the injury pattern can be described by its arthroscopic appearance. The most common type is the degenerative tear that is caused by aging and tissue attrition (Fig. 5–16). As the labrum degenerates, the smooth gliding surface of the normal labrum is replaced by irregular, roughened fibrous tissue. A "kissing lesion" of chondromalacia on the humeral head may occur where the degenerated labrum abrades.

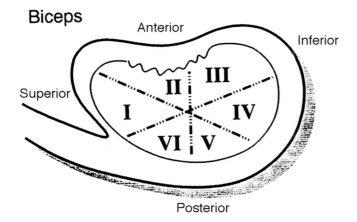

Figure 5–15 • Diagram of the six labral areas. (From Rames RD and Karzel RP: Injuries to the glenoid labrum, including SLAP lesions. Orthop Clin North Am 24:45–53, 1993.)

Other examples of labral tears include flap tears, bucket-handle tears, split nondetached tears, and, in the throwing athlete, SLAP lesions.

Andrews and Carson[18] first described superior labral tears involving the biceps tendon in throwing athletes. These tears were thought to be traction injuries of the biceps tendon on the superior labrum during the throwing motion. Snyder, Karzel, and Del Pizzo[17] coined the term SLAP lesion. Four basic types of SLAP lesions have been described (Fig. 5–17). In the type I lesion, the superior labrum appears frayed and degenerative, but both the labrum and biceps tendon remain firmly attached. With further injury, in the type II lesion, the labral-biceps tendon anchor is detached, rendering the complex unstable. Type III injuries are characterized by a bucket-handle tear of the superior labrum, but with the biceps tendon left intact. Finally, in the type IV pattern, a bucket-handle tear of the superior labrum is accompanied by a split, intrasubstance tear of the biceps tendon.

Glenohumeral Ligaments

Within the circumferential joint capsule of the shoulder are variable thickenings that are defined as the superior, middle, and inferior glenohumeral ligaments (Fig. 5–18). Their names are derived from their attachment on the humerus rather than to the glenoid. Unlike the distinct freestanding ligaments found in other joints, such as the ankle and knee, the glenohumeral ligaments are thickenings of portions of the shoulder capsule. They serve as the primary components of static restraint in the glenohumeral joint. The role of the glenohumeral ligaments in

SLAP lesions

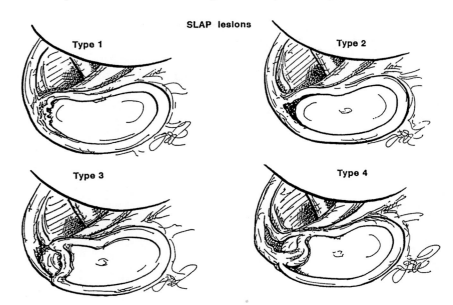

Figure 5–17 • SLAP lesions. (Courtesy of John S. Rogerson, M.D.)

preventing instability is complex and varies with shoulder position and with the direction of the translating force. Considerable variation exists in their size, shape, and insertion to the glenoid. Occasionally, when viewed arthroscopically, they have distinct labral insertions instead of those usually seen to the glenoid. In addition, although the ligaments lie close to the glenoid labrum, with fluid distention during arthroscopic visualization the ligaments appear anteriorly displaced.

The superior glenohumeral ligament is the smallest of the glenohumeral ligaments. Together with the coracohumeral ligament, it functions to stabilize the shoulder joint when the arm is in the adducted dependent position. The superior glenohumeral ligament is the primary static restraint against anteroposterior and inferior translation with the arm in this position.[30] This ligament has two scapular attachments, one to an area near the base of the coracoid process and the other to the region of the supraglenoid tubercle conjoined with the biceps tendon.[31] The ligament then courses laterally to attach to the anterior aspect of the anatomic neck of the humerus near the fovea capitis. Although the superior glenohumeral ligament is almost always identified in cadaveric dissections, it is iden-

tified only occasionally arthroscopically. The ligament may be obscured behind the biceps tendon, or it may be buried deep within the synovium. When it is visualized, it may be identified superior to the subscapularis tendon or near the insertion of the biceps tendon (Fig. 5–19).

The middle glenohumeral ligament assists the inferior glenohumeral ligament in resisting anterior translation when the arm is in 45 degrees of abduction.[30] The middle glenohumeral ligament attaches to the glenoid at the junction of the middle and inferior one-third of the glenoid rim. It then courses anterolaterally to insert on the anterior humerus in the region of the lesser tuberosity and blends with the attachment of the subscapularis tendon. Arthroscopically, the best location for identifying the ligament is in its midportion, where it obliquely crosses posterior to the subscapularis tendon at an angle of approximately 60 degrees (Fig. 5–20).

The inferior glenohumeral ligament complex is the primary static stabilizer resisting anterior, posterior, and inferior translation when the arm is abducted between 45 and 90 degrees.[30] O'Brien et al.[27] have defined the complex as consisting of three components: an anterior band, a posterior band, and an interposed axillary pouch (see

Figure 5–18 • Diagram of joint capsule and ligaments. (Courtesy of John S. Rogerson, M.D.)

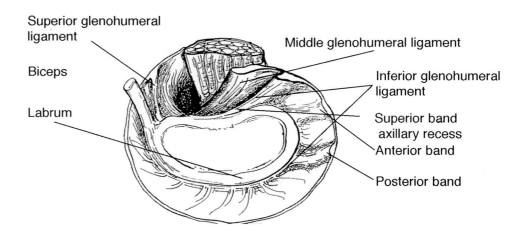

Superior glenohumeral ligament

Biceps

Labrum

Middle glenohumeral ligament

Inferior glenohumeral ligament

Superior band axillary recess

Anterior band

Posterior band

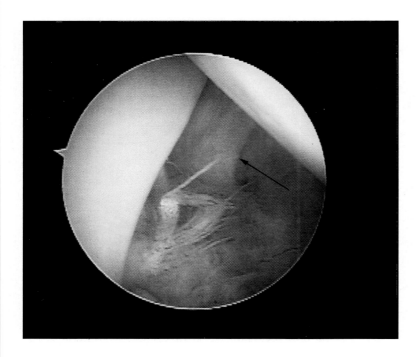

Figure 5–19 • Superior glenohumeral ligament (*arrow*), right shoulder. Biceps tendon left side of figure.

Fig. 5–18). The complex is a hammock-like structure originating from the anterior and posterior glenoid and inserting into the anatomic neck of the humerus in a collar-like or V-shaped fashion. The anterior and posterior bands are thickenings within the capsule, attach to the humerus just inferior to the articular edge, and give the complex most of its strength. Interposed between the bands lies the very thin, patulous axillary pouch, which attaches more distally away from the articular margin of the humerus.

When viewed arthroscopically, the inferior glenohumeral complex is the most prominent of the capsular ligaments. The anterior and posterior bands are most clearly defined by abducting the arm and applying gentle distraction. With external rotation, the anterior band fans out, supporting the humeral head, and the posterior band appears cord-like. Conversely, by rotating the arm internally, the posterior band fans out to support the humeral head, and the anterior band appears more cord-like (Fig.

Figure 5–20 • Middle glenohumeral ligament (*MGHL*) crossing subscapularis tendon (*ST*), right shoulder.

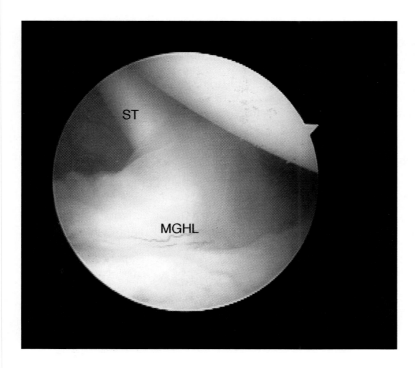

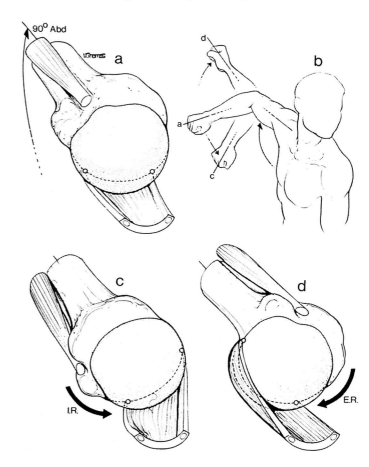

Figure 5–21 • Schematic drawing showing how the inferior glenohumeral ligament complex functions to support the humeral head both anteriorly and posteriorly with the arm in abduction. *A*, The arm is abducted 90 degrees and is in neutral rotation. *B* and *C*, As the arm is rotated internally, the posterior band of the inferior glenohumeral ligament complex fans out to support the humeral head posteriorly. *B* and *D*, When the arm is rotated externally, the anterior band of the inferior glenohumeral ligament complex fans out to support the humeral head anteriorly.

5–21). This reciprocating mechanism aids the inferior glenohumeral complex in providing humeral head support resisting both anterior and posterior translation. The anterior band of the inferior glenohumeral ligament is usually easily identifiable, appearing as a cord-like structure running obliquely inferiorly from the anterior glenoid when viewed through the posterior portal (Fig. 5–22). Morphologically, it appears cord-like due to the obligatory internal rotation of the humerus that occurs with joint distention. The arthroscope can be advanced into the axillary pouch by providing gentle distraction on the humerus and directing the arthroscope inferiorly. The posterior band is most easily assessed from an anterior portal and becomes more distinct with external rotation.

The arthroscopist must bear in mind that there is tremendous variation of the capsular glenohumeral ligaments. The ligaments appear to have varied shape, size, and orientation. Occasionally, the middle glenohumeral ligament blends with the inferior glenohumeral ligament and appears as one continuous structure. At other times, the ligaments are separated by openings or foramina into the subscapularis bursa. The most common foramen is found between the superior and middle glenohumeral ligaments. Rarely, one is visible below the middle glenohumeral ligament or in both positions, the so-called Buford complex[32] (Fig. 5–23).

Pathologic Anatomy

The glenohumeral ligaments are most commonly injured after an acute anterior shoulder dislocation. The ligaments may be detached directly from the glenoid or avulsed with the glenoid labrum. Identifying a separation of the glenohumeral ligaments and labrum is easy when they remain distracted from the glenoid (Fig. 5–24). However, attenuation or stretching of the glenohumeral ligaments is a more difficult diagnostic determination. When an interstitial tear occurs with an intact labrum, the entire anterior capsule and ligaments move away from the glenoid with distention. The humerus appears distracted from the glenoid, and the arthroscope passes easily into the axillary pouch. This has been termed the drive-through sign. When the glenohumeral ligaments have been chronically detached, fibrous tissue may fill the gap between the ligaments and the glenoid, reuniting it in an elongated state, thereby creating ligamentous laxity.

Subscapularis Tendon and Recess

The subscapularis tendon is the anterior rotator cuff muscle that is easily visualized from the posterior portal with the arm in the abducted position. The arthroscopically

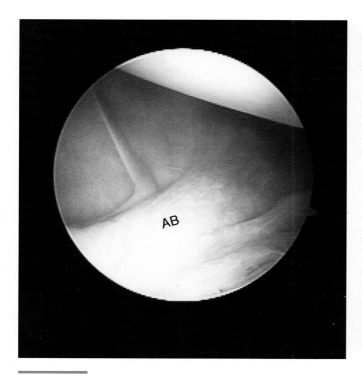

Figure 5–22 • Anterior band (*AB*) of inferior glenohumeral ligament, right shoulder.

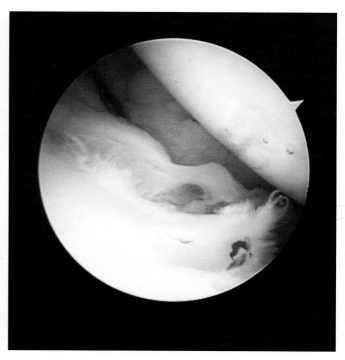

Figure 5–24 • Anterior labral detachment, right shoulder.

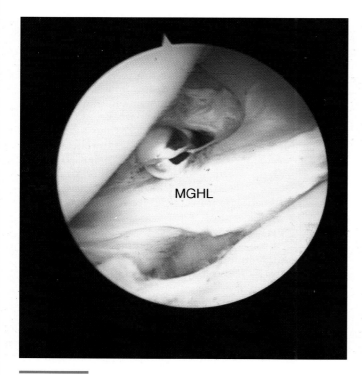

Figure 5–23 • Buford complex, left shoulder. *MGHL*: middle glenohumeral ligament.

viewable portion of the subscapularis tendon represents the posterior superior border. It constitutes only a small percentage of the broad-based subscapularis tendon, which measures 3–5 cm at its humeral insertion. The intra-articular slip of the subscapularis tendon lies between the superior and middle glenohumeral ligaments. At arthroscopy, the subscapularis tendon may occasionally be obscured by, or appear to blend with, the overlying middle glenohumeral ligament. The two can be distinguished as the subscapularis tendon courses perpendicularly to the long axis of the glenoid, whereas the middle glenohumeral ligament crosses obliquely over the subscapularis tendon near the glenoid (see Fig. 5–20). Directly superior to the subscapularis tendon and middle glenohumeral ligaments but inferior to the biceps tendon and superior glenohumeral ligament is the rotator interval. The rotator interval occupies a triangular space with its greatest width located at the base of the coracoid process and its apex at the transverse humeral ligament over the biceps sulcus. It is bordered superiorly by the anterior aspect of the supraspinatus tendon and inferiorly by the superior border of the subscapularis tendon.[33] Several studies have suggested that defects in the rotator interval may contribute to symptomatic shoulder instability.[33–35]

The subscapularis recess or bursa is a potential space that is posterior to the subscapularis tendon and muscle and anterior to the middle glenohumeral ligament. At the attachment of the middle glenohumeral ligament to the glenoid, the posterior wall of the bursa then becomes the scapula. The recess is primarily in the plane between the scapula and the subscapularis muscle and runs from the level of the glenoid to the base of the coracoid process.

Due to the tremendous variation in the glenohumeral ligaments, the subscapularis tendon may be completely obscured, or several foramina may enter into the subscapularis recess. Entrance into the recess is usually superior to the middle glenohumeral ligament but may occasionally occur through a foramen below the ligament as well. Rarely, the middle glenohumeral ligament may be completely absent, resulting in a single large recess. Once again, care should be taken to avoid misinterpreting these normal anatomic variations as pathologic lesions in the anterior shoulder capsule.

Complete arthroscopic visualization of the subscapularis recess is not possible.[10] From the posterior portal, the lateral wall of the recess can be visualized. Generally, the recess can be entered superiorly between the subscapularis tendon and the middle glenohumeral ligaments (Fig. 5–25). The medial wall of the recess is best visualized via the anterior portal allowing visualization of the neck of the glenoid, scapula, and subscapularis muscle.

Pathologic Anatomy

The superior slip of the subscapularis tendon is easily visualized arthroscopically, particularly when the glenohumeral ligaments are absent. Unlike the remaining rotator cuff muscles, the subscapularis is rarely torn or involved with the impingement syndrome. Traumatic tears of the subscapularis have been reported. Clinically, if weakness of internal rotation or a positive lift-off test is noted, the subscapularis and recess must be carefully inspected.

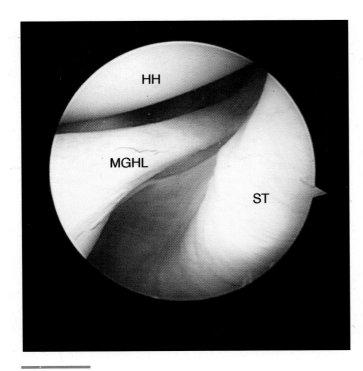

Figure 5–25 • Anterior portal view of left shoulder middle glenohumeral ligament (*MGHL*) and subscapularis tendon (*ST*). *HH*: humeral head.

Loose bodies are most commonly found within the axillary pouch but may also occasionally be located in the subscapularis recess. If a loose body is suspected and the axillary pouch is empty, the recess should be inspected thoroughly from both the posterior and anterior portals.

Rotator Cuff

The rotator cuff functions to dynamically stabilize the glenohumeral joint. It is composed of the four tendinous insertions of the subscapularis, supraspinatus, infraspinatus, and teres minor muscles. The subscapularis muscle is anatomically and functionally distinct from the other cuff muscles. The subscapularis is located anteriorly, and it is separated from the other cuff muscles by the rotator interval. Only a small portion of the subscapularis can be viewed anteriorly, because only its superior edge is intra-articular. The tendinous portions of the supraspinatus, infraspinatus, and teres minor muscles blend at the level of the glenoid and make up the superior and posterior walls of the glenohumeral joint as they continue laterally to insert on the proximal humerus. Functionally, the subscapularis is an internal rotator, and the remaining cuff muscles serve as external rotators.

The rotator cuff may be thoroughly evaluated arthroscopically. The undersurface of the rotator cuff can be inspected from the glenohumeral joint, and the superior surface from the subacromial space. Glenohumeral arthroscopic examination of the supraspinatus, infraspinatus, and teres minor muscles begins with proper orientation. The biceps tendon is identified, and the supraspinatus tendon is located just superior to the biceps as it enters the bicipital groove (Fig. 5–26). The undersurface of the supraspinatus tendon is covered by a thin veil of capsule and synovium that normally appear smooth. Further posteriorly, the infraspinatus and finally the teres minor muscles can be visualized. No distinct division between any of the three muscles can be made because at the level of the glenoid the tendons blend together to form a cuff of tissue. As with the supraspinatus, the undersurface of the infraspinatus and teres minor is covered with smooth synovium with minimal vascularity. Inspection of the more posterior aspect of the rotator cuff can be facilitated by rotating the arthroscope superiorly and towards the humeral head as the arthroscope is slightly retracted posteriorly. If there is difficulty in retracting the arthroscope to view the posterior rotator cuff, an anterior portal that allows easy visualization of the posterior joint can be established (Fig. 5–27).

Pathologic Anatomy

Tear of the rotator cuff most commonly involves the supraspinatus tendon. Normally, the biceps tendon and rotator cuff are separated by fluid distention during arthroscopy. If the rotator cuff does not move away from the biceps tendon with distention, a rotator cuff tear should be suspected. With a complete tear, the joint fluid escapes through the tear into the subacromial space, equalizing the pressure, and the biceps tendon and rotator cuff remain

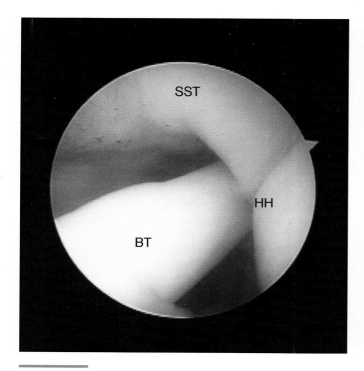

Figure 5–26 • Supraspinatus tendon (*SST*) insertion into humeral head (*HH*), right shoulder. *BT*: biceps tendon.

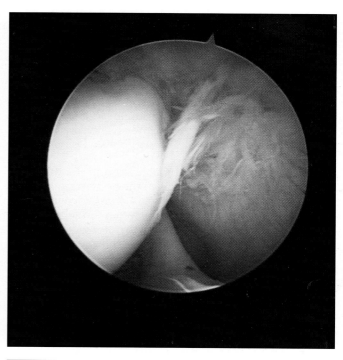

Figure 5–28 • Internal impingement. Undersurface tearing of posterior rotator cuff in a professional baseball pitcher, left shoulder.

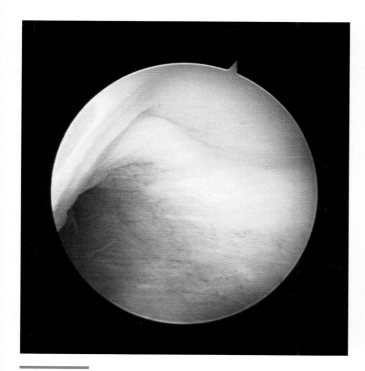

Figure 5–27 • Anterior portal view of posterior rotator cuff and capsule, right shoulder.

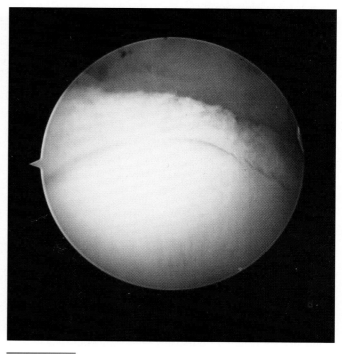

Figure 5–29 • Anterior portal view of posterior labral fraying in the patient in Figure 5–28.

juxtaposed. Careful probing and arthroscopic débridement may be required to determine the depth and extent of a rotator cuff tear.

Overhand athletes occasionally develop internal impingement. Internal impingement occurs with hyperexternal rotation of the shoulder during the late cocking phase of the throwing motion. The posterior rotator cuff is pinched between the humerus and glenoid. Internal impingement is best assessed arthroscopically from the anterior portal. Arthroscopic findings include undersurface tearing of the posterior rotator cuff (Fig. 5–28) as well as degenerative changes in the posterior glenoid labrum (Fig. 5–29).

SUBACROMIAL SPACE

Diagnostic arthroscopy of the shoulder is not complete until the subacromial space has been evaluated thoroughly. Because a significant amount of fluid may extravasate into the soft tissue during arthroscopy of the subacromial space, arthroscopy is usually performed after the examination of the glenohumeral joint has been completed.

The posterior portal is the standard viewing portal for the arthroscopic evaluation of the subacromial space.[36-39] Through the stab incision for the previously made posterior glenohumeral portal, the obturator and arthroscopic sheath are tracked below the posterior acromion into the subacromial space aiming toward the anterolateral corner of the acromion. The tip of the obturator and sheath are then swept medially and laterally within the subacromial space. When properly placed, the tip of the obturator and sheath should have a free excursion, and the undersurface of the acromion should be palpable. The working portal for subacromial arthroscopy is the lateral portal. This portal is located approximately 3 cm distal to the lateral edge of the acromion in line with the anterior edge of the acromion. The placement of the portal parallel to the anterior edge of the acromion ideally positions the portal to facilitate arthroscopic acromioplasties. Often the subacromial space is partially obscured by the gossamer-like bursa. Inserting a resector to remove the bursa greatly improves visualization within the subacromial space.

The borders of the subacromial space as they pertain to arthroscopic evaluation and treatment have been defined by Matthews and Fadale.[39] The roof of the subacromial space is composed of the undersurfaces of the distal clavicle, the acromioclavicular joint, the acromion, and the overlying coracoacromial ligament. The floor is the rotator cuff, which includes primarily the musculotendinous unit of the supraspinatus as well as the superior 20% of the subscapularis and infraspinatus. The anterior limit is the coracoid process. Medially, the base of the coracoid process and the vertical fibrous bands to the supraspinatus epimysium serve as the medial boundary. Finally, the deltoid muscle provides the lateral and posterior borders.

Once within the subacromial space from the posterior portal, the 30 degree oblique lens is directly laterally. The lateral portal is established, and the arthroscope is further oriented off an arthroscopic probe or shaver. Correct orientation is obtained when the angulation of the probe on the video monitor is identical to the arthroscopist's view

with the naked eye. The 30 degree oblique lens is then directed superiorly, and the undersurface of the acromion is visualized (Fig. 5–30). Because the undersurface of the acromion is covered by periosteum and the coracoacromial ligament, the true anterior and lateral borders may be obscured. The borders can be identified by palpating with a probe. Off the anterior edge of the acromion running obliquely medially is the coracoacromial ligament (Fig. 5–31). To identify the acromioclavicular joint and the distal clavicle, the 30 degree oblique lens is now oriented medially. The acromioclavicular joint and distal clavicle are often obscured by osteophytes, fat, and soft tissue.[40] Identification of the acromioclavicular joint is aided by placing an 18 gauge spinal needle from superior to inferior through the acromioclavicular joint into the subacromial space before the commencement of arthroscopy (Fig. 5–32). Also, depressing the clavicle while viewing the undersurface arthroscopically confirms the correct location of the joint. Finally, the 30 degree oblique lens is oriented inferiorly, and the superior surface of the rotator cuff is inspected. The superior aspect of the cuff is covered by a thin lining of bursal tissue and should appear smooth without hypervascularity. A greater expanse of the rotator cuff can be visualized by alternately rotating the brachium internally and externally.

Pathologic Anatomy

Variations in acromial shape have been described by Bigliani, Morrison, and April,[41] and significant correlation between bone shape and rotator cuff disease has been doc-

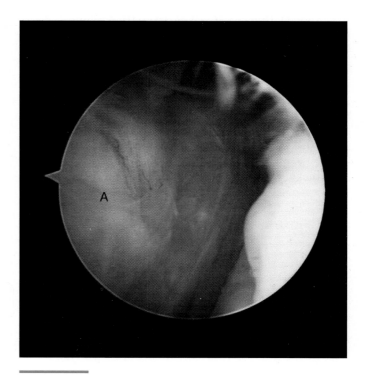

Figure 5–30 • Undersurface of right acromion (*A*) viewed from posterior portal. The bursal side of the rotator cuff is seen on the right.

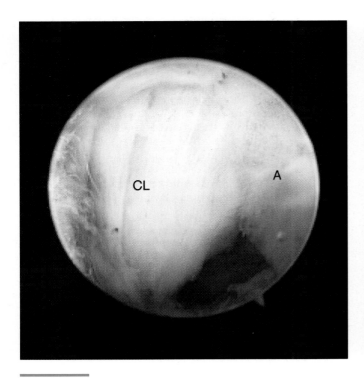

Figure 5–31 • Coracoacromial ligament (*CL*), left shoulder, coursing obliquely from the anterior edge of the acromion (*A*) toward the coracoid process.

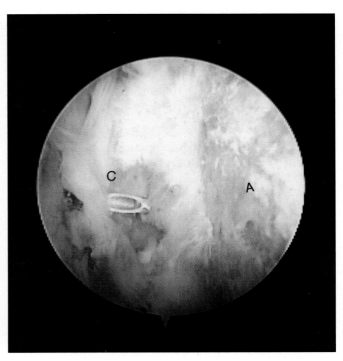

Figure 5–32 • An 18 gauge spinal needle entering the left acromioclavicular joint. The undersurface of the acromion (*A*) is seen on the right. The distal clavicle (*C*) is seen behind the needle tip.

umented. The acromial shape has been classified into three types: type I, flat; type II, gently curving; and type III, hooked (Fig. 5–33). The type III acromion allows for minimal rotator cuff clearance and has the highest incidence of rotator cuff tearing. When the acromion is viewed arthroscopically, hooking and erosion of the acromion may be encountered with cuff disease and the impingement syndrome. A general rule of thumb is that, when viewed arthroscopically, the acromion should have a greater diameter in the medial to lateral plane than the anterior to posterior plane.

With early impingement, the bursa may appear fibrotic or inflamed. Later, the rotator cuff may have a partial-thickness tear involving only the superior surface, or a

complete, full-thickness tear in which the arthroscope may be readily passed from the subacromial space into the glenohumeral joint (Fig. 5–34). With massive tears, the cuff retracts and no anatomic boundary exists between the subacromial space and the glenohumeral joint (Fig. 5–35).

Calcific tendinitis only rarely requires surgical intervention after conservative measures, including needle aspiration, have been exhausted. The calcification is often within the tendon and is not visualized superficially with the arthroscope in the subacromial space. The area can usually be identified by needle puncture and palpation with a probe. After the area has been identified, the superficial tendon tissue is resected, and the calcification may be removed.

Type I   Type II   Type III

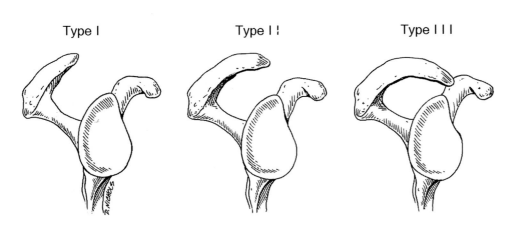

Figure 5–33 • Schematic diagram of a Bigliani type I, II, and III acromion.

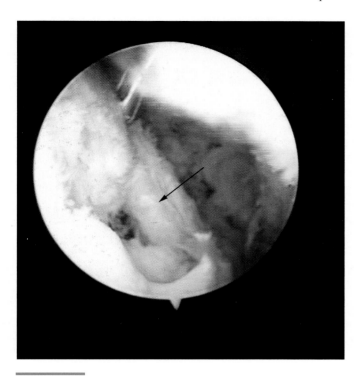

Figure 5–34 • Full-thickness tear (*arrow*), left rotator cuff, viewed from subacromial space.

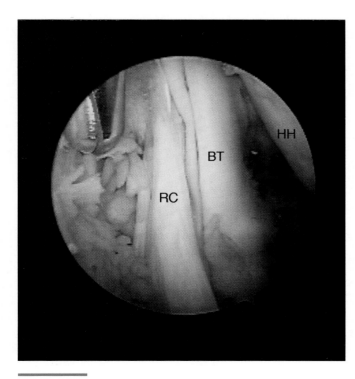

Figure 5–35 • Massive rotator cuff tear, right shoulder. *HH*: humeral head; *BT*: biceps tendon; and *RC*: retracted edge of rotator cuff.

References

1. Burman MS: Arthroscopy or direct visualization of joints: an experimental cadaver study. J. Bone Joint Surg 8:669, 1931.
2. Andrews JR and Carson WG: Shoulder joint arthroscopy. Orthopedics 6:1157–1162, 1983.
3. Andrews JR, Carson WG, and Ortega K: Arthroscopy of the shoulder: technique and normal anatomy. Am J Sports Med 12:1–7, 1984.
4. Andrews JR and Carson WG: Operative arthroscopy of the shoulder in the throwing athlete. In Zarins B, Andrews JR, and Carson WG (eds.): Injuries in the Throwing Athlete. Philadelphia, WB Saunders Co., 1985, pp 89–94.
5. Andrews JR, Heckman MM, and Guerra JJ: Normal arthroscopic examination of the glenohumeral joint. In McGinty JB, Caspari RB, Jackson RW, et al. (eds.): Operative Arthroscopy. Philadelphia, Lippincott–Raven, 1996, pp 647–661.
6. Blachut PA and Day B: Arthroscopic anatomy of the shoulder. Arthroscopy 5:1–10, 1989.
7. Bramhall JP, Scarpinato DF, and Andrews JR: Operative arthroscopy of the shoulder. In Andrews JR and Wilk KE (eds.): The Athlete's Shoulder. New York, Churchill Livingstone, 1994, pp 105–111.
8. Carson WG: Normal arthroscopic anatomy of the shoulder. In Andrews JR and Wilk KE (eds.): The Athlete's Shoulder. New York, Churchill Livingstone, 1994, pp 93–103.
9. Caspari RB: Shoulder arthroscopy: a review of the present state of the art. Contemp Orthop 4:523, 1982.
10. Detrisac DA and Johnson LL: Arthroscopic Shoulder Anatomy: Pathologic and Surgical Implications. Thorofare, N.J., Slack, 1986.
11. Geissler WB and Caspari RB: Arthroscopic techniques of the shoulder. In Andrews JR and Wilk KE (eds.): The Athlete's Shoulder, New York, Churchill Livingstone, 1994, pp 85–91.
12. Johnson LL: Arthroscopy of the shoulder. Orthop Clin North Am 11:197–204, 1980.
13. Johnson LL: The shoulder joint: an arthroscopist's perspective of anatomy and pathology. Clin Orthop 223:113–125, 1987.
14. Johnson LL: Arthroscopic surgical anatomy. In Johnson LL (ed.): Diagnostic and Surgical Arthroscopy of the Shoulder. St. Louis, Mosby-Year Book, 1993, pp 189–230.
15. Ogilvie-Harris DJ and Wiley AM: Arthroscopic surgery of the shoulder: a general appraisal. J Bone Joint Surg Br 68:201, 1986.
16. Skyhar MJ, Altchek DW, Warren RF, et al.: Shoulder arthroscopy with the patient in the beach-chair position. Arthroscopy 4: 256–259, 1988.
17. Snyder SF, Karzel RP, Del Pizzo W, et al.: SLAP lesions of the shoulder. Arthroscopy 6:274–279, 1990.
18. Andrews JR and Carson WG: Glenoid labrum tears related to the long head of the biceps. Am J Sports Med 13:337–341, 1985.
19. Johnson LL, Bays BM, and van Dyk GE: Vincula of the biceps tendon in the glenohumeral joint: an arthroscopic and anatomic study. J Shoulder Elbow Surg 1:162–166, 1992.
20. Steinberg ME and Steinberg DR: Avascular necrosis of the femoral head. In Steinberg ME (ed.): The Hip and Its Disorders. Philadelphia, WB Saunders Co., 1991, pp 623–647.
21. Johnson LL: Pathologic anatomy. In Johnson LL (ed.): Diagnostic and Surgical Arthroscopy of the Shoulder. St. Louis, Mosby-Year Book, 1993, pp 231–275.
22. Hovelius L: Anterior dislocation of the shoulder in teen-agers and young adults. J Bone Joint Surg Am 69: 393–399, 1987.
23. Arciero RA, Wheeler JH, Ryan JB, et al.: Arthroscopic Bankart repair versus nonoperative treatment for acute, initial anterior shoulder dislocations. Am J Sports Med 22:589–594, 1994.
24. Baker CL, Uribe JW, and Whitman C: Arthroscopic evaluation of acute initial anterior shoulder dislocations. Am J Sports Med 18: 25–28, 1990.
25. Bankart ASB: Recurrent or habitual dislocation of the shoulder joint. Br Med J 2:1132–1133, 1923.
26. Saha AK: Mechanics of elevation of glenohumeral joint: its application in rehabilitation of flail shoulder and upper brachial plexus injuries and poliomyelitis and in replacement of the upper humerus by prosthesis. Acta Orthop Scand 44:668–678, 1973.
27. O'Brien SJ, Neves MC, Arnoczky SP, et al.: The anatomy and histology of the inferior glenohumeral ligament complex of the shoulder. Am J Sports Med 18:449–456, 1990.

28. Moseley HG and Overgaard B: The anterior capsular mechanism in recurrent anterior dislocation of the shoulder: morphological and clinical studies with special reference to the glenoid labrum and the glenohumeral ligaments. J Bone Joint Surg Br 44:913, 1962.

29. Snyder SJ, Rames RD, and Wolbert E: Labral lesions. In McGinty JB (ed.): Operative Arthroscopy. New York, Raven Press, 1991, pp 491–499.

30. Warner JJP, Deng XH, and Warren RF: Static casuloligamentous restraints to superior-inferior translation of the glenohumeral joint. Am J Sports Med 20:675–685, 1992.

31. Turkel SJ, Panio MW, Marshal JL, et al.: Stabilizing mechanism preventing anterior dislocation of the glenohumeral joint. J Bone Joint Surg Am 63:1208, 1981.

32. Williams MM, Snyder SJ, and Buford D: The Buford complex—the "cord-like" middle glenohumeral ligament and absent anterosuperior labrum complex: a normal anatomic capsulolabral variant (see comments). Arthroscopy 10:241–247, 1994.

33. Field LD, Warren RF, O'Brien SJ, et al.: Isolated closure of the rotator interval defects for shoulder instability. Am J Sports Med 23:557–563, 1995.

34. Rowe CR and Zarins B: Recurrent transient subluxation of the shoulder. J Bone Joint Surg Am 63:863–872, 1981.

35. Harryman DT, Sidles JA, and Harris SL: The role of the rotator interval capsule in passive motion and stability of the shoulder. J Bone Joint Surg Am 74:53–66, 1992.

36. Ellman H: Arthroscopic subacromial decompression: analysis of one to three year result. Arthroscopy 3:173–181, 1987.

37. Gartsman GM, Blair ME, and Noble PC: Arthroscopic subacromial decompression: an anatomic study. Am J Sports Med 16:48–50, 1988.

38. Laumann V: Decompression of the subacromial space: an anatomical study. In Bayley I and Kessell L (eds.): Shoulder Surgery. Berlin, Springer-Verlag, 1982, pp 14–21.

39. Matthews LS and Fadale PD: Subacromial anatomy for the arthroscopist. Arthroscopy 5:36–40, 1989.

40. Gartsman GM, Combs AH, Davis PF, et al.: Arthroscopic acromioclavicular joint resection: an anatomical study. Am J Sports Med 19:2–5, 1991.

41. Bigliani LU, Morrison DS, April EW: The morphology of the acromion and its relationship to rotator cuff tears. Orthop Trans 10:216–1986.

Arthroscopic Acromioplasty

Michael M. Heckman • *Gordon I. Groh*

Neer's classic description of the diagnosis and treatment of impingement syndrome in 1972[1] increased our understanding of the anatomy and pathophysiology of the impingement process and provided a rationale and technique for treatment of rotator cuff lesions and the impingement syndrome. The anterior acromioplasty has become the procedure of choice for stages II and III impingement lesions, and many investigators have reported high success rates treating both the impingement syndrome and rotator cuff tears by utilizing Neer's techniques.[2–5]

As an alternative to Neer's conventional method of open decompression, Ellman[6] in 1985 provided an initial description for the technique of arthroscopic subacromial decompression. He described the primary objectives of the procedure to be release of a coracoacromial ligament, resection of the undersurface of the anterior acromion, and débridement of the hypertrophic bursa without detachment of the deltoid. His initial results[7] and those of other authors have been comparable to those of open surgical techniques.[8] Arthroscopic subacromial decompression has become an accepted standard in the treatment of patients with stages II and III impingement lesions.

The purpose of this chapter is to describe the surgical technique of arthroscopic subacromial decompression. Because the technique is technically demanding and has a documented steep learning curve,[8–10] a technique for completing the procedure is discussed that attempts to minimize potential operative complications.

SURGICAL INDICATIONS

Neer[1, 11] developed a staging system for grading impingement lesions of the shoulder. A stage I lesion consists of inflammation of the rotator cuff, typically in younger individuals. Treatment with rest, anti-inflammatory medication, and physical therapy resolves the condition. A stage II lesion occurs in the third and fourth decade of life and is treated similarly to a stage I lesion. Unfortunately, some stage II lesions do not respond successfully to conservative treatment. When symptoms persist despite conservative treatment for more than 6–12 months, surgical intervention is warranted. A stage III lesion is associated with rotator cuff disruption; current treatment algorithms were summarized by Iannotti.[12]

Less common surgical indications for acromioplasty exist as well. Massive rotator cuff tears, which are irreparable, are amenable to acromioplasty, with reduction of pain and improvement of function.[13] Acromioplasty has been extended to arthroscopic procedures[14] with similar results. Greater tuberosity fractures, which unite with displacement; calcific tendinitis refractory to conservative management; and acromioclavicular joint spurs may require acromioplasty when conservative management fails.[15, 16]

SURGICAL CONTRAINDICATIONS

Anterior shoulder pain, typical of impingement, is also shared with a variety of other syndromes. Differentiation of impingement from these conditions ensures that unwarranted arthroscopic acromioplasty is not attempted. Cervical disk syndromes associated with radiculopathy at the fifth and sixth interspace are prone to create anterior shoulder pain and are differentiated by history, physical examination, and cervical spine radiographs. Brachial plexus neuritis and suprascapular nerve entrapment[17] may mimic impingement symptoms, based on loss of depressor function of the rotator cuff.

Acromioclavicular arthritis and osteolysis may present in conjunction with impingement or as isolated entities. Distal clavicle osteolysis is more prominent in the weight-training athlete in the second and third decade of life. Both entities are confirmed by localized joint tenderness and by radiographs centered on the joint. Radiographs of the joint, as suggested by Zanca,[18] begin with a 10 degree cephalic tilt and a 50% reduction to the kilovolts utilized in a standard anteroposterior shoulder radiograph (Fig. 6–1).

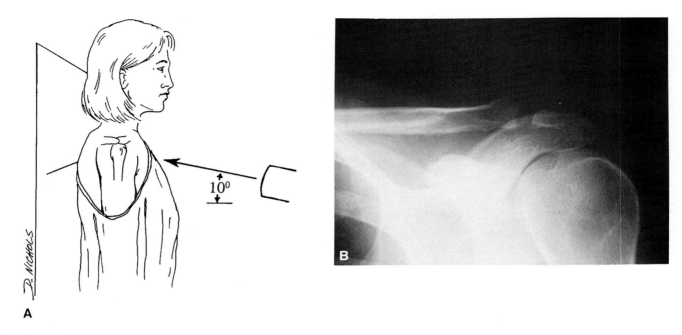

Figure 6–1 • *A*, Ten degree cephalic anteroposterior (AP) view of acromioclavicular joint. *B*, Osteolysis of acromioclavicular joint demonstrated on Zanca view. Radiographic findings are enhanced by reducing standard kilovolts by 50% compared with those utilized in a standard AP view of the shoulder.

Glenohumeral instability with secondary impingement is an important diagnosis to exclude, particularly in the patient with lax connective tissue. The coexistence of multidirectional instability and impingement symptoms is not uncommon. Treatment should be directed at the root cause rather than at the impingement symptoms.[15] A snapping scapula[19] and adhesive capsulitis may present similarly; however, acromioplasty is not indicated in either condition. Patients unable to undergo general anesthesia and surgical treatment secondary to bleeding dyscrasia, pacemakers, or cardiovascular conditions are similarly unfit for arthroscopic acromioplasty.

CLINICAL PRESENTATION

Presentation to the physician typically occurs after the patient's shoulder pain has failed to resolve with time. Pain is typically located over the anterior shoulder and may worsen with sleeping on the affected extremity. Similarly, the pain often increases on utilizing the hand above shoulder level. Tenderness on palpation may be elicited over the coracoacromial arch. It is important to differentiate this pain from the pain of acromioclavicular degenerative joint disease.

Range of motion may be limited in impingement disease and should be carefully documented. Limitation of forward elevation may occur in impingement disease; however, limitation of external rotation should raise the suspicion of adhesive capsulitis. The impingement sign as described by Neer[1] requires stabilization of the scapula and pain on forward elevation of the arm. Hawkins and Kennedy[3] described the maneuver to be elicited by abduc-

tion of the shoulder and internal rotation performed in the plane of the scapula. The impingement sign accentuates the pain by mechanical irritation of the rotator cuff beneath the coracoacromial arch. The impingement sign is associated with rotator cuff disease but may be present in other causes of shoulder pain (Figs. 6–2 to 6–5).

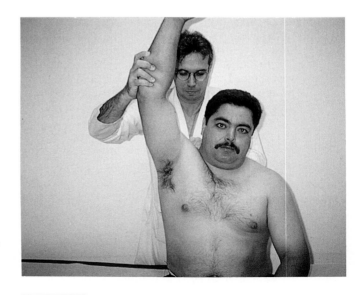

Figure 6–2 • The classic impingement sign noted with stressing the shoulder at maximum elevation with scapular stabilization.

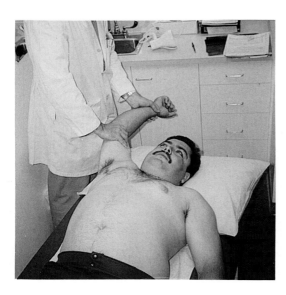

Figure 6–3 • The classic impingement test with the patient in the supine position.

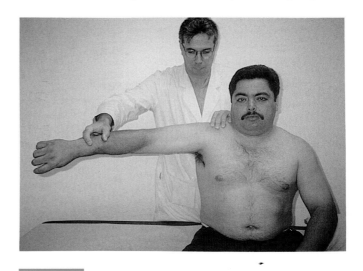

Figure 6–5 • Testing for dysfunction of the supraspinatus musculotendinous unit. Resistance is applied with the arm abducted 90 degrees, with the shoulder flexed foward 30 degrees, and with the forearms pronated, helping to isolate the supraspinatus.

The impingement test is the most useful tool for the clinician. Ten milliliters of 1% lidocaine is injected into the subacromial space via either an anterior or posterior portal. Pain relief in impingement syndrome should always be greater than 50%; otherwise, another source of shoulder pain should be considered. Further, the amount of pain relief should indicate the final pain reduction as a result of rehabilitation or surgical treatment (Fig. 6–6).

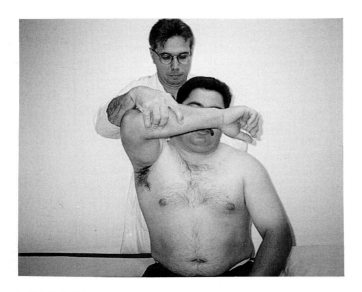

Figure 6–4 • As described by Hawkins and Kennedy,[3] impingement is produced when the arm is flexed forward 90 degrees with forceful internal rotation, causing the supraspinatus tendon to impinge against the coracoacromial ligament.

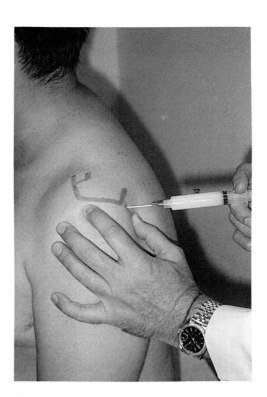

Figure 6–6 • The impingement test. Ten milliliters of local anesthetic is injected into the subacromial space. Subsequent examination to find impingement should elicit no or significantly reduced discomfort, which is considered a normal test result.

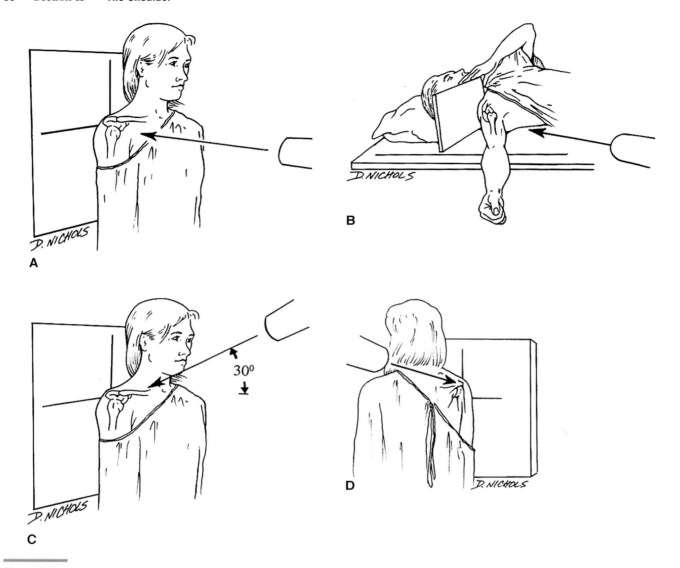

Figure 6–7 • Radiographic evaluation of the shoulder. Radiographic evaluation of the symptomatic shoulder should include *(A)* true anteroposterior, *(B)* axillary lateral, *(C)* anteroposterior view with 30 degree caudal tilt, and *(D)* supraspinatus Y-outlet views in evaluating the patient with suspected impingement.

Radiographic evaluation of the symptomatic shoulder should include an anteroposterior radiograph, an axillary lateral radiograph, a supraspinatus Y-outlet radiograph, and a 30 degree caudal tilt anteroposterior radiograph (Fig. 6–7). Unfused apophyses are best evaluated with axillary lateral radiographs. Further, the extent of proliferative acromion lying anterior to the clavicle is also observed. The degree of proliferative acromion may be characterized by the supraspinatus Y-outlet view as flat (type I), curved (type II), or hooked (type III)[20] (Fig. 6–8). Rockwood and Lyons[5] described an anteroposterior view of the shoulder taken with the beam angled 30 degrees caudally. In this drawing (Fig. 6–7C), proliferative acromion is defined as any protuberance of acromion lying below the smooth line of the clavicle.

Regardless of the view chosen to evaluate the proliferative anterior and inferior acromion, successful arthroscopic decompression must ensure complete resection. A hooked or curved acromion on the supraspinatus outlet view must be converted to a smooth acromion. Similarly, if the 30 degree caudal tilt anteroposterior view is utilized, no bone must lie below the smooth line in the clavicle. Rockwood and Lyons[5] emphasized the importance of removal of acromion anterior to the clavicle. Failure to accomplish this resection results in recurrent impingement.

Many other tools are available to the orthopaedic surgeon, including magnetic resonance imaging (MRI), ultrasonography, and arthrography (Fig. 6–9). Although these tools are of sound foundation in determining the integrity of the rotator cuff, the authors have not found them to be of great assistance in technical planning of bone resection for arthroscopic subacromial decompression. The authors prefer the combination of plain radiographs already described for delineating the amount of acromial resection required.

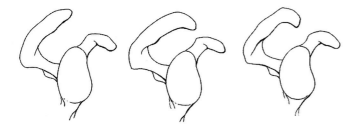

Figure 6–8 • Three shapes of the acromion are recognized on the supraspinatus Y-outlet view: flat (type I), curved (type II), and hooked or angled (type III).

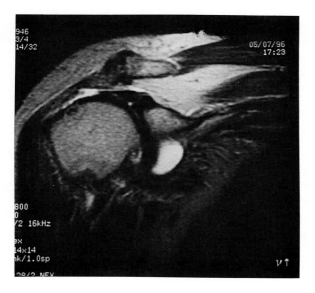

Figure 6–9 • MRI findings consistent with impingement. MRI findings show rotator cuff tendinitis, involving the supraspinatus attachment site with downward impression into the supraspinatus at the level of the acromioclavicular joint, consistent with an impingement process.

OPERATING ROOM SET-UP AND EQUIPMENT

Arthroscopic subacromial decompression of the shoulder is performed on a regular operating room table. If a sitting or beach-chair position is to be utilized, then a headrest and side support are recommended for stabilizing the patient during the procedure. In cases utilizing the lateral decubitus position, a bean bag or kidney rest and shoulder traction device are required. The procedure requires a basic arthroscopic set-up including a camera with a 30 degree arthroscope (4.5–5.0 mm), a powered arthroscopic shaver and bur system, and an electrocautery that functions in the selected irrigation fluid. Distention during the procedure may be provided by the use of either an arthroscopic mechanical pump system or a gravity inflow. If additional arthroscopic procedures are anticipated, for example rotator cuff repair, then the surgeon's equipment of choice should also be available (Fig. 6–10).

After the patient is in the operating room, anesthesic and intravenous antibiotics are administered. Because of the thick subcutaneous tissues and musculature about the shoulder, local anesthesia is rarely if ever utilized. Either a general anesthetic or an interscalene block may be used to anesthetize the shoulder effectively. After induction of anesthesia, the shoulder should be examined to document passive range of motion, to rule out any signs of adhesive capsulitis or stiffness, to determine if instability exists, and more specifically to feel for signs of subacromial crepitation, which may signify underlying rotator cuff disease.

If the procedure is to be performed with the patient in the lateral decubitus position, the patient is supported by a bean bag or kidney rest apparatus. An axillary roll is placed under the unaffected side, and the unaffected arm is well supported with all bony prominences padded. A prefabricated wrist gauntlet made of foam or plastic is then applied to the operative arm with an Ace or Coban bandage. The arm is then placed in longitudinal traction by use of either a rope-and-pulley system or a shoulder suspension device that allows for manipulation of the extremity as needed for visualization. Manual traction on the arm is not recommended for the lateral decubitus position because such traction results in fatigue of the surgical assistant and inability of the surgeon to view the joint in a steady position.[21] Depending on the size of the patient, 10–15 lb of traction is in most cases adequate to afford visualization during surgery.[21-23] Weight greater than 20 lb is not recommended in any case as there is a potential of producing a neuropraxic injury secondary to the increased force applied along the extremity.[24]

After the arm is placed in longitudinal traction, refinements in the arm's position are then completed. The patient's torso is rolled back approximately 15 degrees in relation to the operating table to allow easier access to the anterior aspect of the joint. This prevents the surgeon from operating in a downhill or forward-flexed position, impinging the instruments into the surgical drapes. The arm is then placed in a position of 70 degrees of abduction and 15 degrees of forward flexion, in which it is maintained for the course of the procedure. This position provides adequate visualization of the glenohumeral joint and the subacromial space and in most cases alleviates the need for repositioning the extremity throughout the procedure.[25] Impervious U-drapes are then placed superiorly and inferiorly, covering the patient's torso, neck, and head. These drapes keep irrigation runoff from collecting about the patient's face. The arm and shoulder are then scrubbed and prepared, and a shoulder or hip pack is used for draping. In addition, a sterile towel or plastic Steri-Drape should be applied to the forearm for sterile coverage of the previously applied wrist gauntlet. This allows the surgeon to manipulate the extremity as needed without contamination. The surgeon is positioned directly posterior to the shoulder, with the first assistant toward the patient's feet and the second assistant, if one is necessary, placed toward the patient's head (Fig. 6–11*A*).

The beach-chair and sitting positions offer advantages over the lateral decubitus position in that they facilitate management of the patient's airway under general anesthesia and allow an arthrotomy to be performed either after or in association with the arthroscopic procedure

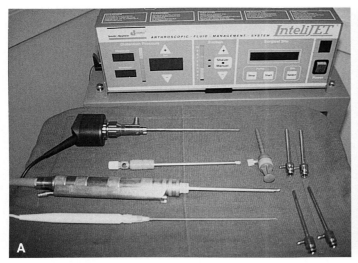

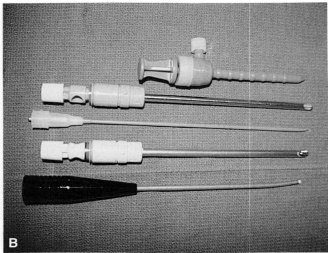

Figure 6–10 • *A*, Basic equipment for completion of acromioplasty includes a standard 30 degree arthroscope, arthroscopic shaving system, standard and disposable cannulae, and an arthroscopic irrigation system. *B*, Standard instrumentation utilized for completion of acromioplasty includes the surgeon's cautery tip of choice, a full-radius resector, and acromionizer bur.

without repositioning and draping the patient. Arthroscopic visualization of the intra-articular structures is in a more anatomic orientation in comparison with a lateral decubitus position without the added effects of distortion of the capsular structures provided by traction on the arm with a shoulder traction device.[26]

If the procedure is to be performed with the patient in the beach-chair or sitting position, compressive wraps should be placed around the patient's lower extremities to prevent venostasis during surgery. The operating table is initially adjusted by reflexing and then raising the back of the table to a position of 80–90 degrees from the horizontal. Final positioning is then adjusted with the assistance of height and reverse Trendelenburg controls. The shoulder may then be positioned off the edge of the table, allowing for complete access to the posterior aspect of the joint. In those cases utilizing a general anesthetic, the head is secured to the table via a McConnell headrest, and the torso is supported with a padded side plate (Figs. 6–11*B* and *C*).

After completion of patient positioning, the instrumentation and equipment needed to perform the procedure are arranged about the operating table. An arthroscopic cart containing the video monitor, video control box, light source, videotape recorder, irrigation pump if needed, shaver power source, and laser imager is placed opposite the surgeon at the level of the shoulder on the opposite side of the patient. This positioning provides for visualization of the video monitor screen and allows the arthroscopy to be performed without the surgeon being handicapped by various cables and tubing entering the operative field from different directions. A Mayo stand is placed just distal to the first assistant at the level of the patient's waist and should contain the basic and most frequently utilized instrumentation necessary to complete the surgery. A back table is then positioned within easy reach

behind the first assistant and should contain equipment that is less frequently utilized but necessary for the procedure (Fig. 6–11*D*)

SURGICAL TECHNIQUE

For operative orientation and accurate portal placement, the bony anatomic landmarks about the shoulder are initially identified and outlined with a surgical skin marker. These landmarks are the anterolateral and posterior borders of the acromion, the distal clavicle and the acromioclavicular joint, and the coracoid process[22, 25] (Fig. 6–12). Routinely, 18 gauge spinal needles are placed into the acromioclavicular joint and at the anterolateral edge of the acromion to aid in visualizing the full width of the acromion and to provide orientation during the course of the subacromial decompression. This is done before the start of the procedure because extravasation of irrigation fluid into the soft tissues may occur upon initiation of the arthroscopy, making later localization of the acromioclavicular joint and the anterolateral portion of the acromion much more difficult.

Portal Placement

Arthroscopic subacromial decompression may be performed utilizing two or three arthroscopic portals.

Posterior Portal

The posterior, or soft-spot, portal is the one most commonly used in diagnostic arthroscopy of the shoulder because it allows for almost complete visualization of the

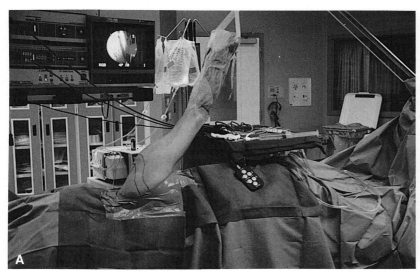
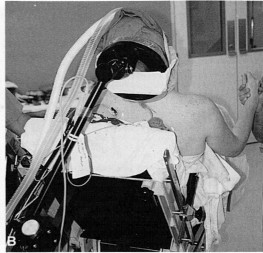
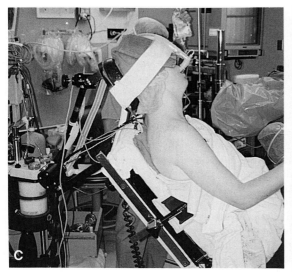
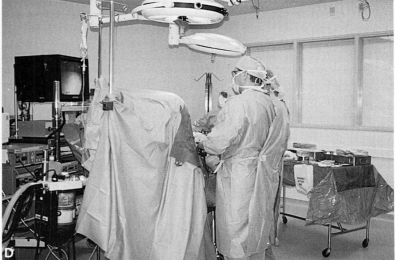

Figure 6–11 • *A*, Patient in the lateral decubitus position with arms supported by a shoulder holder device. *B* and *C*, Patient in the beach-chair position with head, neck, and torso supported by a McConnell device with side plate. *D*, Final position with surgeon, assistant, and equipment for completion of acromioplasty.

glenohumeral joint. Various techniques and locations for placement of this portal have been described but all utilize the posterolateral border of the acromion as a reference. Portal placement, depending on technique and patient positioning, is 1–3 cm inferior to the posterolateral tip of the acromion.[22, 25, 27, 28] With the patient in the beach-chair or sitting position, moving the portal slightly medially, approximately 1 cm, allows somewhat easier access to the glenohumeral joint. Placement of the portal corresponds to the posterior soft spot of the shoulder that represents the interval between the infraspinatus and teres minor muscles. It is the authors' experience that a portal placed approximately 3 cm inferior and 1–1 1/2 cm medial to the posterolateral tip of the acromion allows excellent visualization of the glenohumeral joint and the subacromial space.

Lateral Portal

The lateral portal is most frequently utilized for instrumentation of the subacromial space or, depending on the technique, as a viewing portal. Depending on the surgeon's preference, portal placement may be from a point in line with the posterior edge of the distal clavicle to a level parallel to the anterolateral tip of the acromion.[8, 29] A stab incision placed in the skin at 2–3 cm from the lateral border of the acromion results in splitting the lateral deltoid fibers at approximately 1–2 cm inferior to the lateral acromial edge and minimizes the potential for deltoid denervation. More superior placement of the portal usually results in impingement of the instruments or the shaver being utilized into the edge of the lateral acromion. This impingement may prevent full access to the subacromial

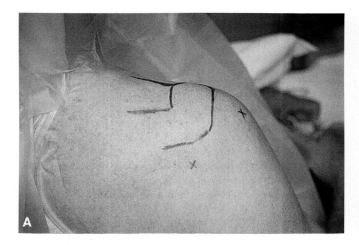
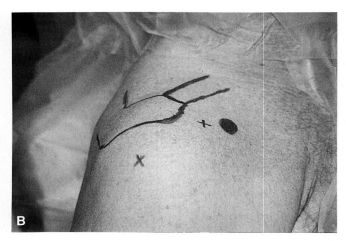

Figure 6–12 • Bony anatomic landmarks are demarcated on initiation of the procedure, as are portal placement sites for anterior, posterior "soft-spot," and lateral arthroscopic portals. *A,* Posterior view. *B,* Anterior view.

space and can limit the surgeon's ability to perform an adequate subacromial decompression.

Anterior Portal

A third anterior or accessory portal may be utilized during the procedure as a primary portal for irrigation inflow, as a second portal for additional instrumentation, or as a portal for gravity outflow. This portal is located just lateral to the coracoid process and half the distance between the coracoid and the anterior edge of the acromion. Cannulae or instruments utilized through this portal pass through the anterior one-third of the deltoid and in proximity to or through the coracoacromial ligament before entering the subacromial space. The musculocutaneous nerve is in the greatest danger of injury when utilizing this approach; care should be taken to keep the approach lateral to the coracoid so as not to endanger the nerve.[27]

Preoperative Preparation

Patients presenting as appropriate candidates for subacromial decompression require preoperative radiographs to assist the surgeon in planning and completing an adequate and safe decompression. Preoperative radiographs of the shoulder should include true anteroposterior, 30 degree caudal tilt anteroposterior, axillary lateral, 10 degree cephalic tilt anteroposterior, and supraspinatus Y-outlet views. If rotator cuff disease is suspected, then the status of the rotator cuff should be documented with the assistance of arthrogram, ultrasound, or MRI techniques. Status of the rotator cuff and, if necessary, its potential for reparability need to be discussed with the patient preoperatively as cuff disease or repair may affect both the postoperative treatment and results of subacromial decompression.[30]

When planning the acromioplasty, the axillary lateral view demonstrates unfused apophyses of the acromion, the os acromiale, and the amount of acromion that is anterior

to the acromioclavicular joint that requires resection at the time of the acromioplasty (Figs. 6–13*A* and *B*). The 30 degree caudal tilt anteroposterior view provides information regarding the shape of the anterior edge of the acromion and assists in allowing the surgeon to concentrate on specific areas where the acromion appears to be more proliferative and protruding inferiorly (Fig. 6–13*C*). The 10 degree cephalic tilt anteroposterior view (Zanca view) helps in defining specific disorders associated with the acromioclavicular joint to determine whether distal clavicular undersurface or complete resection may be required at the time of subacromial decompression. Finally, the supraspinatus Y-outlet view assists the surgeon in defining acromial shape, allowing the acromion to be categorized as a type I, II, or III[20] (Fig. 6–13*D*). The thickness of the acromion can be assessed as well as the amount of bone that needs to be resected to create a smooth, flat decompression (Fig. 6–14). This view offers critical information as overzealous resection can lead to excessive thinning of the acromion and possible fracture. This complication is most prevalent in females with a thin type III acromion and in those patients with osteoporotic bone.[8, 31]

Glenohumeral Arthroscopy

Diagnostic and operative arthroscopy of the glenohumeral joint should be completed before subacromial decompression is initiated. The joint is initially inflated with 30–50 mL of normal saline injected through an 18 gauge spinal needle inserted at the posterior, or soft-spot, portal site. Intra-articular placement of the needle is documented by pressurized backflow of the inserted irrigation fluid. If pressurized backflow is not noted, the surgeon should be suspicious that the needle is placed extra-articularly or that rotator cuff disease exists that is allowing fluid to pass into the subacromial space. Diagnostic arthroscopy of the glenohumeral joint can be completed with inflow on the arthroscope through the posterior portal. If better visualization of the posterior structures is necessary or

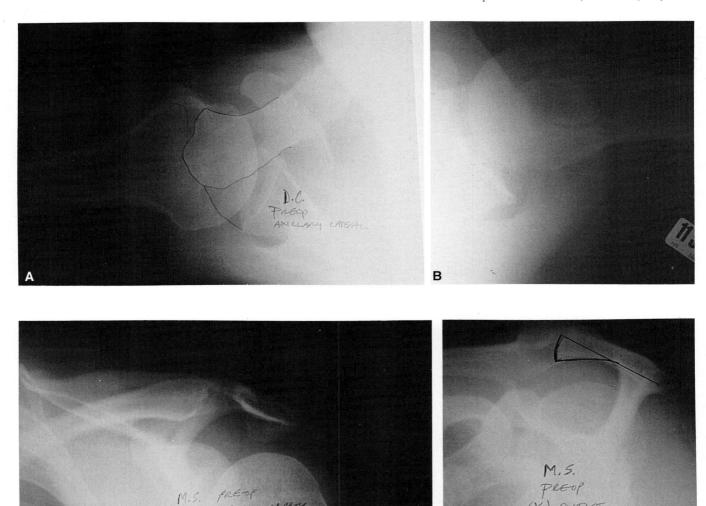

Figure 6–13 • Radiographs for preoperative assessment. *A*, Preoperative axillary lateral radiograph demonstrates proliferative acromion anterior to the distal clavicle. Any bone noted anterior to the distal clavicle requires resection at the time of acromioplasty. *B*, Axillary lateral radiograph demonstrates unfused apophysis or os acromiale. *C*, Preoperative 30 degree caudal tilt anteroposterior view of the shoulder. All bone that is noted inferior to the undersurface of the distal clavicle requires resection for completion of adequate acromioplasty. *D*, Supraspinatus Y-outlet view demonstrates proposed acromial resection level.

instrumentation of the joint is required, then an anterior portal can be created under direct visualization or with a switching-stick technique through the capsular interval just superior to the subscapularis, lateral to the anterior lip of the glenoid, and inferior to the biceps tendon.

Diagnostic arthroscopy of the glenohumeral joint should be performed methodically. The articular surfaces of the glenoid and humerus, glenohumeral ligaments, glenoid labrum, long head of the biceps, and rotator cuff should be viewed and their condition documented.[25, 32] If operative intervention is necessary in treatment of injuries to any of these structures, then that should be completed at this time. Specific attention should be focused on any findings consistent with instability of the glenohumeral joint that may result in secondary impingement of the shoulder. These findings include lesions of the superior labrum from anterior to posterior, labral tearing or Bankart lesions, redundancy of the glenohumeral ligaments, and an abnormal drive-through sign consistent with generalized laxity of the tissues. If documented, such findings may influence the decision to proceed with subacromial decompression.

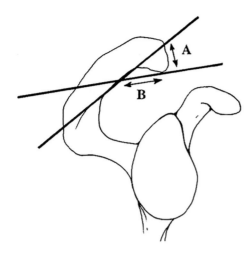

Figure 6–14 • Preoperative planning based on supraspinatus Y-outlet view. Distance *A* denotes the thickness of the proposed resection at the leading edge of the acromion. *B*, Denotes the distance that the acromion must be planed to convert it to a type I or smooth shape.

Subacromial Bursoscopy

On completion of diagnostic and operative arthroscopy of the glenohumeral joint, attention is directed to the subacromial space. By utilizing the original posterior portal, a cannula with trocar is advanced into the space and directed toward the anterior lateral tip of the acromion. If the patient is in the beach-chair position, the authors have found that slight downward distraction on the arm in a position of approximately 20 degrees of abduction allows the subacromial space to be entered, thereby reducing the risk of penetration of the rotator cuff musculotendinous junction or muscular fibers by the cannula. The subacromial space is then distended by utilizing inflow on the arthroscope to improve visualization. Lactated Ringer's solution with 1 cc of 1:1,000 epinephrine for each 3-L bag is recommended as an irrigant solution to assist in controlling hemostasis during the procedure.

If an anterior portal is necessary for inflow or instrumentation of the space, the portal may be established by utilizing a previously placed anterior glenohumeral portal directed superiorly or by using a switching-stick or direct technique through a stab incision placed at the anterolateral edge of the patient's coracoacromial ligament. In those cases in which a prior anterior portal site is utilized, the cannula entering the subacromial space usually penetrates the fibers of the coracoacromial ligament. Fortunately, in most cases, this does not result in the production of significant bleeding.

If necessary, a lateral portal is placed, as previously described, at a level approximately 2–3 cm from the lateral border of the acromion. More proximal placement of this portal usually results in impingement of the instrumentation or arthroscope on the lateral acromial edge and compromises access to the space. This impingement limits the surgeon's ability to perform an adequate subacromial decompression. The location of this portal in the anteroposterior plane depends, to a certain degree, on surgeon preference. It may be located anywhere from the posterior edge of the distal clavicle moving anteriorly toward the anterior acromial edge or anterior lateral acromial corner. If a lateral and an anterior portal are to be utilized concurrently during the procedure, the authors have noted that keeping the lateral portal slightly more posterior prevents difficulties that result from instrumentation being placed in proximity within the limited confines of the space.

After completion of portal placement a subacromial bursoscopy is performed. On entering the space with the arthroscope, the subacromial bursa is usually the first structure encountered. In fact, the arthroscope may be introduced initially into the lining of the bursa, which obscures visualization and prevents adequate distention. If this occurs, then the arthroscope should be removed and redirected medially into the central portion of the bursa, which will allow for distention and improve visualization. In most cases a posterior bursal veil is readily apparent, limiting visualization of the space even after distention. This veil should be cauterized and removed along with any additional bursa tissue that obstructs visualization of the structures within the space at the initiation of the procedure (Fig. 6–15).

A methodical diagnostic arthroscopy of the subacromial space is then performed. Subacromial anatomy, detailing those structures that can be visualized arthroscopically, has been well defined in studies by Matthews and Fadale[33] and Laumann.[34] The superior surface of the rotator cuff, in particular the supraspinatus and infraspinatus, should be examined carefully for any evidence of tearing or abrasion. By rotating the arm internally and externally, a thorough evaluation of each of these tendons can be completed. Abduction of the arm allows for visualization of the insertion site of the rotator cuff into the greater tuberosity. Evidence of cuff irritation or abrasion in this

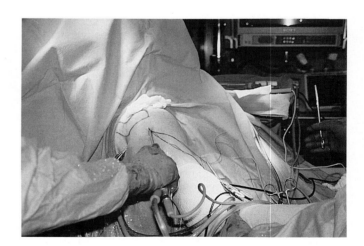

Figure 6–15 • Completing the acromioplasty with the arthroscope in the posterior soft-spot portal and the shaver in the lateral portal.

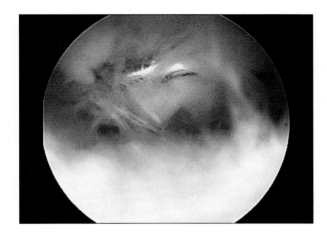

Figure 6–16 • Findings of abrasion on coracoacromial ligament and undersurface of acromion, consistent with impingement.

area would be consistent with the diagnosis of impingement. By redirecting the arthroscope superiorly, the coracoacromial ligament and the undersurface of the acromion are visualized. The degree and extent of acromial hooking can be documented as well as the width and insertion site of the coracoacromial ligament. Again, as with the rotator cuff, abrasion in the area of the anterolateral aspect of the acromion or of the fibers of the coracoacromial ligament would be consistent with a diagnosis of impingement (Fig. 6–16).

Coracoacromial Ligament Release and Acromioplasty

After diagnostic arthroscopy of the subacromial space has been completed and appropriate findings have been documented, coracoacromial ligament release and acromioplasty are performed. With the arthroscope in the posterior portal, an insulated 90 degree angled bipolar electrocautery is placed through the lateral portal to morsalize and coagulate the periosteum and coracoacromial ligament attachment on the undersurface of the acromion. This tissue is then removed by utilizing a full-radius resector, resulting in better visualization of the anterior and lateral margins of the acromion and remaining coracoacromial ligament attachment. The coracoacromial ligament is then released via one of two techniques. The first technique involves direct release of the ligament from the anterior edge of the acromion by utilizing the electrocautery. If this technique is utilized, the electrocautery must be kept directly against the bone as the vessels within the ligament are 5–8 mm from the acromial edge, and derivation into the ligament fibers may result in significant bleeding from the acromioclavicular branch of the coracoacromial artery[35] (Figs. 6–17A and B). The second technique releases the ligament by removing the leading 4–5 mm of the acromion with a bur. This technique is advantageous in that it distances the instrumentation from the fibers of the

ligament and therefore reduces the incidence of bleeding at the time of ligament release[36] (Figs. 6–17C and D). If bleeding is encountered, then anesthetic depression of systolic blood pressure, elevation of the irrigation fluid bags, or increasing irrigation pump flow and pressure will improve hemostasis and visibility so that precise use of the electrocautery may be employed.

The acromioplasty is then performed. By using an acromionizer or a round bur, the anterolateral corner and anterior leading edge of the acromion (usually 5–8 mm) are resected to a level parallel to that of the leading edge of the patient's distal clavicle. Meticulous care is taken during this portion of the procedure to preserve the anterior deltoid attachment. Being able to visualize the attachment of the deltoid signifies the level at which the resection is complete. If deltoid muscular fibers are visualized or are readily apparent along the resection plane, that should raise suspicion that the deltoid insertion has been disrupted and that repair may be necessary.

The posterior margin of the acromioplasty, as calculated from preoperative x-ray films, is then located with a graduated measuring device placed through the anterior portal or by referencing this level in relation to the posterior aspect of the patient's distal clavicle. After this level is determined, an acromionizer is used through the lateral portal to create a trough approximately 3 mm in depth across the full width of the acromion. This trough serves as a reference for the posterior resection level and as a leading edge of bone for the acromionizer, making it much more effective when it is utilized to resect the acromion through the posterior portal (author's conversation with S. Snyder, MD [1995]) (Fig. 6–18).

The acromionizer and arthroscope are now switched, respectively, from the lateral to the posterior portals. The acromionizer is then swept or planed, beginning at the edge of the posterior reference trough, in a mediolateral direction until the undersurface of the acromion has been completely flattened or smoothed[37] (Fig. 6–19). After the resection is complete, the arthroscope is replaced posteriorly for better visualization of any residual spurring of the anterolateral acromial corner, which is difficult to view from the lateral portal (Fig. 6–20).

Finally, the arthroscope is directed toward the acromioclavicular joint and distal clavicle (Fig. 6–21). The capsule of the acromioclavicular joint is released by utilizing the cautery and is resected from the inferior surface of the clavicle. The clavicle can be utilized at this time as a reference for the level of acromioplasty that has been completed. If significant degeneration or downward spurring of the clavicle exists, then the undersurface of the distal clavicle may be resected utilizing a 1/4 in osteotome through the lateral portal or the acromionizer (Figs. 6–22A, B, and D). If necessary, downward pressure over the distal clavicle can aid in the clavicle's visualization and stabilization during the course of undersurface resection. Unless complete distal clavicular excision is indicated, only the inferior clavicular facet should be resected as overaggressive resection may lead to prolonged irritation of the acromioclavicular joint postoperatively, especially in those patients who undergo a more aggressive postoperative rehabilitation program (Figs. 6–22C and E).

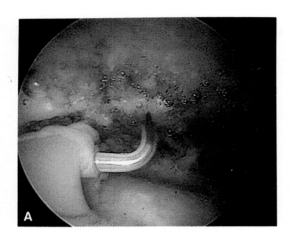

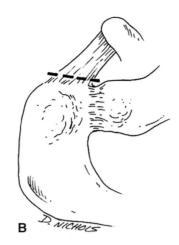

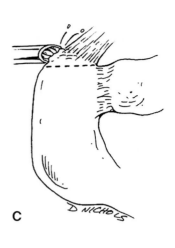

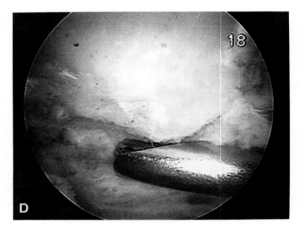

Figure 6–17 • Release of the coracoacromial ligament. *A* and *B*, By direct resection from the anterior acromion utilizing the electrocautery to coagulate the tissue on the acromion undersurface at its leading edge. *C*, By resecting the leading bony edge of the acromion, utilizing the acromionizer bur. *D*, By using the acromionizer to resect the leading edge of the acromion. The deltoid attachment has been protected and is denoted as the white fibrous tissue beyond the acromionizer.

Figure 6–18 • *A* and *B*, Creation of a trough at the posterior edge of acromial resection based on preoperative radiographic calculation with the bur in lateral portal.

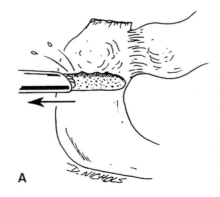

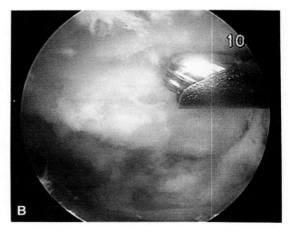

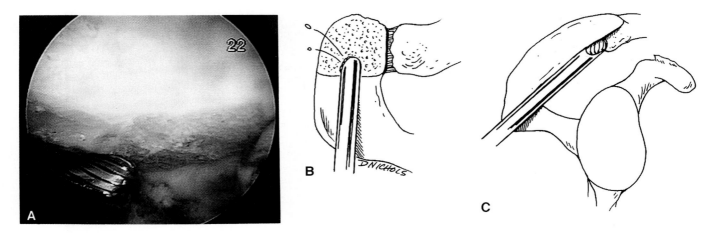

Figure 6–19 • *A*, *B*, *C*, Planing of the acromion from the posterior portal with the acromionizer.

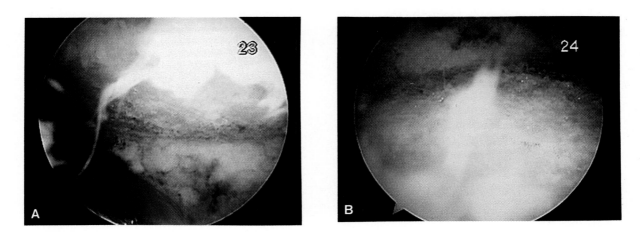

Figure 6–20 • The acromion viewed from the lateral portal on completion of the acromioplasty. *A*, The resection is viewed anatomically with the arthroscope. *B*, The smoothness of the resection is noted with anatomical references flipped 180 degrees.

POSTOPERATIVE CARE AND REHABILITATION

Postoperative Care

After the operative procedure has been completed, the portal sites and subacromial space are routinely injected with local anesthetic to assist in postoperative pain control. The portals are closed with nonabsorbable sutures, and a bulky dressing is placed to absorb any irrigation fluid draining from the incision sites. This dressing is routinely changed to an adhesive bandage dressing on the first postoperative day. This dressing improves the effect of postoperative cryotherapy and provides less restriction to passive motion of the shoulder. A sling is utilized up to the end of the first week postoperatively or until the patient's deltoid can support the shoulder without displaying signs of fatigue. Portal sutures are removed at 7–10 days postoperatively and are replaced with Steri-Strips. The patient is allowed to shower at 2 days postoperatively, but baths that immerse the portal sites are not allowed until the sutures are removed. Normal activities of daily living may be resumed when postoperative discomfort of the shoulder subsides.

Rehabilitation Days 1 to 10

On the day of surgery, pendulum or circumduction exercises are initiated as postsurgical pain is controlled. Passive range-of-motion exercises that stress nonpainful, fully assisted forward flexion and internal and external rotation are demonstrated. These exercises are advanced to active-

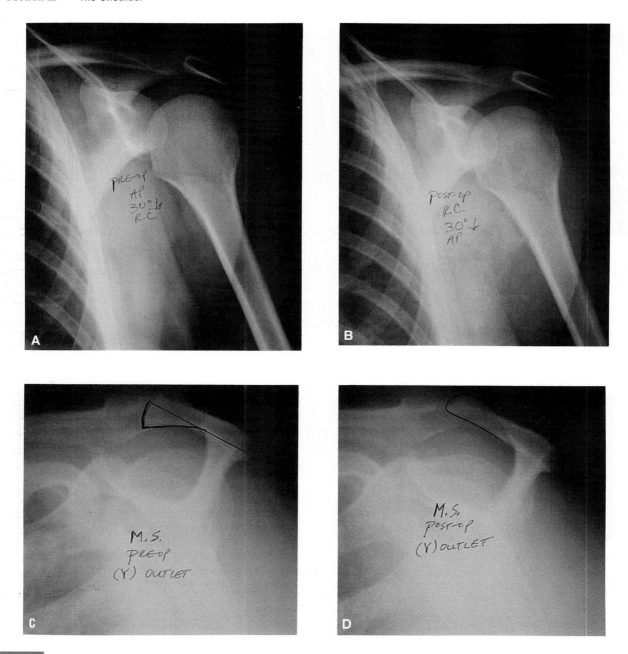

Figure 6–21 • *A* and *B*, Pre- and postoperative 30 degree caudal tilt anteroposterior, *C*, supraspinatus, and *D*, Y-outlet views demonstrate the appropriate resection level for acromioplasty.

assisted exercises with the T-bar or pulley as tolerated by the patient. Nonsteroidal anti-inflammatory medications and modalities including ice, electrical stimulation, and ultrasound are utilized to reduce swelling and the inflammatory effects of the surgery. A scapular stabilization program is begun that emphasizes scapulothoracic mechanics throughout shoulder range of motion. A glenohumeral capsular stretching program is initiated utilizing the opposite arm to create a gentle and nonpainful stretching sensation on the operative side.

Rehabilitation Day 10 to Week 6

Active-assisted activities are continued until a full, painless range of motion is achieved. Capsular stretching and scapular stabilization are stressed, and an isometric program for the rotator cuff and deltoid is initiated (Fig. 6–23*A*). Abduction of the shoulder is avoided because it may result in creating pain and an acute inflammatory response. Patients at this time should be cautioned against overly aggressive activities as their postoperative discom-

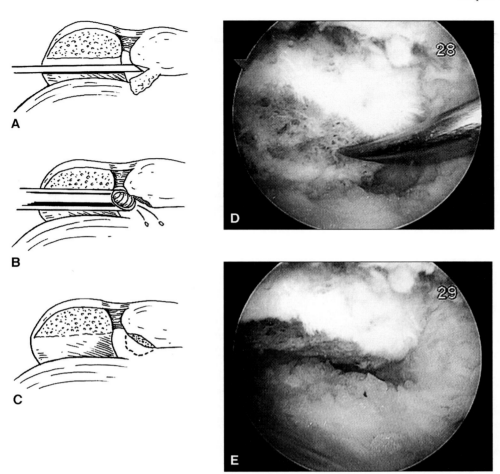

Figure 6–22 • Resection of inferior clavicular spurring utilizing (*A* and *D*) 1/4 in osteotome, (*B*) acromionizer, and (*C* and *E*) final resection level denoting no evidence of downward impingement into the rotator cuff.

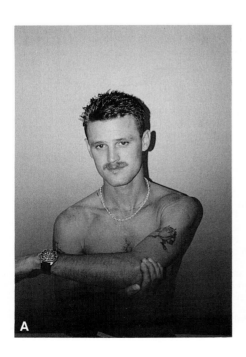
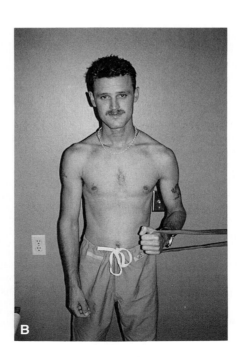

Figure 6–23 • Postoperative rehabilitation. *A*, Posterior capsular stretching is stressed as tightness of the posterior capsule forces the humeral head upward against the acromion as the shoulder is brought into flexion. *B*, Postoperative rehabilitation with initiation of a gentle rotator cuff exercise program with TheraBand for internal and external rotators.

fort subsides because such activities may lead to increased inflammation and loss of function. Inflammation is again controlled with the assistance of physical therapy modalities and nonsteroidal anti-inflammatory medications.

Rehabilitation Week 6 to 12

Submaximal isokinetic exercises in the scapular or subimpingement plane are initiated and are advanced with TheraBand or surgical tubing as long as the shoulder remains nonpainful (Fig. 6–23*B*). Abduction activities may begin but are limited to less than 90 degrees. Light overhead activity may be resumed, including less strenuous sports-related activities. Maximal strengthening activities, heavy overhead work, and strenuous throwing or racquet sports should be avoided until at least 12 weeks after surgery.

RESULTS AND COMPLICATIONS

The results of arthroscopic acromioplasty should not be judged before 6 months postoperatively,[29] and patients may demonstrate continued improvement up to 12 months after surgery. Satisfactory results utilizing the arthroscope for decompression have been reported in 80–90% of patients with stage II disease,[7, 38] but results in patients with stage III disease, those with rotator cuff tears, remain somewhat controversial.[7, 8, 14, 39, 40] Overall, results utilizing the arthroscopic technique compare favorably with those of the traditional open acromioplasty, including Neer's techniques.[3, 11, 30, 41, 42]

The failure of a patient to regain good function after acromioplasty has been attributed to several factors, the foremost among these being an error in diagnosis or an inadequate decompression. Failure to recognize, especially in athletes who are engaged in sports that involve overhead use of the extremity or in patients with generalized laxity and multidirectional instability, that impingement was secondary to instability is the most common diagnostic pitfall. It is important for the physician examining the patient to remember that approximately 20% of patients presenting with generalized laxity and multidirectional instability demonstrate symptoms of impingement.[40, 43] Because acromioplasty is usually ineffective, surgical stabilization of the shoulder may prove necessary in these patients to control their impingement symptoms.

An inadequate acromioplasty may also result in clinical failure.[29, 38] For patients who continue to exhibit pain through the impingement arc, careful radiographic analysis is warranted on 30 degree caudal tilt anteroposterior, supraspinatus Y-outlet, Zanca 10 degree cephalic tilt, and cervical spine views to document the level of acromial bony resection and to note evidence of any acromioclavicular joint or cervical spine disorder. Unfortunately, if a second attempt at surgical decompression is attempted, results utilizing either an open or arthroscopic surgical technique have been reported to correct impingement or eliminate pain in less than 50% of cases.[29, 44] Other reported complications associated with arthroscopic subacromial decompression include overaggressive thinning

of the acromion with fracture,[8, 32] formation of subacromial heterotopic ossification postoperatively,[45] brachial plexus injuries,[8] hypoglossal nerve palsies,[46] deltoid detachment with persistent pain, and reflex sympathetic dystrophy.

SUMMARY

Arthroscopic subacromial decompression has become an accepted standard in the treatment of patients with stages II and III impingement lesions. Results utilizing the technique compare favorably with those of open acromioplasty. The arthroscopic technique offers many advantages when compared with the traditional open acromioplasty, including a significant reduction in postoperative morbidity. The procedure may therefore be performed on an outpatient or overnight-stay basis. Because the deltoid is left attached, potential complications of deltoid rupture with resulting deltoid weakness are not encountered.

Unfortunately, the procedure is somewhat technically demanding surgically. This results in surgeons dealing with a steep learning curve when attempting to perform the procedure utilizing the arthroscope. Careful preoperative clinical and radiographic planning, appropriate operative equipment, a skilled operative staff, and familiarity with the arthroscopic anatomy are essential if an adequate decompression is to be performed with a minimum of complications. As with open acromioplasty, the procedure should be effective in treating patients with primary impingement who have failed a course of conservative management of their condition.

References

1. Neer CS: Anterior acromioplasty for the chronic impingement syndrome in the shoulder: a preliminary report. J Bone Joint Surg Am 54:41–50, 1972.
2. Jackson DW: Chronic rotator cuff impingement in the throwing athlete. Am J Sports Med 4:231–240, 1976.
3. Hawkins RJ and Kennedy JC: Impingement syndrome in athletes. Am J Sports Med 8:151–158, 1980.
4. McShane RB, Leinberry CF, and Fenlin JM: Conservative open anterior acromioplasty. Clin Orthop 223:137–144, 1987.
5. Rockwood CA and Lyons FA: Shoulder impingement syndrome: diagnosis, radiographic evaluation, and treatment with a modified neer acromioplasty. J Bone Joint Surg Am 75:1593–1605, 1993.
6. Ellman H: Arthroscopic subacromial decompression. Orthop Trans 9:49, 1985.
7. Ellman H: Arthroscopic subacromial decompression: analysis of one- to three-year results. Arthroscopy 3:173–181, 1987.
8. Paulos LE and Franklin JL: Arthroscopic shoulder decompression development and application: a five year experience. Am J Sports Med 17:235–244, 1990.
9. Paulos LE, Harner CD, and Parker RD: Arthroscopic subacromial decompression for impingement syndrome of the shoulder. Tech Orthop 3:33–39, 1988.
10. Hawkins RJ: Presented at Meeting of American Academy of Orthopaedic Surgeons, New Orleans, Feb., 1994.
11. Neer CS: Impingement lesions. Clin Orthop 173:70–77, 1983.
12. Iannotti JP: Rotator cuff disorders. Presented at Meeting of American Academy of Orthopaedic Surgeons, Chicago, March, 1991.
13. Rockwood CA and Burkhead WZ: Débridement of massive rotator cuff tears. Presented at Meeting of American Academy of Orthopaedic Surgeons, San Francisco, Feb., 1993.
14. Burkheart SS: Arthroscopic treatment of massive rotator cuff tears. Orthop Trans 14:173, 1990.

15. Burkhead WZ, Jr and Rockwood CA, Jr: Treatment of instability of the shoulder with an exercise program. J Bone Joint Surg 74:890–896, 1992.
16. Matsen FA: Subacromial impingement. In Rockwood CA and Matsen FA (eds.): The Shoulder. Philadelphia, W.B. Saunders Co., 1990, pp 623–646.
17. Post M: Suprascapular nerve entrapment: diagnosis and results of treatment. J Shoulder Elbow Surg 2:190–198, 1994.
18. Rockwood CA and Curtis RJ: X-ray evaluation of shoulder problems. In Rockwood CA and Matsen FA (eds.): The Shoulder. W.B. Saunders Co., 1991, pp 178–207.
19. Groh GI, Heckman MM, Allen TA, et al.: Treatment of snapping scapula with a physical therapy program. Presented at Meeting of American Academy of Orthopaedic Surgeons, Orlando, Fla., Feb., 1995.
20. Morrison DS and Bigliani LU: The clinical significance of variations in acromial morphology. Presented at Meeting of American Shoulder and Elbow Surgeons, San Francisco, Feb., 1987.
21. Johnson LL: Shoulder arthroscopy. In Johnson LL (ed.): Arthroscopic Surgery: Principles and Practice. St. Louis, C.V. Mosby Co., 1986, pp 1301–1445.
22. Andrews JR and Carson WG: Shoulder joint arthroscopy. Orthopedics 12:1157–1162, 1983.
23. Caspari RB: Shoulder arthroscopy: a review of the present state of the art. Contemp Orthop 4:523, 1982.
24. Spinner M: Injuries to the Major Branches of Peripheral Nerves in the Forearm. Philadelphia, W.B. Saunders Co., 1978.
25. Andrews JR, Carson WG, and Ortega K: Arthroscopy of the shoulder: technique and normal anatomy. Am J Sports Med 12:1–7, 1984.
26. Skyhar NJ, Altchek DW, Warren RF, et al.: Shoulder arthroscopy with patient in the beach chair position. Arthroscopy 4:256–259, 1988.
27. Caspari RB: Anatomy and portals for arthroscopic surgery of the shoulder. In McGinty JB (ed.): Arthroscopic Surgery Update: Techniques in Orthopaedics. Rockville, Md., Aspen Systems Corp., 1985, pp 15–24.
28. Caspari RB: Instrumentation and operating room organization for arthroscopy of the shoulder. In McGinty JB (ed.): Arthroscopic Surgery Update: Techniques in Orthopaedics. Rockville, Md., Aspen Systems Corp., 1985, pp 155–160.
29. Ellman H: Arthroscopic acromioplasty. In McGinty JB (ed.): Operative Arthroscopy. New York, Raven Press, 1991.
30. Esch JC, Ozerkis LR, Helgager JA, et al.: Arthroscopic subacromial decompression results according to the degree of rotator cuff tear. Arthroscopy 4:241–249, 1988.
31. Wuh HCK and Snyder SJ: Modified classification of the supraspinatus outlet view based on the configuration and the anatomical thickness of the acromion. Presented at the 59th Meeting of the American Academy of Orthopaedic Surgeons, Washington, D.C., Feb., 1992.
32. Andrews JR and Carson WG: Arthroscopic Anatomy of the Shoulder. In McGinty JB (ed.): Shoulder Surgery in the Athlete: Techniques in Orthopaedics. Rockville, Md., Aspen Systems Corp., 1985, pp 25–30.
33. Matthews LS and Fadale PD: Subacromial anatomy for the arthroscopist. Arthroscopy 36–40, 1989.
34. Laumann V: Decompression of the subacromial space: an anatomical study. In Bayley and Kessell (eds.): Shoulder Surgery. Berlin, Springer-Verlag, 1982, pp 14–21.
35. Esch JC and Baker C: Surgical Arthroscopy: The Shoulder and Elbow. Philadelphia, J.B. Lippincott Co., 1993.
36. Caspari RB and Thal R: A technique for arthroscopic subacromial decompression. Arthroscopy 8:23–30, 1992.
37. Sampson TJ, Nesbit JK, and Glick JM: Precision acromioplasty and arthroscopic subacromial decompression. Arthroscopy 7:301–307, 1991.
38. Paulos LE, Chamberlain S, and Murray S: Arthroscopic shoulder decompression: techniques and preliminary results. Orthop Trans X:222, 1986.
39. Altchek DW, Warren RF, Wickiewicy TL, et al.: Arthroscopic acromioplasty: technique and results. J Bone Joint Surg Am 72:1198–1207, 1990.
40. Levy HA, Gardner RD, and Lemak LJ: Arthroscopic subacromial decompression in treatment of full thickness rotator cuff tears. Arthroscopy 7:8–13, 1991.
41. Raggio CL, Warren RF, and Sculco T: Surgical treatment of impingement syndrome: four year follow-up. Orthop Trans 9:48–49, 1985.
42. Ha'eri GB, and Wiley AM: Shoulder impingement syndrome: results of operative release. Clin Orthop 168:128–132, 1982.
43. Schneider T, Strauss JM, Hoffstetter I, et al.: Shoulder joint stability after arthroscopic subacromial decompression. Arch Orthop Trauma Surg 113:129–133, 1994.
44. Hawkins RJ, Saddemi SR, and Mor JT: Analysis of failed arthroscopic subacromial decompression (abstract). Arthroscopy 7:315–316, 1991.
45. Berg EE, Ciullo JV, and Oglesby JW: Failure of arthroscopic decompression by subacromial heterotopic ossification causing recurrent impingement. Arthroscopy 10:158–161, 1994.
46. Mullins RC, Drez D, Jr, and Cooper J: Hyperglossal nerve palsy after arthroscopy of the shoulder and open operation with the patient in the beach chair position: a case report. J Bone Joint Surg Am 74:137–139, 1992.

Chapter

7

Rotator Cuff Tears

Timothy B. Sutherland

The advent of shoulder arthroscopy has introduced an important new tool for the treatment and diagnosis of rotator cuff injuries in the competitive and recreational athlete. Rotator cuff disorders remain, however, a diagnostic and therapeutic challenge for the sports medicine physician. Timely and accurate diagnosis, coupled with appropriate treatment, allows safe and expedient return to preinjury status.

HISTORY AND PHYSICAL FINDINGS

A complete and accurate history and physical examination are crucial in the evaluation of the athletic rotator cuff injury.[1] The athlete should be questioned regarding the presence of weakness and pain. Pain location, onset, quality, severity, and timing should be indicated. Sports-related and position-specific questions help define the athlete's disability. Questions for the throwing athlete should concern the level of competition (recreational, collegiate, or professional), the position played, the exact activity and motion that reproduce the patient's disability, and the phase of throwing affected (windup, cocking, acceleration, deceleration, or follow-through). The thrower's control, velocity, and endurance (both pitch count and innings pitched) should also be carefully scrutinized to obtain subtle hints as to the underlying problem. The collision athlete should be questioned carefully regarding the location and position of the injured extremity at impact, the presence of any neurologic symptoms (weakness or numbness), and the current functional disability. The player's protective equipment (padding) should be assessed carefully for its role both in preventing injury and in allowing early return to competition. Competitive and highly trained athletes are often able to pinpoint the location and exacerbating activities of their shoulder injuries, thus greatly assisting in diagnosis.

A complete physical examination is essential. Observation of the athlete at rest, disrobing, and reproducing athletic motions can provide subtle information regarding muscle atrophy and abnormal motion patterns. Game films of the athlete, if available, can be reviewed to evaluate both the initial mechanism of injury and current postinjury status. Gentle palpation can reveal specific areas of tenderness and should include the sternoclavicular joint, the acromioclavicular joint, the rotator cuff insertion, and the anterior and posterior glenohumeral joint. Strength testing with manual muscle testing and carefully documented active and passive range-of-motion testing should be done for both shoulders. Range-of-motion tests should be done with the athlete in both the sitting and supine positions. Specific tests for impingement, stability, and labral problems are then done.[2]

After a complete history and physical examination, ancillary tests are conducted if necessary to assist in diagnosis or treatment. For most athletes, a standard set of plain radiographs is obtained. This evaluation includes anteroposterior views in internal and external rotation, a West Point axillary view, and a Stryker notch view. With suspected rotator cuff injury, additional views are utilized to define the anatomy of the acromion and the coracoacromial arch. The supraspinatus outlet[3] and the acromial profile views[4] have been described for this purpose. Additional radiographic studies including magnetic resonance imaging (MRI) scans, contrast-enhanced MRI scans, and arthrograms are ordered on a case-by-case basis. Routine use of these specialized studies is unnecessary; they should be used only if the outcome will alter therapeutic decision-making. Isokinetic muscle testing, at both low and high speeds, can be used to document and diagnose subtle motor deficiencies. Electrodiagnostic testing (electromyograms and nerve conduction velocity studies) is used occasionally if a nerve injury is suspected on the basis of history and physical examination.

INJURIES TO THE ROTATOR CUFF

Rotator cuff disease can be classified by mechanism of injury and morphologic picture. The four major categories of rotator cuff injury in the athlete are primary compressive cuff disease, secondary compressive cuff disease, tensile failure of the cuff, and acute traumatic rotator cuff tears. The overhead athlete most commonly presents with some manifestation of overuse cuff failure, whereas acute traumatic rotator cuff tears are seen more commonly in collision sports and high-energy injuries. Rotator cuff injuries can also be classified morphologically by the tendon involved, the surface involved (bursal, articular, or both), and the percentage of the cuff compromised.

Primary Compressive Cuff Disease

Primary compressive cuff disease is essentially the classic impingement lesion described by Neer.[5] Extrinsic compression on the rotator cuff from the coracoacromial arch combined with age-related degenerative changes within the tendon itself leads to primary compressive disease. Clinically, these patients present with the insidious onset of shoulder pain, radiation to the deltoid muscle, nocturnal pain, and exacerbation of symptoms with overhead activities. Examination generally reveals a positive impingement sign (pain with internal rotation and forward flexion)[6] in a painful arc from 80 to 120 degrees of forward flexion. The impingement test, which is the relief of symptoms with injection of local anesthetic into the subacromial space, often confirms the diagnosis. Primary compressive disease is found most commonly in athletes older than 40 years of age, and these patients are most often involved in overhead sports. The pain can often be localized temporally to the follow-through stages in throwing and racquet sports when the internally rotated arm enters the painful arc of flexion. Variable amounts of rotator cuff weakness can be present secondary to either pain or actual rotator cuff involvement (tendinitis, partial-thickness rotator cuff tearing, or full-thickness tearing).

Weakness should be evaluated during physical examination, with external rotation strength at 0 and 90 degrees of abduction, the "empty can test," and internal rotation at 0 degrees of abduction. Weakness secondary to pain is often alleviated completely with subacromial injection of local anesthetic (the impingement test).

Primary compressive disease is uncommon in athletes younger than 35 years of age. Young patients with true primary compressive cuff disease generally demonstrate bony abnormalities of the coracoacromial arch, either a congenitally hooked (type III) acromion[7, 8] or an os acromiale.[9] Most commonly, athletes younger than 35 years of age with impingement symptoms have underlying anterior glenohumeral instability. History and physical examination reveal evidence of this instability, which should be carefully sought in the young athlete.[10]

Secondary Compressive Cuff Disease

Anterior glenohumeral instability often presents as secondary compressive cuff disease in young athletes.[10] Failure of the glenohumeral ligament capsule complex, the static stabilizer of the shoulder, leads to overuse and progressive fatigue of the dynamic stabilizers of the shoulder,

the rotator cuff. This fatigue allows abnormal translation of the humeral head with impingement under the coracoacromial arch. This abnormal translation can also lead to internal impingement of the posterosuperior rotator cuff on the glenoid in the cocking position of abduction with maximal external rotation.[11] Distinguishing primary from secondary compressive disease is critical because the treatment approaches are radically different. The impingement sign and test can be positive in both primary and secondary compressive disease, and a meticulous examination must be done to delineate the often subtle findings of anterior glenohumeral instability.

Tensile Cuff Failure

Tensile lesions are seen most commonly in overhead athletes and occur as undersurface rotator cuff tears or lesions of the biceps anchor labral complex.[12–14] This tensile failure is due to repetitive microtrauma during the deceleration phase of throwing with eccentric overload of the cuff as it resists the forces of horizontal adduction, internal rotation, anterior translation, and distraction. Partial tears secondary to this repetitive microtrauma are usually seen in the undersurface of the supraspinatus and posterior cuff tendons.[15] Tensile lesions can also be secondary to anterior laxity with increased forces placed on the posterior cuff musculature. On physical examination, athletes with tensile lesions often have minimal weakness, with pain primarily over the supraspinatus and infraspinatus tendons and the posterior capsule. Advanced radiographic imaging with computed tomography arthrograms or contrast-enhanced MRI may reveal partial undersurface tearing.

Acute Traumatic Rotator Cuff Tears

Acute traumatic rotator cuff tears are uncommon in the athlete's shoulder and are most commonly seen in collision sports or as a sequela of high-energy trauma. The usual mechanism of injury is forced adduction or active abduction against resistance. Athletes with this problem present with a single well-defined traumatic episode. Examination reveals variable degrees of discomfort with significant weakness of the rotator cuff musculature. Expedient diagnosis and early treatment with rotator cuff repair seem to offer these athletes the best functional result.

INITIAL TREATMENT

Except for the acute traumatic tear, the initial treatment of most rotator cuff injuries is conservative. This conservative treatment involves a supervised rehabilitation program emphasizing the protection of healing tissues with progression to complete return of motion and strength. All patients enter a carefully supervised interval sports program that is activity- and sports-specific and tailored to each athlete's underlying cuff disease.

The arthroscope is a secondary tool used in the diagnosis of elusive shoulder disorders and for the treatment of many common athletic rotator cuff injuries that prove recalcitrant to conservative treatment. Diagnostic arthroscopy of the shoulder allows enhancement of the clinical assessment of the rotator cuff condition, verification of the suspected clinical lesion, and precise delineation of the location and extent of underlying shoulder disease. The arthroscope can also be used for appropriate decompression and débridement as indicated by the patient's clinical and arthroscopic examination and presentation.

PREOPERATIVE EVALUATION

Surgical arthroscopy should begin in the clinic with the preoperative education and preparation of the athlete. Careful explanation of the proposed procedure greatly facilitates postoperative rehabilitation. Both the goals and limitations of surgery should be reviewed with the athlete, and the postoperative rehabilitation regimen should be outlined and emphasized to ensure compliance.

As intraoperative hemostasis is critical in achieving visualization of the subacromial space, preoperative evaluation should include the assessment of any bleeding tendency or coagulopathy. If any question of a bleeding disorder exists, appropriate laboratory studies (including prothrombin time, partial thromboplastin time, and bleeding time) should be checked. All nonsteroidal anti-inflammatory drugs and other prostaglandin inhibitors should be discontinued 7–10 days before surgery.

The supraspinatus outlet view or acromial profile view should be reviewed before surgery to assess the size of the acromial hook and acromial thickness. This allows estimation of the amount of bone to be resected anteriorly and the total amount of bone that can be removed without increasing the risk of postoperative acromial fracture. Acromions less than 8–10 mm thick on outlet views should be decompressed carefully to avoid overthinning and fracture. Preoperative muscle strength and ancillary studies (MRI scan, arthrograms) should be reviewed to allow for planning of rotator cuff repair if clinically indicated. The possibility of an occult full-thickness rotator cuff repair, missed by preoperative studies but revealed with arthroscopy, should be discussed with the patient. As well, the technique of an open rotator cuff repair, with its implication for postoperative rehabilitation and return to sports, should be discussed.

OPERATIVE TECHNIQUE

After appropriate preoperative preparation, the patient is taken to the operating suite. The author commonly uses general anesthesia for routine shoulder arthroscopy unless contraindicated by the patient's overall medical health. If an open or miniopen rotator cuff repair is planned or probable, an interscalene regional block may be used to supplement general anesthesia. A careful examination under general anesthesia is done on both shoulders. Translation anteriorly, posteriorly, and inferiorly is assessed in neutral rotation, internal rotation, and external rotation and is documented in the operative report. The patient is positioned in the lateral decubitus position and is supported by a bean bag or kidney rest. All bony prominences are padded, and an axillary roll is used if necessary. The arm is suspended from the overhead pulley system in about 60 to 70 degrees of abduction and 15 degrees of forward flexion. The suspension rope is secured to a free-hanging weight of 10–20 lb. The lightest weight that suspends the arm adequately without exerting undue traction is utilized. The operating room table is rotated to allow access to both the anterior and posterior aspects of the shoulder. After the shoulder is sterilely prepared and draped, the essential bony anatomic landmarks are marked with a sterile marking pen: the anterolateral and posterolateral corners of the acromion, the acromioclavicular joint, and the coracoid process.[16]

The author routinely adds epinephrine to the arthroscopic fluid (one ampule of 1:1000 epinephrine per 3 L bag of fluid). At this point the patient's blood pressure is checked and the systolic pressure is reduced to 90 mm Hg or less (if the patient's overall cardiovascular condition permits). These two maneuvers help to obtain hemostasis in the bursal space and ensure adequate visualization for arthroscopy.

The acromioclavicular joint is palpated, and an 18 gauge needle is inserted into the joint. It is useful to visualize the angle of the acromioclavicular joint on the anteroposterior shoulder radiograph before needle insertion. This assists in the localization of the acromioclavicular joint when the arthroscope is in the subacromial space; this localization is most easily accomplished before arthroscopy because the soft tissues may become distended.

Diagnostic Arthroscopy

The posterior portal is established first, and its location is identified by palpating the posterior "soft spot" over the glenohumeral joint. This point is approximately 2–3 cm inferior and 1 cm medial to the posterolateral corner of the acromion and represents the interval between the infraspinatus and the teres minor. Gentle internal and external rotation of the arm can assist in localizing this interval. Care should be taken to avoid being too close to the posterior acromion as this can make visualization of the anterior acromion and acromioclavicular joint difficult. An 18 gauge needle is inserted in the soft spot and advanced toward the coracoid process anteriorly. A gentle pop may be felt as the needle penetrates the posterior capsule. The glenohumeral joint is distended with 40–50 mL of saline, and free backflow from the needle confirms intra-articular placement. As the joint reaches maximal distention, the arm is observed to rotate gently. The spinal needle is removed, and a small stab incision is made in the skin with a No. 11 blade. The arthroscopic cannula and dull trocar are advanced to the glenohumeral joint. Only dull trocars are used, and it is advised that the sharp trocars be removed from the surgical field to avoid inadvertent use. The tip of the dull trocar is used to palpate the posterior rim of the glenoid, and the arthroscopic cannula is inserted just lateral to the posterior rim.

The arthroscope is inserted, and the glenohumeral joint is initially assessed. The biceps tendon is used for orientation and is examined for any degenerative change or

Undersurface tendon

Humeral head

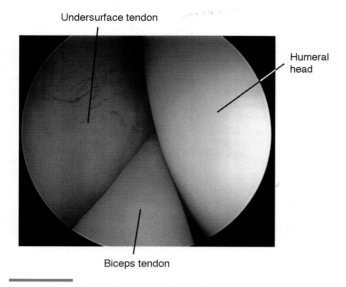

Biceps tendon

Figure 7–1 • Normal undersurface of rotator cuff.

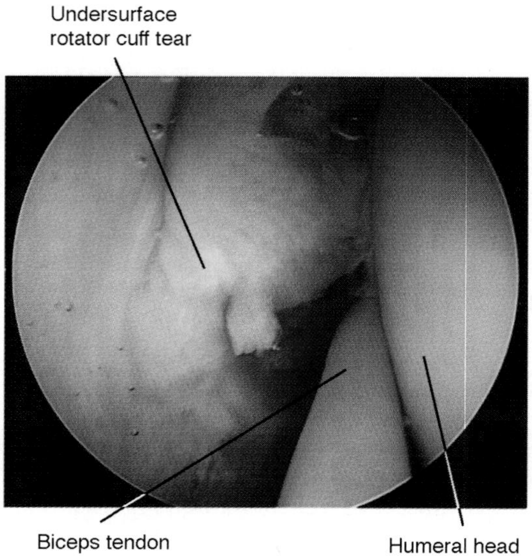

Undersurface rotator cuff tear

Biceps tendon

Humeral head

Figure 7–2 • Undersurface tear of supraspinatus.

detachment of the biceps labral anchor. The anterior capsulolabral complex is evaluated for evidence of a traumatic Bankart lesion, with detachment of the anteroinferior labrum from bone, or the presence of capsular laxity. If the arthroscope can be advanced without difficulty anteroinferiorly between the humeral head and the glenoid, this is considered evidence of abnormal capsular laxity. The articular surfaces of the humeral head and the glenoid are examined for evidence of chondral damage. The anterior and posterior humeral heads are evaluated for the presence of Hill-Sachs or reverse Hill-Sachs lesions consistent with pathologic laxity.

The entire rotator cuff is visualized. The subscapularis and rotator interval are inspected anteriorly. The biceps tendon and the undersurface of the supraspinatus tendon are checked for any evidence of wear or undersurface tearing (Fig. 7–1). The posterior cuff and its attachment to the humeral head just adjacent to the bare area are inspected. Fraying of the undersurface of the supraspinatus and the posterior cuff are seen with tensile failure of the cuff in overhead athletes[13] (Fig. 7–2). Full-thickness tears of the cuff are usually easily identified from the glenohumeral joint. Rotation of the arm allows all of the cuff to be studied and small full-thickness tears to be detected.

An anterior portal is established to allow complete visualization of the joint and the use of operating instruments. This portal is established halfway between the coracoid process and the anterolateral corner of the acromion. A spinal needle is passed from this location into the joint and visualized with the arthroscope. The needle should pass just below the biceps tendon, through the rotator interval, when viewed intra-articularly. If the initial examination revealed a traumatic Bankart lesion and consideration is being given to arthroscopic stabilization, the position of the anterior portal may be altered. In this situation the portal may be moved superiorly to just below the anterolateral corner of the acromion. The intra-articular position should be confirmed with spinal needle placement; the needle is then removed. A small skin incision is made, and the arthroscopic cannula and dull trocar are advanced into the joint under direct visualization. The arthroscope is inserted into the anterior portal, and the diagnostic arthroscopy is completed.

Operative Arthroscopy

The anterior capsuloligamentous structures and the posterior cuff and labrum are evaluated for undersurface tearing or degenerative change. Undersurface tears of the cuff can be débrided sequentially using the anterior and posterior portals utilizing a 5.2 mm motorized débrider. These undersurface tears are found most commonly in young throwing athletes. Débridement of the lesions allows many athletes to return to their preinjury status.[13] Any degenerative labral tears are débrided, taking care to prevent destabilization of the shoulder joint[17, 18] (Fig. 7–3). An additional anterior portal may be established inferior to the original anterior portal, if necessary for additional instrumentation. Large partial-thickness tears should be palpated to avoid missing a full-thickness tear. Internal and external rotation of the arm assists in visualizing the entire undersurface of the rotator cuff. If a large partial-thickness tear is identified and the surgeon suspects a full-thickness tear, the partial-thickness tear can be marked with a small suture. Under direct visualization an 18 gauge needle is passed below the acromion into the tear; a suture is advanced through this needle into the glenohumeral joint. The needle is removed, leaving the suture in place as a marker on the bursal surface of the tear. This area is inspected during the subacromial bursoscopy.

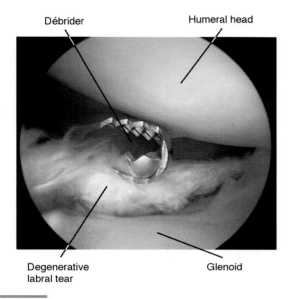

Figure 7–3 • Degenerative labral tear.

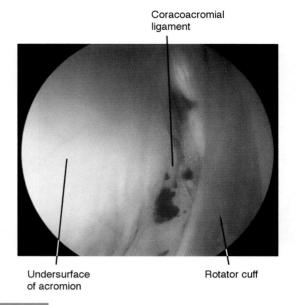

Figure 7–4 • Normal subacromial bursa.

Subacromial Bursoscopy

After the glenohumeral arthroscopy is completed, subacromial bursoscopy is done. Before beginning the bursoscopy, the athlete's blood pressure is checked to ensure adequate hypotension (systolic blood pressure less than 90 mm Hg) has been maintained. Bursal visualization may also be improved by lowering the overhead pulley system to decrease abduction of the shoulder to 15–20 degrees. The arthroscope and the cannula are removed from the glenohumeral joint. The arthroscopic cannula and dull trocar are taken through the posterior skin incision, the posterior acromion is palpated, and the cannula and trocar are advanced into the subacromial space. The coracoacromial ligament can often be palpated anteriorly with the tip of the trocar. Before inserting the arthroscope, the general position of the cannula is checked by lining up a second cannula of identical length on the superior aspect of the shoulder. Care is taken that the tip of the cannula is under the anterior aspect of the acromion, not medially under the acromioclavicular joint or laterally into the deltoid muscle. The arthroscope is inserted into the cannula in the bursal space. Even with bursal adhesions and scarring, a bursal space should be identifiable (Fig. 7–4). If not, often the posterior bursal curtain has not been penetrated, and the arthroscope should be removed and the dull trocar replaced in the cannula and advanced more anteriorly (Fig. 7–5). Occasionally, it may be necessary to establish an anterior bursal portal for outflow to improve visualization. This can be done by passing a blunt-tipped switching stick through the posterior portal. The stick can be passed through the anterior incision made previously, and a cannula is passed retrograde over the rod into the bursal space.

The subacromial space is evaluated. The coracoacromial ligament, undersurface of the acromion, superior sur-

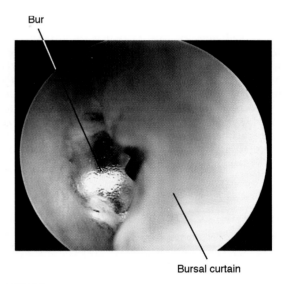

Figure 7–5 • Posterior bursal curtain.

face of the rotator cuff, and acromioclavicular joint are identified (Fig. 7–6). Subacromial adhesions and scarring often make visualization difficult, and a lateral portal must be established. A spinal needle is inserted approximately 1 cm posterior and 3 cm distal to the anterolateral corner of the acromion. This needle is visualized in the bursal space. The needle should be roughly parallel to the undersurface of the acromion. If the needle must be angled too far caudad or cephalad to be identified in the bursal space, then manipulation of instruments in the lateral portal will be difficult. A small skin incision is made, and the cannula with the dull trocar is advanced into the bursa. Débridement of the subacromial adhesions is accomplished with a

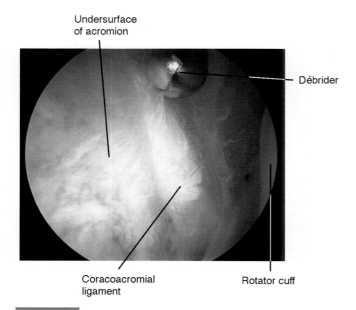

Undersurface
of acromion

Débrider

Coracoacromial
ligament

Rotator cuff

Figure 7–6 • Subacromial bursa.

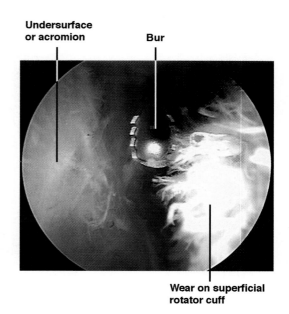

**Undersurface
or acromion**

Bur

**Wear on superficial
rotator cuff**

Figure 7–8 • Superficial rotator cuff wear.

motorized débrider. After débridement the subacromial space is evaluated for any evidence of impingement or rotator cuff tearing. The undersurface of the acromion and the coracoacromial ligament are examined for areas of abrasion or wear (Fig. 7–7). The bursa over the rotator cuff is débrided and examined for any evidence of abrasion or superficial partial-thickness rotator cuff tears (Fig. 7–8). If a marking suture was placed to localize a large partial-thickness articular side tear, this area on the bursa surface is inspected and palpated to ensure that no area of full-thickness tearing exists. The arm is internally and exter-

nally rotated to allow the entire cuff to be inspected. The arthroscope may be placed in the lateral and anterior bursal portals to complete visualization of the subacromial space and rotator cuff. All superficial partial-thickness tears should be débrided to viable tissue.

Visualization in the subacromial space can be problematic secondary to bleeding, and attention must be paid to hemostasis. The electrocautery is used liberally, to coagulate areas of active bleeding as well as prophylactically near the coracoacromial ligament and acromioclavicular joint (Fig. 7–9). Instrumentation of the subacromial space

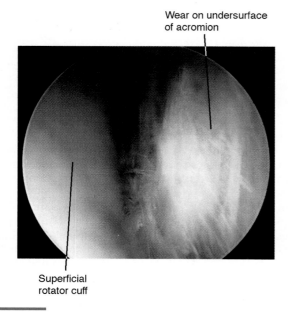

Wear on undersurface
of acromion

Superficial
rotator cuff

Figure 7–7 • Wear on undersurface of coracoacromial ligament.

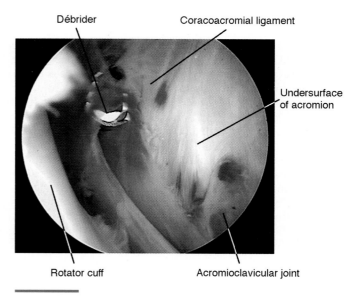

Débrider

Coracoacromial ligament

Undersurface
of acromion

Rotator cuff

Acromioclavicular joint

Figure 7–9 • Coracoacromial ligament.

often causes an increase in the athlete's blood pressure, and the systolic pressure should be maintained below 90 mm Hg. An arthroscopic pump system is routinely used; while in the bursa the pump system increases pressure from 30 mm Hg (used for glenohumeral arthroscopy) to 50–60 mm Hg in the subacromial space. Use of higher pressures does increase the risk of soft tissue distention, and surgery in the subacromial space must be accomplished efficiently and expediently.

Arthroscopic Acromioplasty

If evidence of impingement exists, or a full-thickness rotator cuff tear is identified, the surgeon should proceed with arthroscopic subacromial decompression. With the arthroscope in the posterior portal, a motorized débrider from the lateral portal is used to débride all soft tissues off the undersurface of the acromion. The acromioclavicular joint is visualized. Localization of the acromioclavicular joint is assisted by the previously placed 18 gauge spinal needle. The electrocautery is used liberally in this stage because the soft tissues below the acromion and surrounding the acromioclavicular joint are quite vascular. The electrocautery is used to divide and elevate the coracoacromial ligament from the anterior aspect of the acromion. At this point the anterior hook of the acromion can be identified, and the acromion appears to be longer in its posterior-to-anterior dimension (secondary to the anterior hook) (Fig. 7–10). An oval motorized bur is inserted through the lateral portal, and the anterior edge of the acromion is removed. Difficulty in maneuvering the bur to remove the anterior edge often indicates the presence of osteophytes on the lateral acromion, and these must be removed before removing the anterior acromion. As the anterior acromion is removed medially, the anterior acromioclavicular joint and distal clavicle are identified.

The remainder of the acromion is flattened utilizing the motorized bur. Care must be taken to avoid taking too much bone from the center of the acromion and creating a concavity, or "soup bowl," on the undersurface of the acromion. This occurs most commonly in patients with very soft cancellous bone or very hard cortical bone. The acromion is flattened posteriorly approximately 2–3 cm, and this point can be visualized by withdrawing the arthroscope slightly in the posterior portal.

The depth and the adequacy of the acromioplasty are assessed. The periosteal sleeve anteriorly is used to estimate the amount of bone removed. This layer is easily identifiable, and its depth can be estimated by the outside diameter of the bur cannula (Fig. 7–11). Typically, 8–10 mm from the anterior acromion is excised. The thickness of the acromion and the size of the anterior hook may alter the amount of bone resected. The distal clavicle is visualized, and the anterior resection is checked by the depth of the exposed distal clavicle. Depending on the presence of preoperative infraclavicular osteophytes, the resection should also measure approximately 4–6 mm. If any spurs are present on the undersurface of the distal clavicle, they are resected with a motorized bur at this time. These can be confirmed on preoperative radiographs that should support the presence of large infraclavicular spurs. Finally, the overall configuration of the acromion is examined. After adequate acromioplasty, the long diameter visualized should run in a medial-to-lateral direction secondary to excision of the anterior spur. The arthroscope maybe placed in the lateral portal to confirm that an adequate acromioplasty has been accomplished. The lateral view portal allows direct confirmation of the removal of the anterior hook and flattening of the undersurface of the acromion. With the arthroscope in this position, the motorized bur may be introduced through the posterior portal and used to flatten any remaining irregularities.

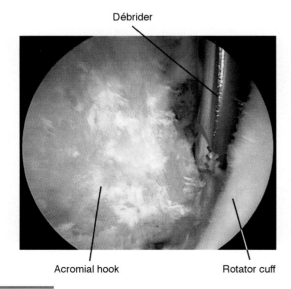

Figure 7–10 • Anterior acromial hook.

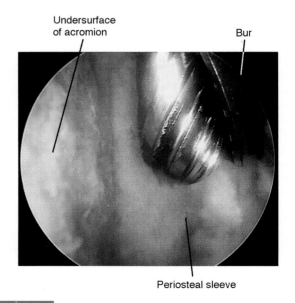

Figure 7–11 • Anterior acromioplasty.

Arthroscopic Distal Clavicle Excision

If the preoperative examination revealed significant acromioclavicular joint pain, arthroscopic distal clavicle excision is performed.[19] Adequate hemostasis and soft-tissue débridement are essential, and the anterior and posterior borders of the undersurface of the clavicle should be clearly visualized from the subacromial space. With the arthroscope in the posterior portal, the motorized bur can be introduced through the lateral bursal portal and the distal clavicle excision initiated. Approximately 1 cm of the inferior clavicle should be resected, from the anterior to the posterior aspect of the clavicle. With gentle downward pressure on the clavicle externally, approximately 50–75% of the inferior clavicle can be resected with the bur in the lateral portal. Ensure that both the anterior and posterior corners of the distal clavicle are excised. When no further clavicle can be excised using the lateral portal, the anterior portal is utilized. Just anterior to the acromioclavicular joint, an 18 gauge needle should be inserted into the joint under direct visualization. A small incision is made, and the dull trocar and cannula are introduced into the acromioclavicular joint. Often, the previously established anterior portal incision may be utilized. The motorized bur is placed in the anterior portal, and the remainder of the superior clavicle is excised. The final excision should be approximately 1 cm of the distal clavicle, with removal of the anterior and posterior borders done evenly. The arthroscope is placed sequentially in the lateral and anterior portals to ensure adequate clavicular excision (Fig. 7–12). The anterior acromioclavicular portal is particularly helpful, and the superior and posterior aspects of the clavicle may be visualized directly and evaluated. If residual superior or posterior clavicle is present, a posterior acromioclavicular portal may be established. The posterior acromioclavicular joint is palpated and, viewed from the anterior portal, an 18 gauge needle is placed, followed by a stab incision and a dull trocar. The motorized bur may be introduced, and the excision is completed under direct vision. Occasionally, a 70 degree arthroscope may be necessary and should be available on the sterile field.

Full-Thickness Rotator Cuff Tears

Full-thickness tears of the rotator cuff are evaluated arthroscopically from both the glenohumeral joint and the subacromial space (Fig. 7–13). Nonviable tissue is carefully débrided utilizing a motorized débrider. With large full-thickness tears, the mobility of the cuff tissue can be assessed by placing a grasper in the lateral portal and gently pulling on the cuff while observing from the posterior portal. The ability or inability to pull the cuff tissue to its attachment site on the greater tuberosity determines the mobility of the cuff. If a rotator cuff repair is planned and the cuff is unable to reach the tuberosity, an intra-articular capsular release is done. Viewing posteriorly from the glenohumeral joint, the capsule is released intra-articularly above the glenoid and labrum from approximately the 10-o'clock to 2-o'clock position. Instrumentation for release is introduced through the lateral bursal portal. Care must be taken to release only the superior capsule necessary to

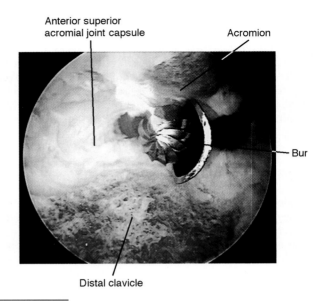

Figure 7–12 • Distal clavicle excision.

avoid creating an iatrogenic Bankart-type lesion. In athletes, significant fixed retraction of the cuff is uncommon.

In athletes with full-thickness tears of the rotator cuff, the author generally proceeds with diagnostic arthroscopy, arthroscopic subacromial decompression, and miniopen rotator cuff repair. The miniopen approach allows mobilization of the tendons, secure fixation of the cuff, and aggressive postoperative rehabilitation. The arthroscopic evaluation and subacromial decompression must be done expediently in this situation to avoid excessive fluid extravasation into the soft tissues, which can make miniopen repair difficult. The miniopen repair can be accomplished either by leaving the patient in the lateral

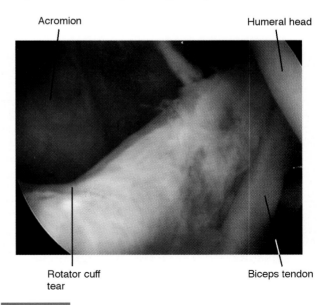

Figure 7–13 • Full-thickness rotator cuff tear.

decubitus position or by putting the patient into the standard beach-chair position. The author utilizes a 4–5 cm incision paralleling the lateral aspect of the acromion. This incision is centered over the anterolateral corner of the acromion in lines of minimum skin tension. This incision is preferred because it is easily extendable either anteriorly or posteriorly to approach the glenohumeral joint, prevents scarring and puckering of the skin incision into the deltoid incision, and is cosmetically pleasing. The incision is taken sharply to the deltoid fascia, hemostasis is obtained, and the raphe between the anterior and middle heads of the deltoid is identified. This interval is then developed, and it is taken up onto the acromion subperiosteally with a limit of extension to 4 cm distal to the acromion to protect the axillary nerve. The subacromial bursa is entered, and the bursa is débrided. The rotator cuff tear is identified, and core grasping sutures with No. 2 nonabsorbable sutures are placed just medial to the edge of the torn tendon. The cuff is mobilized. Intra-articular releases have been previously accomplished arthroscopically, and the superficial adhesions are released utilizing blunt dissection. If necessary, an anterior interval slide can be done in the rotator interval between the supraspinatus and subscapularis to the base of the coracoid process. Occasionally, if the cuff is quite retracted, a posterior interval slide between the superior and posterior cuff may also be necessary. This should be done carefully because the suprascapular nerve is vulnerable to injury with this maneuver. When the cuff has been adequately mobilized to reach its insertion site on the proximal humerus in 20 degrees of abduction, the humerus is prepared. A shallow trough is established just lateral to the articular surface of the humeral head. The cuff is repaired to bone with a belt-and-suspenders approach utilizing both anchors and interosseous sutures. Drill holes are made, and soft-tissue anchors are placed just lateral to the articular margin at intervals of 1 cm. The sutures from these anchors are passed through the cuff 8–10 mm from the free edge in a horizontal mattress fashion. Drill holes are established from the trough through the lateral cortex of the humerus. The previously placed core grasping sutures are passed through those interosseous tunnels and tied down over bone. The anchor sutures are tied, closely approximating the tendon to the prepared cancellous bone of the trough (Fig. 7–14). Absorbable No. 0 sutures are used to approximate the supraspinatus and infraspinatus and the rotator interval anteriorly. The acromioplasty is palpated, and the arm is taken through a complete range of motion to ensure that no impingement of the repaired cuff occurs. The wound is irrigated and closed in layers. The arm is immobilized in a simple sling, and the patient begins a sports-specific therapy regimen.

Arthroscopic débridement alone of full-thickness rotator cuff tears can be considered in certain situations (Fig. 7–15). Débridement is usually considered in the older patient who presents with a complaint of pain without weakness. No weakness should be detectable on physical examination of the cuff. Arthroscopic débridement alone can be considered in this situation but only if the patient is carefully counseled regarding the possibility of an additional procedure (open rotator cuff repair) should the arthroscopic débridement procedure fail. The author's

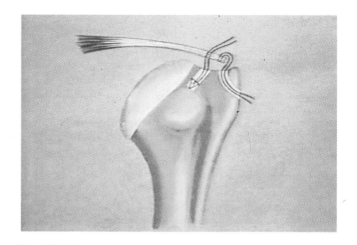

Figure 7–14 • Rotator cuff repair.

preference is to repair all reparable rotator cuff tears in the athletic population, regardless of age. Arthroscopic débridement is used only in the presence of massive, long-standing, irreparable cuff tears. For the tears of those patients, usually elderly, decompression and débridement often provide significant pain relief and surprising improvement in function. Postoperative rehabilitation emphasizes strengthening the anterior and middle deltoid to compensate for the absent rotator cuff. Care should be taken in débridement of these patients with massive cuff defects to avoid destabilization of the coracoacromial arch. For this reason, minimal bone resection is done with the acromioplasty, and the coracoacromial ligament is not excised.

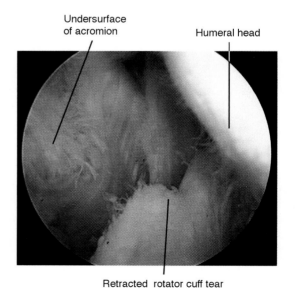

Undersurface of acromion

Humeral head

Retracted rotator cuff tear

Figure 7–15 • Massive rotator cuff tear.

SUMMARY

Appropriate diagnosis and treatment of rotator cuff injuries in athletes allow safe and early return to sports participation. Shoulder arthroscopy provides an additional diagnostic and therapeutic modality when the athlete fails to respond to conservative treatment. Surgical arthroscopy combined with a well-supervised rehabilitation program returns many of those athletes to their preinjury status.[20]

References

1. Scarpinato DF, Bramhall JP, and Andrews JR: Arthroscopic management of the throwing athlete's shoulder: indications, techniques, and results. Clin Sports Med 10:913–927, 1991.
2. Andrews JR and Gillogly S: Physical examination of the shoulder in throwing athletes. In Zarins B, Andrews JR, and Carson WG, (eds.): Injuries to the Throwing Arm. Philadelphia, W.B. Saunders Co., 1985, pp 51–65.
3. Neer CS and Poppen NK: Supraspinatus outlet. Orthop Trans 11:234, 1987.
4. Andrews JR, Byrd JWT, Kupferman SP, et al. The profile view of the acromion. Clin Orthop 263:142–146, 1991.
5. Neer CS: Anterior acromioplasty for the chronic impingement syndrome in the shoulder. J Bone Joint Surg Am 54:41–50, 1972.
6. Hawkins RJ and Kennedy JC: Impingement syndrome in athletes. Am J Sports Med 8:151–158, 1980.
7. Aoki M, Izhii S, and Usui M: The slope of the acromion and rotator cuff impingement. Orthop Trans 10:228, 1986.
8. Bigliani LU, Morrison D, and April EW: The morphology of the acromion and its relationship to rotator cuff tears. Orthop Trans 10:228, 1986.
9. Bigliani LU, Norris RT, and Fischer J: The relationship between the unfused acromial epiphysis and subacromial impingement lesions. Orthop Trans 7:138, 1983.
10. Jobe FW and Kvitne RS: Shoulder pain in the overhead or throwing athlete: the relationship of anterior instability and rotator cuff impingement. Orthop Rev 18:963–975, 1989.
11. Walch G, Boileau P, Noel E, et al.: Impingement of the deep surface of the supraspinatus tendon on the posterosuperior glenoid rim: an arthroscopic study. J Shoulder Elbow Surg 1:238, 1992.
12. Andrews JR and Gidumal RH: Shoulder arthroscopy in the throwing athlete: perspectives and prognosis. Clin Sports Med 6:565–571, 1987.
13. Andrews JR, Brousard TS, and Carson WG: Arthroscopy of the shoulder in the management of partial tears of the rotator cuff: a preliminary report. Arthroscopy 1:117–122, 1985.
14. Andrews JR and Angelo RL: Shoulder arthroscopy for the throwing athlete. Tech Orthop 3:75–81, 1988.
15. Andrews JR, Carson WG, and McLeod WD: Glenoid labral tears related to the long head of the biceps. Am J Sports Med 13:337–341, 1985.
16. Andrews JR, Carson WG, and Ortega K: Arthroscopy of the shoulder: technique and normal anatomy. Am J Sports Med 12:1–7, 1984.
17. Andrews JR, Kupferman SP, and Dillman CJ: Labral tears in throwing and racquet sports. Clin Sports Med 10:901–911, 1991.
18. Pappas AM, Goss TP, and Kleinman PK: Symptomatic shoulder instability due to lesions of the glenoid labrum. Am J Sports Med 11:279–288, 1983.
19. Gartsman GM, Combs AH, Davis PF, et al. Arthroscopic acromio-clavicular joint resection: an anatomical study. Am J Sports Med 19:2–5, 1991.
20. Wilk KE, Arrigo C, and Courson R: Preventive and Rehabilitative Exercises for the Shoulder and Elbow, 3rd ed. Birmingham, Ala., American Sports Medicine Institute, 1991.

Chapter

Shoulder Instability

Yvonne E. Satterwhite

Opinion of arthroscopic treatment of shoulder instability varies among orthopaedic luminaries from embracement to vehement rejection. Many surgeons concur that diagnostic arthroscopy may complement the clinical assessment of instability and that operative arthroscopy is valuable in addressing the associated intra-articular conditions of loose bodies, partial rotator cuff tears, biceps tendon injuries, and lesions of the superior labrum from anterior to posterior[1–7] (Figs. 8–1 and 8–2). However, the controversy lies in one's ability to efficaciously repair capsulolabral injuries arthroscopically rather than by open surgical reconstruction, which is the gold standard. Historically, recurrent shoulder instability has been attributed to a disrupted, dysfunctional labrum or to a capsuloligament complex. Etiologic factors that contribute to the recurrence of instability are age at initial injury (50–95% recurrence in patients younger than 20 years of age), activity level (high recurrence rate associated with collision sports), and the presence of congenital ligamentous hyperlaxity.

Open surgical stabilization procedures have a success rate of 91–96%, with success defined as the elimination of further subluxation or dislocation events.[8–19] These procedures, however, may lead to a loss of shoulder motion (average 10–20 degrees external rotation), which can be detrimental to an athlete's performance, particularly in throwing or overhand sports. In these patients, the preinjury range of motion often exceeds that of the average population. This may afford them a biomechanical advantage but may also increase the likelihood of incurring traumatic or microtraumatic instability. The goals of surgical reconstruction in this population are to correct the instability pattern without eliminating critical motion and with minimal morbidity to the normal, adjacent soft-tissue structures.

Patients who have undergone arthroscopic stabilization procedures of the shoulder have been noted to require a shorter total operative and hospitalization time and less postoperative narcotics and to demonstrate lower blood loss, more rapid return to work activities, less scarring of anterior structures (thus, a minimal loss of external rota-

tion), fewer complications, and a higher percentage return to athletics.[20] However, the recurrence rate of postoperative instability has been reported to be as high as 49%. Although early studies reported a recurrence rate of only 5%, the longer the follow-up period was, the worse the results were.

Admittedly, arthroscopic stabilization has undergone a significant evolution since its inception by Johnson in 1982. Clinical reports on current techniques appear more optimistic, but follow-up is still short-term. Authors agree that the success of arthroscopic stabilization procedures is predicated on preoperative and intraoperative patient selection. Criteria for the "ideal candidate" as well as absolute and relative contraindications have been delineated but not unanimously agreed upon. The contraindications include participation in all collision or high-contact sports or heavy labor, a history of multiple subluxations or dislocations, multidirectional instability, atraumatic or posterior instability, a noncompliant personality, age younger than 20 years, absence of a Bankart lesion, poorly defined capsulolabral tissues (i.e., a significantly degenerated labrum, severe capsular laxity involving the anterior inferior glenohumeral ligament, deficiency in or a transverse tear of the glenohumeral ligaments, or humeral avulsion of the glenohumeral ligaments), and a large Hill-Sachs lesion.[5,21–24]

The importance of surgical restoration of the integrity of the capsulolabral structures cannot be overemphasized. Turkel, Pario, and Marshall[25] established the role of the anterior inferior glenohumeral ligament as the primary restraint to anterior translation of the humeral head with the shoulder in an abducted, externally rotated position.[25] Other authors have demonstrated dysfunction of the inferior glenohumeral ligaments in the presence of a Bankart lesion.[26–28] Rowe, Patel, and Southmayd[18] reviewed patients with recurrent instability who had failed attempts at surgical stabilization procedures. They found 84% to have a Bankart lesion and 85% with excessive capsular laxity. Wolf proposed that it is "reasonable to assume that all types of shoulder instability have some degree of ligamentous attenuation.[29]

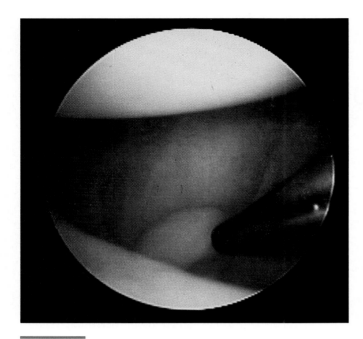

Figure 8–1 • Arthroscopic intraoperative photograph of loose body.

Baker, Uribe, and Witman[30] reported on the acute arthroscopic findings of patients who sustained a traumatic anterior dislocation that required manual reduction. They described three groups of pathologic conditions: group I (6 patients): capsular tear between the middle and anterior inferior glenohumeral ligaments; stable on examination under anesthesia (EUA); group II (11 patients): partial labral detachment from the inferior glenohumeral ligament extending superiorly toward the biceps tendon;

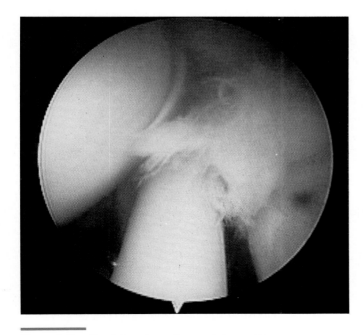

Figure 8–2 • Partial undersurface rotator cuff tear.

anterior subluxation on EUA; and group III (28 patients): complete disruption of the anterior labrum with full detachment of the inferior glenohumeral ligament; grossly unstable on EUA. A similar study, conducted by Norlin,[31] found 24 of 24 acute dislocators to have a Bankart lesion with an associated detachment of the anterior inferior and, occasionally, the middle glenohumeral ligament. All patients were unstable on EUA.

On review of earlier arthroscopic stabilization techniques, it appears that attention was focused primarily on repairing the Bankart lesion. This may explain the ultimately poor long-term results from those procedures. More recent techniques have emphasized a meticulous dissection of the capsulolabrum complex off the glenoid rim and neck, followed by superior translation and fixation at multiple points. Thus, the labrum's role as a "chock block" is restored with relative deepening of the concavity of the glenoid face, and the capsular laxity is addressed through imbrication and plication.[32] Furthermore, gentle synovial and capsular abrasion is recommended to enhance a fibroblastic response with subsequent adherence and improved healing of the plicated capsule.[5,29] Open anterior reconstructions have been referred to as "hot poker techniques" due to the amount of soft-tissue scarring that certainly contributed to postoperative stability but often diminished external rotation. The addition of capsular abrasion to arthroscopic stabilization procedures may improve postoperative stability without increasing motion loss. The avoidance of any significant dissection of the overlying subscapularis muscle with subsequent subscapularis shortening is, in contradistinction to most open procedures, an advantage of the arthroscopic techniques.

FIXATION DEVICES AND TECHNIQUES FOR ARTHROSCOPIC STABILIZATION

During the last 15 years, advances have been made in the types of arthroscopic capsulolabral fixation devices that are available. Clinical experience with formerly used metal implants demonstrated initially adequate intra-articular purchase in the glenoid and adjacent soft tissues. However, complications developed and included loose or migrated hardware, articular injury, persistent pain due to retained hardware, iatrogenic injury to neurovascular structures, and an unacceptable recurrence rate of instability.[33] Newer devices are smaller and often absorbable and obviate the need for transglenoid drilling. A review of fixation devices and techniques for arthroscopic stabilization follows.

STAPLE CAPSULORRHAPHY

In 1982, Johnson[34] revealed his arthroscopic modification of the capsular stapling procedure of duToit and Roux. By utilizing a 4 mm metal staple, the anterior capsulolabral structures are pierced, advanced superiorly, and secured to the anterior glenoid neck. His first series of patients treated in this manner had a 21% redislocation rate at the 2-year follow-up. In the next group of patients, he increased the length of postoperative immobilization to

3 or 4 weeks and noted a reduction of the recurrent instability rate to 4%.[22,35–37] The surgical patients of other authors demonstrated postoperative recurrent subluxation or dislocation rates of 16–44%.[7,24,38–42] Furthermore, hardware complications were abundant, including pain, cutting through or transection of the capsulolabral tissue, and loosening, breakage, or migration of the staple into adjacent soft tissues, the glenohumeral joint, the subacromial space, and the brachial plexus, and between the scapula and the rib cage.[33,41]

REMOVABLE RIVET

In 1988, Wiley[43] reported on the use of a removable rivet—a long, threaded collared pin—for Bankart repairs. The detached labrum was speared with the tip of the rivet, which was then driven into the glenoid neck. The rivet's blunt end was left just deep to the subcutaneous tissue anteriorly. After 4 weeks, the rivet was removed and a rehabilitation program initiated. Wiley's success rate in 10 patients was 90%, with a follow-up of 6 months to 2 years. The rivet is not currently used, and no other published reports are available on this device.

CANNULATED SCREW

In the late 1980s and early 1990s, Snyder, Stafford, Wolf, Warner, and Warren[44–46] discussed their experience utilizing a metal cannulated screw with an incorporated washer for arthroscopic repairs of capsulolabral disruptions. The technique involved piercing the labrum-ligament complex with a guide pin, drilling the pin securely into the glenoid neck, overdrilling the pin with a cannulated drill bit, and introducing a cannulated screw until it was securely seated. The guide pin was removed and a shoulder immobilizer applied. With a follow-up period of 3–40 months, the failure rate due to recurrent instability ranged 15–30%, and 5–20% of patients had complaints of pain secondary to screw irritation. This implant has been largely replaced by cannulated absorbable devices.

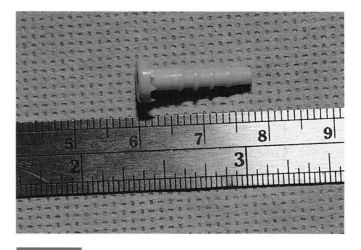

Figure 8–3 • A Suretac II implant.

CANNULATED ABSORBABLE DEVICES

In 1991 Warner and Warren[46] described their arthroscopic technique for repairing Bankart lesions with the Suretac device. The Suretac II (Acufex Microsurgical, Mansfield, Mass.) is a 6 or 8 mm polyglyconate tack that is resorbed approximately 6 weeks after implantation (Fig. 8–3). The repair procedure begins with completion of the Bankart detachment from the 2-o'clock to 6-o'clock position (right shoulder) and includes medial mobilization of the inferior glenohumeral ligament off the glenoid neck. The anterior scapular neck is decorticated down to a bleeding surface. The capsulolabrum complex is grasped, shifted superiolaterally, and pierced with a guide pin that is advanced into the nonarticular glenoid rim before being overdrilled with a cannulated drill (Figs. 8–4 and 8–5). The arm is held in adduction and neutral rotation as a cannulated Suretac tack is slipped over the guide pin and tapped securely into place (Fig. 8–6). Often, two or three Suretacs are necessary to complete the repair (Fig. 8–7). Postoperatively, patients are placed in an immobilizer for 4 weeks.

Figure 8–4 • Introduction of the Suretac guide pin.

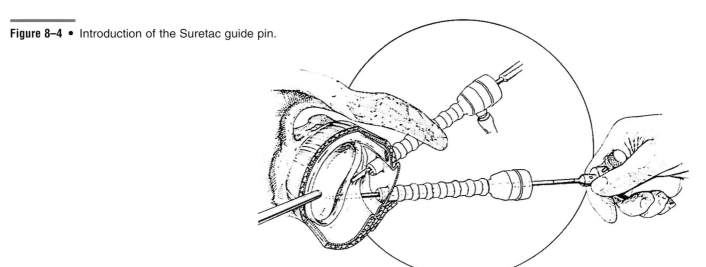

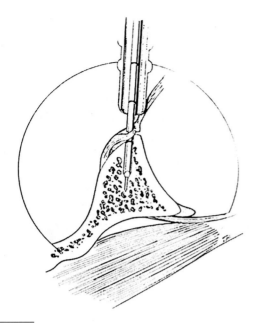

Figure 8–5 • Introduction of the Suretac guide pin.

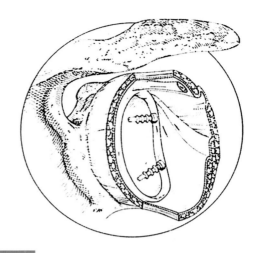

Figure 8–7 • Suretac repair completed.

Light throwing and swimming are permitted after 4 months; however, contact and overhand sports are not allowed for 8 months.

The success of this technique is compromised if an inadequate amount of tissue is purchased by the Suretac or if the implant tears through the capsulolabral structures or is seated too far medially on the glenoid neck. Problems may also develop in the presence of underdeveloped, attenuated, or significantly patulous capsuloligamentous tissue. Warner and Warren[46] described a "drive-through" sign as an indication of anterior inferior glenohumeral ligament laxity wherein the arthroscope can be easily driven through the glenohumeral joint from a posterior portal entry point across and inferiorly to the anterior inferior

capsule. Although initial results with the Suretac were encouraging (recurrent instability rate of 8% and loss of external rotation 7 degrees average), long-term follow-up revealed a recurrent instability rate of 21%. Causes for this deterioration in results were theorized to include inadequate preoperative patient selection, too short an implant tissue half-life, technical errors, and rare severe histiocytic reaction to the Suretac.[47] Currently, Warren emphasizes narrow indications for the use of this fixation device: patients who have sustained fewer than five traumatic anterior instability episodes, are noncollision athletes, have no signs of generalized ligamentous hyperlaxity, and arthroscopically have a Bankart lesion with no labral deterioration or associated capsular attenuation. Overhead athletes are included as possible candidates for the procedure. In 1994 Laurencin[48] reported a 5% recurrence rate when optimal conditions and criteria were observed. Arciero[49] and Wheeler et al.[7] have been involved in a prospective nonrandomized study of cadets from West Point military academy who have sustained acute initial traumatic dislocations requiring a closed reduction. Two groups of patients have been compared: those electing nonoperative treatment and those requesting arthroscopic Bankart repair. The initial arthroscopic fixation methods employed metal staples, followed later in the series by the transglenoid suture repair technique, which has been supplanted by use of the Suretac since 1991. Instability recurrence rates for these three fixation methods were 22%, 14%, and 11%, respectively. Although less satisfactory than results obtained from open stabilization, these results contrast favorably when compared with those for the nonoperative group, in which recurrence rates were 92%, 80%, and 85%, respectively.

SUTURE CAPSULORRHAPHY

Arthroscopic suture repair of capsulolabral injuries has been advocated by several authors and continues to undergo technique modifications. Currently, fixation may involve the use of resorbable or permanent sutures placed anteriorly or in a transglenoid approach.

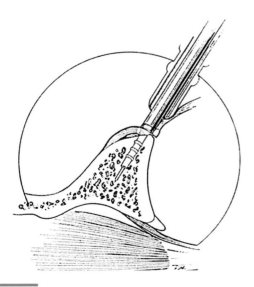

Figure 8–6 • Suretac tapped into place along the glenoid.

Transglenoid Repair

In 1987 Morgan and Bodenstab[50] published their early results on transglenoid Bankart suture repairs. Their arthroscopic procedure required the use of a sharp-tip modified Beath pin to impale the Bankart lesion through an anterior inferior portal and reapproximate the labrum to the glenoid rim. The pin was then drilled across the glenoid neck to exit posteriorly. An absorbable suture was inserted into the eye of the pin anteriorly, and one limb was pulled through the glenoid as the Beath pin was removed posteriorly. In a similar fashion, a second suture was introduced approximately 1.0–1.5 cm proximal to the first, and both anterior limbs were tied into a secure knot. The posterior limbs were pulled taut to secure the knot and adjacent labrum to the glenoid rim. The posterior limbs were tied over the infraspinatus/posterior deltoid fascia while the arm was held in 0 degrees of abduction and neutral rotation. Surgical concerns included potential injury to the suprascapular nerve and the difficulty in adjusting suture tension when tying over muscle tissue posteriorly. Initial reports indicated a 2% recurrent instability rate that was noted to increase to 5%, after a minimum follow-up of 1 year, and then up to 10% with even longer follow-up (17% in contact athletes).[24] Rhee, Ohn, and Lee[51] published encouraging results on their series of eight patients who had a 0% redislocation rate; however, follow-up was only 11 months. Benedetto and Glotzer[35] reported on 22 patients who underwent a Morgan-type repair within 5 months (average 4 weeks) of their initial injury. There were no recurrences of instability after 2–3.5 years. In 1993 Grana, Buckley, and Yates[52] shared their findings on 27 patients with anterior instability who, after an average of 36 months postoperatively, demonstrated a 42% rate of redislocation/subluxation. The proposed reasons for any failure of an arthroscopic suture capsulorrhaphy have included the insertion of fewer than four sutures, lack of suture fixation of the capsule (inferior glenohumeral ligament) along with the labrum, drill hole placement too superiorly on the glenoid rim, absence of a Bankart or a large Hill-Sachs lesion, presence of atraumatic instability or a transverse tear of the labrum-ligament complex, and an insufficiently brief period of postoperative immobilization.

To address the need for multiple suture fixation sites in the capsulolabral tissues, Caspari[53] designed a "suture punch" device (Concept Inc., Clearwater, Fla.) that permits the insertion of as many as 10 sutures anteriorly (Fig. 8–8). The sutures are passed through one transglenoid drill hole and tied posteriorly over the infraspinatus fascia. In 1988 Caspari[54] published a recurrent instability rate of 8% in 49 shoulders inspected at an average of 33 months postoperatively. Long-term follow-up demonstrated an 18% recurrence rate. Savoie[55] reported a 9% recurrence rate in 161 patients with traumatic anterior instability. At the 1996 annual meeting of the American Academy of Orthopaedic Surgeons, Danziger and Neviaser[56] presented their results using the Caspari technique. They had an average 28% redislocation rate; however, when the patients were divided into two groups based on the postoperative immobilization period, they found the reinjury rate to be 41% for those immobilized for 3 weeks as com-

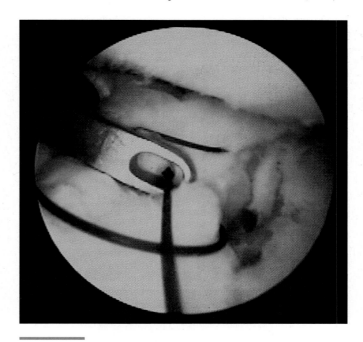

Figure 8–8 • Arthroscopic view as suture is passed through the suture punch.

pared with 11% for those held 6 weeks. The follow-up periods were an average of 30 months and 24 months, respectively. Other surgeons who have utilized the transglenoid techniques (Warren,[46] Wolin, Weber, Walch[57], and Grana[52]) have reported failure rates ranging 19–44%.

Maki[58] modified Morgan's technique by eliminating the need for tying the suture over the infraspinatus fascia. He recommended passing a limb of the labral sutures from anterior to posterior through the transglenoid drill holes followed by tying a mulberry knot in the posterior suture limbs. As tension is applied to the anterior limbs, the posterior knot is pulled back through the soft tissues to reside against the posterior glenoid neck. By using an arthroscopic knot tier and pusher, the anterior suture limbs are advanced as a mattress stitch down to the glenoid while the labrum is held in its corrected position with a tissue grasper. In 1991 Maki[59] published his early results with this technique and noted a 6% recurrence rate in 15 patients. Morgan[24] adopted Maki's modification and found that only 5% of his 175 patients developed recurrent instability after 1–7 year follow-up. Athletes who participated in collision sports had a 16.6% failure rate compared with a 1.5% failure rate in throwers and noncollision athletes.

Suture Anchors

In order to obviate the need for transglenoid drilling and improve soft-tissue fixation strength, Wolf, Wilk, and Richmond[60] advocate implanting, along the edge of the glenoid rim, three or four Mitek-II double-armed suture anchors (Mitek, Norwood, Mass.) loaded with absorbable sutures. The suture limbs are passed with a suture hook through the detached labrum-ligament complex and then tied securely to the anterior glenoid rim with a knot pusher. With less than a 2 year follow-up, Wolf, Wilk, and Richmond documented no recurrences or complications in 30 patients. However, long-term follow-up revealed a failure rate of 10% (15% in contact athletes). Weber[61] reported an 8% recurrence rate in his patients treated arthroscopically as compared with a 2% recurrence rate in patients who underwent an open repair during the same study period.

Snyder[32] has further popularized the use of suture anchors for arthroscopic Bankart repairs, specifically the mini-Revo anchor (Linvatec Corp., Largo, Fla.) (Fig. 8–9). These anchor devices are "retrievable" and can be loaded with a nonabsorbable suture. Snyder advocated freeing up the capsulolabral tissue down to the 6-o'clock position (right shoulder), as necessary, and decorticating the glenoid neck followed by the insertion of three or four anchors anteriorly along the edge of the glenoid articular

cartilage (Fig. 8–10). By using an anterior superior portal, a suture hook is inserted to capture one of the suture limbs of the mini-Revo anchor (Fig. 8–11). A "shuttle relay" device (Linvatec Corp.) is guided through a suture hook or suture punch that, via an anterior midglenoid portal, has pierced the pathologic capsulolabral tissue. The shuttle is then pulled up through an anterior superior or posterior portal cannula (Fig. 8–12). One limb of the suture anchor is passed through the shuttle's eyelet, and the shuttle is pulled back intra-articularly and then out of the cannula

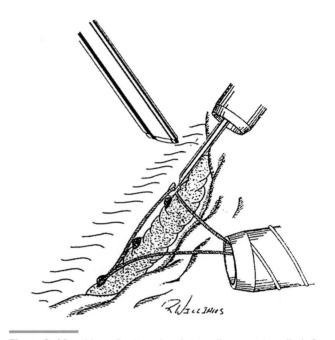

Figure 8–11 • Use of suture hook to pull one suture limb from anchor up through an anterior superior cannula.

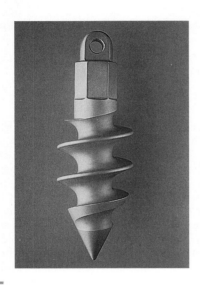

Figure 8–9 • Mini-Revo fixation device.

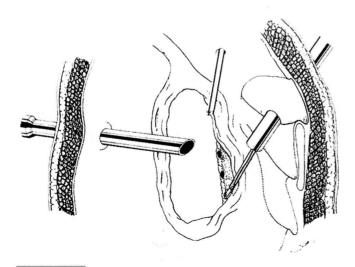

Figure 8–10 • Suture anchor insertion into drill hole on glenoid rim.

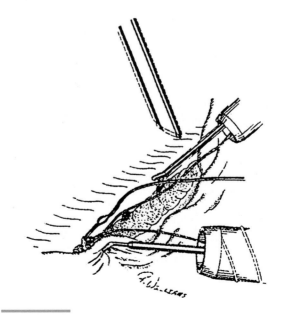

Figure 8–12 • Use of grasper to pass shuttle relay out of the anterior superior cannula.

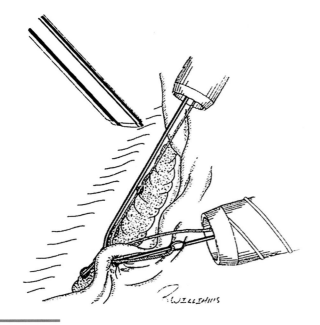

Figure 8–13 • Shuttle relay (loaded with one limb from suture anchor) is pulled back into the joint and out of the anterior midglenoid cannula.

from which it was introduced, thus bringing the single limb of the suture anchor with it through the capsulolabral tissues (Fig. 8–13). This process is repeated for the second limb of the mini-Revo anchor. Three or four sutures are introduced in a similar fashion, and each is tied using an arthroscopic knot tier while the arm is maintained in neutral rotation and adducted to the patient's side (Fig. 8–14). Snyder recommended two types of knots: a Revo knot consisting of five nonidentical half-hitches or a Duncan knot followed by two nonidentical half-hitches. Postoperatively, the shoulder is immobilized for 3–4 weeks.

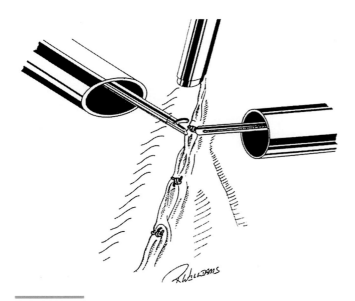

Figure 8–14 • Sutures are tied tautly and ends are cut.

In patients with capsuloligamentous laxity but no Bankart lesion, Wolf[29] and Snyder[32] have performed arthroscopic capsular plication procedures. No suture anchors are utilized. Instead, through an anterior midglenoid portal, a suture hook is used to place multiple "pinch tucks" within the capsule 8–10 mm from the glenoid rim, beginning inferiorly and then continuing superiorly within the capsule. Each time a pinch tuck is created, the shuttle relay is inserted through the suture hook needle and pulled out the anterior superior portal to receive a limb of a nonabsorbable suture. As the shuttle relay is retrieved from its introductory midglenoid portal, the suture limb is brought with it and is tagged. Another shuttle relay pass through a pinch tuck allows for the companion limb of the suture to be pulled through the capsule. A stacked Revo knot is tied, and the process is repeated continuing superiorly, with the end result being a tucked or plicated capsule. Patients are immobilized postoperatively for 3–4 weeks. Return to light sports is allowed at 3–4 months and collision sports at 6 months.[32] Wolf's capsular plication technique is similar; however, he elects to start his sutures in the superior aspect of the middle glenohumeral ligament and then continue as far inferiorly as is deemed necessary.[29]

Multidirectional instability is now being treated arthroscopically by a select group of surgeons. Duncan and Savoie[62] reported their results using the Caspari technique, in which the most inferior capsular attachment is left intact, as a tether, while the anterior and posterior capsuloligamentous structures are detached, advanced superiorly, and secured with sutures. Savoie[63] has performed this procedure in more than 40 patients and, at 2–5 years of follow-up, found that 90% of them had a satisfactory result. This compares with a 97% satisfactory rate in his patients who underwent an arthroscopic inferior capsular shift and a 93% satisfactory rate in those who had an arthroscopic closure of the rotator interval.

In regard to posterior instability, the surgical results of open stabilization procedures often fare no better than 50% for eliminating chronic recurrent instability. Arthroscopically, pathologic changes in the posterior capsule and posterior inferior glenohumeral ligament may be quite difficult to assess and even more challenging to repair. The techniques described in this section may be modified to attempt to address posterior injuries. However, an isolated reverse Bankart lesion appears to be the most amenable to arthroscopic treatment.[64] Long-term studies are pending.

COMPARATIVE STUDIES

Although there are no prospective randomized studies comparing open versus arthroscopic anterior stabilization techniques, there are a few nonrandomized prospective and retrospective studies that deserve review. In 1991, Weber[65] reported on 47 Bankart repairs—24 open and 23 arthroscopic procedures. The recurrence rate of instability was 2% in the open group versus 12% in the arthroscopic patients. Jorgensen et al.[66] published their report in 1992 of 21 open repairs with a 0% failure rate compared with 20 arthroscopic repairs with a 5% failure rate. Of the retrospective studies in 1994, Geiger et al.[67] published their series of 34 patients, of whom 16 were treated with open procedures compared with 18 who were treated arthroscopically. They noted a failure rate of 0% and 44%, respectively. Similarly, Gauche, Buss, and Sodergren[68] quoted a 0% instability recurrence rate in 13 patients treated with open procedures as opposed to a 33% rate in those treated arthroscopically. In 1995, Luetzow, Atkin, and Sachs[69] reported a recurrent instability rate that was three times higher in their arthroscopically treated patients than in their open cases. Notably, many of these studies indicated that patients treated arthroscopically demonstrated better range of motion postoperatively than their open counterparts. Nonetheless, possible reasons for some of the marginal outcomes obtained by arthroscopic stabilization methods may include the following: inadequate elevation of the labrum onto the glenoid rim, difficulty plicating the capsule or shifting it superiorly, technical challenges in rotator cuff interval closures, chronic plastic deformation of the inferior glenohumeral ligament complex, and capsular adhesions to the overlying subscapularis tendon.[70]

CONCLUSIONS

Clinical reports on recent arthroscopic capsulolabral stabilization procedures and newer techniques for fixation are promising; however, long-term follow-up is unavailable. Review of studies involving the earliest techniques is, for the most part, disconcerting, especially when compared with the success rates achievable with open procedures. A routine, honest self-assessment of our own current arthroscopic skill level in conjunction with scrupulous patient selection should help to improve the overall success rate of these relatively new procedures. In other words, arthroscopic shoulder repair and reconstruction is not appropriate for every patient or every surgeon.

References

1. Adolfsson L and Lysholm J: Arthroscopy and stability testing for anterior shoulder instability. Arthroscopy 5:315–320, 1989.
2. Baker CL, Uribe JW, and Witman C: Arthroscopic evaluation of acute initial anterior shoulder dislocations. Am J Sports Med 18:25–28, 1990.
3. Calandra JJ, Baker CL, and Uribe JW: The incidence of Hill-Sachs lesions in initial anterior shoulder dislocations. Arthroscopy 5:254–257, 1989.
4. Hurley JA and Anderson TE: Shoulder arthroscopy: its role in evaluating shoulder disorders in the athlete. Am J Sports Med 18:480–483, 1990.
5. Jobe FW and Bradley JP: The diagnosis in nonoperative treatment of shoulder injuries in athletes. Clin Sports Med 8:419–438, 1989.
6. McGlynn FJ and Caspari RB: Arthroscopic findings in the subluxating shoulder. Clin Orthop 183:173–178, 1984.
7. Wheeler JH, Ryan JB, Arciero RA, et al.: Arthroscopic vs. nonoperative treatment of acute shoulder dislocations in young athletes. Arthroscopy 5:213–217, 1989.
8. Barry TP, Lombardo SJ, Kerlen RK, et al.: The coracoid transfer for recurrent anterior instability of the shoulder in adolescence. J Bone Joint Surg Am 67:383–387, 1985.
9. Collins KA, Capito C, and Cross M: The use of the Putti-Platt procedure in the treatment of recurrent anterior dislocation with special reference to the young athlete. Am J Sports Med 14:380–382, 1986.
10. duToit GT and Roux D: Recurrent dislocation in the shoulder: a 24 year study of the Johannesburg stapling operation. J Bone Joint Surg Am 38:1–12, 1956.
11. Freeman BL: Recurrent dislocations. In Crenshaw AH (ed.): Campbell's Operative Orthopaedics. St. Louis, C. V. Mosby, 1987, pp 2173–2220.
12. Hovelius L, Thorling J, and Fredin H: Recurrent anterior dislocation of the shoulder: results after the Bankart and Putti-Platt operations. J Bone Joint Surg Am 61:566–569, 1979.
13. Karadamis J, Rentis G, and Varouchas G: Repair of recurrent anterior dislocation of the shoulder using transfer of the subscapularis tendon. J Bone Joint Surg Am 62:1147–1149, 1980.
14. Leach RE, Corbett M, Schepsis A, et al.: Results of a modified Putti-Platt operation for recurrent shoulder dislocations and subluxations. Clin Orthop 164:20–25, 1982.
15. Paavolainen P, Bjorkenheim JM, Ahovuo J, et al.: Recurrent anterior dislocation of the shoulder: results of Eden-Hybinette and Putti-Platt operations. Acta Orthop Scand 55:556–560, 1984.
16. Rao JP, Francis AM, Hurley J, et al.: Treatment of recurrent anterior dislocation of the shoulder by duToit Staple capsulorrhaphy: results of long-term follow-up study. Clin Orthop 204:169–176, 1986.
17. Rockwood CA. Subluxations and dislocations about the shoulder: In Rockwood CA and Green DP (eds.): Fractures. Philadelphia, J. B. Lippincott, 1984, pp 722–948.
18. Rowe CR, Patel D, and Southmayd WW: The Bankart procedure: a long-term end-result study. J Bone Joint Surg Am 60:1–16, 1978.
19. Rowe CR and Zarins B: Current transient subluxation of the shoulder. J Bone Joint Surg Am 63:863–872, 1981.
20. Christensen KP: Arthroscopic vs. open Bankart procedures: a comparison of early morbidity and complications. Arthroscopy 9:371–374, 1993.
21. Johnson LL: Symposium on open vs. arthroscopic techniques for shoulder instability. Presented at the Fourth Open Meeting of the American Shoulder and Elbow Surgeons, Atlanta, Feb., 1988.
22. Perry J and Glousman RE: Biomechanics of throwing. In Nicholas JA and Hershman EB (eds.): The Upper Extremity and Sports Medicine. St. Louis, C. V. Mosby, 1990, pp 727–750.
23. Matthews LS, Vetter WL, Oweida SJ, et al.: Arthroscopic staple capsulorrhaphy for recurrent anterior shoulder instability. Arthroscopy 4:106–111, 1988.
24. Morgan CD: Arthroscopic transglenoid Bankart suture repair. Oper Tech Orthop 1:171–179, 1991.
25. Turkel SJ, Pario MW, and Marshall JL: Stabilizing mechanisms preventing anterior dislocation of the glenohumeral joint. J Bone Joint Surg Am 63:1206–1208, 1981.
26. Caspari RB and Guissler WB: Arthroscopic manifestations of shoulder subluxation and dislocation. Clin Orthop 291:54–66, 1993.
27. Howell SA and Galinat BJ: The containment mechanism: the primary stabilizer of the glenohumeral joint. Presented at the Annual Meeting of the American Academy of Orthopedic Surgeons, San Francisco, Jan., 1987.
28. Johnson LL: Diagnostic arthroscopic findings and traumatic anterior dislocation of the shoulder. Presented at the Closed Meeting of the American Shoulder and Elbow Surgeons, Seattle, Sept., 1991.
29. Wolf EM: Capsular plication techniques for anterior, posterior, or multi-directional instability. Presented at the Arthroscopic Association of North America Specialty Day Meeting, Atlanta, Feb., 1996.
30. Baker CL, Uribe JW, and Witman C: Arthroscopic evaluation of acute initial anterior shoulder dislocation. Am J Sports Med 18:25–28, 1990.
31. Norlin R: Intra-articular pathology in acute first time anterior shoulder dislocation: an arthroscopic study. Arthroscopy 9:546–549, 1993.
32. Snyder S: Scoi technique for anterior shoulder stabilization using suture shuttle relay and implantable "mini" Revo sutures anchors ICL. Presented at the Annual Meeting of the American Academy of Orthopaedic Surgeons, Atlanta, Feb., 1996.
33. Zuckerman JD and Matson FA: Complications about the glenohumeral joint related to the use of screws and staples. J Bone Joint Surg Am 66:175–180, 1984.
34. Johnson L: Instrument Maker's Educational Film. Okemos, Mich., Instrument Maker Company, 1982.

35. Benedetto KP and Glotzer W: Arthroscopic Bankart procedure by suture technique: indications, technique, and results. Arthroscopy 8:111–115, 1992.
36. Caspari RB: Arthroscopy of the shoulder. Instructional Course Lectures. New York, Hospital for Joint Disease, 1989.
37. Johnson LL: Techniques of anterior glenohumeral ligament. In Arthroscopic Surgery: Principles and Practice. St. Louis, C.V. Mosby, 1986, pp 1405–1420.
38. Coughlin L, Rubinovich M, Johansson J, et al.: Arthroscopic staple capsulorrhaphy for anterior shoulder instability. Am J Sports Med 20:253–256, 1992.
39. Gross RM: Arthroscopic shoulder capsulorrhaphy: does it work? Am J Sports Med 17:495–500, 1989.
40. Hawkins RB: Arthroscopic stapling repair for shoulder instability: a retrospective study of 50 cases. J Arthroscopy 5:122–128, 1989.
41. Lane JG, Sachs RA, and Riehl B: Arthroscopic staple capsulorrhaphy: a long-term follow up. Arthroscopy 9:190–194, 1993.
42. Morrey BF and Janes JM: Recurrent anterior dislocation of the shoulder: long-term follow-up of the Putti-Platt and Bankart procedures. J Bone Joint Surg Am 58:252–256, 1976.
43. Wiley AM: Arthroscopy for shoulder instability and a technique for arthroscopic repair. Arthroscopy 4:25–30, 1988.
44. Snyder SJ and Stafford BB: Arthroscopic management of instability of the shoulder. Orthopedics 16:993–1002, 1993.
45. Wolf EM: Arthroscopic anterior shoulder capsulorrhaphy. Techniques Orthopaedics 3:66–73, 1988.
46. Warner JP and Warren RF: Arthroscopic Bankart repair using cannulated absorbable fixation device. Op Tech Orthop 1:192–198, 1991.
47. Warner JP, Miller MD, Marks P, et al.: Arthroscopic Bankart repair with the Suretac device. Part I: clinical observations. Arthroscopy 11:2–13, 1995.
48. Laurencin CT et al.: Arthroscopic Bankart repair degradable polymeric tack. Presented at the Annual Meeting of the American Orthopaedic Society for Sports Medicine, Palm Desert, Calif., 1994.
49. Arciero RA: Arthroscopic evaluation of first-time traumatic shoulder dislocations. Presented at the Arthroscopic Association of North America Speciality Day Meeting, Atlanta, Feb., 1996.
50. Morgan CD and Bodenstab AB: Arthroscopic Bankart suture repair: technique and early results. Arthroscopy 3:111–122, 1987.
51. Rhee KJ, Ohn SR, and Lee JK: Arthroscopic capsular suture for anterior instability of the shoulder. Orthopedics 15:217–224, 1992.
52. Grana WA, Buckley PD, and Yates CK: Arthroscopic Bankart suture repair. Am J Sports Med 21:348–353, 1993.
53. Caspari RB: Arthroscopic stabilization for shoulder instability. In Operative Techniques and Shoulder Surgery. Gaithersburg, Md., Aspen, 1991, pp 57–63.
54. Caspari RB: Arthroscopic reconstruction for anterior shoulder instability. Tech Orthop 3:59–66, 1988.
55. Savoie FH III: Arthroscopic stabilization of anterior instability. Presented at American Shoulder and Elbow Surgeons, New Orleans, 1994.
56. Danziger M and Neviaser TJ: The arthroscopic Bankart procedure for anterior glenohumeral instability: effective immobilization on redislocation. Presented at the Arthroscopic Association of North America Specialty Day meeting, Atlanta, Feb., 1996.
57. Weber SC: History of arthroscopic shoulder stabilization. Instructional Course Lecture. Presented at the Annual Meeting of the American Academy of Orthopaedic Surgeons, Atlanta, Feb., 1996.
58. Maki NJ: Arthroscopic stabilization for recurrent shoulder instability. Presented at the Annual Meeting of the American Academy of Orthopaedic Surgeons, Las Vegas, Feb., 1988.
59. Maki NJ: Arthroscopic stabilization: suture technique. Op Tech Orthop 1:180–183, 1991.
60. Weber EM, Wilk RM, and Richmond JC: Arthroscopic Bankart repair using suture anchors. Op Tech Orthop 1:194, 1991.
61. Weber SC: Arthroscopic anterior suture anchor repair versus open Bankart repair in the management of traumatic anterior glenohumeral instability. Presented at the Arthroscopic Association of North America meeting, Washington, D.C., 1996.
62. Duncan R and Savoie FH III: Arthroscopic inferior capsular shift for MDI of the shoulder: preliminary report. Arthroscopy 9:24–27, 1993.
63. Savoie FH III: Arthroscopic management of multi-directional instability of the shoulder. Instructional Course Lecture. Presented at the Annual Meeting of the American Academy of Orthopaedic Surgeons, Atlanta, Feb., 1996.
64. Elrod BF: Indications for arthroscopic posterior instability repair for the suture anchor. Instructional Course Lecture. Presented at the Annual Meeting of the American Academy of Orthopaedic Surgeons, Atlanta, Feb., 1996.
65. Weber SC: A prospective evaluation comparing open and arthroscopic treatment of recurrent anterior glenohumeral dislocations. Orthop Trans 15:763, 1991.
66. Jorgensen U, Svend HH, Back K, et al.: Anterior shoulder instability: open arthroscopic repair. Orthop Trans 16:760, 1992.
67. Geiger DF, Hurley JA, Torey J, et al.: Results of arthroscopic vs. open Bankart suture repair. Orthop Trans 17:973, 1994.
68. Gauche CA, Buss DD, and Sodergren KM: The results of arthroscopic versus open reconstruction of the shoulder in patients with an isolated Bankart lesion. Orthop Trans 18:1125, 1994.
69. Luetzow WF, Atkin DM, and Sachs RA: Arthroscopic vs. open Bankart repair of the shoulder for recurrent anterior dislocation. Presented at the Annual Meeting of the American Academy of Orthopaedic Surgeons, New Orleans, Feb., 1995.
70. Pettrone FA: Indications for arthroscopic vs. open stabilization. Presented at the Arthroscopic Association of North America Specialty Day meeting, Atlanta, Feb., 1996.

Chapter

9 Labral Tears

Stephen J. Snyder • *Stephen L. Kollias*

INTRODUCTION

Injuries to the glenoid labrum have historically been difficult to diagnose. With the use of arthroscopy, knowledge of the labrum, in normal and pathologic variations, has increased rapidly. Radiologic imaging has provided some assistance in the diagnosis of labral lesions and may become more valuable in the future. This chapter discusses the evaluation and management of injuries to the glenoid labrum, emphasizing the benefits of modern arthroscopic techniques.

Gardner and Gray[1] evaluated the prenatal development of the shoulder and the glenoid labrum. Their study involved 65 embryos at 8 weeks' gestation and full-term fetuses. At a crown-rump length of 12 mm, the humerus and glenoid were a mass of precartilage cells without a discernible joint space. Within this mass of cells is a condensed layer called the interzone, which is the precursor of the future joint space. With further development, the interzone differentiates into the glenoid labrum, capsule, subscapularis tendon, and biceps tendon. As the embryo reached a crown-rump length of 38 mm, the joint space was more clearly defined with a typical triangular labrum superiorly, inferiorly, and posteriorly. The anterior labrum was routinely less developed.

Snyder, Rames, and Wolbert[2] examined 21 fresh-frozen cadavers grossly and microscopically. It was apparent that the posterior labrum was more distinct than the anterior. The labrum appears to be formed of dense fibrous material with some elastic fibers intermixed. Centrally, the labrum is continuous with the articular cartilage of the glenoid, and peripherally it is continuous with the fibrous capsule. The capsule covers the labral base broadly, attaching to the scapular neck. Routinely, a fibrocartilage interzone was noted between the glenoid cartilage and labrum superiorly, anteriorly, and posteriorly. No fibrocartilage was noted inferiorly.

Variations in labral anatomy were noted by Detrisac and Johnson.[3] Originally, five variations were described, but more recently Detrisac (oral communication, November 1993) changed his classification to two types. Type A

has a superior labrum that is detached centrally but well attached peripherally. The remainder of the labrum is attached both centrally and peripherally in the posterior, anterior, and inferior portions (Fig. 9–1). The type B labrum is well attached centrally and peripherally at all sites (Fig. 9–2).

According to Snyder, Rames, and Wolbert,[2] the labrum showed similar findings. The inferior labrum had the most consistent appearance, with a triangular shape and attached central edge. Posteriorly, it retained a triangular shape, with attachment of the undersurface to the glenoid. The superior labrum showed consistent peripheral attachment with a variable free central edge. The anterior labrum did not typically show the triangular shape but was consistently attached centrally and peripherally.

Occasionally, labral anomalies may be misperceived as disease by the arthroscopist unfamiliar with normal anatomic variations. Most commonly, the anterior superior labrum is firmly attached to the glenoid rim. In approximately 11% of shoulders, there is a sublabral foramen that separates the labrum from the glenoid rim.[4] This sublabral hole must be differentiated from the lesion of the superior labrum from anterior to posterior (SLAP), which involves the area of the biceps anchor, and the Bankart lesion, which begins below the midglenoid notch. Infrequently, a Buford complex may be encountered. This is also a normal variant that occurs in approximately 1.5% of shoulders.[5] The Buford complex consists of a thick, cord-like middle glenohumeral ligament that crosses the subscapularis tendon at a 45 degree angle and attaches to the superior labrum just anterior to the biceps anchor; there is no labral tissue on the anterior superior labral edge. The Buford complex is often mistaken for a pathologic labral detachment, although it is seldom associated with clinical instability.

Biomechanics of the Labrum

The shoulder has the greatest mobility of any joint in the body. Because it lacks inherent bony congruity, the soft

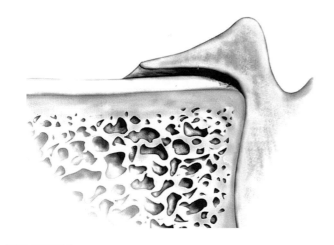

Figure 9–1 • Type A labrum. Leaf-like free edge overhanging the articular surface like the meniscus of the knee. Most frequently found in superior quadrant but may be anterior or posterior.

tissues of the shoulder play a major role in joint stability. There is no single structure that is responsible for the stability of the glenohumeral joint in all shoulder positions. However, the stability is maintained for the most part by the interactions of the muscles and ligaments of the shoulder girdle. The labrum participates in joint stabilization in many ways: it forms a rim around the periphery of the glenoid, giving a suction cup effect with the humerus; it provides an anchor for ligamentous structures; and it deepens the socket of the glenoid and increases surface contact area. The addition of the glenoid labrum increases the surface area 25% in the vertical plane and 57% in the transverse plane.[6] Reeves[7] and Perry[8] have shown that the bonding strength of the labrum to the glenoid increases with age. As one matures, the bonding strength of the labrum eventually becomes greater than the breaking strength of the capsule and subscapularis tendon. This may explain why a patient younger than 25 years of age is more likely to sustain a Bankart lesion with a shoulder dis-

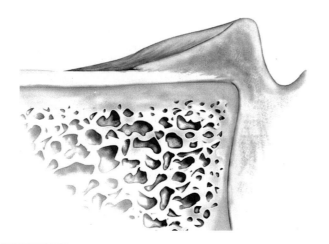

Figure 9–2 • Type B labrum. The more common situation in which the labrum is continuous with the articular surface with no free edge.

location as opposed to middle-aged patients sustaining midsubstance capsular injuries or cuff tears.

Jobe[9] demonstrated impingement of the posterior superior labrum in a cadaveric study. The shoulder specimens were fixed in a position of 70 degrees abduction and maximum external rotation, causing a joint impression where humeral and superior labral contact occurred. The greater tuberosity of the humerus compressed the posterior superior labrum with the rotator cuff interposed. When anterior capsular laxity was created, posterior labral impingement increased. These findings agreed with the common observation of posterior labral tears and articular side cuff tears in throwing athletes.

Karzel, Nuber, and Lautenschlager[10] also performed biomechanical testing in cadaveric specimens. When a compression load was applied with the shoulder in a 90 degree abducted position, the labrum affected distribution of contact forces.

The superior labrum has been shown to have decreased vascularity in comparison with the remainder of the labrum. William Burkhead (oral communication, November 1992, and in unpublished data) showed abundant vasculature to the entire labrum except the superior portion. Cooper et al.[11] showed decreased vascularity in the superior and anterior superior segments as well. The limited vascularity may be related to the development of the SLAP lesion and superior labral degeneration and biceps tears noted with advancing age.[12]

PATIENT SELECTION

Indications for Surgery

In its infancy, shoulder arthroscopy was used primarily for diagnostic purposes. As imaging techniques become more reliable for shoulder disease, the need for diagnostic arthroscopy diminishes. However, labral lesions present a particular dilemma because of the difficulty in imaging this area even with magnetic resonance arthrography. Therefore, if clinical suspicion of a potential labral lesion is high, diagnostic arthroscopy still plays a primary role in defining and, often, treating a potential lesion.

Preoperative Evaluation

History

A patient's complete clinical history should be evaluated in a systematic and logical sequence. An occupational and recreational history should be elicited along with the patient's general state of health. The type and degree of pain are important as well as any activities that may exacerbate the symptoms. The examiner should attempt to define a precise mechanism of injury, whether the injury was caused by an acute event or a chronic repetitive activity.

A patient may relate a fall on an abducted arm and have complaints of pain associated with snapping, locking, cracking, and mechanical-type symptoms. These symptoms are all consistent with, but not diagnostic of, labral injury. Patients may also have other associated conditions, such as impingement syndrome, biceps tendinitis, or instability. In summary, the history may be nonspecific for the diagnosis of labral problems.

Physical Examination

A thorough shoulder examination is essential in the evaluation of a patient with a possible labral injury. Palpation for tenderness, especially in the areas of the biceps tendon and rotator cuff, is important. The biceps tension test is performed by resisting shoulder flexion with the shoulder in a 90 degree forward-flexed position, the elbow extended and forearm supinated. Positive test results may suggest irritation or injury of the biceps tendon or biceps tendon anchor. This test has been the most helpful in the authors' experience for evaluating SLAP lesions. The compression-rotation test may also be useful. It is performed by compressing the humeral head into the glenoid and then rotating the shoulder. This test attempts to trap the torn labrum between the joint surfaces, similar to the way a McMurray test catches and snaps the meniscus in the knee. Some patients may have palpable or audible popping or catching in the joint due to labral damage. Despite these provocative maneuvers, none of these tests are specific for labral injury.

All patients should be evaluated for associated problems such as a rotator cuff injury or glenohumeral instability. Inspection may reveal atrophy of the cuff musculature. Range of motion may be normal, but a "painful arc" may exist between 60 and 120 degrees of forward elevation or abduction. Palpation of the shoulder should include cuff insertion sites as well as the bicipital groove and acromioclavicular joint. Supraspinatus strength should be tested to evaluate pain and weakness in the rotator cuff. Impingement tests should also be performed. The impingement No. 1 test is performed with the patient supine and the shoulder in full forward flexion and internal rotation. Pain indicates a positive result. The impingement No. 2 test is also performed with the patient supine. The arm is positioned in 90 degrees of abduction, with the elbow in flexion. The arm is then gently adducted with further elevation and internal rotation. This compresses the rotator cuff structures beneath the acromial arch and causes pain when disease is present.

Tests for glenohumeral instability should examine the subacromial sulcus sign for inferior subluxation, posterior apprehension, anterior apprehension and apprehension suppression, and anterior and posterior translation laxity.

Radiographic Evaluation

Conventional radiographs are routinely obtained in the patient with shoulder problems. Characteristic findings of impingement syndrome, degenerative arthritis, shoulder instability, and acromioclavicular joint disease may be present. These radiographs may also help to exclude neoplasm and calcium deposits from a diagnosis. Conventional radiography is not generally helpful in diagnosing routine labral lesions. A superior humeral head fracture has been noted in some cases of SLAP lesion caused by forceful joint compression. Ianotti and Wang[13] described a rare situation in which a small fracture of the superior glenoid tubercle was present with a SLAP lesion. These examples appear to be the rare instances in which plain radiographs can suggest a noninstability labral lesion.

Computed tomographic arthrography has improved the detection of labral lesions, primarily in cases in which a Bankart lesion is present.[14, 15] However, such arthrography is better suited to evaluate bony rather than soft tissue abnormalities. Magnetic resonance imaging techniques are better suited for soft tissue abnormalities; however, they are more helpful with the rotator cuff and biceps tendon than the glenoid labrum and capsule. Magnetic resonance arthrography has been used to evaluate labral injuries.[16] This technique involves an intra-articular injection of gadolinium and saline in an attempt to increase the efficacy of magnetic resonance evaluation. This procedure improves the chances of detecting SLAP lesions as well as isolated labral tears when conventional magnetic resonance imaging is not helpful. Overdiagnosis is a potential problem, especially in patients with normal variations such as sublabral holes or a meniscoid labrum. It is not prudent to rely solely on a magnetic resonance image to diagnose or exclude a labral lesion.

As has been discussed, labral injuries are often difficult to diagnose accurately despite a thorough history, physical examination, and the latest in diagnostic imaging. In patients who have persistent shoulder pain and symptoms that do not fit into a common diagnosis, it is important to maintain high clinical suspicion for a labral lesion. Ultimately, diagnostic shoulder arthroscopy may be required to make a definitive diagnosis.

Conservative Treatment

Conservative management is often futile in the patient with a symptomatic labral lesion. Frequently, the diagnosis has been difficult to make and the patient has been symptomatic for some time. Conservative measures such as restriction of activities and modification of work may be tried along with a general shoulder rehabilitation program. These measures, however, may be unsuccessful because of the inherent mechanical nature of the underlying labral injury. Therefore, there appears to be little role for nonoperative management of the patient with a documented, mechanically significant labral lesion.

Patient Education

All patients with labral abnormalities should be advised of treatment options. Frequently, instruction by the physician as well as take-home brochures and videotapes that explain the condition and treatment options are helpful. The patient should also be counseled on the importance of complying with the postoperative immobilization and rehabilitation program. Because labral lesions may also be associated with other abnormalities, such as of the rotator cuff or the biceps tendon, or instability, the patient must also be informed about the possibility of addressing the secondary conditions that might exist.

SURGICAL TECHNIQUES

Patterns of Injury

The labrum is the anchor point of the glenohumeral ligaments and serves as a load-sharing structure. There are several potential mechanisms of injury that can be postulated from a biomechanical standpoint. Potential mechanisms are compression, avulsion, traction, shear, and chronic degeneration. These may be isolated mechanisms or occur in combination, resulting in complex patterns of labral injury. These injuries may occur in any one or more of six arbitrarily designated areas: (1) superior labrum; (2) anterior labrum above the midglenoid notch; (3) anterior labrum below the midglenoid notch; (4) inferior labrum; (5) posterior inferior labrum; and (6) posterior superior labrum.

Labral tear patterns can be described by the arthroscopic appearance of the tear, similar to the description of meniscal tears in the knee. Tears are classified as degenerative lesions, flap tears, incomplete split tears, bucket-handle tears, and SLAP lesions.

Degenerative Lesions

Degenerative tears of the labrum appear as fraying and fragmentation and may occur with degenerative joint disease. These tears may also be related to the normal aging process, according to DePalma, White, and Callery.[12] Some lesions may be related to chronic joint abuse with repetitive compression overload of the joint. The smooth gliding surface of the normal labrum gives way to roughened irregular fibrous elements. Frequently, a "kissing lesion" of chondromalacia on the articular cartilage of the humerus is present. Conversely, in some patients, articular lesions of the humerus may initiate degenerative tearing of the labrum.

Flap Tears

Flap tears of the glenoid labrum may occur in any location. These lesions are thought to be associated with compression of the labral tissues between the humeral head and glenoid. Often, the mechanism is a fall on the outstretched arm or shearing caused by an anterior/posterior subluxation episode. Another cause of flap tears, especially in the posterior superior labrum, is posterior impingement as described by Jobe.[9] Labral flap tears can become mechanically significant, causing clicking, popping, and catching, and occasionally can have symptoms resembling those of instability of the shoulder.[17]

Incomplete Split Tears

Incomplete split labral tears most commonly occur anteriorly or posteriorly. They may be associated with anterior or posterior subluxation of the shoulder and may be related to the traction on the capsule and compression of the labrum. Often, the split tear causes abrasion of the overlying humeral head, resulting in a chondromalacic kissing lesion.

Bucket-Handle Tears

The bucket-handle tear is frequently an extension of an incomplete split tear. These lesions may or may not be associated with instability. The fragment may displace and become incarcerated or may be potentially displaceable. The shoulder remains stable if the peripheral attachment of the glenoid remains intact. Displaced tears may be a cause of pseudoinstability and result in locking, catching, and popping.[18]

Lesions in Throwing Athletes

Andrews and Carson[19] described tearing of the anterior superior labrum seen in elite throwing athletes. The lesions were considered secondary to traction on the biceps tendon and the biceps tendon insertion on the superior labrum. Many of these patients had associated lesions, including supraspinatus tendon tears and partial biceps tendon ruptures. The average duration of symptoms before surgery was 12 months. All patients underwent débridement of the labral tear, the rotator cuff tear, and the partial biceps rupture. Of the 73 throwing athletes, results were excellent or good in 88% of cases, whereby the athletes were able to return to their throwing sports at an average of 13.5 months.

SLAP Lesions

A SLAP lesion is an injury to the superior labrum extending from anterior to posterior. SLAP lesions must always include the area of the biceps tendon anchor onto the superior labrum and glenoid. A meniscoid-type superior labrum is more at risk for a type III or type IV SLAP lesion.

SLAP lesions are classified according to their arthroscopic appearance:[20]

Type I   The superior labrum is frayed and degenerative in appearance, but the attachment of the labrum to the glenoid and the biceps tendon anchor is intact (Fig. 9–3).

Type II   There may or may not be fraying of the superior labrum, but definite pathologic detachment of the labrum and biceps anchor from the glenoid is present. The anchor arches away from the superior glenoid neck, resulting in an unstable biceps-labral complex (Fig. 9–4).

Type III   The superior labrum has a bucket-handle tear analogous to that of the knee meniscus. The biceps tendon remains intact as does the peripheral labral rim attachment (Fig. 9–5).

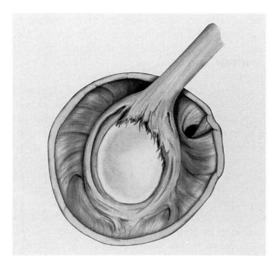

Figure 9–3 • Type I SLAP lesion.

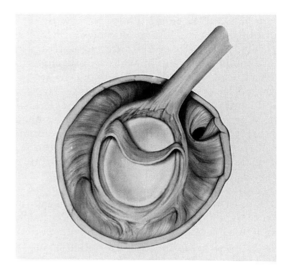

Figure 9–5 • Type III SLAP lesion.

Type IV   A bucket-handle tear of the superior labrum is seen that extends as a split tear into the biceps tendon. The biceps anchor remains intact, but the torn tendon-labral complex may displace into the joint (Fig. 9–6).

Complex   A combination consists of two or more types of SLAP tears, most commonly a type II and type IV.

At our institution, Snyder, Banas, and Karzel[21] completed a retrospective evaluation of a large number of SLAP lesions. Between 1985 and 1993, 2,375 arthroscopic shoulder procedures were performed at the Southern California Orthopedic Institute. Superior glenoid labral injuries were seen in 140 patients, or approximately 6% of all shoulder arthroscopic procedures. The average age of the patients was 38 years, with males predominating at 91% of the patient population. Of all SLAP lesions, 55% were type II, 21% were type I, 10% were type IV, 9% were type III, and 5% were complex lesions. Only 28% of these lesions were isolated, and the remainder were associated with rotator cuff or anterior labral disease. Twenty-two percent of patients had an associated Bankart lesion. The average time from injury to surgery was 20 months for all tears and 13 months for isolated labral lesions.

Maffet, Gartsman, and Moseley[22] also showed a male predominance (88%) of the SLAP lesion. Rotator cuff injury was present in 48% of their patients and Bankart lesions in 19 of 84 shoulders. They described several SLAP lesion patterns in addition to the classification of Snyder and colleagues.

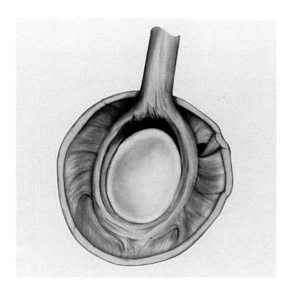

Figure 9–4 • Type II SLAP lesion.

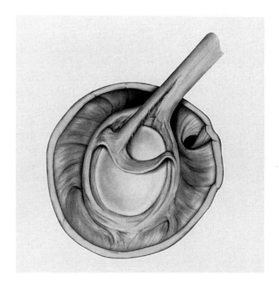

Figure 9–6 • Type IV SLAP lesion.

Etiology of SLAP Lesions. There is presently no laboratory proof to support a distinct etiology for SLAP lesions. Historically, there are several different potential mechanisms.[20] Compression and impaction of the superior joint surface can occur with a fall on an abducted arm, causing the humeral head to subluxate superiorly. There may be chondral damage similar to that of a Hill-Sachs lesion, but on the superior articular surface of the humeral head rather than the posterior lateral. Another potential mechanism is a sudden pull on the arm that causes the biceps tendon anchor to avulse the superior labrum from the glenoid. Similarly, this type of mechanism may also occur with repetitive trauma, such as throwing.

Our most recent study[21] showed that a fall or direct blow to the shoulder was the most common mechanism, occurring in 31% of patients. Nineteen percent of patients had an episode of glenohumeral dislocation or subluxation, and 16% were injured while lifting a heavy object. Fourteen percent had an insidious onset of pain. Patients in overhead racquet sports accounted for only 6% and repetitive throwers for 6%. Eight percent had unspecified injury patterns.

Rodosky and co-workers[23] showed the role of the biceps-superior labrum complex in augmenting the anterior stability of the shoulder. When the superior labrum was detached from the glenoid in the cadaveric model, anterior capsular stress was increased. There is a significant association of shoulder instability with SLAP lesions, especially type II. Frequently, successful surgical treatment requires repair of both the SLAP lesion and anterior instability.

Diagnosis of the Type II SLAP Lesion. Many times, it is difficult arthroscopically to distinguish a type II SLAP lesion from a normal anatomic variation. The authors believe that the type II SLAP lesion is frequently overdiagnosed. The superior labrum often has a meniscoid appearance with a free edge that may be misinterpreted as a pathologic detachment. The meniscoid labrum may have its attachment below the level of the glenoid articular surface, leading to the misdiagnosis of a labral avulsion. Acute traumatic cases are more easily diagnosed because of the concomitant hemorrhage around the labral tissue similar to an acute Bankart lesion. The chronic cases, however, are more difficult to diagnose because of the tendency for fibrous healing, which mimics a normal variant and can mask a pathologic detachment. The glenoid articular cartilage extends down to the labral attachment in the normal shoulder; in a chronic type II SLAP lesion, a space exists between the glenoid articular cartilage and the attachment of the biceps anchor. On viewing with the arthroscope, the superior labrum arches away from the underlying bone by approximately 3–4 mm when tension is applied to the biceps tendon.

Treatment of Labral Lesions

Because labral tears are often associated with glenohumeral laxity, shoulder stability should be examined in the office preoperatively and with the patient under anesthesia before proceeding with shoulder arthroscopy. Labral tears that are truly isolated in the stable shoulder may be treated with débridement of the tear alone. Damaged tissue is removed, the surgeon taking care to preserve the peripheral attachment of the labrum and its capsular attachment to the glenoid. Vertical split tears may be treated similarly to bucket-handle tears of the meniscus. A combination of basket forceps, motorized shavers, and, possibly, electrosurgery may be used. If instability is present, the damaged labral tissues should be débrided to prevent mechanical symptoms postoperatively; a stabilization procedure should then be performed.

Glasgow et al.[24] reported results of arthroscopic glenoid labral resection in 28 overhead athletes. Shoulder stability appeared critical for good results. Ninety-one percent of patients with normal stability had good to excellent results at 2-year follow-up. On the contrary, if glenohumeral instability was present, 75% of patients showed fair or poor results when débridement was performed without stabilization. Altchek et al.[25] studied 40 patients after labral débridement. At the time of surgery, 40% had instability, but 72% of patients reported significant improvement of pain at 1-year follow-up. These authors' results deteriorated steadily with time, with only 7% of patients achieving long-term relief. Both groups of authors concluded that labral débridement alone does not achieve satisfactory results in the overhead athlete and that it is essential to focus on the underlying glenohumeral instability.

Payne and Jokl[26] evaluated 14 patients who underwent labral débridement. All patients had shoulder pain with overhead activity and showed no evidence of glenohumeral instability preoperatively. At 6 months, 93% of patients had good or excellent results. However, at an average of 2 years postoperatively, only 71% had good or excellent results. The best results in this study were noted for the superior and anterior inferior labral segments. Patients who had the anterior superior labrum débrided were at risk for delayed glenohumeral instability. It is important to be aware, especially in the elite overhead athlete, that glenohumeral instability may be present when a labral lesion is noted at the time of arthroscopy and that successful treatment may require attention to both problems.

Treatment of Type I and Type III SLAP Lesions

Treatment of SLAP lesions depends on the type of problem. A type I SLAP lesion should be débrided back to a stable rim in the same fashion as a degenerative tear of the knee meniscus. A type III SLAP lesion is treated similarly to the bucket-handle meniscus tear, with resection of the torn fragment. It is important to evaluate the stability of the biceps anchor in type I and type III lesions. Occasionally, the middle glenohumeral ligament may attach to a type III SLAP lesion. It may be necessary to suture repair ligament labral complex to prevent progressive glenohumeral instability. As with isolated labral tears, SLAP lesions may occur with glenohumeral instability; the instability, when present, must be treated at the same time the SLAP lesion is treated.

Treatment of Type II SLAP Lesions

The type II SLAP lesion is characterized by superior labral detachment from the superior glenoid tubercle, resulting in an unstable biceps anchor. The biceps anchor requires reattachment to the glenoid not only to ensure normal biceps function but also to restore normal shoulder stability. Initially, our management of type II SLAP lesions included débridement of interposed fibrous tissues and decortication of the glenoid neck to promote healing. With prolonged immobilization in an arm sling, many of these patients healed. However, healing was sometimes incomplete, and early motion was more desirable, especially if the patient had an associated problem, such as a partial rotator cuff tear. Currently, we use suture anchors to fix the superior labral tissue to attain more reliable healing and allow for early motion.

Field and Savoie[27] used the transglenoid fixation technique in 20 patients with type II and type IV SLAP lesions. At an average follow-up time of 21 months, all 20 patients had good or excellent results. Yoneda and colleagues[28] treated 10 athletes with type II SLAP lesions. All patients were treated with abrasion followed by arthroscopic staple fixation. A second-look arthroscopic procedure was performed at 3–6 months for staple removal. At the time of second look, all 10 lesions were stable, 4 showed complete healing, and 6 incomplete healing. At a minimum follow-up time of 2 years, 80% of patients had good or excellent results.

Resch et al.[29] have reported the results of SLAP repairs in 14 patients. They used absorbable tacks or cannulated titanium screws. At a minimum follow-up time of 6 months, eight patients were able to return to full overhead activities. Four patients were improved but unable to return to such activity, and two were unimproved.

Authors' Preferred Treatment

At the Southern California Orthopedic Institute, it is preferable to fix SLAP lesions by utilizing nonabsorbable braided suture and implantable suture anchors. Either the 2.7 or 4.0 mm threaded Revo suture anchor (Linvatec Inc., Largo, Fla.), which allows firm fixation but can be removed if the suture fails during knot tying, is preferred.

Surgical Technique. Standard anterior and posterior arthroscopic portals are established (the anterior directly behind the biceps tendon), and a third portal, the anterior midglenoid portal (AMP), is established just above the subscapularis tendon. The second anterior portal is essential when we use the suture Shuttle Relay. This portal is 2 cm inferior to the anterior superior portal. To create the AMP, an incision is made through the skin only, and an outside-in technique is used with a blunt obturator to place the cannula just superior to the leading edge of the subscapularis tendon. The degenerative biceps and labral tissue is débrided with a small motorized shaver. The shaver is then used to débride the fibrous tissue attached to the superior glenoid neck via the anterior superior portal (Fig. 9–7). A 4 mm round bur lightly decorticates the exposed superior glenoid neck, and a target hole is created

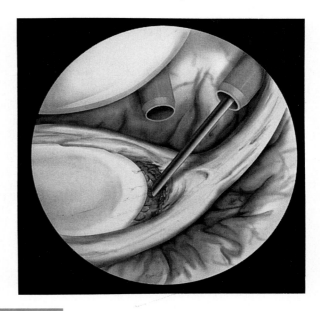

Figure 9–7 • The bone beneath the superior labrum and biceps anchor is lightly decorticated with a 4 mm ball tip bur.

just below the cartilage to prevent skiving of the punch. With the superior glenoid neck prepared, a Revo punch is placed via the anterior superior portal into the target spot directly below the biceps tendon insertion (Fig. 9–8). The punch is angled 45 degrees below the articular cartilage and 45 degrees posteriorly, and it is inserted up to its hub.

A Revo suture anchor loaded with No. 2 nonabsorbable braided suture is inserted into the pilot hole (Fig. 9–9) via the anterior superior cannula. The anchor is tested for stability, and the suture is visualized to pass

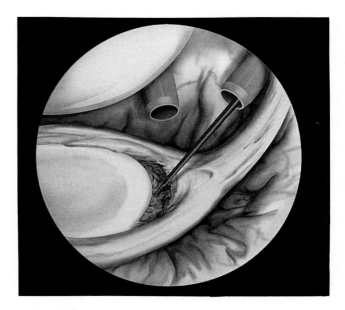

Figure 9–8 • A Revo drill bit or punch is used to create a hole for suture anchor placement. This hole is directed 45 degrees posteriorly and 45 degrees medially.

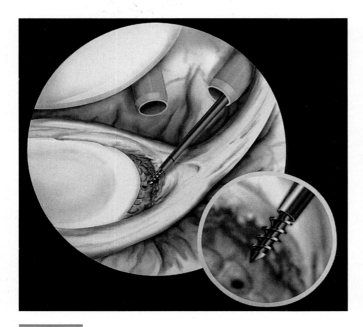

Figure 9–9 • A Revo suture anchor loaded with No. 2 Ethibond suture is placed into the predrilled hole.

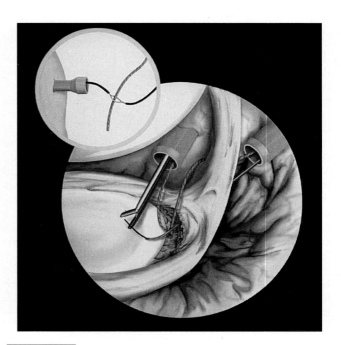

Figure 9–11 • An epidural needle is passed through the superior labrum. A suture Shuttle Relay is advanced through the needle and retrieved through the AMP portal.

easily within the eyelet. One limb of the suture is retrieved out of the AMP with a crochet hook (Fig. 9–10).

A 6 inch 17 gauge epidural needle or a crescent-shaped suture hook is passed down the anterior superior cannula, piercing the posterior aspect of the biceps anchor (Fig. 9–11). A suture Shuttle Relay is passed through the needle and retrieved via the AMP with a grasper. The limb of the suture outside the AMP is loaded into the eyelet of

the Shuttle Relay (Fig. 9–12), and the Shuttle Relay is then pulled back down the AMP, up through the labrum and biceps anchor, and out through the anterior superior cannula (Fig. 9–13). The process is repeated, first by retrieving the second suture out of the AMP and then by passing the needle into the anterior portion of the biceps anchor. The Shuttle Relay is passed through the needle and retrieved via the AMP. The second suture limb is loaded

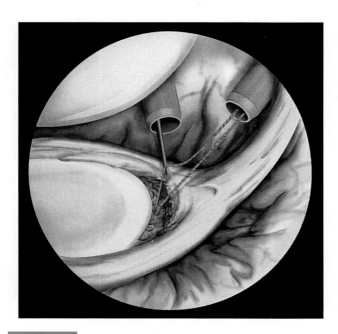

Figure 9–10 • A crochet hook is used to retrieve one or both limbs of the suture through the AMP portal.

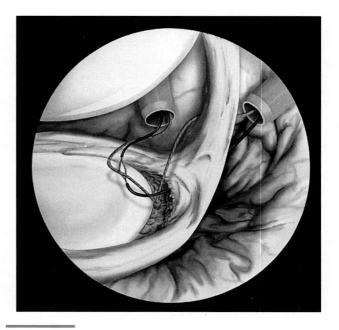

Figure 9–12 • One limb of the suture is threaded through the eyelet of the Shuttle Relay and carried with the Shuttle Relay back through the labrum exiting the anterior superior portal.

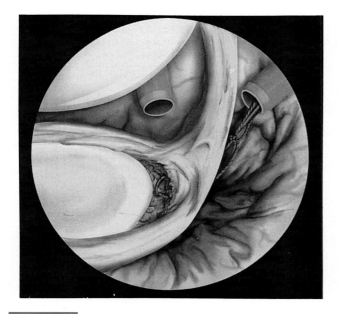

Figure 9–13 • The two limbs of the suture are tied with an arthroscopic knot pusher, and a mattress stitch is completed.

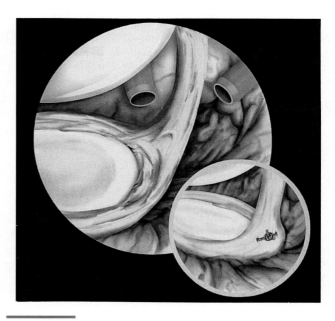

Figure 9–14 • A completed repair showing a well-approximated labrum and a stable knot.

into the Shuttle Relay eyelet and pulled in a retrograde fashion down the anterior midglenoid cannula, through the labrum and biceps anchor, and out the anterior superior cannula.

Both limbs of the suture are now out the anterior superior cannula and are on the capsular side of the superior labrum. The arthroscopic knot pusher is then utilized to check for twists in the suture limbs. If the knot pusher passes easily without twists, the labrum is held in a reduced position while sequential half-hitch knots are stacked with the knot pusher (Fig. 9–14). Generally, five half-hitch sutures are placed, alternating suture posts after the third and fourth throws. An arthroscopic punch is used to clip the suture tails, and a probe is used to test security of the knot and stability of the biceps anchor.

Treatment of Type IV SLAP Lesions

In a type IV SLAP lesion, there is tearing into the biceps tendon and the superior labrum. Most often, the biceps tendon is still firmly anchored to the superior glenoid. If the amount of biceps involved is small, the torn labrum and biceps can be resected. If the tear encompasses 30% or more of the biceps tendon in an older patient, this may be an indication to proceed with a primary biceps tenodesis. Frequently, the remaining biceps tendon of the older patient is degenerative. Young patients present a dilemma when they have a significant biceps tear in connection with a superior labral tear. The authors' preference is to preserve the superior labrum and biceps with suture repair. Mattress sutures are placed directly through the tissues. Suture anchors are not required because the biceps anchor is well attached to the glenoid, and the superior labral root is still stable.

Standard anterior and posterior portals are established. The suture repair is initiated with the arthroscope in the posterior operating portal. A 6 inch 17 gauge epidural needle is passed through the skin along the lateral border of the acromion. The needle is passed through the intact portion of the biceps, then through the split portion. A suture Shuttle Relay is passed down the epidural needle and retrieved with a grasping clamp via the anterior portal. The needle is withdrawn, and a nonabsorbable suture is loaded into the eyelet of the Shuttle Relay on the percutaneous side. The Shuttle Relay is then pulled out the anterior cannula, pulling the suture through the tendon. The epidural needle is reinserted, puncturing the biceps and superior labrum 4–5 mm from the first suture site. Again, the Shuttle Relay is passed through the needle and retrieved out of the anterior cannula. The Shuttle Relay is then loaded on the anterior cannula side and passed retrograde through the labrum and biceps tendon out the capsular side.

Both suture tails are now on the capsular side, and a crochet hook is inserted through the anterior cannula to retrieve both limbs of the suture. An arthroscopic knot pusher first checks for twists in the suture and then is used to tie alternating half-hitch knots. Again, the posts are switched after the third and fourth throws. As the knot is tied, the tear closes between the biceps and labrum. Suturing continues in the manner previously described to repair the labrum anterior and posterior to the biceps tendon anchor until the labrum is repaired. Frequently, the arthroscope must be switched to the anterior portal to repair the posterior extension of the SLAP lesion. The posterior portal is used as the operating portal for retrieval of the Shuttle Relay.

The bucket-handle tear of a type III SLAP lesion may be repaired in the fashion previously described for type IV lesions if the middle glenohumeral ligament is unstable. Infrequently, a complex SLAP lesion, usually a type II and type IV together, must be reattached. The labral tear is débrided or repaired after the anchor is stabilized.

POSTOPERATIVE CARE

The postoperative treatment of type II and type IV SLAP lesions is similar. Patients are protected in a neutral rotation sling (UltraSling, DonJoy Inc., Carlsbad, Calif.) for 3 weeks. They are allowed gentle elbow, wrist, and hand range-of-motion exercises in this early period. After the first week, they may remove the sling periodically, but they must avoid forceful external rotation or extension of their arm behind the body, and they must avoid biceps strain. At 4 to 5 weeks postoperatively, rehabilitation is advanced to protected biceps strengthening. No stressful biceps activity is allowed for 3 months.

Two patients with type II SLAP lesions and two patients with type IV SLAP lesions have undergone repeated arthroscopy. All four demonstrated secure reattachment of the labrum and biceps tendon and healing of the superior labrum.

SUMMARY

As shoulder arthroscopy is performed more routinely, labral disease has been increasingly recognized as a cause of shoulder dysfunction. A high degree of suspicion must be maintained for a patient whose mechanical symptoms do not fit a usual pattern of shoulder disease. Labral lesions are difficult to diagnose without arthroscopic evaluation. If a labral lesion is present, one should recognize preoperatively if the patient has associated instability. If instability is present in conjunction with a labral tear, the instability must also be repaired to obtain the most favorable result. Without instability, the labral tear can be arthroscopically treated by débridement, suture anchor fixation, or repair of SLAP lesions. As the understanding of labral lesions grows and surgical techniques and imaging are refined, earlier diagnosis and treatment should reduce the morbidity and progressive disability that currently accompany these injuries.

References

1. Gardner E and Gray DJ: Prenatal development of the human shoulder and acromioclavicular joint. Am J Anat 92:219–276, 1953.
2. Snyder SJ, Rames RD, and Wolbert E: Labral lesions. In McGinty JB (ed.): Operative Arthroscopy. New York, Raven Press, 1991, pp 491–499.
3. Detrisac DA and Johnson LL: Arthroscopic Shoulder Anatomy: Pathologic and Surgical Implications. Thorofare, N.J., Slack, 1986.
4. Morgan C, Rames RD, and Snyder SJ: Anatomical variations of the glenohumeral ligaments. Presented at the Annual Meeting of the American Academy of Orthopaedic Surgeons, Anaheim, Calif., 1991.
5. Snyder SJ, Buford D, Wuh HCK: The Buford complex—the loose anterior superior labrum-middle glenohumeral ligament complex: a normal anatomical variant. Presented at the Annual Meeting of the American Academy of Orthopaedic Surgeons, Boston, 1992.
6. Howell SM and Galinat BJ: The glenoid-labral socket: a constrained articular surface. Clin Orthop 243:122–125, 1989.
7. Reeves B: Experiments on the tensile strength of the anterior capsular structures of the shoulder in man. J Bone Joint Surg Br 50:858–865, 1968.
8. Perry J: Anatomy and biomechanics of the shoulder in throwing, swimming, gymnastics and tennis. Clin Sports Med 2:247–270, 1983.
9. Jobe CM: Evidence linking posterior superior labral impingement and shoulder instability. Presented at the Meeting of the American Shoulder and Elbow Surgeons, Seattle, Wash., September 1991.
10. Karzel R, Nuber G, and Lautenschlager E: Contact stresses during compression loading of the glenohumeral joint: the role of the glenoid labrum. Proc Inst Med Chicago 42:64–65, 1989.
11. Cooper DE, Arnoczky SP, O'Brien SJ, et al.: Anatomy, histology, and vascularity of the glenoid labrum: an anatomical study. J Bone Joint Surg Am 74:46–52, 1992.
12. DePalma AJ, White JB, and Callery G: Degenerative lesions of the shoulder joint at various age groups which are compatible with good function. AAOS Instr Course Lect 7:168–180, 1950.
13. Iannotti JP and Wang ED: Avulsion fracture of the supraglenoid tubercle: a variation of the SLAP lesion. J Shoulder Elbow Surg 1:26–30, 1992.
14. Deutsch AL, Resnick D, Mink JH, et al.: Computed and conventional arthrotomography of the glenohumeral joint: normal anatomy and clinical experience. Radiology 153:603–609, 1984.
15. Rafii M, Firooznia H, Golimbu C, et al.: CT arthrography of capsular structures of the shoulder. Am J Roentgenol 146:361–367, 1986.
16. Karzel RP and Snyder SJ: Magnetic resonance arthrography of the shoulder: a new technique of shoulder imaging. Clin Sports Med 1:123–136, 1993.
17. Kohn D: The clinical relevance of glenoid labrum lesions. Arthroscopy 3:223–230, 1987.
18. Pappas A, Goss T, and Kleinman P: Symptomatic shoulder instability due to lesions of the glenoid labrum. Am J Sports Med 11:279–288, 1983.
19. Andrews JR and Carson WG: The arthroscopic treatment of glenoid labrum tears: the throwing athlete. Orthop Trans 8:44, 1984.
20. Snyder SJ, Karzel RP, Del Pizzo W, et al.: SLAP lesions of the shoulder. Arthroscopy 6:274–279, 1990.
21. Snyder SJ, Banas MP, and Karzel RP: An analysis of 140 consecutive injuries to the superior glenoid labrum. J Shoulder Elbow Surg 4:243–248, 1995.
22. Maffet MW, Gartsman GM, and Moseley B: Superior labrum-biceps tendon complex lesions of the shoulder. Am J Sports Med 23:93–98, 1995.
23. Rodosky MW, Harner CD, Fu FH: The role of the long head of the biceps muscle and superior glenoid labrum in anterior stability of the shoulder. Am J Sports Med 22:121–130, 1994.
24. Glasgow SG, Bruce RA, Yacobucci GN, et al.: Arthroscopic resection of glenoid labral tears in the athlete: a report of 29 cases. Arthroscopy 8:48–54, 1992.
25. Altchek DW, Warren RF, Wickiewicz TL, et al.: Arthroscopic labral debridement: a three-year follow-up study. Am J Sports Med 20:702–706, 1992.
26. Payne LZ and Jokl P: The results of arthroscopic debridement of glenoid labral tears based on tear location. Arthroscopy 9:560–565, 1993.
27. Field LD and Savoie FA: Arthroscopic suture repair of superior labral detachment lesions of the shoulder. Am J Sports Med 21:783–790, 1993.
28. Yoneda M, Hirouka A, Saito S, et al.: Arthroscopic stapling for detached superior glenoid labrum. J Bone Joint Surg Br 73:746–750, 1991.
29. Resch H, Golser K, Thoeni H, et al.: Arthroscopic repair of superior glenoid labral detachment (the SLAP lesion). J Shoulder Elbow Surg 2:147–155, 1993.

Chapter

Throwing Shoulder

Laura A. Timmerman

INTRODUCTION

The throwing motion places tremendous stresses on the soft tissues and bony structures of the athlete's shoulder. The injuries that occur as a result of throwing are different from what is commonly seen in patients with shoulder pain who are not involved in overhead sports. For an athlete to throw successfully, the shoulder complex must be capable of achieving the excessive external rotation required to throw while maintaining a stable glenohumeral joint. Injuries to the throwing shoulder can result from acute trauma, such as a fall with a resulting dislocation or fracture, but a more common occurrence is overuse injuries resulting from repetitive throwing.[1] Imbalance in the muscles and soft tissues about the shoulder can result in an injury secondary to abnormal biomechanics of the glenohumeral complex.

History and Epidemiology of Throwing Injuries

In 1941 Bennett[2] first reported on shoulder and elbow lesions of the professional baseball pitcher. He divided the pathologic changes into two groups, the anterior group and the posterior group. The anterior group included inflammatory and traumatic lesions of the supraspinatus tendon, the subacromial space, and the biceps tendon. The posterior lesions were described as an exostosis that developed on the posterior inferior margin of the glenoid secondary to the constant strain during the deceleration portion of the pitch. In 1969 King, Brelsford, and Tullos[3] reported that more than 50% of the professional pitchers examined had a flexion contracture in their elbow and 30% had a valgus deformity of their elbow, and there was a rather uniform finding of an increase in external humeral rotation with a concomitant decrease in internal shoulder rotation in the pitching arm.

In 1978 Barnes and Tullos[1] reported on an analysis of 100 symptomatic baseball players. Of the 100 players, 56 had shoulder problems, with 29 anterior lesions, 24 poste-

rior lesions, and 3 miscellaneous lesions. The anterior lesions included bicipital tendinitis, supraspinatus tendinitis, pectoralis major tendinitis, latissimus dorsi tendinitis, and acromioclavicular joint injuries. All 24 of the posterior lesions were described as posterior capsular syndrome, with an exostosis seen on radiographs in eight patients.

As arthroscopy has developed during the last two decades, the nature of diagnosis in the throwing shoulder has changed. Initially, bicipital tendinitis and bursitis were common diagnoses.[4, 5] This was replaced with the diagnosis of impingement syndrome.[6–8] Despite relief of pain due to treatment of impingement syndrome, the return to the previous level of performance with an acromioplasty alone was poor in some series[9, 10]; for example, in one series only 4 of 18 athletes involved in pitching and throwing returned to their former preinjury status after acromioplasty.[9]

The concept of recurrent shoulder instability as a cause of chronic shoulder pain began to develop in the early 1980s. In 1981 Rowe and Zarins[11] reported on the results of utilizing the Bankart procedure to treat recurrent transient subluxation of the shoulder; although their series reported 70% excellent results, only four of eight pitchers were able to return to throwing. Garth, Allman, and Armstrong[12] reported on a series of patients with occult anterior subluxation in noncontact sports who, at arthroscopic examination of their shoulder, were noted to have conditions consistent with anterior subluxation. With increased use of shoulder arthroscopy, previously unrecognized lesions of the capsule, of the undersurface of the rotator cuff, and of the labrum became important diagnoses.[13–15]

A dynamic electromyographic (EMG) analysis[16] in throwers with anterior instability demonstrated a marked reduction in activity of the pectoralis major, subscapularis, and latissimus dorsi. This in turn added to the anterior instability by decreasing the normal internal rotation force that is required during the late cocking and acceleration phases of the pitch. The activity of the serratus anterior was also decreased in the throwers with anterior instability, which is associated with decreased protraction of the scapula and increased anterior laxity. The neuromuscular imbalance seen in the throwing athletes with anterior shoulder instability was considered to be either a part of the primary condition or a secondary phenomenon.

Current concepts regarding shoulder pain in the throwing athlete are based on early instability of the glenohumeral joint, which can lead to muscular imbalance and abnormal demands on the muscles about the shoulder, including the scapular stabilizers and the rotator cuff. Rotator cuff irritation can result because the cuff is attempting to stabilize the humeral head. With persistent instability, labral tears and capsular laxity can develop. With subluxation of the shoulder, secondary impingement can develop.[17]

Knowledge of the biomechanics of the throwing motion is crucial to the clinician involved in treating shoulder injuries of throwing athletes. By understanding the anatomy of the shoulder complex and the mechanics involved in throwing, one has a framework for diagnosis and treatment of shoulder disorders, which can be approached in a systematic fashion.

BIOMECHANICS OF THROWING

The throwing motion is used in various activities, including racquet sports, the javelin toss, and basketball. Analysis of the baseball pitch allows the most comprehensive understanding of throwing mechanics; this information can then be applied to other forms of throwing.[18, 19]

Pappas, Zawacki, and Sullivan[20] analyzed 15 major league pitchers with high-speed cinematography. They divided the pitch into three phases: cocking, acceleration, and follow-through. They found that the shoulder had an average peak angular velocity for internal rotation of 6,180 degrees/sec just prior to ball release. The movement about the shoulder is impressive. The authors reported that the entire excursion of the arm through space occurred within a range of 225 degrees with respect to the horizontal plane. This motion is not confined just to the glenohumeral joint; rather, it is the result of the composite action of the glenohumeral and scapulothoracic joints, along with trunk extension, flexion, and rotation.

At the Biomechanics Laboratory of the American Sports Medicine Institute in Birmingham, Ala., data have been collected using motion analysis of the pitching motion of more than 230 baseball pitchers. On the basis of the analysis of this information, the baseball pitch is divided into five phases of throwing: wind-up, cocking, acceleration, deceleration, and follow-through.

Wind-Up Phase

The wind-up phase (Fig. 10–1) starts with a two-legged stance and ends in a position of a one-legged stance. In the one-legged stance position, the ipsilateral leg is planted while the contralateral leg is brought up into a tucked position, with the hip and knee flexed to approximately 90 degrees. This phase is complete when the ball is removed from the glove. The pitcher prepares for delivery of

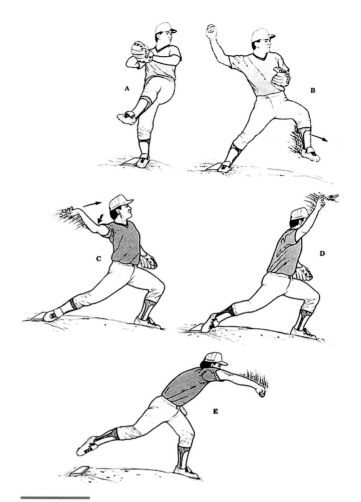

Figure 10–1 • The five phases of pitching: *A*, Wind-up. *B*, Cocking. *C*, Acceleration. *D*, Deceleration and ball release. *E*, Follow-through. (From Nicholas JA and Hershman EB: The Upper Extremity in Sports Medicine, St. Louis, Mosby-Year Book, 1995, p 751.)

the ball by obtaining correct body posture and balance. This is a smooth preparation phase of throwing, and no excessive strain is placed across the pitcher's shoulder or elbow. EMG analysis of the muscles about the shoulder shows minimal activity during this phase, and there is little difference in the activity of muscles in professional as compared with amateur pitchers.[21]

Cocking Phase

During the cocking phase (see Fig. 10–1), the acceleration generated for ball delivery is a result of correct and optimal body position. The contralateral leg is taken from a tucked position and is planted in front of the body. The pelvis and trunk are rotated internally to face the plate, and the internal rotation of the shoulder follows with maximum external rotation of the humerus while the arm is in a 90 degree abducted position. The elbow is flexed approximately 90 degrees, and as the humerus reaches the point of maximum external rotation, the elbow begins to extend. During this position, there is very little forward motion of the ball. Consequently, at the end of this phase, the shoulder has advanced, and the hand and ball remain positioned behind the body. This results in an eccentric load applied to the humeral adductors (including the pectoralis major and the subscapularis) and the internal rotators (latissimus dorsi and teres major). This extrinsic muscle tension allows the body to become "coiled" to impart energy to the ball.

With EMG analysis Gowan and co-workers[21] identified two groups of muscles that are active during the pitching act. The first group included the supraspinatus, infraspinatus, teres minor, deltoid, trapezius, and biceps brachii. They found that this group was responsible primarily for positioning the shoulder and elbow for delivery of the pitch; a second group of muscles, including the pectoralis major, serratus anterior, subscapularis, and latissimus dorsi, displayed stronger activity during the propulsive phase of the pitch. EMG analysis of muscle activity during the early cocking phase showed increased activity of the biceps, with increased activity of the subscapularis and supraspinatus during late cocking.[22, 23]

Acceleration Phase

The acceleration phase (see Fig. 10–1) of the pitch is that time between the end of the cocking phase to the point of ball release. This is an extremely short period; the term acceleration refers to the energy imparted to the ball, not to the action of the arm segments during the pitch. During approximately 50 to 80 milliseconds, the ball is accelerated from a stationary position to a speed in excess of 80 miles per hour.[24] The pitcher moves forward and transfers weight onto the forward-planted contralateral foot and leg. This allows for the transfer of the anterior momentum from the legs to the trunk and then to the shoulder. As the trunk is rotated anteriorly during the cocking phase, the anterior motion of the shoulder is stopped to allow the transfer of the forward momentum from the trunk to the arm, thereby providing acceleration of the ball. The momentum is carried in a chain reaction from the shoulder to the humerus, elbow, and forearm, and eventually the momentum reaches the hand, where the energy is imparted to the ball at release.

In addition to this extrinsic load that is applied to the arm, intrinsic acceleration in the horizontal plane results from contraction of the anterior muscles of the shoulder, including the pectoralis and subscapularis. The shoulder internal rotators (subscapularis, latissimus dorsi, and teres major) contract to initiate internal rotation of the humerus. There are tremendous forward forces generated at the shoulder, and during the second half of the acceleration phase the rate of humeral adduction is decreased by the firing of the teres minor, infraspinatus, and supraspinatus. This deceleration of the humerus allows the momentum to be transferred to the forearm and increases the rate of internal rotation, thereby accelerating the ball further. This period of forward hand and ball propulsion is critical for the transfer of energy to the baseball.[21]

Just before the point of maximum external rotation of the arm, the elbow begins to extend. This rapid elbow extension just before ball release is due primarily to the angular velocity of the upper arm and the trunk, not to the elbow extensor muscles.[25, 26] The end of the acceleration phase occurs just before ball release. The shoulder external rotators, including the posterior deltoid and the teres minor, begin to contract to stop the arm. This allows a transfer of momentum to the hand and the ball, and the ball is released. The phase between stopping the acceleration of the arm and complete extension of the wrist with subsequent ball release is called the release point. From this moment on, the relative arm motion is decelerated, and this marks the beginning of the deceleration phase.

Deceleration Phase

The deceleration phase (see Fig. 10–1) lasts from the point of ball release to the end of maximum humeral internal rotation. This is the most violent phase in the pitching mechanism because the momentum generated during the acceleration phase results in an outward force on the arm of approximately the body weight of the athlete,[24] which must be opposed by muscle contraction at the shoulder to maintain stability of the glenohumeral joint. The forces during deceleration are much higher but much shorter than the forces during acceleration. The combination of these compressive forces and the abnormal anterior or posterior subluxation of the humeral head that is seen with glenohumeral joint instability can result in labral tearing.

Follow-Through Phase

During the follow-through phase (see Fig. 10–1), the body moves forward with the arm, thereby reducing the distraction forces applied to the shoulder, and allows the pitcher to regain balance. The follow-through allows for the energy generated during the pitching motion to be dissipated. By utilizing a long follow-through pathway, with the arm combined with forward trunk flexion, extension of the front leg, and swing of the back leg forward, the load across the arm can be transferred to the larger body parts, resulting in a reduction of tension to the posterior side of the arm.

PATHOMECHANICS OF THROWING INJURIES

The forces generated during the throwing motion result in adaptive physiologic changes. These adaptations include an alteration in the range of motion, with a gain in external rotation and a loss of internal rotation of the shoulder. The humerus may become hypertrophic in response to exercise.[27] The repeated stress on the rotator cuff and biceps tendon can result in inflammation with eventual tendinitis and tearing. The labrum is subject to repeated stress and can detach or tear. Repeated stress to the ligamentous capsule can result in instability. More rarely, chondromalacia of the humeral head and glenoid can result.[28] In the skeletally immature, a stress reaction (apophysitis) or separation of the proximal growth plate may occur.[29]

An alteration in the normal muscular balance about the shoulder can result in distraction and subluxation of the glenohumeral joint, which can lead to injury of the involved soft tissue and bony structures. The types of injury can be related to the phases of throwing: anterior impingement; posterior tension; avulsion; and anterior laxity.

Anterior Impingement Injuries

During the throwing motion, the humeral head and the overlying soft tissue sleeve of the rotator cuff and biceps tendon must pass rapidly under the coracoacromial arch. The arch consists of the anterior acromion and the coracoacromial ligament. Impingement of the soft tissues under this arch can result from several different mechanisms. The actual space may decrease secondary to osteophyte formation of the acromion and fibrosis of the subacromial space. Actual weakness or incompetence of the rotator cuff may allow the humerus to ride up and impinge against the coracoacromial arch. Less commonly, an increase in the bulk of the muscles of the rotator cuff secondary to strengthening or inflammation can cause impingement.

Posterior Tension Injuries

The most severe insult to the soft tissues about the shoulder occurs during the deceleration of the pitch. During this phase, the posterior shoulder muscles must contract eccentrically to counteract an outward glenohumeral distraction force equal to the body weight of the thrower. These deceleration torques are nearly twice as great as the acceleration torque on the arm. During deceleration, the rotator cuff muscles may fail under tension and result in posterior rotator cuff tears. These tears are the result of tension overload and commonly occur on the undersurface of the rotator cuff tendons.

Avulsion Injuries

Avulsion of the anterosuperior labrum[30] at the insertion[31] of the biceps tendon is well described in throwers.[30, 31] The biceps contracts during the late cocking phase in order to flex the elbow, and then during the deceleration phase the biceps is actively contracting eccentrically to oppose extension of the elbow.[22] Andrews, Carson, and McLeod[30] demonstrated that with stimulation of the long head of the biceps muscle, the tendinous portion became taut near its attachment to the glenoid labrum and actually lifted the labrum off the glenoid. As the humerus is rapidly rotated internally, additional forces are placed on the biceps tendon between its position in the bicipital groove and its attachment to the glenoid tubercle. The combination of these two forces can result in avulsion of the anterosuperior labrum at the site of insertion of the tendon of the long head of the biceps.

Anterior Laxity Injuries

For an athlete to throw successfully, laxity in the shoulder joint is required to allow for the extreme amount of external rotation of the arm. This external rotation places a tremendous amount of tension on the anterior stabilizing structures of the shoulder, including the anterior capsulolabral complex and the rotator cuff. During the deceleration phase of throwing, the muscles about the shoulder contract to oppose the outward distraction and internal rotation of the humerus, resulting in anterior translation of the humerus on the glenoid. Howell and co-workers[32] demonstrated that with anterior instability the humeral head glides anteriorly when the arm is flexed or rotated from the cocking stage of the throwing motion, producing a shearing stress on the glenoid and labrum. In the normal shoulder, the center of the humeral head rested approximately 4 mm posterior to the center of the glenoid cavity during the cocked stage of the throwing motion; otherwise the humeral head remained centered in the glenoid. The anterior translation of the humerus on the glenoid results in repetitive microtrauma to the anterior labrum and capsular structures, which over time can result in anterior labral tears and capsular laxity.

EVALUATION OF THE THROWER'S SHOULDER

History

Taking the patient's history is the first and usually the most important step in evaluating an injury. The primary complaint is usually a painful shoulder. It is important to determine whether the injury is acute or chronic, whether there have been any recent changes in equipment or throwing style, and what aggravates or relieves the pain. Ascertaining during what phase of the pitch the symptoms occur is useful in localizing the problem. The occurrence of other associated injuries, including those of the elbow, back, and lower extremities, which may have altered the biomechanics of the throwing motion, should be sought out. History of previous treatment, including rehabilitation, medication, injections, and surgery is important. The specific type of previous rehabilitation exercises should be defined to determine whether an adequate course of conservative treatment has been followed.

Physical Examination

The physician should perform a consistent examination of the throwing shoulder on every patient. This avoids missing positive findings and allows the physician to relate the functional phases of throwing to the findings of the physical examination. With experience, the physician becomes familiar with normal physical findings in a throwing shoulder. The uninjured shoulder should always be included for comparison.

Initially, the shoulder is inspected. Any signs of atrophy or swelling should be noted. The scapular motion and contour of the scapular stabilizing muscles should be examined, as those are often missed on physical examination. The scapula plays a pivotal role in the stability and motion of the glenohumeral joint.[33] A simple test for this is to have the patient perform a sitting lift off the table and then observe the scapula while the patient elevates both arms overhead. The posterior musculature of the shoulder is examined to determine the development and strength of the external rotators. The shoulder should then be palpated for areas of tenderness or crepitus. These areas include not only the glenohumeral joint but also the sternoclavicular and acromioclavicular joints, the clavicle, the scapulothoracic joint, and the soft tissues about the shoulder. The best position for examining the posterior capsule and external rotators is with the patient prone and the arm relaxed over the side of the table. While the patient is in this position, the quadrilateral space can be palpated inferior to the teres minor muscle, a rare site of axillary nerve and posterior humeral circumflex artery compression.

Range of motion should be carefully assessed in the sitting, supine, and prone positions. Sitting internal rotation is noted by recording the spinous process the patient can touch with the thumb. In a comparison of both sides of a throwing athlete, the throwing side usually lacks internal rotation. External rotation at both 0 and 90 degrees of abduction should be noted. The throwing side will most likely have an increase in external rotation at 90 degrees of abduction. Brown and co-workers[34] reported on range-of-motion findings in 41 professional baseball players. They noted that pitchers demonstrated 9 degrees more external shoulder rotation and 15 degrees less internal rotation with the arm abducted, 5 degrees more forearm pronation, 5 degrees less shoulder flexion, and 9 degrees less shoulder extension on the dominant side. The amount of forward flexion and abduction should be noted; a painful shoulder often lacks the last few degrees in this plane of motion. True glenohumeral external rotation can be evaluated with the patient in the prone position by fixing the scapula and rotating the humerus in 90 degrees of abduction.

Determining the strength of the muscle groups is a critical part of the examination. Weakness in one portion of the shoulder musculature can result in an imbalance and subsequent injury. The strength of the scapular stabilizers, internal and external rotators, deltoid and supraspinatus, triceps, and biceps are all compared with that of the non-throwing arm.

Stability testing of the shoulder is at times the most difficult part of the physical examination, especially in individuals with a large musculature. It is necessary to compare the stability findings with those of the uninjured shoulder to determine the amount of baseline laxity present. Initially, one can evaluate glenohumeral translation in the sitting position with the arm relaxed. The sulcus sign, or inferior translation of the humeral head, is assessed. The humeral head can be gently pushed in the anterior and posterior planes in this position. Then, while the patient is supine with the shoulder abducted approximately 130 degrees and externally rotated 90 degrees, an anterior translation force is directed to the shoulder by grasping the humeral head with one hand while stabilizing the distal humerus with the other and lifting up on the humerus. This is similar to the Lachman test of the knee. Posterior

instability can be determined by bringing the arm across the chest in 90 degrees of adduction and then placing a posterior force across the humerus while palpating the humeral head posteriorly. Any apprehension with anterior or posterior translation can be determined. Having the patient prone is one of the best positions for detecting anterior instability in the throwing athlete. The arm is externally rotated at 90 degrees of abduction, and a forward force is applied to the humerus. If there is any apprehension with anterior translation, it will be detected with this test, and the symptoms will be relieved with posterior translation of the humerus.

An important part of the physical examination in throwing shoulders is a careful assessment of the labrum. Andrews and Gillogly[35] described this as a "clunk test." The test is performed with the patient in the supine position. The examiner's hand is placed posteriorly on the humeral head, and the opposite hand holds the humeral condyles at the elbow to provide a rotating motion. The patient's arm is brought into full overhead abduction, and the examiner's hand on the humeral head provides an anterior force while the opposite hand rotates the humerus around the glenoid. A clunk or grinding can be felt in the shoulder as the humerus hits or snaps on the labral tear. The location of the labral tear, either superior, anterior, or posterior, is determined by the position of the humeral head at the time the grinding is felt. This clunk can also be felt with the patient in the prone position and anterior force directed on the humeral head as it contacts an anterior labral tear.

It is often difficult to determine whether pain with abduction and external rotation of the humerus is due to instability or to rotator cuff tendinitis. Impingement is elicited by internal rotation of the forward-flexed arm. This can be done with the patient in either the sitting or supine position; in large athletes the latter may be easier. Throwers with undersurface rotator cuff tears may not have obvious signs of impingement, and subtle clues indicating irritation of the rotator cuff should be noted. By internally rotating and adducting the arm across the patient's chest, the supraspinatus tendon is placed on a stretch, and it can be palpated just anterior to the acromion process, with the infraspinatus tendon palpated posteriorly.

Ancillary Tests

Radiographs of the shoulder, including internal and external rotation anteroposterior views, a modified Stryker view (Fig. 10–2) (humerus abducted 45 degrees to allow visualization of the glenoid rim and acromioclavicular joint), and an axillary view, are useful in the throwing athlete. An outlet view and occasionally a profile view of the acromion are both useful in evaluating the subacromial space.[36]

In the past, arthrograms were used to evaluate the rotator cuff, and the arthrogram-computed tomography scan of the shoulder allowed for evaluation of glenoid and labral conditions. Magnetic resonance imaging studies are now commonly used in evaluation of shoulder pain. In the throwing shoulder, the structures most commonly affected

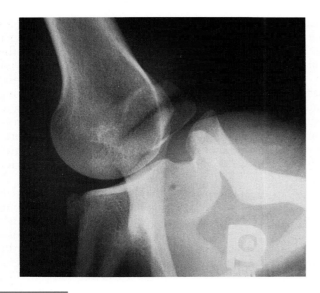

Figure 10–2 • A modified Stryker view of the shoulder. The humerus is abducted 45 degrees and the glenoid rim is visualized. A posterior exostosis is seen.

(partial rotator cuff tears and labral tears) are often difficult to visualize without using contrast media, either saline solution or gadolinium medium.[37] The contrast outlines the labrum and rotator cuff, and tears can be detected more easily. Isokinetic testing of muscle strength is helpful in determining the strength of specific muscle groups. Not only can this testing delineate specific pathologic conditions but it may also assist in developing a rehabilitation program for the injured thrower.[38, 39]

Diagnostic testing with local anesthetic is useful in determining the source of pain. The subacromial space can be injected as well as the acromioclavicular joint. This can help to separate intra-articular problems such as labral tears and anterior laxity from impingement or acromioclavicular joint plan.

Finally, diagnostic arthroscopy is considered the last step in evaluating the injured thrower's shoulder. Every effort is made to reach a diagnosis before surgery, with appropriate conservative treatment instituted. Often a properly performed strengthening program relieves the athlete's symptoms. Arthroscopy should be considered for the athlete who fails to respond to a conservative treatment course. At times, the diagnosis is not confirmed until the shoulder is examined under anesthesia and then systematically inspected arthroscopically.[15, 40, 41]

Rotator Cuff Pathology

Rotator cuff disease in the thrower consists of three main entities: tensile failure, impingement "compressive" disease, and instability. Acute traumatic tears can occur, but these are less common than the injuries due to repetitive activity.

In the thrower, a common rotator cuff lesion is a tensile failure of the undersurface of the rotator cuff, most commonly found in the region of the supraspinatus and infraspinatus tendons. This tensile failure is due to repetitive microtrauma with eccentric overload during the deceleration phase of throwing. This lesion can also be found isolated to the infraspinatus tendon and the posterior glenohumeral capsule. The athlete complains of pain with overhead motion and may complain of pain only with throwing. On physical examination tenderness to palpation over the rotator cuff may be exhibited. Obvious weakness or visible atrophy of the rotator cuff is usually not present. A contrast magnetic resonance image may demonstrate a partial undersurface tear of the rotator cuff. Initially, the athlete is placed in a rehabilitation program with an emphasis on rotator cuff strengthening. If there is no improvement after 2–3 months, arthroscopic débridement of the tear is performed with the rationale that this will stimulate a fibroblastic healing response. The tear is carefully inspected at arthroscopy to rule out a full-thickness defect. The frayed edges are then débrided to a smooth surface, and the defect is lightly débrided back to bleeding tissue (Fig. 10–3). Andrews, Broussard, and Carson[42] reported on 34 athletes with partial tears treated with athroscopic débridement: 85% of the patients had good or excellent results and were able to return to their previous athletic activities; 15% of the patients had poor results and were not able to return to competitive throwing.

If an undersurface tear is present, underlying instability should be ruled out, because this tear can lead to secondary impingement or compressive rotator cuff disease. To rule out instability, a careful examination of the shoulder under anesthesia and a careful arthroscopic examination of the glenohumeral joint for other signs of instability, including a Hill-Sachs lesion and anterior labral and capsular detachments, are required.

Compressive, or impingement, rotator cuff disease can also result in primary rotator cuff problems. The hallmark finding of this mechanism is extra-articular superior surface tears (outside to inside) with evidence of subacromial erosion (Fig. 10–4). This impingement can be caused by a type III hooked acromion, os acromiale,[43] degenerative acromial spurs, or congenital thickening of the coracoacromial ligament.[15]

On physical examination, the patient's pain is relieved with an injection of anesthetic into the subacromial space. Treatment consists of stretching the tight posterior capsule often seen in throwers to help prevent the anterior migration of the humeral head and strengthening the rotator cuff musculature. Surgical decompression may be necessary if conservative treatment fails.

A particular finding in the throwing shoulder involves impingement of the undersurface of the supraspinatus in the position of 90 degrees of abduction and maximum external rotation. In this position, the posterior superior labrum is caught between the posterior rotator cuff and the humeral head. This is also proposed as a mechanism of injury for the posterior cuff tears and labral tears that are seen in throwing athletes.[44, 45]

Full-thickness rotator cuff tears are not often reported in the young throwing athlete, but they can occur. A repair is warranted, but the return to previous level of play is often not successful. In one large series,

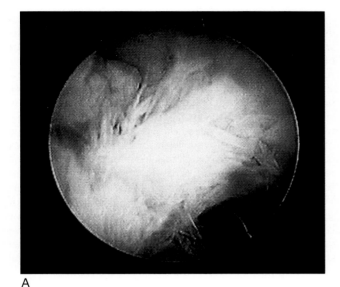

A

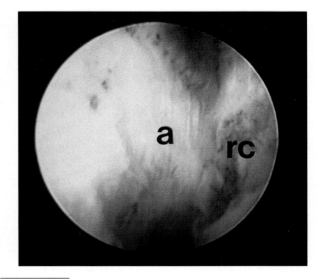

Figure 10–4 • An example of impingement superiorly. This view is of the right shoulder from the posterior portal. a: acromion; rc: rotator cuff.

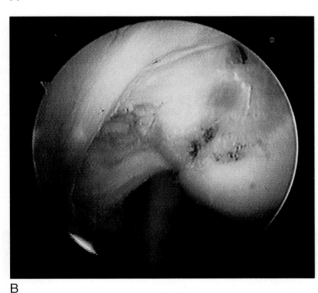

B

Figure 10–3 • An undersurface tear of the rotator cuff in a pitcher. This is the right shoulder as viewed from the posterior portal with the patient in the lateral position. *A,* Predébridement. *B,* Postdébridement.

only 7 of 22 professional or collegiate-level pitchers and throwers with complete or partial rotator cuff tears were able to return to the same competitive level.[10] With arthroscopic decompression of the subacromial space and arthroscopic débridement of the tear, followed by repair through a small deltoid splitting incision, early results are encouraging as compared with an open acromioplasty and rotator cuff repair.[46]

Instability

Instability in the throwing shoulder can be in either the anterior or posterior direction. Instability may result from primary capsular laxity or stretching or be secondary to rotator cuff disease. The diagnosis is usually made based on the history and the physical findings. The athlete may complain of apprehension, feeling of slipping or looseness in the joint, and pain or clicking in the shoulder. The most reliable finding on physical examination is pain with stressing of the humeral head in either the anterior or posterior direction, or a positive apprehension test. The mainstay in treatment of instability is strengthening of the muscles about the shoulder to provide dynamic stability to the glenohumeral joint. If labral problems are present, surgical intervention may be required. If the athlete fails a conservative rehabilitation program, surgery is considered.

After a careful examination of the shoulder under anesthesia, diagnostic arthroscopy is performed. The glenoid labrum is evaluated for evidence of detachment or tears. Under direct visualization, the humeral head is pushed in the anterior, posterior, and inferior directions and the amount of subluxation is noted (Fig. 10–5). Evidence of erosion of the humeral head can indicate minor repetitive subluxation of the humeral head. Once the degree of instability is noted, a decision is made regarding treatment. Mild instability is usually best treated with a conservative strengthening program.

With more severe instability, an open procedure may be indicated for repairing the labrum and capsular structures. The athlete needs to be aware that a return to the previous level of throwing is at times difficult after this procedure. In one series of 12 pitchers who underwent an open anterior capsulolabral reconstruction, only 6 (50%) returned to their former competitive level for at least one season, with an average time to return to competition of 15 months.[47] A report by Bigliani et al.[48] describing an inferior capsular shift procedure for anterior inferior instability offers similar results: only 50% of the throwing athletes returned to their same level of competition, and only 33% of the professional or varsity-level players had this success. Montgomery and Jobe[49] described an anterior capsulo-

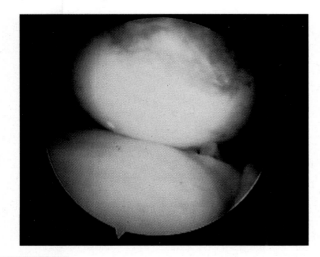

Figure 10–5 • An example of excessive capsular laxity, a large Hill-Sachs lesion, and an anterior Bankart lesion. This patient suffered a traumatic dislocation of the right shoulder. At arthroscopy 5 years after initial injury, the humeral head is seen sitting out of the glenoid, with no stress applied. The patient is in the lateral position, and the view is from the posterior portal.

labral reconstruction that involved a horizontal capsulotomy and suture anchors. They reported 97% good or excellent results in the entire series, and 75% of the baseball players were able to return to their prior level of competition.

Arthroscopic repair of labral detachment has been described.[50] The procedure can be used selectively in athletes with early, true Bankart lesions or early detachment of the anterior capsule and labrum. One technique for repair of anterior lesions involves placement of arthroscopic sutures in the labrum, then passing these sutures posteriorly through a drill hole in the glenoid, where they are tied down over the infraspinatus fascia. The development of biodegradable screws (Fig. 10–6) that can be placed arthroscopically through the capsulolabral complex is advantageous in that anterior early detachments can be repaired without the concerns of transglenoid drilling, but no long-term results are yet available in throwing athletes. Warner, Kann, and Marks[51] reported on a limited series of seven patients with a combined Bankart and superior labral detachment treated with biodegradable screws. Five of these patients were able to return to recreational-level sports, one patient suffered a redislocation, and the remaining patient required a second arthroscopy for stiffness.

Posterior instability can occur in throwers and batters. Most athletes improve with a stengthening program, followed by an interval throwing program. As with anterior instability, arthroscopy is considered after failure with conservative treatment. The experience with arthroscopic treatment of posterior instability is limited. Débridement of some labral tears may allow the athlete to return to competition, and reverse Bankart lesions may require arthroscopic or open repair. In case of severe instability, open stabilization with a capsular shift employing suture anchors into bone may be necessary.

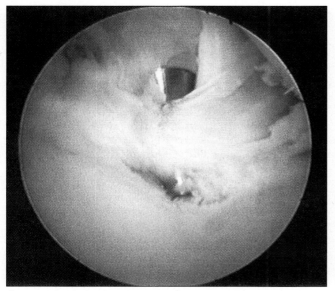
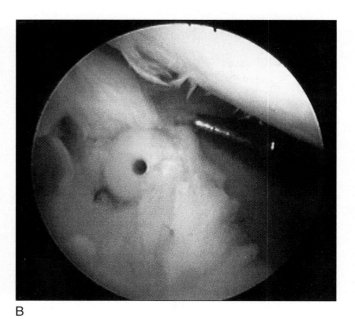

A

B

Figure 10–6 • An example of a biodegradable screw used to repair an early anterior labral detachment. *A,* A drill placed over a guide pin that is reattaching the anterior labrum to the glenoid. The view is from the posterior portal in the right shoulder with the patient in the lateral position. *B,* The view from the anterior portal, after the screw is in place.

Labral Tears

Labral tears can occur in the shoulder secondary to the large compressive and shear forces that are seen in the shoulder during throwing (Figs. 10–7 to 10–9). A significant percentage of labral tears involves the anterosuperior portion near the insertion of the biceps tendon and is not associated with instability[41]; in one series, labral tears occurred without anatomic instability in 72% of the patients.[14] Posterior labral tears can also occur in the lead arm with batting. The labrum can also become entrapped between the humerus and glenoid during a fall and tear, as is often seen when the player dives to catch a ball.

The thrower usually complains of pain during a certain motion and may also have catching, clicking, or locking in the shoulder. Physical examination may yield positive results for a clunk test. Labral tears can sometimes be seen with either a computed tomography-arthrogram or contrast magnetic resonance imaging study of the shoulder. The tear can be visualized at arthroscopy and a treatment option selected.

For a degenerative or flap-type tear, arthroscopic débridement with a motorized shaver is usually indicated. Débridement should be done with caution. A stable peripheral rim of labrum is desired, and glenohumeral instability may be aggravated or created with excessive labral débridement. Andrews and Carson[13] reported on the results of arthroscopy in 73 athletes with labral tears. The most common tear was anterosuperior, and after arthroscopic débridement 88% had good-to-excellent results with follow-up more than 1 year later.

Glasgow et al.[14] reported on arthroscopic resection of glenoid labral tears in athletes and found a statistically significant difference in the functional outcome at 2 years between patients with stable joints and those with unstable joints. In the patients with a stable joint, there was 91% good or excellent outcome, as opposed to a 75% fair or poor functional outcome in the unstable shoulder. No

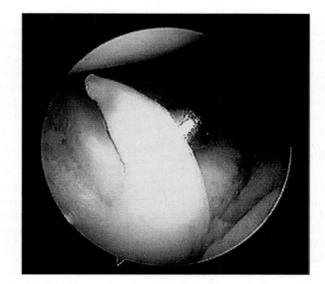

Figure 10–8 • A superior flap labral tear as seen from the anterior portal of a right shoulder. The flap was débrided back to a smooth rim.

patient with a stable shoulder developed subsequent instability after débridement.

Terry, Friedman, and Uhl[52] analyzed the factors influencing the outcome of arthroscopically treated labral tears. They noted that transverse tears, like radial meniscal tears, were the most common and that glenohumeral ligament injury was present in 58% of the patients. A subtle increase in glenohumeral translation was noted in 24% of the patients. Patients with a complete avulsion of the glenohumeral ligaments correlated with a poor result. Whereas 82% of athletes returned to their primary sport, only 48% returned to their previous level of play.

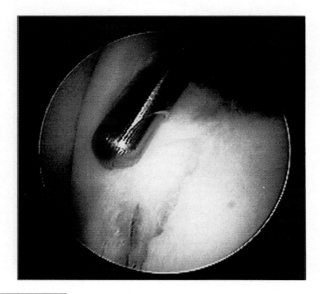

Figure 10–7 • The right shoulder of a baseball player. A posterior superior labral tear is seen from the posterior portal.

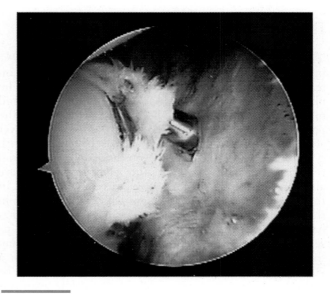

Figure 10–9 • A posterior labral tear as seen from the anterior portal of a right shoulder.

These studies all support the concept that it is extremely difficult to re-establish the stability of the glenohumeral joint while allowing an athlete to resume the previous level of play. It remains to be seen whether the newly developing arthroscopic techniques for capsular repair, including capsular shifts and laser capsulorrhaphy, will be associated with a higher rate of return to competition for throwing athletes.

Biceps Tendon Injuries

The biceps is active in the cocking and acceleration phase and has its highest level of activity during the follow-through phase.[22] With the eccentric contraction during the follow-through phase, biceps tendinitis may develop, although, as mentioned previously, this is not diagnosed as frequently as before the advent of shoulder arthroscopy.

The biceps tendon can easily be located on physical examination by placing the patient supine and abducting the shoulder 90 degrees, with internal rotation of 30 degrees; the biceps tendon is then located directly in front of the shoulder. At arthroscopy a longitudinal split in the intra-articular portion of the biceps tendon is sometimes observed, and fraying with subsequent rupture can also occur. If a probe is inserted through the anterior cannula, the biceps tendon can be pulled into the glenohumeral joint, and the portion of the tendon not usually visible at arthroscopy is examined for tendinitis. Rupture in a young throwing athlete is rare; if it occurs, it is usually due to chronic inflammation, attrition, or a mechanical spur in the groove. Treatment of biceps tendinitis is usually conservative, with the same protocol used to treat impingement. Arthroscopy can be useful in treatment of this disorder as the tendon can be carefully inspected, and if it is torn the stump can be débrided. If the tendon is nearly ruptured, the rupture can be completed arthroscopically, and then the long head of the biceps tendon can be openly tenodesed in the bicipital groove.

Throwers' Exostosis

The term throwers' exostosis was first described in 1941 by Bennett,[2] who described an ossification occurring on the posterior glenoid in professional baseball players. The players complain of persistent posterior shoulder pain, and on a modified Stryker view a bony exostosis is seen off the posterior inferior glenoid (see Fig. 10–2). Lombardo et al.[53] reported on four professional baseball players with symptomatic ossification in the posterior inferior glenoid region treated with open excision; all four players were able to return to satisfactory competitive levels of play. In the past, the exostosis was thought to be a calcification in the long head of the triceps, but open surgical inspection has shown that the lesion is not located in the triceps insertion.[54] The exostosis is extracapsular, but by viewing the posterior shoulder from the anterior portal with a 70 degree arthroscope the posterior inferior capsule can be reflected with a motorized débrider and the exostosis located. A motorized bur can then be used to remove the bony lesion.[55] Andrews has resected this lesion in several

pitchers and allowed them to return to competitive pitching.

Ferrari et al.[54] describe a series of seven throwing athletes who presented with posterior shoulder pain and evidence of posterior ossification of the shoulder on imaging studies preoperatively. At arthroscopy, all seven of the athletes had an identifiable posterior labral injury, and six of the seven had undersurface posterior cuff tearing. The ossification was not identifiable intra-articularly, and the only treatment was débridement of the intra-articular labral and cuff defects. Six of the seven athletes returned to play after 4–6 months of rehabilitation. The authors were concerned about disrupting the posterior capsule arthroscopically in order to remove the lesion, and they thought by addressing the intra-articular lesions, the symptoms resolved. They also supported the concept that the exostosis not a traction lesion, because it is not located in the region of the triceps insertion.

Osteochondritis Dissecans

A common lesion seen at arthroscopy in the throwing shoulder is an erosion of the center of the glenoid, at times to the subchondral bone. This appears to be a normal finding in the throwing shoulder as it is seen quite frequently in both young and mature throwers (Fig. 10–10). However, osteochondral defects of both the humerus and glenoid can occur in throwers, either from direct trauma or by insidious onset (Fig. 10–11). This is not a common diagnosis, and, unless a loose body is seen on radiographs, the defect is usually first diagnosed at arthroscopy. Treatment consists of burring or drilling the defect, if possible, to stimulate the formation of fibrocartilage.

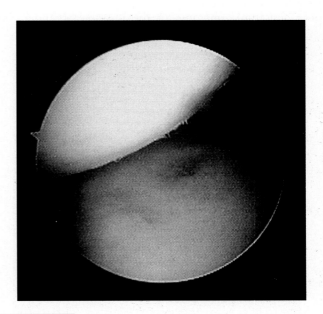

Figure 10–10 • An example of a normal "centering" lesion in the glenoid as seen from the anterior portal in the right shoulder of a thrower.

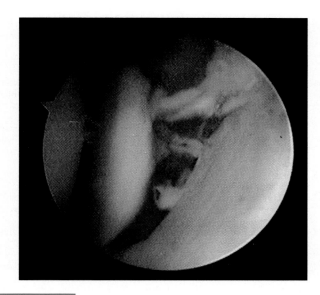

Figure 10–11 • An osteochondral fragment from the glenoid of the right shoulder as viewed from the anterior portal.

Neurovascular Syndromes

Neurovascular disorders about the shoulder are seen rarely, but they may be a source of shoulder pain that is difficult to diagnose. These patients often undergo an extensive work-up, including an unremarkable arthroscopic examination of the shoulder. These syndromes can include quadrilateral space (through which the axillary nerve and posterior humeral circumflex artery pass) syndrome, suprascapular nerve entrapment, thoracic outlet syndrome, and axillary artery occlusion.[56]

In 1986 Redler, Ruland, and McCue[57] reported on a case of quadrilateral space syndrome in a pitcher who complained of an ache in his shoulder on pitching and the development of weakness and a dead feeling in his shoulder. His EMG and nerve conduction studies were normal, but an arteriogram with the arm in full abduction and external rotation showed occlusion of the posterior humeral circumflex artery. The patient altered his pitching style to a three-quarter overhand throw; this change resulted in relief of his symptoms.

The suprascapular nerve innervates both the supraspinatus and infraspinatus muscles. The nerve can be damaged secondary to stretching from the high speed of pitching, or from compression at several sites, most commonly in the suprascapular notch by the superior transverse scapular ligament.[58] An interesting anatomic and clinical study revealed that otherwise asymptomatic baseball pitchers may exhibit slowing of suprascapular nerve conduction as the season progresses and that denervation of the infraspinatus and supraspinatus muscles is not always due to entrapment of the nerve at the suprascapular or spinoglenoid notches.[59]

Once diagnosed, this condition should be treated conservatively with emphasis on strengthening the involved muscles and the scapular stabilizers. The authors observed this abnormality on several occasions in professional-level baseball pitchers, and on isokinetic evaluation their strength parameters were within an acceptable range. They were able to pitch without difficulty or evidence of altered body mechanics.

Acromioclavicular Joint

Injuries to the acromioclavicular joint are often the result of acute trauma from a fall. The type III acromioclavicular joint sprain, or complete rupture, presents a diagnostic dilemma to the treating physician. Although most athletes do well with conservative treatment of type III dislocations,[60] surgical repair of the ligaments should be considered in the throwing athlete.

Degenerative changes in the acromioclavicular joint are seen more commonly in the baseball thrower. Any athlete who lifts weights or engages in repeated throwing is at risk of developing degenerative changes, including bony spurs, osteolysis, and osteophyte formation. Conservative treatment, including nonsteroidal anti-inflammatory medication, modification of physical activity, and steroid injection into the joint, is tried initially. If this fails, arthroscopic débridement of the joint is indicated.

Skeletally Immature Thrower

Similar conditions affect the mature and young throwing shoulder, but the presence of epiphyseal plates creates the opportunity for specific predictable injuries.[29] Adams[61] first described Little League shoulder as an osteochondrosis of the proximal humeral epiphysis. This is associated with proximal shoulder pain, and radiographs show a widening of the proximal humeral epiphysis with demineralization.[62] This heals with rest; however, subsequent proximal growth alterations have been reported.[63]

Other reported shoulder injuries in the skeletally immature include a spiral oblique fracture of the proximal humerus and epiphyseal avulsion fractures of the coracoid process with concomitant acromioclavicular separation.[29]

SUMMARY

The act of throwing requires the coordination of the entire body, including the lower extremities, back, and upper torso. Although common injuries in baseball usually involve the upper extremity, it is important to remember that an alteration in body mechanics can result in a change in pitching style and possible injury. The most critical preventive measure an athlete can take to maintain a healthy throwing shoulder is to participate in a regular shoulder-strengthening program. It is when the muscles about the shoulder become imbalanced, secondary to injury or to relative weakness that instability and injury can occur. By understanding the biomechanics of the throwing motion and the relative contribution of the muscles, the treating physician has a framework on which to build knowledge regarding physical findings and diagnosis of shoulder injuries in athletes. Once a diagnosis is made, a successful treatment plan may be developed for the player, including both conservative and, at times, surgical means.

References

1. Barnes DA and Tullos HS: An analysis of 100 symptomatic baseball players. Am J Sports Med 6:2, 1987.
2. Bennett GE: Shoulder and elbow lesions of the professional baseball pitcher. JAMA 117:7, 1941.
3. King J, Brelsford JH, and Tullos HS: Analysis of the pitching arm of the professional baseball player. Clin Orthop 67: 116, 1969.
4. Neviaser RJ: Lesions of the biceps and tendinitis of the shoulder. Orthop Clin North Am 11:2, 1980.
5. Norwood LA, Del Pizzo W, Jobe FW, et al.: Anterior shoulder pain in baseball pitchers. Am J Sports Med 6:3, 1978.
6. Jackson DW: Chronic rotator cuff impingement in the throwing athlete. Am J Sports Med 4:6, 1976.
7. Penny JN and Welsh RP: Shoulder impingement syndromes in athletes and their surgical management. Am J Sports Med 9:1, 1981.
8. Neer CS II: Impingement lesions. Clin Orthop 173:70, 1983.
9. Tibone JE: Shoulder impingement syndrome in athletes treated with an anterior acromioplasty. Clin Orthop 188:134, 1985.
10. Tibone JE, Elrod B, Jobe FW, et al.: Surgical treatment of tears of the rotator cuff in athletes. J Bone Joint Surg AM 68:6, 1986.
11. Rowe CR and Zarins B: Recurrent transient subluxation of the shoulder. J Bone Joint Surg Am 63:863, 1981.
12. Garth WP, Allman FL, and Armstrong WS: Occult anterior subluxations of the shoulder in non-contact sports. Am J Sports Med 15:6, 1987.
13. Andrews JR and Carson WG: The arthroscopic treatment of glenoid labrum tears in the throwing athlete. Orthop Trans 8:44, 1984.
14. Glasgow SG, Bruce RA, Yacobucci GN, et al.: Arthroscopic resection of glenoid labral tears in the athlete: a report of 29 cases. Arthroscopy 8:48–54, 1992.
15. Scarpinato DF, Bramhall JP, and Andrews JR: Arthroscopic management of the throwing athlete's shoulder: indications, techniques, and results. Clin Sports Med 10:4, 1991.
16. Glousman R, Jobe F, Tibone J, et al.: Dynamic electromyographic analysis of the throwing shoulder with glenohumeral instability. J Bone Joint Surg Am 70:2, 1988.
17. Jobe FW, Kvitne RS, and Giangarra CE: Shoulder pain in the overhand or throwing athlete: the relationship of anterior instability and rotator cuff impingement. Orthop Rev 18:963, 1989.
18. Albright JA, Jokl P, Shaw R, et al.: Clinical study of baseball pitchers: correlation of injury in the throwing arm with method of delivery. Am J Sports Med 6:1, 1987.
19. Gainor BJ, Piothrowski G, Puhl J, et al.: Biomechanics and acute injury. Am J Sports Med 8:2, 1980.
20. Pappas AM, Zawacki RM, and Sullivan TJ: Biomechanics of baseball pitching: a preliminary report. Am J Sports Med 13:4, 1985.
21. Gowan ID, Jobe FW, Tibone JE, et al.: A comparative electromyographic analysis of the shoulder during pitching: professional versus amateur pitchers. Am J Sports Med 15:6, 1987.
22. Jobe FW, Moynes DR, Tibone JE, et al.: An EMG analysis of the shoulder in pitching: a second report. Am J Sports Med 12:3, 1984.
23. Jobe FW, Tibone JE, Perry J, et al.: An EMG analysis of the shoulder in throwing and pitching: a preliminary report. Am J Sports Med 11:1, 1983.
24. Fleisig GS, Dillman CJ, Andrews JR: Proper mechanics for baseball pitching. Clin Sports Med 1:151–170, 1989.
25. Feltner ME: Three-dimensional interactions in a two-segment kinetic chain. Part II: Application to the throwing arm in baseball pitching. Int J Sports Biomech 5:420–450, 1989.
26. Feltner ME, Dapena J: Dynamics of the shoulder and elbow joints of the throwing arm during a baseball pitch. Int J Sports Biomech 2:235–259, 1986.
27. Jones HH, Priest JD, Hayes WC, et al.: Humeral hypertrophy in response to exercise. J Bone Joint Surg Am 59:2, 1977.
28. Warren RF: Instability of shoulder in throwing sports. Instr Course Lect 34:337, 1985.
29. Ireland ML and Andrews JR: Shoulder and elbow injuries in the young athlete. Clin Sports Med 7:3, 1988.
30. Andrews JR, Carson WG, and McLeod WD: Glenoid labrum tears related to the long head of the biceps. Am J Sports Med 13:6, 1985.
31. Andrews JR, Kupferman SP, and Dillman CJ: Labral tears in throwing and racquet sports. Clin Sports Med 14:4, 1991.
32. Howell SM, Galinat BJ, Renzi AJ, et al.: Normal and abnormal mechanics of the glenohumeral joint in the horizontal plan. J Bone Joint Surg Am 70:2, 1988.
33. Kibler WB: Role of the scapula in the overhead throwing motion. Contemp Orthop 22:5, 1991.
34. Brown LP, Niehues SL, Harrah A, et al.: Upper extremity range of motion and isokinetic strength of the internal and external shoulder rotators in major league baseball players. Am J Sports Med 16:6, 1988.
35. Andrews JR and Gillogly S: Physical examination of the shoulder in throwing athletes. In Zarins B, Andrews JR, and Carson WG (eds.): Injuries to the Throwing Arm. Philadelphia, WB Saunders Co., 1985, 51–65.
36. Andrews JR, Byrd JWT, Kupferman SP, et al.: The profile view of the acromion. Clin Orthop 263:142–146, 1991.
37. Tirman PF, Stauffer AE, Crues JV III, et al.: Saline magnetic resonance arthrography in the evaluation of glenohumeral instability. Arthroscopy 9:550–559, 1993.
38. Pappas AM, Zawacki RM, and McCarthy CF: Rehabilitation of the pitching shoulder. Am J Sports Med 13:4, 1985.
39. Wilk KE, Arrigo CA, and Andrews JR: Isokinetic testing of the shoulder abductors and adductors: windowed vs nonwindowed data collection. J Orthop Sports Phys Ther 15:2, 1992.
40. Andrews JR, Carson WG, and Ortego K: Arthroscopy of the shoulder: technique and normal anatomy. Am J Sports Med 12:1, 1984.
41. Andrews JR and Gidumal RH: Shoulder arthroscopy in the throwing athlete: perspective and prognosis. Clin Sports Med 6:3, 1987.
42. Andrews JR, Broussard TS, and Carson WG: Arthroscopy of the shoulder in the management of partial tears of the rotator cuff: a preliminary report. Arthroscopy 1:117, 1985.
43. Bigliani LU, Morrison DS, and April EW: The morphology of the acromion and its relationship to rotator cuff tears. Orthop Trans 10:216, 1986.
44. Liu SH and Boynton E: Case report: posterior superior impingement of the rotator cuff on the glenoid rim as a cause of shoulder pain in the overhead athlete. Arthroscopy 9:697–699, 1993.
45. Walch G, Boileau P, Noel E, et al.: Impingement of the deep surface of the supraspinatus tendon on the posterosuperior glenoid rim: an arthroscopic study. J Shoulder Elbow Surg 1:238–245, 1992.
46. Paulos LE and Kody MH: Arthroscopically enhanced "miniapproach" to rotator cuff repair. Am J Sports Med 22:19–25, 1994.
47. Jobe FW, Giangarra CE, Kvitne RS, et al.: Anterior capsulolabral reconstruction of the shoulder in athletes in overhand sports. Am J Sports Med 19:5, 1991.
48. Bigliani LU, Kurzweil PR, Schwartzbach CC, et al.: Inferior capsular shift procedure for anterior-inferior shoulder instability in athletes. Am J Sports Med 22:578–584, 1994.
49. Montgomery WH III, and Jobe FW: Functional outcomes in athletes after modified anterior capsulolabral reconstruction. Am J Sports Med 22:352–358, 1994.
50. Caspari RB: Arthroscopic reconstruction for anterior shoulder instability. In Paulos LE, Tibone JE (eds.): Operative Techniques in Shoulder Surgery. Gaithersburg, Md., Aspen Publishers, 1991, 57–63.
51. Warner JJP, Kann S, and Marks P: Arthroscopic repair of combined Bankart and superior labral detachment anterior and posterior lesions: technique and preliminary results. Arthroscopy 10:383–391, 1994.
52. Terry GC, Friedman SJ, and Uhl TL: Arthroscopically treated tears of the glenoid labrum. Am J Sports Med 22:504–512, 1994.
53. Lombardo SJ, Jobe FW, Kerlan RK, et al.: Posterior shoulder lesions in throwing athletes. Am J Sports Med 5:3, 1977.
54. Ferrari JD, Ferrari DA, Coumas J, et al.: Posterior ossification of the shoulder: the Bennett lesion. Am J Sports Med 22:171–176, 1994.
55. Andrews JR and Angelo RL: Shoulder arthroscopy in the throwing athlete. Techniques Orthop 3:75–81, 1988.
56. Tullos HS, Erwin WD, Woods GW, et al: Unusual lesions of the pitching arm. Clin Orthop 88:169, 1972.
57. Redler MR, Ruland LJ, McCue FC: Quadrilateral space syndrome in a throwing athlete. Am J Sports Med 14:6, 1986.
58. Post M and Mayer J: Suprascapular nerve entrapment. Clin Orthop 223:126, 1987.

59. Ringel SP, Treihaft M, Carry M, et al.: Suprascapular neuropathy in pitchers. Am J Sports Med 18:1, 1990.
60. Tibone J, Sellers R, and Tonino P: Strength testing after third-degree acromioclavicular dislocations. Am J Sports Med 20:3, 1992.
61. Adams JE: Little league shoulder: osteochondrosis of the proximal humeral epiphysis in boy baseball pitchers. Calif Med 105:22, 1966.
62. Tullos HS and King JW: Lesions of the pitching arm in adolescents. JAMA 220:2, 1972.
63. Cahill BR, Tullos HS, and Fain RH: Little league shoulder. Am J Sports Med 2:150, 1974.

Adhesive Capsulitis

Stephen R. Soffer • *John Guido, Jr*

INTRODUCTION

Adhesive capsulitis, or frozen shoulder, has been the subject of intensive investigation for more than 120 years. Duplay[1] in 1872 is generally credited with initially describing this condition as "periarthrite scapulohumeral." Codman[2] in 1934 coined the term frozen shoulder, and Neviaser[3] in 1945 described adhesive capsulitis. Several physicians have attempted to understand this complex syndrome. Grey[4] concluded that, in the majority of patients, idiopathic frozen shoulder is a self-limiting condition in which symptoms subside and full shoulder movement returns within a maximum of 2 years from the onset of symptoms. Physicians know that this may not be the case for many patients, who continue to suffer a permanent loss of motion. A functional limitation may also be evident, manifested as an inability to perform activities of daily living or work without difficulty. There are significant differences in opinion regarding the exact cause and treatment of adhesive capsulitis. In this chapter, we examine adhesive capsulitis as it relates to shoulder arthroscopy, including a brief review of its epidemiology, cause, and history, and discuss clinical examination. Due to the inconsistencies in the literature, the terms adhesive capsulitis and frozen shoulder are used interchangeably in this chapter. We also discuss patient selection, surgical technique, and postoperative care.

DEFINITION

Adhesive capsulitis can be defined as a condition of the shoulder in which active and passive shoulder motion is restricted. Adhesive capsulitis is usually associated with pain, but pain subsides in the subacute phase and becomes limited to the extremes of available motion. Lundberg[5] divided this condition into two main groups with similar clinical presentations but with markedly different histories. He labeled these groups primary and secondary frozen shoulder, and he developed specific criteria for each. Primary frozen shoulder is considered an insidious and idiopathic condition, and secondary frozen shoulder is the result of a clear, precipitating traumatic event.

EPIDEMIOLOGY

The epidemiologic factors of adhesive capsulitis have been examined extensively. Several predisposing factors have been identified that may increase the risk of developing primary frozen shoulder. Age, gender, arm dominance, and diabetes mellitus may all play a role in the development of this condition. Age at onset has been reported by several authors to be from 40 to 70 years,[5, 6] with women tending to be more susceptible than men.[7] Neviaser and Neviaser[7] reported common involvement in the nondominant arm. However, Bulgen et al.[6] reported a 50% prevalence in the dominant extremity in their series. Common sense dictates that increased use of the dominant upper extremity during work and activities of daily living may decrease the risk of developing primary adhesive capsulitis in this limb. Bridgman[8] reported a higher incidence of this condition in the diabetic as compared with the nondiabetic population. Blood glucose screening may be performed to rule out diabetes in patients with adhesive capsulitis.

Secondary frozen shoulder may develop in connection with a host of contributing factors. Any condition that causes pain and immobilization increases an individual's risk of developing secondary frozen shoulder. Some examples include cervical disk disease, intrathoracic disease, and central nervous system disorders.[5, 9, 10] Trauma to the shoulder complex itself, such as a humeral fracture or a rotator cuff abnormality, lends itself to decreased movement or immobilization.

ETIOLOGY

The etiologic factors of adhesive capsulitis are unknown. Diverse theories include anatomic dysfunction, genetic predisposition, and trauma. Decreased joint volume is a common pathologic finding. Kaltsas[11] found histologic examination of the capsule revealed fibrosis, although the synovial lining of the joint appeared normal. Interestingly, Neviaser and Neviaser[7] found capsular adhesions on open exploration of the joint capsule. Several others have denied their existence.[5, 12, 13] Neviaser also described reparative and inflammatory changes in the capsule on histologic examination. Ozaki et al.[14] described contracture of the rotator interval and coracohumeral ligament as the cause of adhesive capsulitis. Obliteration of the inferior capsular recess, fibrosis, and chronic inflammatory changes have been reported by several investigators.[5, 13] Electron microscopy revealed no changes in the collagen structure of the joint capsule.[5] Immunologic and histocompatibility studies have been performed without a clear-cut conclusion.[15] It remains unclear whether changes in the capsule are the cause or the result of adhesive capsulitis. Although a specific set of pathologic factors have not been determined, it is most probable that the causes are many, whether related to pericapsular soft tissues or to a more generalized systemic process.[16]

NATURAL HISTORY

Symptoms of pain usually resolve in 8–24 months; however, residual loss of motion is often present.[4, 17, 18] Patients adapt to their motion loss and are functional despite significant stiffness in some cases.

PREOPERATIVE EVALUATION

Clinical Presentation

The insidious onset of a gradual loss of shoulder motion, accompanied by pain, is a common presentation of adhesive capsulitis. There is usually no history of antecedent trauma. Examination reveals limited passive and active motion, especially abduction and external rotation. Pain at the extremes of motion is common.

Imaging

Plain radiographs are usually normal; however, they are obtained to rule out other shoulder conditions, such as arthritis, tumors, and infection. Other imaging studies are usually not required to make the diagnosis of adhesive capsulitis. Bone scans have been reported to be positive for adhesive capsulitis when obtained.[17] Arthrography usually shows reduced capsular volume. The radiologist often notes increased back pressure during injection of dye into the glenohumeral joint because of the diminished volume and compliance of the joint capsule.

CONSERVATIVE TREATMENT

Conservative treatment usually involves the use of nonsteroidal anti-inflammatory drugs (NSAIDs), physical therapy, and corticosteroid injections into the glenohumeral joint. A physical therapy program must be contoured to each patient and depends on the degree of inflammation.

The key to determining the degree of inflammation present in a joint is the utilization of a pain limitation sequence.[19] During passive range of motion of the shoulder, pain felt before resistance to motion indicates the presence of an acute inflammatory process. If pain is synchronous with resistance, cautious progression of the treatment plan may be indicated. If resistance of the joint is reached before symptoms of pain are experienced, the need for more progressive treatment may be indicated. In the acute phase, the physician may provide the patient with pendulum-and-pulley exercises, NSAIDs, and referral to physical therapy for passive modalities for pain relief. These modalities may include phonophoresis, iontophoresis, transcutaneous electrical nerve stimulation (TENS), and cryotherapy. The goals for the acute phase include minimizing subjective complaints of pain by alleviating the inflammation, reducing repeated irritation, and preventing undesirable tissue shortening.[20]

In the subacute phase, the inflammation and pain have significantly decreased, and an active and progressive physical therapy program may be initiated. The goals of this phase include restoring full active and passive range of motion and normal joint mobility, increasing shoulder girdle muscle strength, and returning to full activities of daily living and work. During this phase, the patient is better able to tolerate the rigors of progressive stretching and joint mobilization that are needed to lengthen connective tissue. Mobilization may be directed at the anterior, inferior, and posterior capsule, followed by passive range of motion. Posterior mobilizations are important initially, because limitation in this area causes impingement on active elevation of the arm. Clinical practice has demonstrated that use of continuous ultrasound, when performed in the axilla, can also help increase the extensibility of the inferior redundancy. There have been several studies examining the outcome of various treatment plans. Rizk et al.[21] reported a significant improvement in all directions of motion following prolonged pulley traction accompanied by TENS. This treatment plan takes advantage of two phenomena associated with connective tissue. Low-load long-duration stretching utilizes the creep-and-load relaxation properties of the joint capsule. Nicholson[22] reported on the effects of passive joint mobilization on pain and hypomobility associated with adhesive capsulitis. The results of this study showed that joint mobilization and exercises increased range of motion in the shoulder but that only abduction was statistically significant when compared with control groups. Tippett[23] advocated prone long-axis distraction with a weight, coupled with internal/external rotation as an effective exercise for stretching the posterior capsule. He also recommended strengthening the shoulder girdle in the new range of motion that is gained with stretching and joint mobilizations so that new motion is not lost.

PATIENT EDUCATION

Patient education should be a significant part of the treatment plan. In the case of primary frozen shoulder, the patient can become depressed because of the lack of a definitive cause for the problem, an inability to perform activities of daily living or work, and slow progress with treatment. Patients fear that, once resolved, frozen shoulder may return or affect the opposite shoulder. This leads to further anxiety and depression.

By educating patients about their condition, one may not only increase their compliance with the treatment plan but also allay their fears. Introducing them to other patients with the same condition creates a mini–support group that helps these individuals take responsibility for the outcome of their treatment.

INDICATIONS AND CONTRAINDICATIONS FOR SURGERY

Lack of progress in an adequately designed and well-supervised conservative treatment program, coupled with good patient compliance, may indicate the need for surgical intervention. Most patients with adhesive capsulitis are treated successfully with the conservative program already discussed. Lack of improvement of pain symptoms and lack of increase in range of motion for several months indicate the patient is failing conservative treatment and that manipulation or surgery may be considered.

The main advantage of manipulation and arthroscopy is to shorten the time course of adhesive capsulitis.[5] The main advantage of manipulation with arthroscopy rather than manipulation alone is to rule out additional pathologic lesions. If subacromial bursitis is associated with adhesive capsulitis, for example, such bursitis is easily treated with an arthroscopic bursectomy.[24]

Manipulation is rarely contraindicated. Relative contraindications include severe proximal humeral osteopenia, history of fracture or dislocation of the shoulder, and recurrence following manipulation.[7]

SURGICAL TECHNIQUES

Manipulation

Brisement is a technique rarely used at present to treat adhesive capsulitis. It involves capsular distention by glenohumeral injection of fluids. Scientific evidence of its results is lacking in the literature.

When a well-supervised course of conservative treatment yields meager results, mechanical manipulation of the shoulder under anesthesia often helps alleviate symptoms. The exact technique of manipulation varies from clinician to clinician.

The authors prefer to grasp the arm with one hand near the axilla and flex the shoulder while holding the scapula down with the opposite hand (Fig. 11–1). This action is performed with a constant and gentle force without any abrupt or jerking motions. If firm resistance is met, we then work on regaining abduction and external rota-

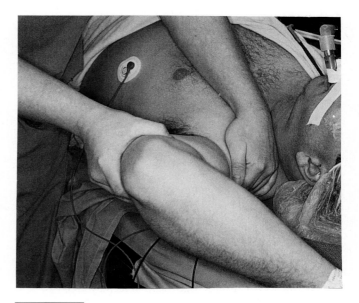

Figure 11–1 • Manipulation of the shoulder. Grasp the arm near the axilla and flex the shoulder while holding the scapula down with the opposite hand.

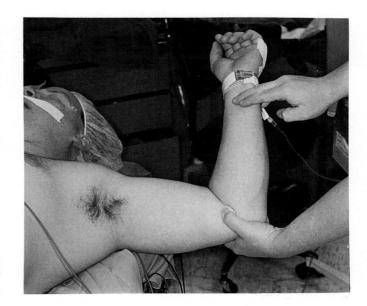

Figure 11–2 • External rotation with two-finger force.

tion. External rotation is performed with two-finger force so as not to cause fracture (Fig. 11–2). When firm resistance is met, manipulation is switched back toward regaining flexion. This technique is continued until full range or close to full range of motion is achieved. One can feel the capsule stretching with manipulation.

Arthroscopy

Manipulation may be performed before or after or before and after arthroscopy. Usually manipulation before arthroscopy allows for easier penetration of the trocar into the joint. There is less chance of scuffing and greater visibility with this approach. Often the glenohumeral joint is extremely tight, and there is difficulty introducing the trocar between the glenoid and the humeral head safely without prior manipulation. Even with prearthroscopy manipulation, it may be difficult to gain access to the joint space.

Usually, one may distend the joint initially with saline solution through an 18 gauge spinal needle. The capsule is more difficult to distend than the usual shoulder, and more pressure on the syringe is necessary. The joint space accepts less fluid volume as well, perhaps only 10 mL. After distention, a trocar is placed through a standard posterior portal and into the glenohumeral joint. If it is difficult to enter into the center of the glenohumeral articulation because of capsular tightness, one may need to aim toward the superior aspect of the joint, that is, the area between the supraspinatus and superior labrum, to gain access to the joint. Once into this superior recess, one may rotate, abduct, flex, or extend the arm to introduce the arthroscope safely between the humeral head and glenoid. One should then establish an anterior portal in standard fashion and perform a diagnostic examination with the arthroscope in both portals. Subacromial bursoscopy is also performed.

Arthroscopic studies and our own experience have shown an absence of intra-articular adhesions and degenerative changes.[12, 25] There is usually no obliteration of the infraglenoid recess. Usually, a patchy vascular synovitis is present in various aspects of the shoulder (Fig. 11–3). The subscapularis bursa and biceps tendon are often involved. Occasionally, a partial rotator cuff tear is seen and may be débrided with a shaver. There are usually no frank labral tears or articular cartilage lesions. The subacromial space is often normal; however, it may show either an acute or chronic bursitis. This bursitis may also be débrided with a shaver. An arthroscopic Bovie should be used to coagulate bleeders. Acromioplasty or removal of acromial undersurface periosteum is avoided because this causes further trauma, stimulates bleeding, and causes pain postoperatively. This in turn interferes with aggressive postoperative physical therapy and ability to achieve normal range of motion.

Occasionally, one may need to perform arthroscopic capsular release for an extremely contracted shoulder. An arthroscopic Bovie may be used to release the inferior capsule (Fig. 11–4).

After arthroscopic surgery is completed, an injection of 20 mL of 0.5% Marcaine without Epinephrine should be made into either the subacromial space or the glenohumeral joint, depending on where the majority of the surgery was performed. This procedure aids in pain control postoperatively and thus aids rehabilitation.

Open Surgery

Open surgery is rarely indicated for most cases of adhesive capsulitis. Usually, manipulation and arthroscopy achieve

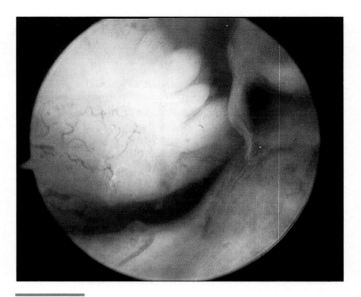

Figure 11–3 • Patchy vascular synovitis.

the desired result. Incisional surgery creates more trauma and pain and inhibits postoperative therapy. In an uncommon case in which manipulation and arthroscopy fail, an open release is performed. This is usually in a patient who has had a previous open-shoulder surgery (e.g., after an instability procedure). One may need to lengthen the subscapularis tendon, release the capsule from the inferior aspect of the humerus or glenoid, release the coracohumeral interval, and lyse adhesions in the subacromial space.

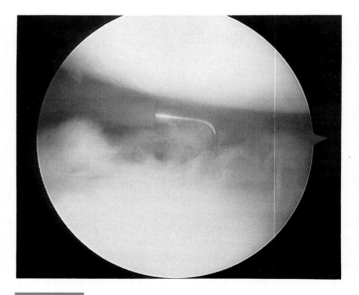

Figure 11–4 • Arthroscopic Bovie releasing inferior capsule.

POSTOPERATIVE CARE

After manipulation and arthroscopic surgery for adhesive capsulitis, we utilize an aggressive postoperative program involving NSAIDs, ice, daily physical therapy, and, possibly, continuous passive motion of the shoulder. The day after surgery, the dressings and a sling are removed, and physical therapy begins.

The goals are to prevent adhesion formation, to minimize pain and inflammation, and to achieve immediate gains in passive range of motion.

TENS, combined with passive and active assisted range of motion, may prove beneficial early on. Postoperative care should follow the same guidelines as those discussed under conservative treatment.

References

1. Duplay ES: De la periarthrite scapulohumeral et des raideurs de l'epaule qui en son la consequence. Arch Gen Med 20:513–542, 1872.
2. Codman EA: The Shoulder. Boston, Thomas Todd Co., 1934.
3. Neviaser JS: Adhesive capsulitis of the shoulder. J Bone Joint Surg 27:211–222, 1945.
4. Grey RG: The natural history of idiopathic frozen shoulder. J Bone Joint Surg 60:564, 1978.
5. Lundberg BJ: The frozen shoulder. Acta Orthop Scand 119(suppl):1–59, 1969.
6. Bulgen DY, Binder AI, Hazleman BL, et al.: Frozen shoulder: prospective clinical study with an evaluation of three treatment regimens. Ann Rheum Dis 43:353–360, 1984.
7. Neviaser RJ and Neviaser TJ: The frozen shoulder: diagnosis and management. Clin Orthop 223:59–64, 1987.
8. Bridgman JF: Periarthritis of the shoulder and diabetes mellitus. Ann Rheum Dis 31:69–71, 1972.
9. Neviaser JS: Arthrography of the shoulder joint. J Bone Joint Surg 44:1321–1330, 1962.
10. Bohannon RW, Larkin PA, Smith MB, et al.: Shoulder pain in hemiplegia: statistical relationship with five variables. Arch Phys Med Rehabil 67:514–516, 1986.
11. Kaltsas DS: Comparative study of the properties of the shoulder joint capsule with those of other joint capsules. Clin Orthop 173:20–26, 1983.
12. Ha'eri GB and Maitland A: Arthroscopic findings in the frozen shoulder. J Rheumatol 8:149–152, 1981.
13. Olgilvie-Harris DJ and Wiley AM: Arthroscopic surgery of the shoulder. J Bone Joint Surg 68:201–207, 1986.
14. Ozaki J, Nakagawa Y, Sakurai G, et al.: Recalcitrant chronic adhesive capsulitis of the shoulder. J Bone Joint Surg Am 71:1511–1515, 1989.
15. Rizk TE and Pinals RS: Histocompatibility type and racial incidence in frozen shoulder. Arch Phys Med Rehabil 65:33–34, 1984.
16. Andrews JR and Wilk KE: The Athlete's Shoulder. New York, Churchill Livingstone, 1993.
17. Binder AI, Bulgen DY, Hazleman BL, et al.: Frozen shoulder: a long-term prospective study. Ann Rheum Dis 43:361–364, 1984.
18. Reeves B: The natural history of the frozen shoulder syndrome. Scand J Rheumatol 4:193–196, 1976.
19. Cyriax J: Textbook of Orthopaedic Medicine, 8th ed. London, Bailliere Tindall, 1982, pp 130–134.
20. Nitz AJ: Physical therapy management of the shoulder. Phys Ther 66:1912–1919, 1986.
21. Rizk TE, Christopher RP, Pinals RS, et al.: Adhesive capsulitis (frozen shoulder): a new approach to its management. Arch Phys Med Rehabil 64:29–33, 1983.
22. Nicholson GG: The effects of passive joint mobilization on pain and hypomobility associated with adhesive capsulitis of the shoulder. J Orthop Sports Phys Ther 6:238–246, 1985.
23. Tippett S: Adhesive capsulitis: pathology, prevention, and treatment. Presented at the Advances in Clinical Education Meeting, Cleveland, May, 1995.
24. Uitvlugt G, Detrisac D, and Johnson L: The pathology of the frozen shoulder: an arthroscopic perspective. Arthroscopy 4:137, 1988.
25. Johnson LL: Diagnostic and Surgical Arthroscopy of the Shoulder. St. Louis, Mosby Year-Book, 1993, pp 353–358.

12 Degenerative Arthritis of the Shoulder

Gary Anderson • James R. Andrews

INTRODUCTION

Although osteoarthritis is the most common cause of joint disease, the shoulder is much less commonly involved than the joints of the lower extremities and back. The characteristic pathologic findings of degenerative joint disease, including progressive loss of articular cartilage surface, sclerosis and cyst formation in the subchondral region, and formation of marginal osteophytes, are the same in degenerative glenohumeral arthritis as in other degenerative joints.[1] The spectrum of degenerative glenohumeral arthritis can be divided in several ways; Neer, Craig, and Fukuda described the important difference between glenohumeral arthritis with an intact rotator cuff versus "cuff tear arthropathy," a severe form of degenerative arthritis that develops in association with a complete rotator cuff tear and is much less amenable to surgical intervention.[2] And, more generally, a distinction can be made between the idiopathic or primary form of glenohumeral arthritis versus secondary forms of osteoarthritis due to a variety of primary diseases; idiopathic osteoarthritis is less common than the secondary forms of degenerative arthritis (see Table 28–1). One possible mechanism for early development of degenerative joint disease is repeated minor trauma leading to an overuse phenomenon, but even in lower extremity joints exposed to higher joint reaction forces, a strong causal relationship is difficult to establish.[3]

Degenerative arthritis about the shoulder is most common in the acromioclavicular (AC) joint, in which arthritic changes develop idiopathically, with an age-related increase in incidence. This degenerative arthritis is often accompanied by inferior AC joint osteophyte formation associated with subacromial rotator cuff impingement disease. Arthritic changes of the glenohumeral joint are much less common, and although age-related degenerative changes of the soft tissues about the shoulder have been observed, the effect of aging on the development of arthritic changes is less clear; specifically, age did not affect articular cartilage thickness of the glenohumeral joint.[4, 5] This chapter reviews arthroscopy for glenohumeral degenerative disease, and Chapter 13 is devoted to AC joint disease.

PATIENT SELECTION

As with other osteoarthritic joints, the primary symptom of glenohumeral degenerative arthritis is pain in the involved shoulder. Pain is frequently accompanied by a gradual loss of motion, particularly external rotation and abduction. Frequently, patients complain of pain at night with inability to sleep on the affected side, and may sometimes complain of crepitation in the shoulder as well. Because glenohumeral arthritis is often associated with other shoulder disease, including subacromial problems (Table 12–1), selective injection can be a useful adjunct in pinpointing the source of a patient's symptoms. Significant muscle atrophy about the shoulder may also be noted as the patient's pain and limited motion contribute to disuse of the shoulder. As with other shoulder conditions, the patient's pain is often most pronounced with overhead activities.

On examination the patient may also have some tenderness and crepitus in the posterior shoulder near the joint line. Significant loss of motion, particularly in abduction and external rotation, and some loss of internal rotation can often be noted. The essential test for diagnosing osteoarthritis of the shoulder, as with other joints, is radiographic evidence of joint-space narrowing, subchondral sclerosis, osteophyte formation, and subchondral cysts. A true anteroposterior radiograph of the glenohumeral joint and an axillary lateral view are particularly helpful in delineating the extent of the disease. In addition, an anteroposterior radiograph of the shoulder in external rotation may help bring out the osteophytes of the inferior humeral neck.

Indications

There are many indications for arthroscopy of the shoulder, as noted in other chapters, including subacromial impingement syndrome with associated rotator cuff disease of varying degrees, shoulder instability, glenoid labral tears, and arthrofibrosis. The indications for arthroscopic débridement for primary osteoarthritis of the shoulder

Table 12–1 | **Secondary Causes of Glenohumeral Degeneration**

Inflammatory arthritis (e.g., rheumatoid arthritis)
Post-traumatic arthritis
Cuff-tear arthropathy
Chronic instability
Poststabilization arthritis
Osteonecrosis
Radiation necrosis
Tumor
Septic arthritis
Neuropathic (Charcot) arthropathy
Metabolic disease (e.g., hemochromatosis, ochronosis)

are still evolving. The nonoperative treatment for glenohumeral arthritis with nonsteroidal anti-inflammatory drugs and physical therapy to preserve motion is only of limited benefit. For more severe disease, the most reproducible treatment is shoulder joint replacement with either a humeral head hemiarthroplasty or a total shoulder replacement. Arthroscopic débridement of the shoulder can be considered an intermediate step between these two extremes, especially for younger, more active patients who have persistent pain in spite of aggressive nonoperative treatment. Throwing athletes with early osteophyte formation may also form a unique subset of this group.

Several small series[6–8] have shown some improvement of shoulder symptoms in patients who had arthroscopic débridement for early degenerative joint disease of the glenohumeral joint. A review of the database at the American Sports Medicine Institute revealed that in a sample of 2,530 shoulder arthroscopies performed during the last 8 years, 175 patients (7%) were identified with grade III and IV changes of the humeral head or glenoid articular surfaces. The majority of these arthroscopic procedures were performed for other primary diagnoses, principally impingement syndrome with rotator cuff tendinitis or rotator cuff tearing, shoulder instability, and arthrofibrosis. This percentage is remarkably similar to the prevalence of degenerative joint disease (6%) noted by Ellman, Harris, and Kay[7] in their patients undergoing arthroscopy for impingement syndrome. Even when patients are not specifically selected for arthroscopic treatment of glenohumeral arthritis, it is not rare to identify degenerative changes at the time of arthroscopy, and these patients appear to respond well to arthroscopic removal of loose bodies and débridement of the joint. Young patients with inferior humeral osteophytes may lose abduction and external rotation, and an attempt can be made to remove the osteophytes arthroscopically to improve motion.

Contraindications

The general contraindications to surgical arthroscopy for glenohumeral arthritis are the same as the contraindications for other arthroscopic procedures; they include medical illnesses that prevent the safe administration of anesthesia and soft-tissue infection in the region of the shoulder that might seed the shoulder joint. Relative con-

traindications include situations in which arthroscopic débridement is less likely to provide a successful result. Patients with more severe disease, including those with advanced joint-space narrowing associated with large osteophyte formation and decreased shoulder motion or "cuff tear arthropathy," are less likely to be satisfied with the results of arthroscopic débridement. In addition, with more severe disease the technical difficulty of the procedure can be greatly increased because of the presence of significant deformity and limited joint motion.

PREOPERATIVE EVALUATION

History

The preoperative history and physical examination remain the primary diagnostic tools for evaluating degenerative disease of the shoulder. Pain with shoulder motion, often referred down the shaft of the proximal humerus, and loss of glenohumeral joint motion are the most common presenting symptoms. There are many associated shoulder conditions that may also be present, including rotator cuff disease, AC joint disease, shoulder instability, a history of prior shoulder surgery, and neurologic conditions affecting the shoulder region. Patients should be specifically questioned about prior trauma, chronic shoulder instability, and prior anterior stabilization because these have been associated with degenerative changes. Although a multitude of systemic diseases can rarely be found to cause degeneration of the glenohumeral joint, three diseases account for the majority of glenohumeral degenerative arthritis: osteoarthritis, rheumatoid arthritis, and post-traumatic arthritis.

Physical Examination

Examination begins with inspection for evidence of muscular atrophy. Evaluation of glenohumeral motion is important because gradual loss of external rotation and abduction is associated with degenerative changes and often leads to substitution with scapulothoracic motion. With progressive wear of the posterior glenoid, posterior subluxation of the shoulder can occur, leading to a mild change in contour of the shoulder. Motor strength can also be diminished as joint pain leads to decreased use of the affected shoulder. Examination of the cervical spine may also be necessary to rule out other causes of pain in the shoulder region.

One of the diagnostic difficulties in evaluating the arthritic shoulder is the nonspecific nature of the symptoms of glenohumeral degeneration, which overlap with other shoulder problems. The compression-rotation test as described by Ellman, Harris, and Kay[7] may serve as a useful adjunct in discriminating between glenohumeral arthritis and some of these associated conditions. Briefly, the patient is placed in the lateral decubitus position with the affected side up. The examiner then loads the glenohumeral joint with downward pressure on the humeral head, and the patient attempts to rotate the humerus. The test result is considered positive if it reproduces the patient's pain. Selective injection of the subacromial space with local anesthetic may improve the specificity of this test by eliminating another source of shoulder pain. Selective injection of the glenohumeral joint, the AC joint, and the subacromial space may be used to help delineate the principal cause of pain in shoulders with multiple problems.

Diagnostic Imaging

The most specific diagnostic test for glenohumeral arthritis is radiographs of the shoulder, including a true anteroposterior view of the glenohumeral joint and an axillary lateral view. An anteroposterior view in external rotation can also be used to demonstrate early osteophyte formation, known as a "goat's beard" deformity, in the region of the inferior humeral neck (Fig. 12–1). A supraspinatus outlet view can be used to evaluate the coracoacromial arch and identify hooking of the anterior acromion, which may contribute to associated subacromial impingement-type symptoms. Rotator cuff arthropathy with a high-riding humeral head and humeroacromial articulation can also be detected on plain radiographs. The essential elements of glenohumeral joint arthritis remain joint-space narrowing and osteophyte formation of the glenohumeral joint as demonstrated on plain x-ray films.

Competitive-throwing athletes may also present with shoulder pain and abnormal radiographs. A Stryker notch view of the throwing arm can demonstrate a Bennett lesion or thrower's exostosis on the posterior inferior glenoid.[9]

Magnetic resonance imaging (MRI) has been used with increasing frequency to evaluate shoulder problems. Although MRI has proved fairly reliable for the diagnosis of rotator cuff disease in the shoulder (and meniscal and ligament injury in the knee), it is less consistent in demonstrating articular surface problems. In Ellman, Harris, and

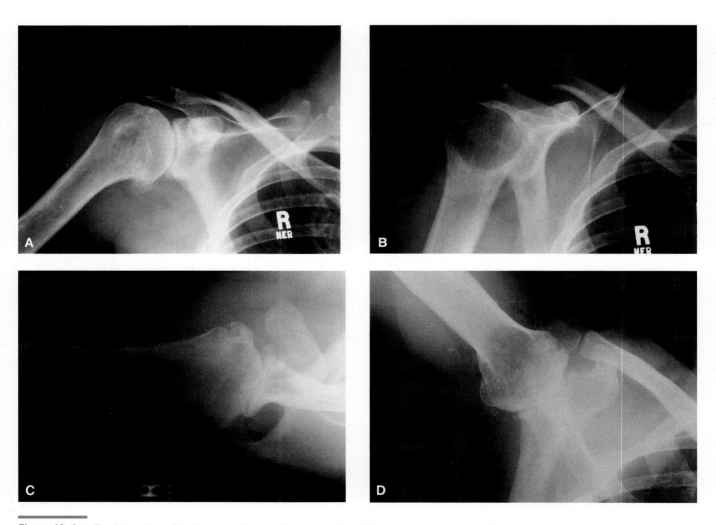

Figure 12–1 • Radiographs of a 56 year old man demonstrating joint-space narrowing, sclerosis, and osteophyte formation. Mild posterior subluxation can also be seen in the lateral view. *A,* Anteroposterior view in internal rotation. *B,* Anteroposterior view in external rotation. *C,* Axillary lateral view. *D,* Stryker notch view.

Kay's series of 18 patients with arthroscopic evidence of osteoarthritis, 11 had preoperative MRI, but articular cartilage damage was noted only on MRI in 6 of the 11.[7] These patients had MRI performed for impingement syndrome, but as noted degenerative changes were seen on the MRI scan in some of these patients. As has been shown with the knee, plain films are more specific than MRI for revealing degenerative changes of the articular surface, and the value of MRI is probably greatest for demonstrating other coexisting disease of the affected shoulder.

NONOPERATIVE TREATMENT

The initial management of glenohumeral joint arthritis is nonoperative and is directed at maintaining shoulder motion and decreasing painful symptoms. The use of nonsteroidal anti-inflammatory drugs was the first form of intervention, and currently mild analgesics such as acetaminophen are also frequently used in the early stages of osteoarthritis. A physical therapy program directed at strengthening the muscles of the affected shoulder to help preserve joint function and maintain joint motion is a useful adjunct in the early phases of osteoarthritis. Intra-articular corticosteroid injections can be used in more severe cases or during acute exacerbations of milder disease. The duration of relief with intra-articular steroid injections is limited and variable and seems to decrease with greater numbers of injections into the same joint. If the patient's shoulder symptoms continue to interfere with occupational or recreational activities of daily living in spite of nonoperative treatment, surgical treatment may be considered.

Patient Education

The authors use illustrations and anatomic models to educate patients about the relevant shoulder anatomy and treatment options. Initially, the benefits of nonoperative treatment are emphasized, and patients are instructed in activity modification to minimize loading of the glenohumeral joint. If in spite of nonoperative treatment the patient continues to have disabling shoulder pain due to arthritis, then the possible surgical treatment options are discussed.

Arthroscopy specifically for degenerative arthritis of the shoulder is extremely rare, and published data on the results are meager. Because of the limited data available regarding the efficacy of arthroscopy for treatment of glenohumeral degeneration, patients should be cautioned about the limitations of this technique. When there is radiographic evidence of joint-space narrowing and osteophyte formation, suggesting more severe degeneration, patients can be informed that only one-third of patients had good results in the only published series.[6]

The majority of patients in the authors' experience who were found to have glenohumeral degenerative changes at the time of arthroscopy underwent shoulder arthroscopy for treatment of another primary diagnosis. In this setting, postoperative patient education is important

to inform patients about their additional diagnosis and its potential effect on joint function.

SURGICAL TECHNIQUE

Different Methods of Surgical Technique

The surgical options for degenerative glenohumeral arthritis include arthroscopic débridement, osteotomy, arthrodesis, humeral head hemiarthroplasty, total shoulder replacement, and resection arthroplasty. Surgical arthroscopy is the least invasive of the surgical options for glenohumeral arthritis that has been refractory to nonoperative treatment methods. The value of arthroscopy can be both diagnostic and therapeutic. Direct visualization of the joint surface can help to delineate the extent of the osteoarthritis and to ascertain the presence of other pathologic conditions of the shoulder. The therapeutic benefits of arthroscopy seem to be greatest in the mild-to-moderate stages of the disease and less so in more advanced cases. If other concomitant conditions, including rotator cuff disease, loose bodies, biceps tendon or labral tears, and subacromial disease, are identified, arthroscopy can often be used to treat these conditions as well at the same sitting.

Shoulder arthroscopy is commonly performed with the patient in either the semireclined (beach-chair) position or the lateral decubitus position, with the affected arm in axial traction as described in Chapter 4. Either of these techniques is quite suitable for diagnostic arthroscopy and arthroscopic débridement for degenerative arthritis.

Authors' Preferred Treatment

First, with the patient under anesthesia and in the supine position, an examination of both shoulders is carried out, documenting range of motion and any evidence of instability. Gentle manipulation is performed if there is a component of arthrofibrosis with loss of shoulder motion. Care is taken not to exert any undue force in case of more severe arthritis where there is potentially a mechanical block to shoulder motion. The patient is then placed in the lateral decubitus position, with the arm in axial traction and suspended in approximately 70 degrees of abduction and 15 degrees of flexion. The operative shoulder and arm are prepared and draped, and the suspended hand and wrist are wrapped with sterile towels and an adhesive drape.

The surface anatomy, including the acromion, the AC joint, and the coracoid, is marked with a skin marker; the arthroscopy portal sites are similarly identified with the marker. Diagnostic arthroscopy of the glenohumeral joint is initiated through a standard posterior arthroscopy portal at the posterior soft spot of the shoulder approximately 3 cm inferior and 1 cm medial to the posterolateral corner of the acromion. An 18 gauge spinal needle is placed through the soft spot into the glenohumeral joint, and the joint is distended with 30–50 mL of normal saline. As the joint nears maximal distention, the suspended arm slowly rotates internally, confirming intra-articular placement of the needle. Free backflow of saline also confirms correct placement. The needle is removed, and a No. 11 blade is used to make the stab incision. An arthroscopy cannula with a blunt obturator is then placed into the joint, with care taken to palpate the back of the glenoid with the obturator before entering the joint to ensure entry as close to the glenoid rim as possible to minimize trauma to the posterior rotator cuff. Joint entry may be difficult in arthritic joints because the posterior capsule may be contracted. Care must be taken not to plunge into the humeral head with the trocar.

Systematic inspection of the posterior glenohumeral joint is conducted. An anterior portal is established under direct arthroscopic vision, using an 18 gauge spinal needle midway between the coracoid and the anterolateral corner of the acromion and directed to enter the shoulder joint in the rotator interval just below the biceps tendon. Instruments, including a motorized shaver, can then be placed in the anterior portal to carry out a débridement and removal of any loose bodies. The arthroscope and instruments can

be reversed, with the arthroscope placed through the anterior portal and the instruments placed through the posterior portal, to complete the arthroscopic examination and débridement. In general, the authors do not perform a chondroplasty of the articular surface but remove any cartilaginous flaps that are identified (Fig. 12–2). Posterior glenoid osteophytes in throwing athletes can be débrided using a bur through the posterior portal. The bur is directed inferiorly beneath the capsule and labrum, and the exostosis is then removed without disturbing the labrum or the articular surface. An additional posterior-inferior portal can be placed to also allow access to inferior humeral neck osteophytes, which can be removed with a bur.

Because there are frequently concomitant subacromial problems, the arthroscope is then inserted into the subacromial space through the posterior portal. If necessary, a subacromial decompression can then be performed. If there is significant AC joint arthritis with osteophyte formation, the osteophytes can also be débrided from the

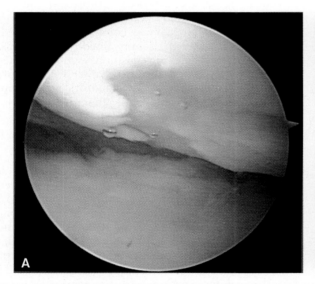

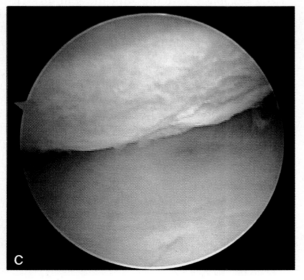

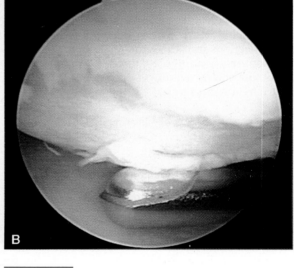

Figure 12–2 • *A,* Arthroscopic view of the shoulder of a 39 year old professional baseball player demonstrating loss of articular surface on the humeral head, with associated cartilage flaps at the edges of the lesion. *B,* Débridement of loose articular cartilage with full-radius resector. *C,* Articular surface after arthroscopic débridement. The patient returned to regular play in major league baseball 6 months postoperatively.

lateral portal. In addition, if the AC joint is severely arthritic, a distal clavicle resection can be performed through the anterior portal. The patient's arm is placed in a sling postoperatively for comfort.

POSTOPERATIVE CARE

Arthroscopic débridement of the shoulder is usually performed on an outpatient basis. Patients are maintained in a sling for comfort for the first several postoperative days. Physical therapy emphasizing range-of-motion exercise is begun on the first postoperative day and is advanced rapidly as tolerated by the patient. The sling is discontinued a couple of days later, and the patient is encouraged to use the affected arm for activities of daily living. Patients are then instructed in a home therapy program to assist them in maintaining their range of motion. After 2 weeks patients are begun on rotator cuff exercises, particularly if they have associated rotator cuff tendinitis and concomitant weakness in abduction and external rotation. At 6 weeks patients are allowed to begin overhead activities, and at 3 months they are gradually allowed to return to functional athletic activities.

SUMMARY

Although the authors only rarely perform arthroscopy for primary osteoarthritis of the shoulder, grade III or IV chondrosis of the glenoid or humeral articular surface has been noted in 175 (7%) of 2,530 shoulder arthroscopies performed during the last 8 years. The preliminary results parallel those reported in the literature,[6, 7] namely, that patients with mild-to-moderate osteoarthritis appear to do quite well in short-term follow-up.

In summary, the value of arthroscopy for osteoarthritis of the shoulder can be diagnostic and therapeutic, with few complications and no compromise of future treatment options. Arthroscopy of the shoulder can give direct visual evidence of osteoarthritic changes, especially in patients who are having arthroscopy for other primary diagnoses. The therapeutic benefits of arthroscopy in the degenerative shoulder are limited, but some symptomatic improvement has been observed in early follow-up of arthroscopic débridement of the glenohumeral joint in patients with milder degrees of osteoarthritis and an intact rotator cuff.

References

1. Neer CS: Replacement arthroplasty for glenohumeral osteoarthritis. J Bone Joint Surg Am 56:1–13, 1974.
2. Neer CS, Craig EV, and Fukuda H: Cuff-tear arthropathy. J Bone Joint Surg Am 65:1232–1244, 1983.
3. Schumacher HR Jr, Klippel JH, and Koopman WJ (eds.): Primer on the Rheumatic Diseases, 10th ed. Atlanta, The Arthritis Foundation, 1993.
4. Meachim G: Effect of age on the thickness of adult articular cartilage at the shoulder. Ann Rheum Dis 30:43–46, 1971.
5. Peterson CJ: Degeneration of the glenohumeral joint: an anatomical study. Acta Orthop Scand 54:277–283, 1983.
6. Olgivie-Harris DJ, and Wiley AM: Arthroscopic surgery of the shoulder. J Bone Joint Surg Br 68:201–207, 1986.
7. Ellman H, Harris E, and Kay SP: Early degenerative joint disease simulating impingement syndrome: arthroscopic findings. Arthroscopy 8:482–487, 1992.
8. Johnson LL: The shoulder joint. Clin Orthop 223:113, 1987.
9. Bennett GE: Elbow and shoulder lesions of the professional baseball pitcher. JAMA 8:510, 1941.

Arthroscopic Resection of the Acromioclavicular Joint

Scott David Martin

The acromioclavicular (AC) joint is a diarthrodial synovial joint. It consists of articular cartilage that covers the distal convex clavicle and medial concave acromion and an intra-articular fibrocartilaginous meniscus, or disc. The intra-articular disk is variable and usually divides the joint cavity incompletely.[1] Capsule and AC ligaments invest the joint and provide anteroposterior stability. Vertical stability is provided by the coracoclavicular ligaments. In addition, the attachments of the deltoid and trapezius to the superior aspect of the clavicle and acromion provide dynamic stability to the AC joint.[2-6]

The AC joint inclines medially from the sagittal plane in a superior-to-inferior direction.[3] Mobility of the AC joint consists of a gliding movement of the distal clavicle on the medial acromion and a rotational movement of the scapula on the clavicle.[4, 7]

The AC joint is a common source of shoulder pain. Acute causes of AC joint pain are often related to direct trauma to the affected shoulder. This may result in a type III distal clavicle injury with an intra-articular chondral fracture or in AC joint instability from ligament disruption.[6]

In addition, post-traumatic distal clavicle osteolysis may ensue as soon as 4 weeks after a shoulder injury, leading to AC joint pain.[8, 9] Osteolysis may be due to microfractures of the subchondral bone with subsequent attempts at repair.[10] Some researchers believe osteolysis is caused by an autonomic nerve dysfunction affecting the blood supply to the clavicle. The increased blood supply leads to resorption of bone from the distal clavicle.[8, 11]

More commonly, osteolysis occurs chronically, due to repetitive microtrauma to the AC joint from activities such as weight-lifting, gymnastics, and swimming.[10, 12, 13] The underlying pathophysiology is believed to be an inflammatory process from stress fractures of the subchondral bone with hyperemic resorption of the distal clavicle.[10, 14] Other causes of osteolysis include rheumatoid arthrosis, hyperparathyroidism, and sarcoidosis, all of which should be considered in the differential diagnosis, especially in bilateral cases.[8, 9] Chronic causes of AC pain include idiopathic intra-articular disc disorders, post-traumatic degenerative arthrosis from joint incongruity, primary degenerative arthrosis, and rheumatoid arthrosis.

Most patients with AC pain respond to conservative treatment, with surgical options reserved for refractory cases. Open resection of the distal clavicle as a treatment option for chronic AC joint pain was initially independently reported by Gurd[15] and Mumford,[16] with good results. Since then, other authors have reported similar good results with open resection; however, significant morbidity can occur, such as disruption of the deltotrapezial fascia and anterior deltoid rupture.[8, 9, 17-19]

Arthroscopic resection of the distal clavicle has been described with results similar to those of open resection.[2, 7, 14, 20-24] Advantages include absence of a surgical scar and preservation of the AC ligaments, capsule, and deltotrapezial fascial attachments to the clavicle. This resection allows for accelerated rehabilitation with immediate motion, shorter hospital stay, and quicker return to functional and athletic activities.[2, 20, 21, 23] In addition, glenohumeral and rotator cuff evaluation may be performed to rule out concomitant disease.[14, 22] When performed by an experienced arthroscopist, the procedure can be done quickly with minimal risk of morbidity.

CONSERVATIVE TREATMENT

Patients with AC joint pain usually respond well to nonoperative treatment; however, complete relief of symptoms may take an extended period. Conservative therapy includes heat, nonsteroidal anti-inflammatory medications, steroid injections, shoulder rehabilitation, and avoidance of painful positions and activities. Steroid injections are repeated at 3-month intervals if painful conditions persist.

Physical therapy emphasizes maintenance of shoulder motion and muscle strength. A standard protocol includes supine, passive range-of-motion exercises along with capsular stretching and isometric strengthening exercises in the acute painful period.[25] As pain lessens, patients go on to isotonic muscle strengthening with continuation of light resistance and stretching exercises. Rotator cuff and periscapular strengthening exercises are done to maintain shoulder strength, especially in those patients with an underlying impingement syndrome. After shoulder strength returns with a painless full range of motion, patients are advanced to an interval sports program with more vigorous overhead activity. Ice is utilized after strenuous activity if pain returns.

The clinical symptoms of AC joint disease and rotator cuff disease may be similar, and the two conditions may coexist. The AC joint and subacromial space may have to be injected on separate occasions to determine the true source of the symptoms. Patients who have failed a minimum of 6 months of appropriate conservative treatment and continue to have AC joint pain that interferes with daily activities, work, or sports may be considered for surgery.

PATIENT EDUCATION

AC disorders usually respond well to conservative treatment; however, this response may take a minimum of 6 months. Patients should be informed that a prolonged treatment course is not unusual and that good results are usually achievable with nonsurgical methods. Patients with atraumatic osteolysis of the distal clavicle should be warned that bilateral involvement may occur, with an occurrence of 70% on one long-term follow-up.[26]

Anatomic shoulder models are used to help patients understand the underlying pathophysiology of their shoulder pain. Strengthening and range-of-motion exercises of the shoulder are emphasized through physical therapy, and a home rehabilitation program is provided.

Clinical follow-up is performed at 3-month intervals, and injections of lidocaine and steroid are offered to those patients experiencing little symptomatic relief. Patients are instructed in proper stretching and warm-up techniques before upper-extremity activities, and they are advised to apply ice after any strenuous activity. Nonsteroidal anti-inflammatory medication is utilized as needed. Activities or positions that exacerbate AC pain are avoided.

If there is little or no improvement in symptoms after 6 months of conservative therapy, surgical options are discussed with the patient.

PREOPERATIVE EVALUATION

History

Preoperative evaluation should always include a detailed history, physical examination, and radiographic evaluation. There may be a history of trauma to the AC joint from a direct fall on or blow to the ipsilateral shoulder. Less commonly, the AC joint may be injured indirectly such as during a fall on the outstretched arm, with the forces being transmitted through the arm to the AC joint.[5, 6] Patients with osteolysis of the distal clavicle sometimes give a history of acute trauma, although the more common cause is repetitive microtrauma to the AC joint from activities such as weight-lifting or gymnastics.[8, 9, 12, 13] Other possible causes of shoulder pain should be excluded, such as cervical spondylosis, cervical radiculopathy, rotator cuff disease, and glenohumeral disorders, which may produce similar clinical signs or symptoms that may be missed on cursory examination.

Patients frequently complain of pain over the AC joint when adducting the ipsilateral shoulder such as during a golf swing or when buckling a seat belt. Often, there is pain when sleeping on the affected shoulder. In addition, athletes may experience AC joint pain on bench-pressing, pushups, and dips.[7, 26, 27] Pain and weakness of the affected shoulder may also be noted with forward flexion and adduction of the arm.[8]

Physical Examination

On physical examination, there may be a visible stepoff between the medial acromion and the distal clavicle, indicating a probable AC separation. Pain can usually be elicited on direct palpation of the AC joint and is made worse by a cross-arm adduction maneuver. This test is performed by internally rotating the arm, which is then adducted maximally across the chest. Test results are considered abnormal if pain is produced in the AC joint. Pain may also be elicited by motion of the arm from a horizontally abducted position to the extended position and on maximum internal rotation of the shoulder.[7, 22] These tests cause rotation and compression of the AC joint and are sensitive but less specific. These test results may also be abnormal with other disorders of the shoulder, such as posterior capsular stiffness.[20] Therefore, the examiner needs to be sure that the location of pain produced during the test corresponds to that of the AC joint. In chronic cases of AC joint pain, there may be associated trapezius muscle spasm from shoulder splinting secondary to pain.[2, 10, 18]

Frequently, AC joint pain coexists with subacromial impingement and rotator cuff disease. In these cases impingement signs are positive, and rotator cuff weakness may be present. Otherwise, there should be no detectable muscle weakness on manual resistance testing and no evidence of muscle atrophy.[20, 21, 26] Some authors have noted an association of AC joint symptoms with shoulder instability.[26] Glenohumeral motion can be variable depending on the chronicity and isolation of the problem to the AC joint. In isolated cases there may be some loss of internal rotation of the affected shoulder secondary to pain.

The lidocaine test is invaluable in differentiating isolated AC joint disorders and in predicting the response to surgical decompression. An injection is given of 2–3 mL of 1% lidocaine, which is inserted superiorly into the AC joint.[19] Examination of an anteroposterior radiograph of the AC joint before injection is helpful in determining the inclination of the AC joint. Corticosteroid may be added for extended relief of symptoms in established cases of AC joint pain. Care must be taken to avoid inadvertent injection of the subacromial space instead of the AC joint.[8] After injection, shoulder examination is repeated, and the results are compared with those of the preinjection examination.

Radiographs and Imaging

Radiographs should include an anteroposterior view of the shoulder in the scapular plane in neutral, internal, and external rotation; a transcapular Y view, an axillary view, and a 15 degree cephalic tilt view of the AC joint at 50% penetrance as described by Zanca (Fig. 13–1).[28] Stress views may be obtained by strapping 5–10 lb of weight to the patient's forearms and determining AC separation. In addition, comparing the coracoclavicular distance of both shoulders may be helpful. When clinically indicated, cervical spine radiographs should be obtained to rule out cervical spondylosis.

Radiographic evaluation may reveal AC joint arthrosis with microcystic changes in the subchondral bone, sclerosis, osteophytic lipping, and joint space narrowing (Fig. 13–2).[19] In the case of osteolysis, a radiograph may reveal a loss of subchondral bone detail with microcystic appearances in the subchondral region of the distal clavicle and osteopenia of the lateral one-third of the clavicle (Fig. 13–3).[9, 10, 12, 13] In the late stages of osteolysis, resorption of the distal end of the clavicle results in marked widening of the AC joint and, at times, complete resorption of the distal clavicle (Fig. 13–4). There may be evidence of AC

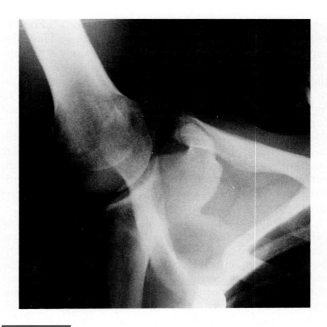

Figure 13–2 • Stryker notch view of a right shoulder showing cyst formation in the distal superior aspect of the clavicle in a patient with previous grade I AC joint separation. (From Rockwood CA, Jr and Young DC: Disorders of the acromioclavicular joint. In Rockwood CA, Jr and Matsen TA III [eds.]: The Shoulder. Philadelphia, W.B. Saunders Co., 1985, pp 413–476.)

separation with widening of the coracoclavicular distance and post-traumatic ossification of the coracoclavicular ligaments. The work of Rockwood, Williams, and Young[6] demonstrated that the major deformity is not the elevation of the clavicle but a downward displacement of the scapula and upper extremity.

AC symptoms do not always correlate with the radiographic appearance of the joint. DePalma[1] found AC

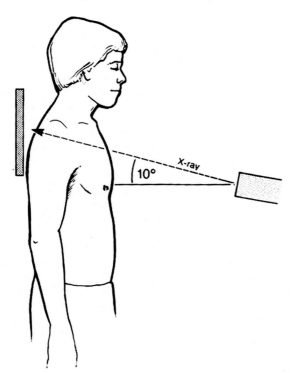

Figure 13–1 • Proper positioning of x-ray tube for a Zanca view with a 10–15 degree cephalic tilt to the AC joint. (From Rockwood CA, Jr and Young DC: Disorders of the acromioclavicular joint. In Rockwood CA, Jr and Matsen TA III [eds.]: The Shoulder. Philadelphia, W.B. Saunders Co., 1985, pp 413–476.)

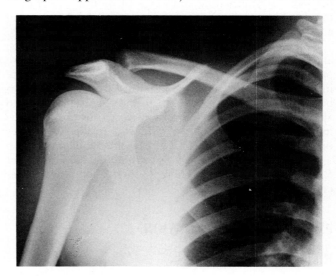

Figure 13–3 • Anteroposterior radiograph of a 26 year old weight-lifter with a painful AC joint revealing distal clavicle osteolysis. (From Rockwood CA, Jr and Young DC: Disorders of the acromioclavicular joint. In Rockwood CA, Jr and Matsen TA III [eds.]: The Shoulder. Philadelphia, W.B. Saunders Co., 1985, pp 413–476.)

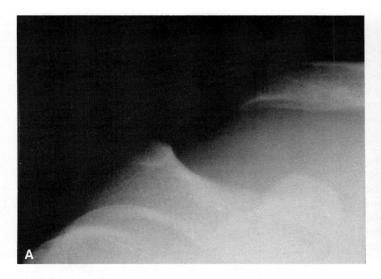
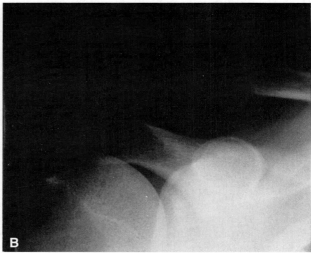

Figure 13–4 • *A*, Zanca radiographic view of symptomatic distal clavicle osteolysis in a 25 year old professional pitcher. *B*, Same patient 4 months later revealing complete resorption of the distal one-third of the clavicle.

joint degeneration to be an age-related process with symptoms not always correlating with radiographic findings of AC joint arthrosis.[28] Also, AC joint pain may persist despite normal radiographic findings.[18]

A technitium Tc 99m bone scan may assist in the diagnosis, revealing increased uptake in the distal clavicle and medial acromion.[10] In the case of atraumatic osteolysis of the distal clavicle, increased uptake may be isolated to the distal clavicle; however, approximately 50% of the time there is increased scintigraphic activity of the adjacent medial acromion.[26] In addition, the bone scan may reveal pathologic changes of the AC joint when plain radiographs appear normal.

In selected cases, magnetic resonance imaging scans can be valuable in determining a diagnosis and evaluating the glenohumeral and subacromial regions for coexisting disorders. AC joint involvement may reveal increased fluid with synovitis, soft-tissue enlargement, and periarticular ossifications with encroachment on the underlying bursal and cuff tissue.

SURGICAL INDICATIONS

Indications for surgery include continued pain that is refractory to proper conservative therapy for a minimum of 6 months, abnormal crossover adduction test results, tenderness on palpation of the AC joint, and a good response to the lidocaine injection test. Radiographic evidence of AC joint degeneration, distal clavicle osteolysis, and AC joint separation (types I and II) are considered relative indications for surgery when associated with AC joint pain. A type II separation is a relative indication if it is determined that AC pain is caused by joint incongruity rather than by joint instability.

Contraindications for surgery include AC joint dislocations of types III through VI, cellulitis of the skin overlying the AC joint or surrounding tissues, and patients without pain on palpation of the AC joint with normal

crossover adduction test results. Relative contraindications include type II AC separations with primary AC instability causing pain, patients who have not undergone a minimum of 6 months of conservative therapy, and patients who have not responded to a lidocaine injection of the AC joint.

SURGICAL TECHNIQUE

Subacromial Versus Superior Approach

Two arthroscopic approaches to AC joint resection have been described. The transcutaneous superior or direct approach is usually performed for those patients with isolated AC joint disease and no inferior clavicular osteophytes (e.g., osteolysis).[29] Many of these patients are young and athletically active, such as weight-lifters and gymnasts. For these patients the superior approach is ideal in that the AC ligaments and capsule are not excised, and the deltotrapezial fascial attachments to the clavicle are not disrupted, allowing a more aggressive postoperative rehabilitation. Usually, the AC joint is not narrowed, which facilitates instrumentation of the joint. After surgery, the patient can be placed in an accelerated rehabilitation program and can return to competition after 4–6 weeks.

The subacromial or bursal approach is recommended for those patients with concomitant subacromial disorders, such as impingement and rotator cuff disease, and for patients with moderate to severe AC joint arthrosis that makes instrumentation of the AC joint difficult.[30, 31] This procedure requires excision of the soft tissue and fat around the AC joint and necessitates the removal of most of the AC joint capsule and ligaments; however, the superior AC ligaments and the deltotrapezial fascial integrity are maintained. Usually, acromioplasty is carried out initially, aiding in the visualization and access to the distal clavicle, which can then be resected through routine portals used for acromioplasty.

Variations of Surgical Technique

Gartsman and colleagues[7, 22] resected the AC joint through a subacromial approach, rather than a direct approach, even in cases of isolated AC joint symptoms. The arthroscope was inserted through a lateral portal for a more direct "end-on" view of the AC joint. The authors recommended removing 10–15 mm of bone from the distal clavicle and 5 mm of bone from the medial acromion (Fig. 13–5).

Kay, Ellman, Esch, and Harris[23, 30, 31] resected the AC joint through the subacromial approach, utilizing posterior, posterolateral, and anterior portals as described by Ellman.[23, 30] The anterior portal was placed just superior to the coracoid tip, as opposed to directly inferior to the AC joint, to facilitate burring of the AC joint. The arthroscope was switched from the posterior to the anterior portal to verify resection.[23]

Bigliani and Flatow[2, 20, 21] resected the AC joint through a superior transcutaneous approach in cases of isolated AC joint disease. The authors recommended starting the procedure with a 2.7 mm arthroscope and changing to the 4 mm arthroscope as the procedure progressed. They recommended removing only 5–7 mm of bone and reported no deterioration of their results at short-term follow-up. They emphasized making an even bony resection and did not recommend the procedure if there were any instability involved, in which case they would consider open resection with ligament reconstruction.

Tolin and Snyder[24] utilized a subacromial approach to gain access to the distal clavicle. Their technique involved enucleation of the distal clavicle to a depth of 1.5 cm and then removal of the surrounding cortical shell of bone with a suction punch (Fig. 13–6). The procedure was performed by using routine anterior, lateral, and posterior portals. The arthroscope was switched from the posterior to the anterior portal for better visualization of the resected area as the procedure progressed. The procedure was carried out with the aid of a claviculizer (Smith-Nephew Dyonics, Andover, Mass.) end- and side-cutting

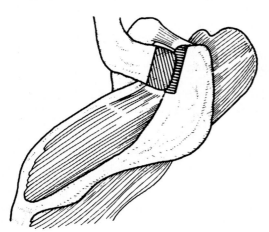

Figure 13–5 • Recommended area of removal for AC joint resection (hatched region). (From Gartsmann GM: Arthroscopic resection of the acromioclavicular joint. Am J Sports Med 21:71–77, 1993.)

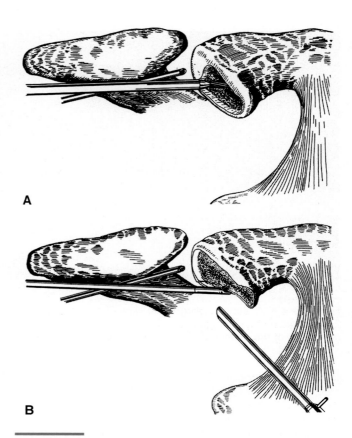

Figure 13–6 • *A*, Enucleation of the distal clavicle with a claviculizer bur. *B*, Removal of the remaining bony rim with a suction punch. (From Tolin BS and Snyder SJ: Our technique for the arthroscopic Mumford procedure. Orthop Clin North Am 24:143–151, 1993.)

bur. The amount of bone removed was determined by using two needles placed through the resected region from above and then measuring the distance with a ruler.

Authors who perform the subacromial approach to AC joint resection point out that this method affords the opportunity to evaluate and treat any concomitant glenohumeral and rotator cuff disease and to perform a decompression if necessary.[22–24] Authors who prefer a direct transcutaneous approach to the distal clavicle for isolated AC disorders believe that the subacromial and glenohumeral joint should not be entered for fear of causing unnecessary inflammation, which may inhibit rehabilitation.[2, 20, 21]

Patient positioning for arthroscopic AC joint resection is a matter of personal preference, with the lateral decubitus position preferred by some authors[7, 14, 22–24, 29] and the beach-chair position by others.[2, 20, 21, 32]

SURGICAL TREATMENT (AUTHOR'S PREFERRED METHOD)

Arthroscopic Examination

After induction of general anesthesia, physical examination of both shoulders is carried out to document range of motion, shoulder laxity, and AC joint stability. The patient is placed in the lateral decubitus position, with the torso supported by a vacuum bean bag. The arm is suspended at 70 degrees of abduction and 15 degrees of forward flexion and held in position with a prefabricated wrist gauntlet or soft wrap. Arm position is maintained by means of an overhead pulley system using a counterweight of 15 or 20 lb. Alternatively, the beach-chair position may be utilized. After the patient is securely positioned, the operative shoulder and arm are aseptically prepared and draped; the wrist gauntlet is covered with a sterile towel and plastic drape. The operating surgeon is positioned behind the operative shoulder, and the surgical table is at a comfortable operating height. The video monitor should be placed directly across from the operating surgeon in front of the patient, with the surgical technician and necessary equipment toward the patient's feet.

Before the start of the procedure, bony landmarks of the shoulder are outlined with a surgical marking pen. Prominent landmarks include the AC joint; the coracoid, anterolateral, and posterolateral borders of the acromion; and the scapular spine. Arthroscopic portal sites are marked before the procedure begins because extravasation of fluid can make anatomic landmarks difficult to identify later in the operation.

Even in cases of isolated AC joint disease, the glenohumeral joint is examined arthroscopically to rule out occult disorders that may have been missed on clinical examination and diagnostic evaluation. This is done through a posterior portal, with inflow through the arthroscope and an 18 gauge spinal needle placed through the site of the anterior portal for outflow.

Diagnostic arthroscopy is begun through a posterior portal located approximately 3 cm inferiorly and 1 cm medially to the posterolateral tip of the acromion. This portal may vary slightly according to the patient's size but is located through the interval of the infraspinatus and teres minor muscles; the interval corresponds to the palpable "soft spot" of the posterior shoulder. An 18 gauge spinal needle is inserted through the soft spot and is directed anteriorly toward the coracoid process. Approximately 40–50 mL of saline is injected into the joint, with free egress of fluid from the needle verifying placement into the glenohumeral joint. The needle is removed, and a small skin incision is made at the point of entry of the needle. A blunt 4.5 mm trocar with sleeve is inserted through the subcutaneous tissues and muscle interval, along the same path as the needle. The glenohumeral interval is identified by palpating the posterior glenoid rim and humeral head with the blunt trocar, which is then introduced into the joint. It is important to enter the joint as closely as possible to the posterior glenoid rim, which can be palpated with the trocar as a "stepoff," to avoid penetrating the tendinous portion of the rotator cuff.

The arthroscope is inserted through the posterior sheath, and inflow is provided through the arthroscope. An arthroscopic fluid pump may be used to maintain a constant fluid pressure for improved visualization. Outflow is established with an 18 gauge needle inserted through the anterior portal site located midway between the coracoid and the anterolateral edge of the acromion. With the arthroscope inserted through the posterior portal, the needle is observed to penetrate the anterior capsule just inferior to the biceps tendon and superior to the subscapularis

tendon, in the area referred to as the "safe triangle." An anterior portal can be established, if needed, through this same site by making a small skin incision around the needle and directing a blunt trocar and sleeve into the joint parallel to the path of the needle. This same anterior skin incision can be utilized to establish an anterior portal for AC joint resection by redirecting the inclination of the portal to the AC joint region.

Arthroscopic examination of the glenohumeral joint should be conducted in a thorough, systemic fashion, identifying and inspecting all intra-articular structures regardless of the preoperative diagnosis.

Subacromial Decompression with Concomitant AC Joint Resection

After completion of the glenohumeral joint evaluation and treatment, subacromial bursoscopy is carried out utilizing the same skin portals. The 4.5 mm cannula and blunt trocar are redirected through the posterior skin incision toward the posterolateral edge of the acromion. The undersurface of the posterolateral acromion is palpated with the trocar, and the cannula and trocar are then advanced into the anterolateral aspect of the subacromial space to avoid bleeding from branches of the thoracoacromial artery that are located medially around the AC joint area. During this maneuver the trocar is kept as close as possible to the undersurface of the acromion so as to stay above the bursal tissue. An arthroscopic fluid pump is utilized to improve visualization and maintain hemostasis; the pump eliminates the need for a separate inflow portal.

A lateral instrument portal is established approximately 3 cm from the lateral edge of the acromion in approximately the midcoronal plane of the acromion. An 18 gauge needle is inserted into the subacromial space and, after the needle is visualized, a small skin incision is made at the point of insertion. Instruments can be inserted directly through the lateral skin portal; alternately, a 5.5 mm plastic blunt trocar and sheath may be introduced into the subacromial space through the lateral portal. If there is difficulty locating instruments through the lateral portal, an anterior portal can be established at this time. The anterior portal is placed just superior and lateral to the coracoid tip to facilitate resection of the AC joint. The posterior cannula and obturator can be invaginated into an anterior cannula placed through the anterior portal. This step ensures that both the inflow cannula and the arthroscope cannula are within the same plane as the subacromial space and are not separated by bursal tissue. The obturator is removed from the posterior cannula and replaced by the arthroscope. The arthroscope is slowly withdrawn from the anterior cannula, and the cannula is assessed to determine adequate placement with access to the AC joint region. Diagnostic arthroscopy of the subacromial space is then carried out, followed by a formal subacromial decompression. The exact technique is described elsewhere in this book.

On completion of the subacromial decompression, the 30 degree arthroscope remains in the posterior portal, and an electrocautery is introduced through the lateral portal to remove soft tissue and fat from around the undersurface of the AC joint, including the inferior capsule of the AC joint. An electrocautery is also used to strip periosteum from the distal clavicle, exposing the area to be resected. As a caveat, the area underneath the AC joint is extremely vascular, and before any bone or soft-tissue resection commences, the area should be cauterized. In addition, hemostasis must be maintained throughout the procedure to facilitate the resection.

The AC joint is identified with an 18 gauge spinal needle passed from above the joint; this needle also identifies the medial border of the acromion. The soft-tissue shaver is used to remove all fibrous tissue from the medial border of the acromion and AC joint region. Next, a 5.5 mm bur is introduced through the lateral portal to begin the distal clavicle resection. Ideally, 8–10 mm of bone is resected from the distal clavicle. If more bony resection is needed, bone can be removed from the medial acromion. The 5.5 mm acromionizer bur and sheath measure 8 mm and can be used as an intraoperative guide to the amount of bone resected. The undersurface of the distal clavicle is made level, using a bur, with the subacromial decompression. If the distal clavicle is unstable, a downward pressure allows even more bone to be resected. At this point, the bur is introduced into the anterior portal, and the 30 degree arthroscope is exchanged for a 70 degree arthroscope for improved upward visualization of the distal clavicle during resection. Exposure is further enhanced by manually depressing the distal clavicle during resection and switching the arthroscope to the lateral portal for a more direct view of the AC joint region (Fig. 13–7). Great care is taken to remove all bone within the resected area, especially over the posterosuperior aspect of the distal clavicle, where bone is often missed and may fail to relieve pain symptoms.

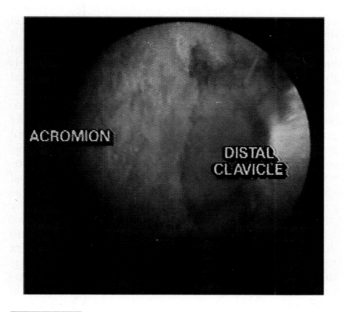

Figure 13–7 • Arthroscopic view of a distal clavicle resection viewed from a 70 degree lens (lateral decubitus position).

Direct Transcutaneous Distal Clavicle Resection (Superior Approach)

The superior or direct approach to the AC joint was first described by Johnson[29] and is ideal for arthroscopic resection of the outer end of the clavicle in patients with isolated AC disorders, such as osteolysis. Therefore, when the AC joint is identified preoperatively as the source of a patient's complaints and when no glenohumeral or subacromial disease is identified at the time of arthroscopy, a direct AC joint débridement and a distal clavicle resection are performed. For this technique the arthroscope and instruments are introduced through a direct transcutaneous approach into the AC joint. The direct resection of the distal clavicle preserves the capsule and AC ligaments, which allows for acceleration of postoperative rehabilitation and quicker return to functional activities and competition. Even in cases of isolated AC joint disease, the glenohumeral and subacromial regions are examined arthroscopically to provide a complete shoulder evaluation. This takes little operative time and adds minimal morbidity to the procedure.

Skeletal landmarks are noted with a marking pen, and the area of the AC joint is delineated. Preoperative radiographs are examined to determine the inclination of the AC joint. The AC joint is identified by direct palpation, and two 18 gauge spinal needles are introduced into the joint. One needle is introduced approximately 5 mm anterior to the anterosuperior edge of the AC joint, and the other needle is introduced about 5 mm posterior to the posterosuperior edge of the joint. These positions allow the proper inclination for easy passage of the arthroscope and instruments into the AC joint. The needles should form an angle of 90 degrees with each other. By using a 25 mL syringe, approximately 3 mL of saline is injected through the posterior spinal needle. Flow through the AC joint is confirmed by egress of fluid from the anterior spinal needle. A third 18 gauge spinal needle is introduced directly into the center of the AC joint to indicate the orientation of the joint (Fig. 13–8). Outflow is confirmed through this third spinal needle as fluid is injected through the posterior needle. After all three needles are determined to be within the AC joint, the posterior portal is established by using a No. 11 blade scalpel that is guided along the spinal needle to the posterior capsule. The obturator and cannula for the 2.7 mm arthroscope are introduced through the posterior skin portal and into the AC joint. Good return of fluid from the cannula verifies the position of the cannula within the AC joint. An arthroscopic fluid pump, which greatly improves visibility, is utilized to maintain pressure, flow, and hemostasis.

The anterior needle is visualized from within the AC joint, and an anterior portal is established parallel to the anterior spinal needle (Fig. 13–9). A 3.5 mm full-radius shaver is introduced through the anterior portal, and any remnant of a meniscoid disk is excised. As the procedure progresses the 2.7 mm arthroscope is exchanged for a 4.0 mm arthroscope to improve visibility. After soft tissue and meniscus have been removed, a bur is introduced through the anterior portal to facilitate bony resection of the distal clavicle. The area of resection can be gauged

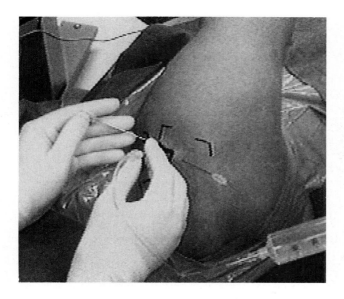

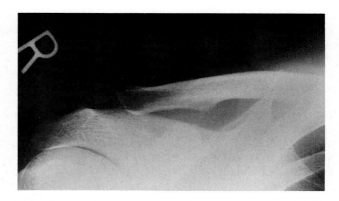

Figure 13–10 • Anteroposterior radiograph of the right shoulder after distal clavicle resection from direct approach with approximately 8 mm of bone resected.

Figure 13–8 • Positioning of 18 gauge needles for isolating the AC joint and insufflation with saline solution.

by the size of the bur, or spinal needles can be introduced into the resected area and the distance can be measured directly. Ideally, 8 mm of distal clavicle should be resected (Fig. 13–10). If a more extensive resection is required, bone is removed from the acromial side of the joint (Fig. 13–11). As the resection proceeds the arthroscope and instruments can be switched from the posterior to anterior portals for improved visualization and access to the joint and to ensure a level bony resection.

On completion of the procedure a meticulous examination is carried out to ensure the resected surface is flat without any bony prominences or residual peripheral bone that may lead to continued impingement.

POSTOPERATIVE MANAGEMENT

AC joint resection is usually performed on an outpatient basis. Steri-Strips are applied to the arthroscopic portals, and the operative extremity is placed in a sling. The patient is discharged home with anti-inflammatory and narcotic medications. The sling is removed on the first postoperative day, and physical therapy is initiated. Because the deltoid and trapezius muscles have not been detached from the clavicle as in open procedures, strength is minimally affected, and rehabilitation can be accelerated. Patients are seen for clinical follow-up at 1 week, 6 weeks, and 3 months or until full function returns.

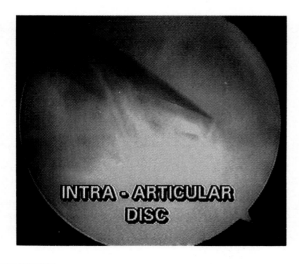

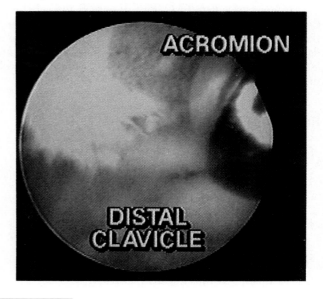

Figure 13–9 • Direct transcutaneous posterior arthroscopic view of AC joint showing anterior needle pointing to degenerative meniscoid intra-articular disk.

Figure 13–11 • Direct arthroscopic view of AC joint demonstrating additional bone resection from acromion.

Rehabilitation is divided into four phases postoperatively. Progression from one phase to the next is allowed when pain-free range of motion and minimal pain during exercises have been achieved. The main goals of phase 1 (postoperatively to 2 weeks) are to decrease pain and inflammation, prevent muscular atrophy, and restore full, nonpainful range of motion. Pain and inflammation are controlled with ice, narcotics, and nonsteroidal anti-inflammatory medication. Motion is initiated with pendulum exercises, rope-and-pulley flexion, and capsular stretching exercises. T-bar active assisted range-of-motion exercises are added, with flexion, abduction, and rotation advanced as tolerated. During this phase abduction is restricted to 90 degrees, and adduction and internal rotation are allowed as tolerated. Isometric strengthening exercises are performed, whereas, resistance against motion is avoided.

Phase two (weeks 2 to 6) is entered when the patient has full, nonpainful range of motion and minimal pain and tenderness during exercises. The goals of this phase are to regain and improve strength, normalize arthrokinematics, and improve neuromuscular control of the shoulder complex. Range-of-motion exercises are continued, and strengthening exercises via isotonic strengthening with light resistance are begun.

Phase three (weeks 6 to 12) is entered when the patient has regained 70% of strength as compared with that of the contralateral side and has no pain or tenderness during exercise. The goals of this phase are to improve strength, power, and endurance and to prepare the patient for overhead activity. During this phase, scapular strengthening exercises are added.

The final phase (week 12) is entered when the patient can perform isotonic exercises without pain and when strength has returned and is equal to that of the contralateral shoulder. The goal of this final phase is to increase activities progressively and prepare the patient for full functional return to activities.

In cases of isolated AC joint resection, the rehabilitation protocol remains the same but is accelerated because the AC ligaments are not excised. Full functional return to daily activities is expected by 4–6 weeks, and return to athletic competition is expected by 6–8 weeks postoperatively in most patients.

References

1. DePalma AF: The role of the disks of the sternoclavicular and acromioclavicular joints. Clin Orthop 13:222–231, 1959.
2. Bigliani LU, Nicholson GP, and Flatow EL: Arthroscopic resection of the distal clavicle. Orthop Clin North Am 24:133–141, 1993.
3. DePalma AF: Surgical anatomy of the acromioclavicular and sternoclavicular joints. Surg Clin North Am 43:1540–1550, 1963.
4. Fukuda K, Craig EV, An K, et al.: Biomechanical study of the ligamentous system of the acromioclavicular joint. J Bone Joint Surg 68:434–440, 1986.
5. Rockwood CA, Jr: Disorders of the acromioclavicular joint. In Rockwood CA, Jr and Matsen FA III (eds.): The Shoulder. Philadelphia, W.B. Saunders Co., 1985, p 449.
6. Rockwood RA, Jr, Williams GR, and Young CD: Injuries to the acromioclavicular joint. In Rockwood CA, Jr, Green DP, and Bucholz RW (eds.): Fractures in Adults. Philadelphia, J.B. Lippincott Co., 1991, pp 1118–1251.
7. Gartsman GM, Combs AH, Davis PF, et al.: Arthroscopic acromioclavicular joint resection: an anatomic study. Am J Sports Med 19:2–5, 1991.
8. Jacobs P: Post-traumatic osteolysis of the outer end of the clavicle. J Bone Joint Surg Br 46:705–707, 1964.
9. Murphy OB, Bellamy R, Wheeler W, et al.: Post-traumatic osteolysis of the distal clavicle. Clin Orthop 109:108–114, 1975.
10. Cahill RB: Osteolysis of the distal part of the clavicle in male athletes. J Bone Joint Surg Am 64:1053–1058, 1982.
11. Maden B: Osteolysis of the acromial end of the clavicle following trauma. Br J Radiol 36:822–828, 1963.
12. Scavenius M and Iversen BF: Nontraumatic clavicular osteolysis in weight lifters. Am J Sports Med 20:463–467, 1992.
13. Slawski DP and Cahill BR: Atraumatic osteolysis of the distal clavicle. Am J Sports Med 22:267–271, 1994.
14. Meyers JF: Arthroscopic débridement of the acromioclavicular joint and distal clavicle resection. In McGinty JB, Caspari RB, Jackson RW, et al. (eds.): Operative Arthroscopy. New York, Raven Press, 1991, pp 557–560.
15. Gurd FB: The treatment of complete dislocation of the outer end of the clavicle: a hitherto undescribed operation. Ann Surg 63:1094–1098, 1941.
16. Mumford EB: Acromioclavicular dislocation: a new operative treatment. J Bone Joint Surg 23:799–801, 1941.
17. Cook FF and Tibone JE: The Mumford procedure in athletes: an objective analysis of function. Am J Sports Med 16:97–100, 1988.
18. Novack PJ, Bach BB, Romeo AA, et al.: Surgical resection of the distal clavicle. J Shoulder Elbow Surg 4:35–40, 1995.
19. Worcester JN and Green DP: Osteoarthritis of the acromioclavicular joint. Clin Orthop 58:69–73, 1987.
20. Flatow EL, Cordasco FA, and Bigliani LU: Arthroscopic resection of the outer end of the clavicle from a superior approach: a critical, quantitative, radiographic assessment of bone removal. Arthroscopy 8:55–64, 1992.
21. Flatow EL, Duralde XA, Nicholson GP, et al.: Arthroscopic resection of the distal clavicle with a superior approach. J Shoulder Elbow Surg 4:41–49, 1995.
22. Gartsman GM: Arthroscopic resection of the acromioclavicular joint. Am J Sports Med 21:71–77, 1993.
23. Kay SP, Ellman H, and Harris E: Arthroscopic distal clavicle resection: technique and early results. Clin Orthop 301:181–184, 1994.
24. Tolin BS and Snyder SJ: Our technique for the arthroscopic Mumford procedure. Orthop Clin N Am 24:143–151, 1993.
25. Donatelli RA: Mobilization of the shoulder. In Andrews JR and Wilk KE (eds.): The Athlete's Shoulder. New York, Churchill Livingstone, 1994, pp 467–482.
26. Cahill BR and Lee MT: Atraumatic osteolysis of the distal clavicle. In Torg JS and Shephard RJ (eds.): Current Therapy in Sports Medicine. St. Louis, Mosby-Year Book, 1995, pp 177–181.
27. Fink EP: Injuries to the acromioclavicular joint. In Torg JS and Shephard RJ (eds.): Current Therapy in Sports Medicine. St. Louis, Mosby-Year Book, 1995, pp 174–177.
28. Zanca P: Shoulder pain: involvement of the acromioclavicular joint (analysis of 1000 cases). Am J Roentgenol 112:493–506, 1971.
29. Johnson LL (ed.): Arthroscopic Surgery: Principles and Practice, 3rd ed. St. Louis, C.V. Mosby, 1986, pp 1356–1359.
30. Ellman H: Arthroscopic subacromial decompression: analysis of one- to three-year results. Arthroscopy 3:173–181, 1987.
31. Esch JC, Ozerkis LR, Helgager JA, et al.: Arthroscopic subacromial decompression: results according to the degree of rotator cuff tear. Arthroscopy 4:241–249, 1988.
32. Skyhar ML, Altcheck DW, Warren RF, et al.: Shoulder arthroscopy with the patient in the beach-chair position. Arthroscopy 4:256–259, 1988.

Chapter

Complications of Shoulder Arthroscopy

Scott D. Gillogly

14

Shoulder arthroscopy has evolved significantly during the past 15 years, from a diagnostic procedure initially to the current complex of surgical procedures. The majority of traditional open-shoulder procedures available to the orthopaedic surgeon have been developed as arthroscopic techniques. In many cases, these arthroscopic techniques offer distinct advantages over corresponding open-shoulder procedures in that they minimize involvement of normal structures while focusing on the specific abnormality, thereby often reducing the morbidity of shoulder surgery. This has been particularly relevant to the treatment of shoulder problems in athletes. As the complexity of arthroscopic shoulder procedures has expanded, so has the potential for intraoperative and postoperative complications.

The complications of shoulder arthroscopy can be divided into three categories. The first category includes the complications associated with standard shoulder arthroscopy related to portal placement, patient positioning, and arthroscopic technique. The second consists of the complications that occur systemically or about the chest wall. The third consists of the complications directly related to advanced arthroscopic techniques designed to address specific shoulder conditions with arthroscopic or arthroscope-assisted procedures. This last category has undergone the greatest development in recent years as improved technology and arthroscopic techniques have expanded the indications for arthroscopic shoulder surgery and thus the potential risk for complications. These complications are often directly related to the specific shoulder abnormality and the arthroscopic techniques designed for specific treatment.

COMPLICATIONS OF STANDARD ARTHROSCOPIC PROCEDURES

Portal Placement

Portal placement for shoulder arthroscopy has been well defined and includes the posterior portal, superior portal,

various anterior portals, and lateral portal, each designed to enhance specific techniques.[1-5] The specific placement of these portals is described in detail elsewhere in this book. However, errant placement of these portals can place neurovascular and tendinous structures at risk. Edelson and Taitz[6] have demonstrated that coracoacromial arch morphology variations can influence portal placements. They recommend assessment of the bony morphology preoperatively to avoid potentially compromised portal placement, which limits visualization or produces iatrogenic damage.

Posterior Portal

The standard posterior portal passes through the deltoid muscle and the "soft spot" created between the infraspinatus and teres minor. This placement ranges from 2 to 4 cm superiorly to the axillary nerve and posterior humeral circumflex artery and 1 cm laterally to the suprascapular nerve and artery.[7, 8] Deviation of the standard posterior portal inferiorly or medially may risk injury to these structures. The posterior portal has also been implicated as a potential source for producing a nonhealing incomplete or full-thickness rotator cuff tear when the trocar is inserted through the tendinous portion of the infraspinatus or teres minor.[9] Norwood and Fowler[9] theorized that forward flexion, abduction, and external rotation of the shoulder during portal placement would contribute to bringing the tendinous portion of the rotator cuff directly in line with the path of the portal aimed at the coracoid, thereby increasing the risk of entering the joint through the tendinous avascular zone of the rotator cuff rather than through the muscular portions of the cuff. They suspected that these "holes" in the tendinous portion of the cuff failed to heal and contributed to continued shoulder symptoms. Therefore, it is important to take into account the arm position as well as the superior-inferior and medial-lateral positioning of the posterior portal. This potential complication would seem more likely in the lateral decubitus position for shoulder arthroscopy, as was the case in

Norwood and Fowler's report. The same problem has not been reported with the beach-chair position. Another unusual complication reported with the posterior portal is the development of a posterior synovial cyst requiring open excision.[10]

Superior (Supraclavicular) Portal

The superior portal traverses the supraclavicular fossa 1 cm medial to the medial acromion and just posterior to the clavicle. Although this portal was initially used as an inflow portal, the advent of the arthroscopic pump has made this portal more of an accessory portal for access to the superior labrum and biceps-labral complex. This portal is aimed from medial to lateral, thus avoiding the suprascapular nerve running on the inferior surface of the supraspinatus muscle 2 cm medial to the path of the portal. Directing the portal more medially than laterally could risk this nerve.[8] The musculotendinous junction and tendinous portion of the supraspinatus portion of the cuff are also potentially in the path of this portal. Arm position is directly related to the risk of trocar placement through the supraspinatus tendon. At abduction of 90 degrees, the supraspinatus tendon is always violated by this portal, whereas at 30 degrees of abduction or less, the portal passes through the muscular portion of the supraspinatus tendon.[11] Like the posterior portal, this portal seems to have greater risk of penetrating the tendon in the lateral decubitus position than in the beach-chair position.

Anterior Portals

There have been several different anterior portals described, particularly as more advanced surgical techniques required an additional anterior working portal.[1, 3, 5, 12] With particular concern for the anterior neurovascular structures, a safe zone has been described for anterior portal placement.[12] This roughly triangular area is bounded by the biceps tendon, the glenoid, and the superior edge of the subscapularis tendon. These structures provide the intra-articular landmarks, and the coracoid and anterior acromion provide important extra-articular reference points in protecting the surrounding neurovascular structures. Placement of all anterior portals should pass superiorly and laterally to the coracoid to prevent any possible injury to the musculocutaneous nerve, brachial plexus, and axillary artery, which lie inferiorly and medially to the coracoid. Abduction of more than 30 degrees moves the musculocutaneous nerve more proximally and laterally and reduces the normal 1.5–4 cm safety margin when using an anteroinferior portal.[5] These portals should also remain superior to the leading edge of the subscapularis tendon, which will avoid the axillary nerve at least 2 cm inferiorly.[7] Deviating from these standard portals or aiming medially or inferiorly to the coracoid and subscapularis can result in neurologic injury as has been described to occur in the brachial plexus.[12] The cephalic vein coursing superficially in the deltopectoral groove is just inferior to the anteroinferior portal. The cephalic vein or its deltoid branches may be lacerated while this portal is

established. Although this complication may cause an anterior hematoma and allow an ecchymosis to extend down the arm, no long-term deleterious effects have been noted.[13]

Lateral (Subacromial) Portals

Lateral portals have been designated posteriorly, centrally, and anteriorly about the lateral acromion, and they are used primarily for addressing abnormalities in the subacromial region.[8] Accommodating the natural lateral curve of the acromion, these portals are made 1–2 cm lateral to the acromion and traverse the deltoid muscle in entering the subacromial space. The axillary nerve is at risk if these portals extend more laterally from the acromion as the nerve comes within 3–5 cm from the acromion. The nerve is closest to the lateral acromion near its anterolateral border.[14, 15]

Patient Positioning

Positioning the patient for shoulder arthroscopy was initially described using the lateral decubitus position with continuous traction on the arm.[1–3, 5] Included in these initial as well as subsequent reports has been the complication of neurapraxia of various portions of the brachial plexus associated with the traction applied to the arm in this position necessary for distraction of the joint. Andrews and colleagues[1, 3] noted three cases of transient neurapraxia involving one musculocutaneous and two ulnar nerves. Paulos and Pitman et al.[16, 17] reported a 20% prevalence of transient neurapraxia usually resolving within 24 hours of shoulder arthroscopy, except for one axillary injury that resolved during 2 months. Ogilvie-Harris and Wiley[18] noted only one case of transient neurapraxia that involved the musculocutaneous nerve in 439 shoulder arthroscopic procedures. They theorized that the low incidence of neurapraxia injuries was related to their use of manual traction rather than a fixed suspended weight. Gross and Fitzgibbons[19] recommended a method for traction on the arm perpendicular to the long axis, with weights of no more than 5–10 lb to minimize the stretch on the brachial plexus. Small[20] reviewed more than 14,300 shoulder arthroscopic procedures in a survey of experienced surgeons and found only four nerve injuries, including one axillary and three brachial plexus injuries, attributable to a stretch mechanism from traction. Ellman[21] found three cases of neurapraxia involving the radial nerve among 50 patients undergoing arthroscopic subacromial decompression.

Several studies have evaluated the effect of arm traction, position, joint distention, and fluid extravasation during shoulder arthroscopy on the brachial plexus. Noting an almost 10% clinical prevalence of transient paresthesia and neurapraxia with shoulder arthroscopy in the lateral decubitus position, Klein et al.[22] studied the effects of arm position on brachial plexus strain in cadavers. They found that the commonly used position of 30 degrees of forward flexion and 70 degrees of abduction produced significant strain on the brachial plexus. The least strain on the plexus was at positions of 45 degrees of forward flexion and 90 degrees of abduction and 45 degrees of forward flexion and 0 degrees of abduction. Pitman et al.[23] used intraoperative somatosensory evoked potentials for detection of neurapraxia during shoulder arthroscopy in the lateral decubitus position in 20 patients. They found abnormal somatosensory evoked potentials of the musculocutaneous nerve in all 20 patients, occurring with initial joint distention in 16 of them and improving with establishment of outflow from the joint. This involvement was further aggravated by traction. In 10 patients, they found varying degrees of median, ulnar, and radial nerve involvement. There were just two with clinical evidence of neurapraxia postoperatively, one involving the musculocutaneous nerve and the other involving the radial nerve, and both cases resolved within 48 hours. Pitman and colleagues noted the musculocutaneous nerve to be most sensitive to the effects of position, traction, and distention due to the course of the nerve through the coracobrachialis, producing stretch on the nerve with abduction and traction. They recommended reducing the weights used for traction to less than 12 lb for the 70 degree abducted position and less than 7 lb for the minimal abduction position.[23]

With concern for the effects of traction and arm position on producing either subclinical or clinical injury to the brachial plexus, Skyhar and associates[24] developed the technique for performing shoulder arthroscopy in the sitting (beach-chair) position, obviating the need for continuous traction and abduction. In over 50 reported procedures with this technique, there were no nerve palsies. Skyhar et al.[24] reported further advantages with this technique, including faster positioning, ease in proceeding to an open procedure without reprepping or draping, and a more anatomic positioning of the capsular ligaments. This positioning method has become more popular as techniques for arthroscopic shoulder stabilization expand.

Extravasation of Fluid

Extravasation of fluid into the surrounding soft tissues during shoulder arthroscopy can occur to an alarming extent. This tense soft-tissue swelling may contribute to stretch injury of the brachial plexus and its proximal branches but does not seem to produce sustained pressures within the deltoid muscle to produce compartment syndrome. Lee, Cohn, and Tooke[25] measured the intramuscular pressure of the deltoid during shoulder arthroscopy using a slit catheter. They found that although the pressures became markedly elevated during extra-articular procedures (subacromial decompression) to as high as 48 mm Hg with gravity inflow and 91 mm Hg with pump infusion, these elevations were transient. Each of 24 patients returned to normal intramuscular pressures within 10–30 minutes after cessation of the procedure, although swelling remained clinically apparent. In pure intra-articular procedures, there was very little transient increase in deltoid pressure. Ogilvie-Harris and Boynton[26] found elevations of the deltoid muscle pressures due to extravasation of fluid during arthroscopic acromioplasty using an inflow pump. The recorded pressures were as high as 120 mm Hg from a baseline of 12 mm Hg. The

pressures were noted to return to baseline within 4 minutes of completion of the procedure. No patient showed evidence of muscle damage during electromyograms performed 4–6 weeks postoperatively.

Infection

Infection and septic arthritis following shoulder arthroscopy are rare; the reported occurrence has been extremely low. Nonetheless, it is imperative to maintain strict aseptic technique throughout the procedure and to follow the same guidelines for prophylactic antibiotics used in other arthroscopic procedures. A broad-spectrum antibiotic is given 30–60 minutes before the procedure is initiated, and a postoperative dose is given.

D'Angelo and Ogilvie-Harris[27] showed a fourfold decrease in infection rates for clean arthroscopy cases with a protocol of preoperative intravenous antibiotics continued as an oral dose 24 hours postoperatively. They noted nine cases of septic arthritis following 4,000 arthroscopic procedures of the knee and shoulder, for an overall infection rate of 0.23%. Two of the nine infections involved the shoulder following arthroscopic rotator cuff débridement and acromioplasty. Both cases were treated with repeated arthroscopic débridement and suction irrigation. The offending organisms were *Staphylococcus epidermidis* and *Staphylococcus aureus*. One patient resolved without sequelae and the other patient had persistent pain and decreased shoulder motion. Small[20] noted just two cases of infection among 14,329 shoulder arthroscopy procedures reported in a survey of members of the Arthroscopy Association of North America.

Miscellaneous

There are general procedural pitfalls that need to be avoided to offer the best possible results with various arthroscopic shoulder procedures. These include avoiding chondral damage to articular surfaces and maintaining adequate inflow for visualization at all times. Bleeding within the joint or particularly in the subacromial space can be troublesome, extending surgical time or even compromising the procedure. Intra-articular electrocautery is available for use with the commonly used arthroscopic fluids, normal saline solution, and Ringer lactate solution. The electrocautery instrument is specially designed with a plastic coating covering all but the very tip of the unit to make its use safe within the joint. The use of 1.5% glycine as a nonconducting fluid medium for intra-articular electrocautery is strongly discouraged due to reports of transient blindness associated with glycine toxicity.[28]

Another relatively isolated complication associated with shoulder arthroscopy is reflex sympathetic dystrophy or sympathetically mediated pain.[29] Certainly no patient with evidence of a more diffuse upper extremity problem or other signs of vasomotor disturbance should undergo shoulder arthroscopy before proper evaluation and treatment.

The instrumentation used in shoulder arthroscopy has greatly improved as technology has met demand.

Although now much less common than in the early period of shoulder arthroscopy, instrument breakage can occur during procedures, usually resulting in intra-articular or subacromial loose pieces. It is imperative that the shoulder arthroscopist have special retrieval instruments available at all times. Magnetized retrieval instruments are particularly helpful in removing small metallic fragments or needle tips from around the shoulder. During more specialized procedures requiring sophisticated integrated instrumentation, back-up instruments should be available in the event of breakage during a critical stage of the procedure. This prevents aborting the procedure or changing to a suboptimal alternative procedure.

SYSTEMIC AND RESPIRATORY COMPLICATIONS

As with any surgical procedure, systemic complications can occur in shoulder arthroscopy. Fortunately, these complications are exceedingly rare and are noted only as isolated case reports. Deep venous thrombosis of the lower extremity has been reported after knee arthroscopy but has not been noted following thousands of reported shoulder arthroscopy procedures.[20] However, a case of deep venous thrombosis affecting the operative upper extremity was recorded in a patient with a previously undetected mass of the mediastinum, which was later confirmed to be Hodgkin's disease.[30] This patient required long-term anticoagulation.

There are reports of pneumomediastinum and potentially life-threatening tension pneumothorax caused by subcutaneous emphysema associated with shoulder arthroscopy.[31, 32] Lee, Dewan, and Crosby[32] reported three cases of excessive subcutaneous emphysema following arthroscopic subacromial decompression under general anesthesia performed with the patient in the sitting position and with an infusion pump in which two patients had pneumothoraces requiring emergent insertion of chest tubes. All three cases resolved without sequelae. Although the exact mechanism of air entry into the subcutaneous tissues is unknown, the theory has been postulated that air is drawn into the subacromial space through the lateral portal. When the suction is off, the positive pressure from the arthroscopic pump may force the air into the subcutaneous tissue, producing subcutaneous emphysema. Further dissection of the air into the axillary sheath and extension to the prevertebral space surrounding the trachea and esophagus result in a pneumomediastinum. Positive pressure ventilation and expiration may lead to rupture of the mediastinal pleura and pneumothorax. These two reports[31, 32] call attention to these potentially serious complications and the importance of early recognition and prompt treatment.[31,32]

Another severe respiratory compromise occurred in a patient undergoing subacromial decompression under interscalene block in the sitting position and with use of an arthroscopic pump.[33] This patient complained of coughing and fullness in the throat just before respiratory compromise. During immediate intubation, there was massive swelling of the pharyngeal tissue, making visualization difficult and requiring blind passage of the endotracheal tube.

Subsequent laryngoscopy revealed a large retropharyngeal fluid collection. The patient remained intubated until the swelling decreased during the next 12 hours; the patient was discharged on the first postoperative day without sequelae. This complication was directly related to the extra-articular migration and accumulation of arthroscopy fluid in the prevertebral and airway tissues.[33]

COMPLICATIONS OF SPECIFIC ARTHROSCOPIC PROCEDURES

It is important to distinguish between failures of a procedure and true complications, although there can be overlap. A poor result following an arthroscopic subacromial decompression caused by an inadequate resection of an anterior acromial spur is a failure due to technically inadequate surgery rather than a complication. However, if the inadequate resection is a result of poor visualization due to excessive subacromial bleeding, then the inadequate resection could be considered a complication as well. A poor result due to a persistent neurapraxia injury would also be a complication. Failures may also result from improper or incomplete preoperative diagnosis, such as performing subacromial decompression in a young athlete with anterior instability, only to have recurrent subluxation symptoms postoperatively. The efficacy of the various procedures is beyond the scope of this chapter.

Subacromial Decompression

Arthroscopic subacromial decompression (SAD) has been reported to have the lowest complication rate, less than 1%, of the commonly performed arthroscopic shoulder procedures.[20, 29, 34] Small,[29] in a review of complications among experienced arthroscopists, noted two cases of reflex sympathetic dystrophy of the involved upper extremity among 175 procedures. Gartsman[35] noted three complications in 165 patients undergoing this procedure, two involving neurapraxia in the arm and one involving transient neurapraxia of the lateral femoral cutaneous nerve due to positioning. Ellman[36] reported three cases of neurapraxia involving the dorsal digital nerve to the thumb, which were considered secondary to the traction holding device on the hand and wrist. Increased padding has eliminated this problem.[21] Ellman[21]; Bigliani, Flatow, and Deliz[34]; Gartsman[35]; and Altchek, Warren, and Wickiewicz[37] reported no infections in their reviews of, collectively, 225 patients undergoing arthroscopic acromioplasty. Ellman[36] further reported no infections in more than 250 cases. Ryu[38] reported a case of deltoid detachment during arthroscopic acromioplasty. Seltzer, Wirth, and Rockwood[39] noted deltoid detachment to be a significant cause of failure after open acromioplasty; they believe this complication may be under-recognized after arthroscopic acromioplasty. Other reports of complications have included isolated hematomas, instrument breakage, and excessive bleeding obscuring visualization. With improved techniques and more advanced equipment, many of these problems seem to have been almost eliminated.

Rotator Cuff Tears

Arthroscopic treatment of rotator cuff tears has included débridement of the cuff tear edges alone or in conjunction with arthroscopic placement of sutures and minideltoid-splitting approach to secure the sutures to bone.[40, 41] Ellman, Kay, and Wirth[40] reported one complication of a wound seroma that resolved without sequelae among 40 patients with full-thickness rotator cuff tears treated with arthroscopic SAD and cuff tear débridement without repair. They noted overall poorer results in this treatment method for large reparable tears when compared with results of open repair. Levy, Uribe, and Delaney[41] noted no postoperative complications in 25 patients treated with SAD, arthroscopically placed sutures, and the minideltoid-splitting incision for full-thickness rotator cuff tears.

Distal Clavicle Resection

Arthroscopic resection of the distal clavicle has been described with a bursal approach and a superior approach. When resection of the distal clavicle is indicated for acromioclavicular joint arthritis in conjunction with rotator cuff disease and impingement, the resection is typically accomplished from the bursal side as part of the SAD. The complications accompanying this resection are included as part of the arthroscopic acromioplasty. When isolated acromioclavicular joint arthritis or osteolysis of the distal clavicle is present, the superior approach is utilized.[42, 43] Flatow and colleagues reported a high failure rate (42%) among patients with acromioclavicular joint instability, although satisfactory results were seen in 93% of patients without acromioclavicular joint instability. In 41 patients, few other complications were noted with isolated resection of the distal clavicle. One case of reflex sympathetic dystrophy was exacerbated by surgery. There were no cases of infection, wound problems, or neurologic injury.[44]

Arthroscopic Anterior Stabilization

Arthroscopic stabilization procedures have developed greatly during the past decade. Various methods have been utilized to achieve fixation of the detached anterior labrum to the glenoid rim and advance the inferior glenohumeral ligament and capsule during fixation. Fixation devices have included staples, screws, direct sutures, suture anchors, and bioabsorbable tacks. The indications, techniques, and recurrence rates are covered elsewhere in this book.

The procedure of arthroscopic anterior staple capsulorrhaphy has the highest complication rate of the commonly performed arthroscopic shoulder procedures. Small[20] noted that staple capsulorrhaphy had a 5.3% complication rate due mostly to hardware problems, including loose, impinging, and bent staples. Among experienced arthroscopists, the complication rate with this procedure fell to only 3.3%.[29] Hawkins,[45] in a review of 50 arthroscopic stapling repairs, reported two cases of loose staples requiring reoperation and one case of transient neuropathy involving the musculocutaneous and median nerves.

He noted that technical difficulty with staple insertion could be avoided by careful technique and greater experience. Detrisac and Johnson[46] reported on 148 staple capsulorrhaphies and noted that 15 staples required removal for pain, looseness, or poor position. They noted no neurovascular complications and one infection requiring staple removal and arthroscopic irrigation and débridement. Lane, Sachs, and Riehl[47] reported on 41 stapling procedures; they found loosening in five and pain from the staple in four others.

In an attempt to avoid the high complication rate with staple procedures, the technique of passing transglenoid sutures was developed to treat anterior instability arthroscopically.[48] Morgan[49] has reported on 175 patients treated with this technique, noting an only 5% recurrence rate and no complications. Caspari and Savoie[50] reported on 49 patients who had reconstruction with the arthroscopic transglenoid Bankart repair and noted a 4% recurrence rate with only one complication involving development of a synovial fistula through the glenoid to the posterior incision over the infraspinatus fossa. This resolved without sequelae after débridement and removal of the suture knot posteriorly. Duncan and Savoie[51] reported two cases of pain associated with the posterior suture knot out of 10 patients treated with transglenoid sutures for multidirectional instability. The symptoms resolved in both these patients after surgical removal of the knot 3 months after the stabilization procedure. Shea and Lovallo[52] described a complication during passage of a transglenoid Beath pin using this technique. The Beath pin bent during passage and entered the scapulothoracic joint; subsequent attempts at removal broke off the pin below the skin. The pin required open removal by taking down the rhomboids from their scapular attachment. It was recommended that a power drill be used to pass the transglenoid pin rather than a mallet to prevent this type of errant passage. Arciero et al.[53] reported on 21 patients at the United States Military Academy undergoing arthroscopic transglenoid Bankart repair for first-time shoulder dislocations. The authors found that 86% were able to return to preinjury sports activity levels. They noted three complications, including one posterior subcutaneous suture abscess in which the knot had been tied over the fascia and two cases of transient hypesthesia in the median nerve distribution. The neurapraxia of the median nerve was thought to be the result of the hand holder used to secure the extremity to the traction device for the lateral decubitus position. Both cases resolved within three weeks.

Landsiedl[54] described three complications among 65 patients undergoing transglenoid fixation. He found one case of posterior synovial fistula, one case of anterior glenoid articular cartilage disruption caused by the pin, and one case of suprascapular nerve injury caused by the pin exiting near the scapular spine. The passage of transglenoid pins (for sutures) can place the suprascapular nerve at risk as the nerve passes the scapular spine on its course to the infraspinatus muscle. For this reason, it is recommended that the course of the pins be directed medially to exit within the infraspinatus fossa. Green and Christensen[55] have reported on 60 patients undergoing arthroscopic Bankart repair using the transglenoid suture technique. They noted an overall failure rate of 42% at an average follow-up of 37 months. The recurrence rate correlated directly with the degree of degeneration and extensiveness of the glenoid labrum–inferior glenohumeral ligament complex lesion. The recurrence rate was only 4% in 22 cases with simple anterior labral detachment. Reported complications included two cases of intra-articular broken Beath pin eyelets, two superficial wound problems, and three cases of posterior knot erosion through the skin over the infraspinatus fossa. These posterior knot problems required the knot to be removed and all healed with local wound care. These authors recommended placement of the posterior knot deep at the level of the infraspinatus fascia to minimize this potential complication. There were no cases of suprascapular nerve injury.

Another means of stabilizing the anterior labrum–ligament complex is using suture anchors placed in the anterior glenoid. This is one of the methods designed to obviate the need to pass transglenoid sutures. Wolf[56] reported on more than 50 patients treated with anterior suture anchors with only one recurrence and no complications associated with the procedure.

Another promising technique of arthroscopic anterior stabilization is the use of bioabsorbable tacks.[57–59] Arciero[58] has reported on 33 patients undergoing this procedure for first-time anterior shoulder dislocations. He noted one case of recurrent instability and two cases of a single recurrent traumatic dislocation. There were no perioperative complications in these procedures performed in the beach-chair position. Warner and Warren[57] reported on 23 patients treated with bioabsorbable tacks and noted two recurrences at 2-year follow-up. They also found that 9 of 12 overhead athletes were able to return to their preinjury level of competition. This technique and the suture anchor technique offer the advantage of avoiding the potential complication of a posterior suture knot abscess or fistula and possible injury to the suprascapular nerve with passage of transglenoid pins and sutures.[58] Edwards et al.[60] identified adverse reactions of pain and stiffness to bioabsorbable tacks in six shoulders requiring repeated arthroscopy 8–24 weeks after insertion. The patients showed mild elevations in sedimentation rate and C-reactive protein with normal white blood cell counts. In all six cases, the labrum was found to be healed, and the shoulders showed synovitis and a nonspecific granulomatous inflammatory response. One case showed the head of the tack free in the anterior joint at 8 weeks. All six cases resolved without pain or motion deficit following arthroscopic lavage and débridement.[59]

Bioabsorbable tacks have also been used in the treatment of tears of the superior labrum from anterior to posterior (SLAP lesions) as described by Snyder et al.[61] The authors did not report any complications with a limited number of these procedures. One patient with attempted repair of a SLAP lesion with a metal staple had intra-articular impingement from the staple, requiring its removal 2 days postoperatively.[61] Field and Savoie[62] addressed appropriate SLAP lesions in 20 patients, with intra-articular sutures passed posteriorly with a transglenoid Beath pin and tied over the infraspinatus fossa. The patients had one complication of adhesive capsulitis requiring closed manipulation.

Miscellaneous Shoulder Procedures

The advancement of shoulder arthroscopic technique has expanded indications for arthroscopy for both diagnosis and treatment of a wide variety of shoulder diseases. Bonutti, Hawkins, and Saddemi[63] reported on nine patients undergoing standard shoulder arthroscopy to assess pain and loosening following total shoulder arthroplasty. Other than some initial difficulty encountered with adjusting to the reflection of light off the polished humeral component, they noted no complications with the procedure and found it valuable for determining glenoid loosening, rotator cuff tears, and resection of adhesions. Morgan and Casscells[64] reported a case of arthroscopic glenohumeral arthrodesis using percutaneous screws without complication. Matthews and LaBudde[65] found shoulder arthroscopy helpful in the treatment of synovial diseases of the shoulder. They recommended its use for synovial biopsy and synovectomy. They reported the risks associated with arthroscopic procedures were lower than for corresponding open procedures. They recommended having blood replacement available for rheumatoid patients due to the risks of excessive bleeding after synovectomy. Synovial fistulae were also noted and usually responded to immobilization but rarely required open excision and joint closure.

SUMMARY

Complications in standard shoulder arthroscopy have clearly been reduced through a greater understanding of portal anatomy and improvements in arthroscopic instrumentation, technique, and positioning. Although they are rare, it is essential that the surgeon be aware of the potentially life-threatening complications involving the airway. Despite the development of more advanced arthroscopic surgical procedures directed at expanded indications for shoulder surgery, the complications associated with these often innovative procedures have been few. Shoulder arthroscopy has become the treatment of choice for a broad spectrum of shoulder problems and has proved to be a safe, consistent, and reliable procedure.

References

1. Andrews JR, Carson WG, and Ortega K: Arthroscopy of the shoulder: Technique and normal anatomy. Am J Sports Med 12:1–7, 1984.
2. Johnson LL: Arthroscopy of the shoulder. Orthop Clin North Am 11:197, 1980.
3. Andrews JR and Carson WG: Shoulder joint arthroscopy. Orthopedics 6:1157, 1983.
4. Neviaser TJ: Arthroscopy of the shoulder. Orthop Clin North Am 18:361–372, 1987.
5. Wolf EM: Anterior portals in shoulder arthroscopy. Athroscopy 5:201–208, 1989.
6. Edelson JG and Taitz C: Bony anatomy of the coracoacromial arch: Implications for arthroscopic portal placement in the shoulder. Arthroscopy 9:201–208, 1993.
7. Detrisac DA and Johnson LL: Arthroscopic Shoulder Anatomy: Pathologic and Surgical Implications. Thorofare, N.J., Slack, 1986.

8. Nottage WM: Arthroscopic portals: anatomy at risk. Orthop Clin North Am 24:19–26, 1993.

9. Norwood LA and Fowler HL: Rotator cuff tears: A shoulder arthroscopy complication. Am J Sports Med 17:837–841, 1989.

10. Moran MC and Warren RF: Development of a synovial cyst after arthroscopy of the shoulder. J Bone Joint Surg Am 71:127–129, 1989.

11. Souryal T and Baker CL: Anatomy of the supraclavicular fossa portal in shoulder arthroscopy. Arthroscopy 6:297–300, 1990.

12. Matthews LF, Zarins B, Michael RH, et al.: Anterior portal selection for shoulder arthroscopy. Arthroscopy 1:33–39, 1985.

13. Caspari RB: Complications of shoulder arthroscopy. In Sprague NF (ed.): Complications of Arthroscopy. New York, Raven Press, 1989, pp 179–197.

14. Bryan WJ, Schauder K, and Tullos HS: The axillary nerve and its relationship to common sports medicine shoulder procedures. Am J Sports Med 14:113–116, 1986.

15. Burkhead WZ, Scheinberg RR, and Box G: Surgical anatomy of the axillary nerve. J Shoulder Elbow Surg 1:31–36, 1992.

16. Paulos L: Arthroscopic shoulder decompression technique and preliminary results. Presented at the Annual Meeting of the Arthroscopy Association of North America, April, 1985.

17. Pitman MI, Nainzadeh N, Ergas E, et al.: The use of somatosensory evoked potentials for detection of neuropraxia during shoulder arthroscopy. Arthroscopy 4:250–255, 1988.

18. Ogilvie-Harris DJ and Wiley AM: Arthroscopic surgery of the shoulder: a general appraisal. J Bone Joint Surg Br 68:201, 1986.

19. Gross RM and Fitzgibbons TC: Shoulder arthroscopy: A modified approach. Arthroscopy 1:156, 1985.

20. Small NC: Complications in arthroscopy: The knee and other joints. Arthroscopy 2:253, 1986.

21. Ellman H: Arthroscopic subacromial decompression: Analysis of one- to three-year results. Arthroscopy 3:173–181, 1987.

22. Klein AH, France JC, Mutschler TA, et al.: Measurement of brachial plexus strain in arthroscopy of the shoulder. Arthroscopy 3:45–52, 1987.

23. Pitman MI, Nainzadeh N, Ergas E, et al.: The use of evoked potentials for detection of neuropraxia during shoulder arthroscopy. Arthroscopy 4:250–255, 1988.

24. Skyhar MJ, Altchek DW, Warren RF, et al.: Shoulder arthroscopy with the patient in the beach-chair position. Arthroscopy 4:256–259, 1988.

25. Lee YF, Cohn L, and Tooke SM: Intramuscular deltoid pressure during shoulder arthroscopy. Arthroscopy 5:209–212, 1989.

26. Ogilvie-Harris DJ and Boynton E: Arthroscopic acromioplasty: extravasation of fluid into the deltoid muscle. Arthroscopy 6:52–54, 1990.

27. D'Angelo GL and Ogilvie-Harris DJ: Septic arthritis following arthroscopy, with cost-benefit analysis of antibiotic prophylaxis. Arthroscopy 4:10–14, 1988.

28. Burkhart SS, Barnett CR, and Snyder SS: Transient postoperative blindness as a possible effect of glycine toxicity. Arthroscopy 6:112–114, 1990.

29. Small NC: Complications in arthroscopic surgery performed by experienced arthroscopists. Arthroscopy 4:215–221, 1988.

30. Burkhart SS: Deep venous thrombosis after shoulder arthroscopy. Arthroscopy 6:61–63, 1990.

31. Lau KY: Pneumomediastinum caused by subcutaneous emphysema in the shoulder: A rare complication of shoulder arthroscopy. Chest 103:1606–1607, 1993.

32. Lee HC, Dewan N, and Crosby L: Subcutaneous emphysema, pneumomediastinum and potentially life-threatening tension pneumothorax: pulmonary complications from arthroscopic shoulder decompression. Chest 101:1265–1267, 1992.

33. Hynson JM, Tung A, Guevara JE, et al.: Complete airway obstruction during arthroscopic shoulder surgery. Anesth Analg 76:875–878, 1993.

34. Bigliani LU, Flatow EL, and Deliz ED: Complications of shoulder arthroscopy. Orthop Rev 20:743–751, 1991.

35. Gartsman GM: Arthroscopic acromioplasty for lesions of the rotator cuff. J Bone Joint Surg Am 72:169–180, 1990.

36. Ellman H: Arthroscopic acromioplasty. In McGinty JB (ed.): Operative Arthroscopy. New York, Raven Press, 1991, pp 543–555.

37. Altchek DW, Warren RF, and Wickiewicz TL: Arthroscopic acromioplasty: technique and results. J Bone Joint Surg Am 72:1198–1207, 1990.

38. Ryu RK: Arthroscopic subacromial decompression: A clinical review. Arthroscopy 8:141–147, 1992.

39. Seltzer DG, Wirth MA, and Rockwood CA: Complications and failures of open and arthroscopic acromioplasties. Oper Tech Sports Med 2:136–150, 1994.

40. Ellman H, Kay SP, and Wirth M: Arthroscopic treatment of full-thickness rotator cuff tears: 2- to 7-year follow-up study. Arthroscopy 9:195–200, 1993.

41. Levy HJ, Uribe JW, and Delaney LG: Arthroscopic assisted rotator cuff repair: Preliminary results. Arthroscopy 6:55–60, 1990.

42. Johnson LL: Diagnostic and Surgical Arthroscopy. St. Louis, CV Mosby, 1981.

43. Flatow EL, Cordasco FA, and Bigliani LU: Arthrosopic resection of the outer end of the clavicle from a superior approach: A critical, qualitative, radiographic assessment of bone removal. Arthroscopy 8:55–64, 1992.

44. Flatow EL, Duralde XA, Nicholson GP, et al.: Arthroscopic resection of the distal clavicle with a superior approach. J Shoulder Elbow Surg 4:41–50, 1995.

45. Hawkins RB: Arthroscopic stapling repair for shoulder instability: A retrospective study of 50 cases. Arthroscopy 5:122–128, 1989.

46. Detrisac DA and Johnson LL: Arthroscopic shoulder capsulorrhaphy using metal staples. Orthop Clin North Am 24:71–88, 1993.

47. Lane JG, Sachs RA, and Riehl B: Arthroscopic staple capsulorrhaphy: A long-term follow-up. Arthroscopy 7:324–328, 1991.

48. Morgan CD and Bodenstab AB: Arthroscopic Bankart suture repair: Technique and early results. Arthroscopy 3:111–112, 1987.

49. Morgan CD: Arthroscopic transglenoid Bankart suture repair. Op Tech Orthop 1:171–179, 1991.

50. Caspari RB and Savoie FH: Arthroscopic reconstruction of the shoulder: the Bankart repair. In McGinty JB (ed.): Operative Arthroscopy. New York, Raven Press, 1991, pp 507–515.

51. Duncan R and Savoie FH III: Arthroscopic inferior capsular shift for multidirectional instability of the shoulder: A preliminary report. Arthroscopy 9:24–27, 1993.

52. Shea KP and Lovallo JL: Scapulothoracic penetration of a Beath pin: An unusual complication of arthroscopic Bankart suture repair. Arthroscopy 7:115–117, 1991.

53. Arciero RA, Wheeler JH, Ryan JB, et al.: Arthroscopic Bankart repair versus nonoperative treatment for acute, initial anterior shoulder dislocations. Am J Sports Med 22:589–594, 1994.

54. Landsiedl F: Arthroscopic therapy of recurrent anterior luxation of the shoulder by capsular repair. Arthroscopy 8:296–304, 1992.

55. Green MR and Christensen KP: Arthroscopic Bankart procedure: two- to five-year follow-up with clinical correlation to severity of glenoid labral lesion. Am J Sports Med 23:276–281, 1995.

56. Wolf EM: Arthroscopic capsulolabral repair using suture anchors. Orthop Clin North Am 24:59–69, 1993.

57. Warner JP and Warren RF: Arthroscopic Bankart repair using a cannulated, absorbable fixation device. Op Tech Orthop 1:192–198, 1991.

58. Arciero RA: Acute stabilization of initial anterior shoulder dislocations. Presented at the American Orthopaedic Society for Sports Medicine Specialty Day, Orlando, Fla., February, 1995.

59. Pagnani MJ and Warren RF: Arthroscopic shoulder stabilization. Op Tech Sports Med 1:276–284, 1993.

60. Edwards DJ, Hoy G, Saies AD, et al.: Adverse reactions to an absorbable shoulder fixation device. J Shoulder Elbow Surg 3:230–233, 1994.

61. Snyder SJ, Karzel RP, Del Pizzo W, et al.: SLAP lesions of the shoulder. Arthroscopy 6:274–279, 1990.

62. Field LD and Savoie FH: Arthroscopic suture repair of superior labral detachment lesions of the shoulder. Am J Sports Med 21:783–790, 1993.

63. Bonutti PM, Hawkins RJ, and Saddemi S: Arthroscopic assessment of glenoid component loosening after total shoulder arthroplasty. Arthroscopy 9:272–276, 1993.

64. Morgan CD and Casscells CD: Arthroscopic-assisted glenohumeral arthrodesis. Arthroscopy 8:262–266, 1992.

65. Matthews LS and LaBudde JK: Arthroscopic treatment of synovial diseases of the shoulder. Orthop Clin North Am 24:101–109, 1993.

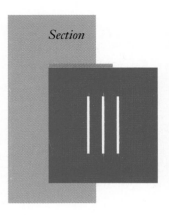

The Elbow

15

Diagnostic Arthroscopy of the Elbow

Stephen R. Soffer

Burman first performed arthroscopy of the elbow in 1931.[1] After performance of arthroscopy on cadaveric elbow specimens, he concluded that the elbow is unsuitable for examination. During the last 60 years, a great deal has been learned about elbow arthroscopy. The anatomy of the elbow with respect to specific arthroscopic portals has been elucidated by Andrews and Carson,[2] Angelo and Soffer,[3] and others. Improvements in fiberoptics and arthroscopic equipment and techniques have provided the surgeon with reliable and safe arthroscopic procedures to relieve various conditions of the elbow.

In this chapter we discuss patient selection and evaluation, current indications and contraindications of elbow arthroscopy, operating room set-up, and general technique of elbow arthroscopy.

PATIENT SELECTION

Indications

As the equipment for arthroscopic surgery and our arthroscopic skills and experience with the elbow continue to improve, so the indications for elbow arthroscopy expand. Currently, the indications for elbow arthroscopy include:

1. Loose bodies

2. Treatment of osteochondritis dissecans

3. Osteoarthritis, post-traumatic arthritis

4. Chronic synovitis (e.g., rheumatoid arthritis, synovial osteochondromatosis)[4]

5. Synovial plica[5, 6]

6. Adhesions and contractures[2, 7–9]

7. Valgus extension overload syndrome[10]

8. Fractures[2, 8, 11, 12]

9. Diagnosis of medial collateral ligament laxity[13]

10. Septic arthritis[8, 9]

11. Diagnosis of symptomatic elbow (e.g., elbow snapping, elbow pain, new onset flexion contracture, biopsy)

Contraindications to Elbow Arthroscopy

Conditions in which the joint space is inaccessible to arthroscopic instrumentation and visualization or conditions in which the neurovascular structures are at increased risk are contraindications to elbow arthroscopy. For example, a severe contracture of the elbow from scarring and adhesions makes instrumentation and visualization difficult or impossible. This is especially evident in patients who have had a previous elbow arthrotomy or extensive casting. The neurovascular structures are also at increased risk in this situation, because distention of the elbow prior to instrumentation is difficult and the neurovascular structures may be closer in proximity to the portal sites. Previous ulnar nerve transposition also increases the risk of neurologic injury with medial portal placement. Distortion of the bony architecture as sometimes seen in severe rheumatoid arthritis, osteoarthritis, or ankylosis alters the anatomy and may result in an increased chance of neurovascular injury.

Lastly, lack of knowledge of the normal arthroscopic anatomy and pathologic lesions of the elbow are contraindications to elbow arthroscopy.

OPERATING ROOM SET-UP

Anesthesia

The most commonly used anesthesia for elbow arthroscopy is a general anesthetic. It allows for both patient comfort and total muscle relaxation to improve visualization of the elbow joint. Intravenous regional anesthesia may be implemented in place of a general anesthetic; however, the use of dual tourniquets about the upper arm limits the ability for the surgeon to have access to the anterolateral and anteromedial portals, especially in the patient with a very short humerus. Intrascalene or axillary blocks may also be implemented. This does, however, rely on the expertise of the particular anesthesiologist. Furthermore, a postoperative neurovascular evaluation is difficult with this type of anesthesia. Local anesthesia may also be used for elbow arthroscopy[14]; however, the problems of patient comfort, muscle relaxation, and tourniquet pain may all contribute to difficulty during arthroscopy. In addition, the local anesthetic may result in a temporary sensory or motor deficit making postoperative neurologic evaluation of the elbow difficult. Given the difficulty of elbow arthroscopy and the close proximity of neurovascular structures, the use of general anesthesia is recommended.

Equipment

Instrumentation for elbow arthroscopy is similar to equipment used for arthroscopy of other joints. Fluid inflow can be either gravity or an arthroscopic pump system. The arthroscopic pump systems are advantageous for several reasons. The shaving apparatus is used frequently in elbow arthroscopy. The pump is useful in allowing an increased flow of fluid into the joint when utilizing a debrider. This allows for rapid filling of the joint as the instrument removes the fluid and debris. The capsule is thus less likely to "collapse" while one is using the shaver with the pump system than with gravity fluid flow. During arthroscopy and shaving in the difficult lateral compartment, the pump system is very helpful in keeping the joint inflated with fluid.

An interchangeable cannula system is extremely helpful during elbow arthroscopy. This allows for interchange of arthroscope and motorized shavers through the cannulas without repeated punctures into the elbow joint. Multiple capsular rents from repeated punctures of the capsule can increase fluid extravasation about the soft tissues of the elbow. Furthermore, with each repeated pass there is an increased risk to the neurovascular structures.

The 4.0 mm 30 degree angled videoarthroscope is used in both the anterior and posterior compartments of the elbow. This allows an excellent panoramic view of the elbow with a large inflow of fluid into the joint and thus affords optimal visualization for these compartments. The lateral compartment, however, is quite small and it is often difficult to utilize the 4.0 mm arthroscope in addition to another instrument in a second accessory portal to allow for instrumentation. The smaller 2.7 mm or 2.9 mm arthroscope allows for improved access to this compartment. In addition, a smaller diameter shaver is also helpful in the lateral compartment.

Elbow arthroscopic equipment includes:

1. Marking pen
2. 50 mm syringe
3. Intravenous connecting tubing
4. 18 gauge spinal needles
5. No. 11 knife blade
6. Small curved hemostat
7. Basic arthroscopic equipment including probes, punches, and graspers with teeth
8. Arthroscopic pump system
9. 4 mm 30 degree angled arthroscope
10. 2.7 or 2.9 mm 30 degree arthroscope
11. Interchangeable cannula systems for 2.7 and 4.0 mm arthroscopes
12. Large motorized shavers and burrs
13. Small motorized shavers and burrs (optional)

Patient Positioning

Elbow arthroscopy may be performed with the patient in either the supine or prone position. In 1985, Andrews and Carson described elbow arthroscopy with the patient in the supine position on the operating room table (Fig. 15–1). This position is comfortable for the surgeon and anesthesiologist, the operating room personnel, and also the patient. The potential for skin pressure–related injuries to the face, trunk, or legs that may occur with improper prone positioning is avoided. Access to all of the elbow compartments is possible with this position. Arthroscopic anatomy of the elbow, which may sometimes be confusing to the less experienced arthroscopist, is in a more anatomic orientation with the supine position. This position also allows anesthesia to have excellent access to the airways and head and neck structures. One also need not be concerned with cumbersome chest rolls or pelvic and facial rolls to protect the patient's soft tissues from compression if the patient is placed in the prone position.

The prone position has been used by several elbow arthroscopists since it was introduced in 1989[15] (Fig. 15–2). The prone position may allow for easier access to the posterior compartment. It allows gravity to move the neurovascular structures in antecubital fossa anteriorly and away from the entering instruments. The arm is moved easily and does not require a traction suspension system. Lindenfeld has described the use of this position along with an initial proximal medial arthroscopic portal.[16] He believed that this was a safer approach to entry into the elbow joint because the instruments enter the joint in a more parallel relationship to the neurovascular structures. He also described an improved view of the anterior compartment with this prone position and proximal medial portal.[16]

In this chapter we describe the operating room set-ups for both the prone and supine positions. We utilized the supine position, which is reflected in the text and illustrations.

GENERAL TECHNIQUE

Portal Anatomy

A thorough knowledge of the bony anatomy as well as the important neurovascular structures relative to the arthroscopic portals is critical to the elbow arthroscopist. This allows for safe and efficient elbow arthroscopy.

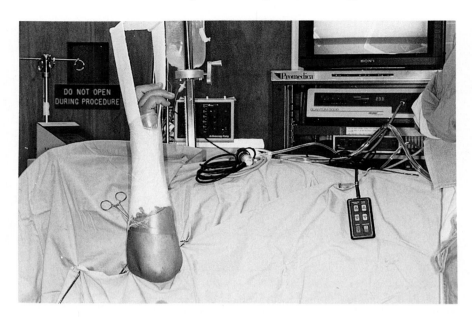

Figure 15–1 • Supine position for elbow arthroscopy.

Bony landmarks are usually palpable about the elbow. These landmarks include the lateral epicondyle, medial epicondyle, and the olecranon. On the lateral aspect of the elbow, the lateral epicondyle, olecranon, and radial head form a triangle (Fig. 15–3). At the center of this triangle is the "soft spot." It is through this area that a needle is introduced into the joint to allow for distention of the elbow with fluid just prior to elbow arthroscopy.

It is important to realize that the articular surfaces of the distal humerus are not in line with the shaft of the humerus. There is a 30 degree anterior projection of the condyles to the shaft of the humerus. The trochlea medially and the capitellum laterally make up the articular surface of the distal humerus. The coronoid fossa and radial fossa lie just proximal to the trochlea and the capitellum respectively and accept the coronoid process and the radial head during deep flexion (Fig. 15–4). These fossa may be visualized during arthroscopy of the anterior compartment and may be filled with fibrous tissue or bony spurs, preventing full flexion of the elbow. Posteriorly and just prox-

imal to the trochlea lies the olecranon fossa, which accepts the olecranon tip of the ulna during full extension (Fig. 15–5).

The trochlea articulates with the trochlear notch of the proximal ulna. The trochlear notch, which is also called the greater sigmoid notch, the greater semilunar notch, or the incisura semilunaris, is formed by four articular facets that blend. An area devoid of articular cartilage is commonly seen in the center of the trochlear notch and is a normal arthroscopic finding. It is located between the proximal and distal articular facets in the center of the notch. This is similar to the bare area seen on the posterior aspect of the humeral head during shoulder arthroscopy, which is also a normal finding. The radial notch or lesser semilunar notch is lateral to the coronoid process and articulates with the radial head during pronation and supination.

Unlike arthroscopy in other joints, neurovascular structures about the elbow lie in close proximity to arthroscopic portals. One must have a thorough knowledge, not

Figure 15–2 • Prone position for elbow arthroscopy. (From Andrews JR and Soffer SR [eds.]: Elbow Arthroscopy. St. Louis, Mosby–Year Book, 1994, p 53.)

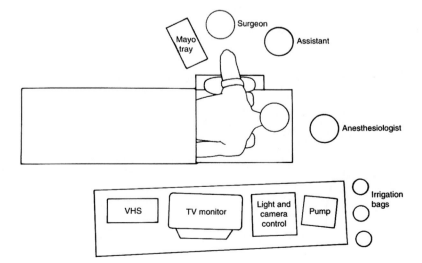

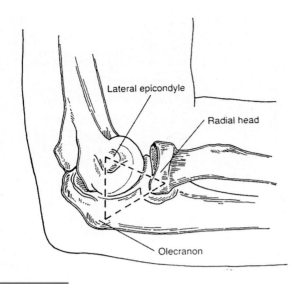

Figure 15–3 • Triangle formed by the radial head, olecranon, and lateral epicondyle. (From Andrews JR and Soffer SR [eds.]: Elbow Arthroscopy. St. Louis, Mosby–Year Book, 1994, p 15.)

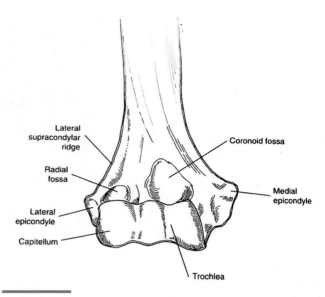

Figure 15–4 • The coronoid fossa and the radial fossa lie proximal to the trochlea and the capitellum. (From Andrews JR and Soffer SR [eds.]: Elbow Arthroscopy. St. Louis, Mosby–Year Book, 1994, p 16.)

Figure 15–5 • Olecranon fossa. (From Andrews JR and Soffer SR [eds.]: Elbow Arthroscopy. St. Louis, Mosby–Year Book, 1994, p 17.)

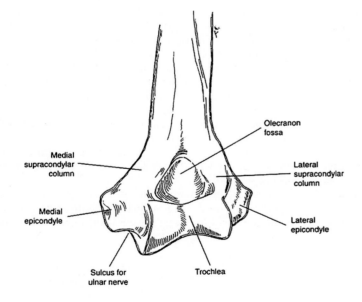

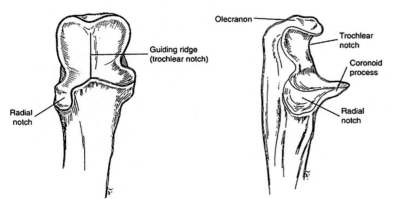

Table 15–1   **Average Portal Distance from Neurovascular Structures***

		Distance (mm)		
Portal	*Nerve/Vessel*	*Andrews and Carson*[2]	*Lynch et al.*[12]	*Lindenfeld*[16]
Anterolateral	Posterior antebrachial cutaneous nerve	—	2	—
	Radial nerve	7	11	3
Anteromedial	Medial antebrachial cutaneous nerve	—	1†	—
Andrews and Carson‡	Median nerve	6	14	—
	Brachial artery	17	—	—
Lindenfeld§	Median nerve	—	—	23
Poehling et al.[15]¶	Median nerve	—	—	—
Posterolateral	Medial brachial cutaneous nerve	—	20	—
	Posterior antebrachial cutaneous nerve	—	25	—
Straight posterior	Ulnar nerve	20	—	—

*All distances from median, radial, and ulnar nerves are with joint distention.
†Nerve in one of five specimens was cut.
‡Portal 2 cm distal and 2 cm anterior from the medial epicondyle.
§Portal 1 cm proximal and 1 cm anterior to the medial epicondyle.
¶Portal (patient prone) 2 cm proximal to medial epicondyle, just anterior to intermuscular septum.
From Andrews JR and Soffer SR (eds.): Elbow Arthroscopy, St. Louis, Mosby-Year Book, 1994, p 26.

only of the major arteries and nerves about the elbow but also of the cutaneous neurovascular pattern to avoid injury to these structures. Distention of the elbow with saline solution prior to establishing arthroscopic portals increases the margin of safety and helps the arthroscopist to avoid injury to the neurovascular structures.[2] The exact distances from portal to neurovascular structures have been described by several authors (Table 15–1). During elbow arthroscopy, it is important to visualize the neurovascular structures in three-dimensional planes as each portal is established in order to decrease the neurovascular risk.

Anterolateral Portal

The anterolateral portal should be placed just anterior and proximal to the capitular-radial articulation, which is often approximately 2–3 cm distal and 1 cm anterior to the lateral humeral epicondyle (Fig. 15–6). The measurement may vary depending on the size of the patient, and the portal placement should depend on locating the capitular-radial articulation. The anterolateral portal passes through the extensor carpi radialis brevis and the deep part of the supinator muscles before it punctures the joint capsule. The posterior antebrachial cutaneous nerve branches from the radial nerve in the arm. The radial nerve lies on the lateral aspect of the arm and supplies the posterolateral aspect of the elbow in the posterior aspect of the forearm.

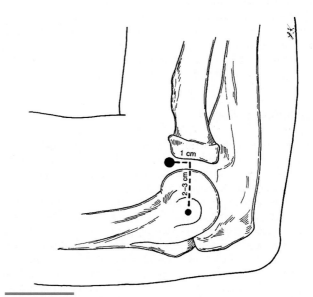

Figure 15–6 • Anterolateral portal. (From Andrews JR and Soffer SR [eds.]: Elbow Arthroscopy. St. Louis, Mosby–Year Book, 1994, p 40.)

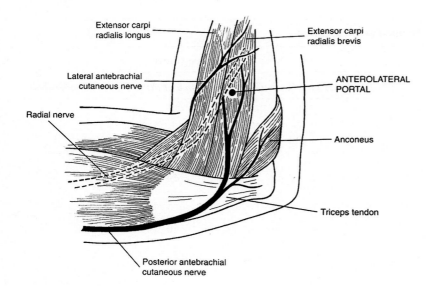

Figure 15–7 • The posterior and lateral antebrachial cutaneous nerves. (From Andrews JR and Soffer SR [eds.]: Elbow Arthroscopy. St. Louis, Mosby–Year Book, 1994, p 42.)

It may be damaged with establishment of the anterolateral portal (Fig. 15–7). The radial nerve crosses the lateral intermuscular septum in the distal one-third of the arm and lies anterior to the lateral epicondyle between the brachioradialis and brachialis muscles. The nerve divides into the superficial branch and the deep branch in the antecubital area. The superficial branch is a sensory branch that lies beneath the brachioradialis muscle. It innervates the dorsoradial aspect of the wrist and the posterior aspect of the lateral 3 1/2 digits. The deep motor branch wraps around the posterior aspect of the neck of the radius and enters the supinator muscle. It forms the posterior interosseous nerve, which innervates the muscles on the posterior aspect of the forearm. The anterolateral portal usually passes posterolateral to the radial nerve by approximately 7–11 mm.[2] Lindenfeld describes the distance as being shorter by approximately 2.8 mm.[16]

The lateral antebrachial cutaneous nerve, a branch of the musculocutaneous nerve, innervates the anterolateral aspect of the elbow and the lateral aspect of the forearm: It is less likely to be injured than the aforementioned nerves during placement of the anterolateral portal.

Anteromedial Portal

The anteromedial portal is placed approximately 2 cm anterior and 2 cm distal to the medial epicondyle[2] (Fig. 15–8). Placement of the anteromedial portal is established under direct visualization with a spinal needle at arthroscopy. The portal passes through the area between the flexor carpi radialis and the flexor digitorum superficialis and then transgresses the deep portion of the pronator teres before entering into the joint capsule. The portal lies approximately 6–14 mm posteromedial to the median nerve and on average 17 mm posteromedial to the brachial artery.[2, 16] The medial antebrachial cutaneous nerve is also in danger during establishment of the anteromedial portal because it may be as close as 1 mm to the portal (Fig. 15–9).

Proximal Medial Portal

The proximal medial portal is located 1 cm anterior and 1 cm proximal to the medial epicondyle.[16] This portal passes through a tendinous portion of the flexor pronator group. Lindenfeld found that there is less fluid extravasation when using this portal since the tissue is more rigid in this area of puncture. In Lindenfeld's study, the average distance from the proximal medial portal to the median nerve is 22.3 mm.[16] Lindenfeld recommended that this proximal medial portal be established initially because it offers more security with regard to the neurovascular structures.

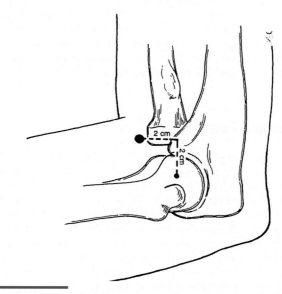

Figure 15–8 • Anteromedial portal. (From Andrews JR and Soffer SR [eds.]: Elbow Arthroscopy. St. Louis, Mosby–Year Book, p 44.)

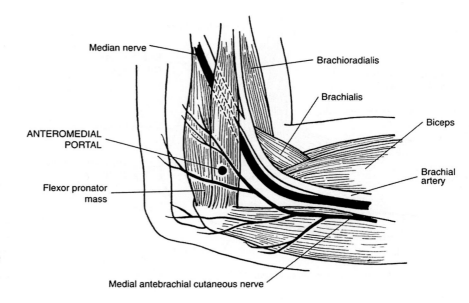

Figure 15–9 • Medial antebrachial cutaneous nerve. (From Andrews JR and Soffer SR [eds.]: Elbow Arthroscopy. St. Louis, Mosby–Year Book, 1994, p 45.)

Poehling has also described a proximal medial portal that lies 2 cm proximal to the medial epicondyle just anterior to the intermuscular septum[15] (Fig. 15–10).

Direct Lateral Portal

The direct lateral portal, also called straight lateral or "soft spot" portal, lies in the center of the triangle formed by the lateral epicondyle radial head and olecranon (see Fig. 15–3). The portal passes through the anconeus muscle before puncturing the capsule. There are no neurovascular structures at risk in this area.

An accessory lateral portal may be placed if débridement is necessary in the lateral compartment. This portal is usually placed 1.5–2 cm distal to the direct lateral portal.

It also passes through the anconeus muscle, and no neurovascular structures are at significant risk.

Posterolateral and Straight Posterior Portals

The posterolateral portal lies 3 cm proximal to the olecranon tip and just lateral to the lateral border of the triceps muscle (Fig. 15–11). The portal passes through the subcutaneous tissue and transgresses the edge of the triceps

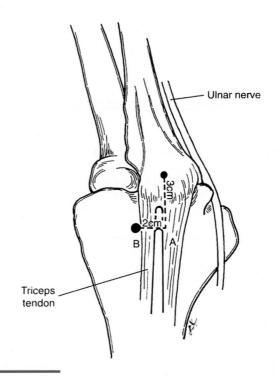

Figure 15–11 • Straight posterior portal (*A*) and posterolateral portal (*B*). (From Andrews JR and Soffer SR [eds.]: Elbow Arthroscopy. St. Louis, Mosby–Year Book, 1994, p 52.)

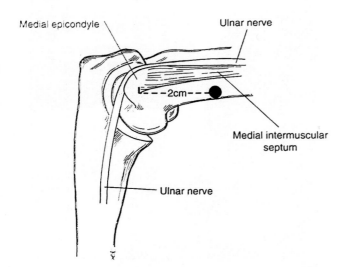

Figure 15–10 • Proximal medial portal. (From Andrews JR and Soffer SR [eds.]: Elbow Arthroscopy. St. Louis, Mosby–Year Book, p 54.)

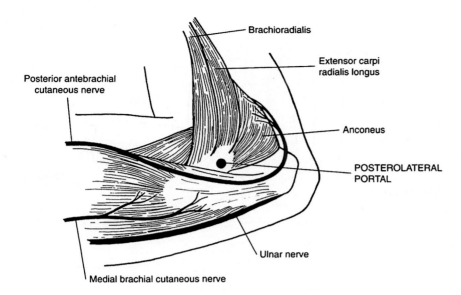

Brachioradialis

Extensor carpi radialis longus

Posterior antebrachial cutaneous nerve

Anconeus

POSTEROLATERAL PORTAL

Ulnar nerve

Medial brachial cutaneous nerve

Figure 15–12 • The posterior antebrachial cutaneous nerve and the medial brachial cutaneous nerve. (From Andrews JR and Soffer SR [eds.]: Elbow Arthroscopy. St. Louis, Mosby–Year Book, 1994, p 51.)

before entering the posterior capsule. The straight posterior trans-triceps portal is located over the center of the triceps tendon, 2 cm medial to the posterolateral portal and 3 cm proximal to the tip of the olecranon (see Fig. 15–11). The posterior antebrachial cutaneous nerve is a branch of the radial nerve that lies on the lateral aspect of the upper arm and innervates the posterolateral aspect of the elbow and the posterior aspect of the forearm (Fig. 15–12). The medial brachial cutaneous nerve lies on the medial side of the upper arm and innervates the posteromedial aspect of the arm and olecranon (see Fig. 15–12). The posterior antebrachial cutaneous nerve lies approximately 25 mm medial to the posterolateral portal, and the medial brachial cutaneous nerve lies approximately 20 mm from the posterolateral portal.[17] The ulnar nerve lies around 15 to 20 mm medial to the straight posterior portal and is usually not in danger.[2]

SURGICAL TECHNIQUE FOR DIAGNOSTIC ARTHROSCOPY

After general endotracheal intubation, the tourniquet is placed as high as possible on the upper arm. This usually necessitates placement of the tourniquet near the axilla. Total tourniquet time should not exceed 90–120 minutes.[18] With the patient in the supine position, the arm is abducted 90 degrees and the elbow is flexed 90 degrees. A wrist gauntlet or finger trap is connected to the forearm or fingers in order to suspend the arm. The arm is suspended by a pulley and weight system with 5 lb of traction. We use the same pulley system that is used for shoulder arthroscopy in the lateral decubitus position (Fig. 15–13).

After preparing and draping the extremity, the surgeon sits on a rolling stool slightly to the radial side of the elbow with the nurse or first assistant sitting on the medial side of the elbow. A metal stand is placed over the trunk of the patient upon which the arthroscopic equipment is secured. All video equipment is placed on the opposite side of the patient such that it is easily visible to the surgeon. The bony landmarks, lateral epicondyle, radial head,

olecranon tip, and medial epicondyle are outlined with a marking pen. The ulnar nerve is also outlined. Next the anterolateral, anteromedial, direct lateral, accessory lateral, posterolateral, and straight posterior portals are appropriately marked (Fig. 15–14).

At this point the limb is exsanguinated with an Esmarch bandage, and the tourniquet is elevated. An 18

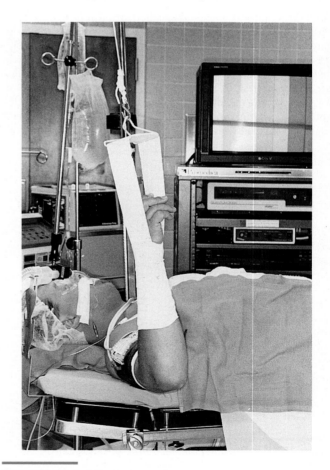

Figure 15–13 • Arthroscopy set-up.

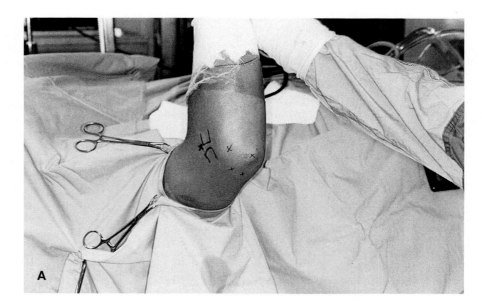

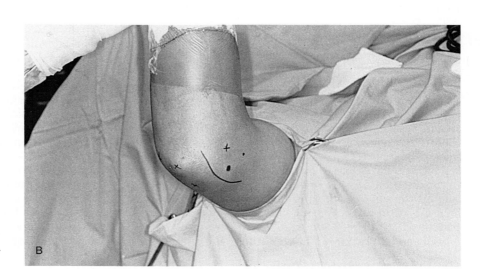

Figure 15–14 • *A*, Lateral bony land-marks and portals. *B*, Medial bony land-marks and portals.

gauge spinal needle is placed through the triangular area (soft spot) on the lateral aspect of the elbow, bordered by the radial head, lateral humeral epicondyle, and olecranon tip. A needle is placed in the center of this triangle, and the elbow is distended with approximately 15–20 mL of saline (Fig. 15–15). Distention of the elbow aides entry into the joint through the initial portal site: It also serves to increase the distance between the portal sites and important neurovascular structures, thus making elbow arthroscopy safer. After the elbow is distended with saline, free backflow from the needle verifies proper placement into the elbow joint.

ANTEROLATERAL PORTAL

The anterolateral portal is established first. This portal lies approximately 2–3 cm distal and 1 cm anterior to the lat-eral humeral epicondyle. This is an *estimation* of the location of this portal and varies in different elbows. The key to proper placement of this portal is to palpate the articulation of the capitellum with the radial head while supinating and pronating the forearm. The proper placement of the portal is just anterior and proximal to this articulation.

As previously mentioned, after proper distention of the elbow joint with saline through the soft spot portal, a second 18 gauge spinal needle is placed at the previously marked anterolateral portal site. The needle is directed towards the center of the joint. The stylette is removed, and free backflow through the anterolateral needle confirms the intra-articular location of this needle. All of this is done with the elbow flexed at 90 degrees (Fig. 15–16).

A No. 11 blade is used to incise the skin only. One must not go through the subcutaneous tissue with the No. 11 blade and cause possible injury to the superficial sensory nerves. After the skin alone is incised with the No. 11

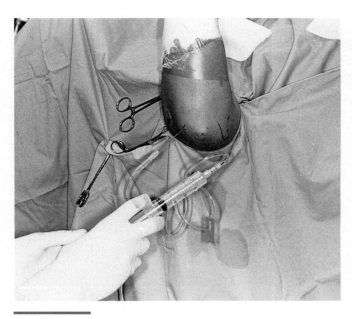

Figure 15–15 • Needle in the "soft spot" distending the elbow with fluid.

blade, a curved hemostat is then used to deepen the portal through the subcutaneous tissue. A blunt trocar with a sheath is then inserted through this portal site. The trocar should be directed towards the center of the elbow. The capsule and synovium must be "trapped" against the distal humerus to puncture it and enter into the elbow joint (Fig. 15–17). It is important to trap the capsule against the bone of the distal humerus in order to avoid skiving of the capsule off the top capsule and plunging the trocar into the anterior neurovascular structures. After the capsule is punctured with the trocar and sheath, the trocar is removed and free backflow of fluid through the cannula ver-

ifies entry into the elbow joint. The arthroscope is then placed through this cannula, and diagnostic arthroscopy is begun.

We utilized an arthroscopic pump system with normal saline solution rather than gravity distention as mentioned previously in this chapter. Maximum pump pressure for elbow arthroscopy should never exceed 50 mm Hg. We maintain elbow distention throughout the elbow arthroscopy, especially during placement of subsequent portal sites. This allows constant distention in the elbow, causing further displacement of the neurovascular structures away from the entering arthroscopic instruments.[17] Through the anterolateral portal, the medial capsule, coronoid process, trochlea, coronoid fossa, and medial aspect of the radial head are visualized.

ANTEROMEDIAL PORTAL

We usually establish the anteromedial portal as our second portal. This is done by direct intra-articular visualization of a localizing needle. Prior to exsanguination of the limb, the anteromedial portal is identified 2 cm anterior and 2 cm distal to the medial humeral at the condyle. This area is marked with a marking pen. With the arthroscope in the anterolateral portal, an 18 gauge spinal needle is then inserted in the previously marked anteromedial portal site (Fig. 15–18). The needle can be visualized entering into the joint. Fine adjustments in the placement of this needle can then be made with direct visualization. The position of the needle should just be proximal to the humeral ulnar joint articulation and just anterior to the distal humerus. The needle passes just anterior to the medial epicondyle and posterior to the antecubital neurovascular structures.

The stylette may be removed from the spinal needle. This allows removal of air bubbles that interfere with visualization. After fine adjustments in needle placement are made, a small incision is made with a No. 11 blade, cutting the skin only. Again a curved hemostat is used to spread

Figure 15–16 • Needle in the anterolateral portal.

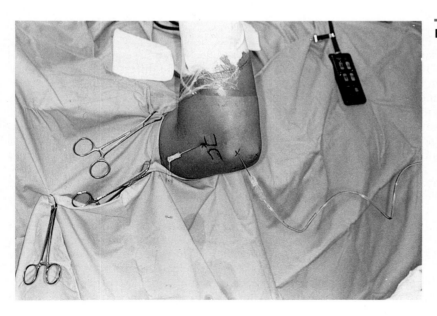

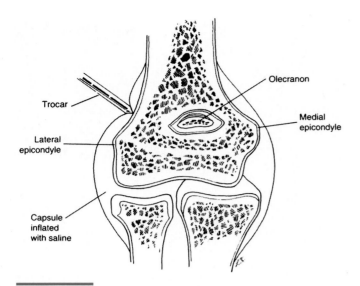

Figure 15–17 • A trocar trapping the capsule against the distal humerus. (From Andrews JR and Soffer SR [eds.]: Elbow Arthroscopy. St. Louis, Mosby–Year Book, 1994, p 43.)

deeper into the subcutaneous tissue to avoid injury to the superficial nerves. The arthroscopic trocar and cannula are then introduced through this portal into the elbow joint. An interchangeable cannula system is used so that the arthroscope may be switched between the anteromedial and anterolateral cannulas. This allows full visualization of both the medial and lateral aspects of the entire anterior compartment. With the arthroscope in the anterolateral cannula, the anteromedial aspect of the joint is well seen. Appropriate arthroscopic débridement may be performed using the anteromedial portal. After completion of surgery on the anteromedial side of the elbow, the arthroscope is

then placed through the anteromedial cannula, and full visualization of the anterolateral aspect of the joint is then allowed. A shaver may be placed into the anterolateral cannula to perform surgery on this side of the joint. The forearm should be rotated to visualize the radial head and note any articular cartilage damage.

After completion of arthroscopic surgery in the anterior compartment of the elbow, both cannulas are left in the portal sites. As the arthroscope and other instruments are placed in subsequent portals, the cannulas in the anterolateral and anteromedial portals prevent extravasation of fluid into the soft tissues. The lateral capsule, radial head, capitellum, and radial fossa are visualized through the anteromedial portal.

DIRECT LATERAL PORTAL

After arthroscopic surgery is completed in the anterior compartment, the lateral compartment is then inspected. The soft spot portal or direct lateral portal is established where the 18 gauge spinal needle was placed to distend the joint: the center of the triangle, which is bordered by the lateral epicondyle, radial head, and olecranon. An incision is made with a No. 11 blade, and the small trocar system for a 2.7 arthroscope is then passed into the joint (Fig. 15–19). The cannulas pass through the skin, subcutaneous tissue, anconeus muscle, and capsule. There is little danger of injuring any neurovascular structures with this portal.

A 2.7 arthroscope is utilized in this area because the lateral compartment is quite small. This is especially helpful with an accessory lateral portal and is necessary for arthroscopic débridement in this area. Occasionally, in the case of a large elbow, we will utilize the 4 mm arthroscope. Through this portal the radial head, capitellum, trochlear notch, and trochlear ridge are well seen.

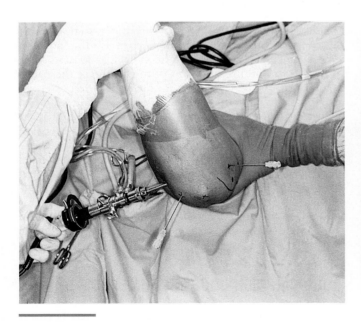

Figure 15–18 • Needle in the anteromedial portal.

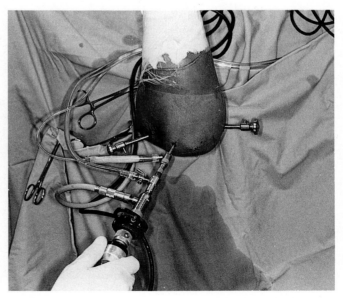

Figure 15–19 • Small arthroscope in the direct lateral portal.

ACCESSORY LATERAL PORTAL

If débridement or other arthroscopic surgery is necessary in the lateral compartment, an accessory lateral portal may be used. An 18 gauge localizing needle is inserted through the skin approximately 1.5–2 cm distal to the direct lateral portal. Once the needle is visualized, the portal is established with a knife and blunt trocar. If débridement or chrondroplasty is necessary, such as with osteochondritis dissecans of the capitellum, a small arthroscopic shaver device may be used. It is not uncommon to inadvertently pull the arthroscope or shaver out of the joint, thus one must be attentive in order to avoid this situation. The arthroscope may be placed in the accessory lateral portal and the shaver into the direct lateral portal to aide arthroscopic débridement.

POSTEROLATERAL PORTAL

After lateral compartment surgery is completed, the posterolateral portal is established to visualize the posterior compartment of the elbow. With the arthroscope in the direct lateral portal, the trochlear notch is followed distally to proximally until the posterolateral capsule adjacent to the olecranon tip is visualized. An 18 gauge spinal needle is then placed through the previously marked posterolateral portal site (Fig. 15–20). After visualization of this needle, the skin may be incised with a No. 11 blade, again under direct vision. A 4.0 blunt trocar and cannula are then placed through this portal site. The posterior antebrachial and lateral brachial cutaneous nerves are at risk for injury with establishment of this portal.

The posterior compartment may also be established without direct arthroscopic visualization. The portal is

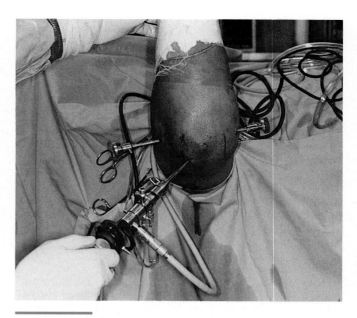

Figure 15–21 • Arthroscope in the posterolateral portal.

approximately 3 cm proximal to the tip of the olecranon along the lateral border of the triceps muscle. The elbow may be kept in 20–30 degrees of flexion, and an incision is then made over the portal site. A blunt trocar is then placed aiming towards the olecranon tip. Free backflow of fluid through the cannula demonstrates entry into the joint, and the arthroscope may now be placed (Fig. 15–21). The tip of the olecranon fossa may be palpated with the blunt tip of the trocar as the posterior compartment is entered.

STRAIGHT POSTERIOR PORTAL

The straight posterior triceps-splitting portal is established if arthroscopic instrumentation of the posterior compartment is necessary. The portal is located 3 cm proximal to the olecranon tip in the center of the triceps tendon, approximately 1.5–2 cm medial to the posterolateral portal. The portal is established under direct visualization with the arthroscope in the posterolateral portal using a localizing spinal needle. After the spinal needle is visualized, a No. 11 knife blade is used to incise the triceps muscle longitudinally in line with the muscle fibers. This portal is useful for the removal of loose bodies and impinging osteophytes from the posterior compartment of the elbow. Utilizing the posterolateral and the posterior portals, olecranon tip, olecranon fossa, posterior trochlear, and proximal aspect of the ulnar collateral ligament are visualized.

SURGICAL TECHNIQUE IN PRONE POSITION

The prone position for elbow arthroscopy has been utilized by some arthroscopists.[15, 16, 19, 20] When this tech-

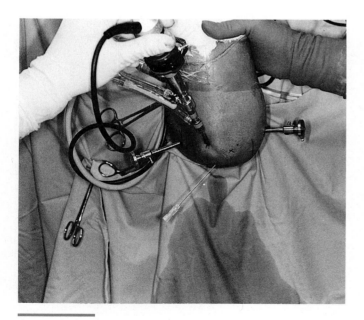

Figure 15–20 • Small arthroscope in the direct lateral portal visualizing the needle in the posterolateral portal.

nique is used, one must pay careful attention towards placing appropriate padding over the head and face, chest, pelvis, and legs to prevent pressure injury from this position. The upper arm is elevated on pillows or a sandbag on an arm board adjacent to the operating room table. The entire arm is prepared and draped free. No traction devices are utilized. The landmarks are marked with a marking pen. The joint is distended through the soft spot portal as mentioned earlier. Poehling has utilized the proximal medial portal as the first portal site of entry. It is located 2 cm proximal to the medial humeral epicondyle and just anterior to the intermuscular septum. The intermuscular septum may be palpated. A No. 11 scalpel blade is utilized to make an incision through the skin only. A hemostat is used to spread through the subcutaneous tissue to protect the medial brachial as well as the medial antebrachial cutaneous nerves. The 4 mm blunt trocar and sheath are then placed through this portal site, with the cannula directed anterior to the intermuscular septum in order to protect the ulnar nerve. The trocar is directed toward the radial head during insertion. As the trocar is advanced to the radial head, the trocar is in contact with the anterior surface of the humerus, thus protecting the ulnar nerve and also the anterior neurovascular structures, the median nerve, and the brachial artery. Backflow fluid through the cannula confirms entry into the joint capsule.

From this portal, the radial head, capitellum, trochlea, coronoid process, medial condyle, and anterior joint capsule are visualized.

POSTOPERATIVE CARE

After the arthroscopic surgery is completed and the elbow has been lavaged copiously with irrigation fluid to remove intra-articular debris, the arthroscopic portals are closed. An intra-articular local long-acting anesthetic is not recommended in the elbow. The anesthetic may leak out through capsular rents at the portal sites and cause transient nerve blocks that make postoperative neurovascular evaluation difficult.[2, 21] Occasionally, if an extensive abrasion arthroplasty or extensive removal of spurs or débridement of the soft tissue is performed, a drain may be used. The patient is quickly started on a physical therapy rehabilitation program with emphasis on active range of motion immediately after surgery. In the case of a contracted elbow, a continuous passive motion may be utilized as part of the postoperative routine at home. The patient may return to athletics when full range of motion, strength, and proprioception are achieved.

References

1. Burman MS: Arthroscopy of the direct visualization of joints. J Bone Joint Surg 13:669, 1931.
2. Andrews JR and Carson WG: Arthroscopy of the elbow. Arthroscopy 1:97, 1985.
3. Angelo RC and Soffer SR: Elbow anatomy relative to arthroscopy. In Andrews JR and Soffer SR (eds.): Elbow Arthroscopy. St. Louis, Mosby–Year Book, 1994, pp 11–32.
4. Amis AA, Hughes SJ, Miller JH, et al.: A functional study of the rheumatoid elbow. Rheumatoid Rehab 21:151, 1982.
5. Porter BB, Richardson C, and Vainio R: Rheumatoid arthritis of the elbow: the results of synovectomy. J Bone Joint Surg Br 56:427, 1974.
6. Clarke RP: Symptomatic lateral synovial fringe (plica) of the elbow joint. Arthroscopy 4:112, 1988.
7. Carson WG: Arthroscopy of the elbow. Instr Course Lect 37:195, 1988.
8. O'Driscoll DW and Money BF: Arthroscopy of the elbow: diagnostic and therapeutic benefits and hazards. J Bone Joint Surg Am 74:84, 1992.
9. Shepard JE, Marion JD, and Hurst DI: Arthroscopic elbow surgery: five year experience and observations in 48 cases. Am J Arthroscopy 1:13, 1991.
10. Wilson FD, Andrews JR, Blackburn TA, et al.: Valgus extension overload in the pitching elbow. Am J Sports Med 11:83, 1983.
11. Guhl JF: Arthroscopy and arthroscopic surgery of the elbow. Orthopedics 8:1290, 1985.
12. Woods GW: Elbow arthroscopy. Clin Sports Med 6:557, 1987.
13. Soffer SR and Andrews JR: The Ulnar Collateral Ligament Arthroscopic Stress Test. American Academy of Orthopaedic Surgeons Annual Meeting, Mar. 1994, and Arthroscopy Association of North America Meeting, May, 1994.
14. Ito K: Arthroscopy of the elbow joint. In Watanabe M (ed.): Arthroscopy of Small Joints. New York, Igaku-Shoin, 1985, pp 57–84.
15. Poehling GG, Whipple TL, Sisco L, et al.: Elbow arthroscopy: a new technique. Arthroscopy 5:222, 1989.
16. Lindenfeld TN: Medial approach in elbow arthroscopy. Am J Sports Med 18:413, 1990.
17. Lynch GJ, Myers JR, Whipple TL, et al.: Neurovascular anatomy and elbow arthroscopy: inherent risks. Arthroscopy 2:191, 1986.
18. Schonholtz GJ: Arthroscopic Surgery of The Shoulder, Elbow, and Ankle. Springfield, IL, Charles C. Thomas, 1986, pp 73–78.
19. Hempfling H: Endoscopic examination of the elbow joint from the dorsoradial approach. Z Orthop 121:331, 1983.
20. Baker CL and Shalvoy RM: The prone position for elbow arthroscopy. Clin Sports Med 10:623, 1991.
21. Morrey BF: Arthroscopy of the elbow. Instr Course Lect 35:102, 1986.

16 Operative Arthroscopy of the Elbow

Laura A. Timmerman

Arthroscopic surgery offers tremendous advantages in the treatment of elbow disorders in throwing athletes.[1, 2] The surgical dissection is minimal in comparison with an arthrotomy of the elbow, and the visualization of the joint is improved. The rehabilitation can proceed more rapidly after surgery. Initially elbow arthroscopy was used as a diagnostic tool, but as arthroscopic surgical techniques have developed the indications for operative arthroscopy have increased.[3, 4] However, elbow arthroscopy is difficult due to the close proximity of neurovascular structures and the small size of the joint, and consequently widespread use of the procedure has been limited.

GENERAL TECHNIQUE

The general technique for a diagnostic arthroscopic examination of the elbow, including both the supine and prone positions, is included in Chapter 15. The following serves as a brief review. The patient is placed in the supine position with the arm suspended overhead. After the elbow is injected with fluid with a spinal needle placed in the soft spot, or the straight lateral portal, the anterolateral portal is then made initially to visualize the elbow joint. A 4.0 mm arthroscope video camera with a pump system allowing fluid inflow through the arthroscopic sheath is used. The medial compartment can be then carefully evaluated, and any valgus instability of the ulnohumeral joint can be assessed. If an open medial procedure is anticipated, the anteromedial portal is not made. If only an arthroscopy is to be performed, then the anteromedial portal is then made under direct visualization. The anteromedial portal allows viewing of the radial head and the capitellum. The straight lateral portal is then made, usually with a small 2.7 mm arthroscope, which allows viewing of the radio-capitellar joint and the lateral compartment. The postero-lateral portal can then be made under direct visualization, and the regular 4.0 mm arthroscope can be introduced into the posterior compartment. The straight posterior compartment can then be made under direct visualization and used as a working portal posteriorly.

SPECIFIC OPERATIVE ARTHROSCOPIC PROCEDURES

Loose Bodies

The removal of symptomatic loose bodies is one of the most common arthroscopic procedures performed on the elbow.[5, 6] Osteocartilaginous loose bodies are usually the result of an osteochondrotic lesion of the capitellum, osteochondral fragments of the radial head, fragments from the impingement posteriorly of the olecranon and trochlea, and as a result of synovial chondromatosis. Arthroscopic removal of loose bodies from the elbow joint has been shown in several studies to be beneficial, especially in the elbow free of degenerative changes.[1, 3–6]

The patient usually complains of locking and catching in the elbow, and he or she may develop a joint effusion after a painful episode. A careful preoperative evaluation by radiographs and a computed tomography (CT) arthrogram or magnetic resonance imaging (MRI) is usually undertaken, but at times the results of all of these studies are negative.[7] The loose bodies may be cartilaginous and noncalcified and may not be visible on a radiograph. In a study,[8] a review was made of 72 professional baseball players who had elbow surgery. The researchers reported that loose bodies occurred in 39% of the players. Of interest, the results of the preoperative radiographs were negative in 71% of these patients, and the CT arthrogram was also negative preoperatively in 38% of the patients. It is important to clarify with the patient prior to surgery that even if a loose body is seen on radiographs, it may not be removable arthroscopically and an arthrotomy may be required.

A complete inspection of the elbow joint is necessary when searching for loose bodies, because they can float from one compartment to another. The loose body may be drawn into view by placing the shaver in the joint with full suction applied. These loose bodies may float to the lateral and posterior compartments, especially with the inflow of fluid and the dependent position of the elbow. If one loose body is found, a careful exploration for additional loose bodies in the joint should be undertaken. It is generally easier to remove loose bodies anteriorly through the anterolateral portal because of less interposed soft tissue. If a loose body is too large to remove through the arthroscopic portal, it can either be broken down using the débrider or removed in a piecemeal fashion by breaking it up into several smaller pieces with a grasper (Fig. 16–1).

After removal of loose bodies from the elbow, the patient should be cautioned that other loose bodies may have been left behind in the joint and furthermore that new loose bodies may reform in the elbow.[9] This is especially true in the throwing athlete, who continues to subject his or her elbow to repetitive microtrauma. The patient can be started on an early range of motion and strengthening program once the portals heal. The athlete is usually ready to begin throwing at 6–8 weeks after surgery.

Posterior Impingement

A common cause of pain in the elbow in throwing athletes is the formation of posteromedial osteophytes on the olecranon with secondary chondromalacia of the trochlea at the area of impingement.[10–12] The forces of throwing place a valgus force across the medial elbow, and after the athlete releases the ball, an extension force occurs posteriorly.[13] The combination of these two actions creates a valgus extension overload phenomenon at the elbow.[12] The extension overload results in osteophyte formation at the tip of the olecranon with fibrous tissue deposition in the olecranon fossa and loose body formation. The valgus stress results in abutment of the medial aspect of the olecranon process against the medial olecranon fossa with formation of posterior medial osteophytes (Fig. 16–2).[10] In a review of elbow surgery on 72 professional baseball players, 65% of the patients had posterior olecranon osteophytes removed, this being the most commonly performed operative procedure.[8]

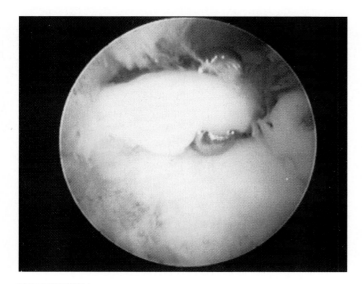

Figure 16–1 • Arthroscopic view of a loose body in the anterior compartment of the elbow.

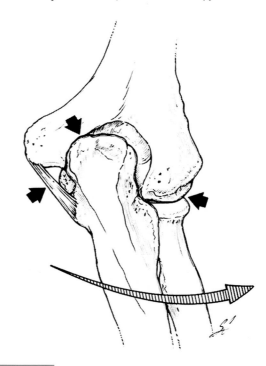

Figure 16–2 • Illustration of valgus extension overload, or the forces that occur at the elbow with throwing: medial tension, lateral compression, and posterior extension. (From Nicholas JA and Hershman EB: The Upper Extremity in Sports Medicine. St. Louis, CV Mosby, 1995, p 759.)

Patients with posteromedial osteophytes present with pain posteromedially, and on physical examination they lack full extension. They also usually have pain with forced extension and valgus loading (a positive valgus extension overload test). Ulnar nerve symptoms can also develop secondary to the close relationship of the nerve. The ulnar collateral ligament must be evaluated carefully in these patients, because medial elbow pain can be difficult to locate on physical examination.[13] Also, patients can have injuries to the ulnar collateral ligament and posteromedial olecranon osteophytes occurring together. The osteophyte may help to buttress the olecranon and reduce the stress on the ulnar collateral ligament, or laxity in the ligament may create enough repetitive microtrauma posteriorly to result in the formation of the posterior osteophytes. A normal radiograph preoperatively does not exclude the presence of a posterior olecranon osteophyte.[8] An axial view is useful in an evaluation of the medial olecranon, but imaging of this area of the elbow is difficult.[12] The diagnosis is usually based on a clinical history and physical examination.

Posterior impingement of the elbow can be treated arthroscopically, with the advantage of improved visualization and decreased morbidity compared with the open surgical approach. Chondromalacia on the posterior trochlea can be very difficult to see without the aid of the arthroscope.

With arthroscopy performed in the supine position, the arthroscope is placed in the posterolateral portal. The elbow is placed in approximately 30 degrees of flexion to relax the posterior structures and increase the working space in the posterior compartment. This is easily accomplished by increasing the traction on the overhead holding device, which will straighten the arm out and place the elbow in more extension. With this position, the arthroscopic camera is below the joint, and the fluid tends to run down into the camera. This can result in fogging, and a coupled videoarthroscope helps to prevent this. A spinal needle is then introduced in the midline of the elbow posteriorly, through the triceps tendon. The location of the straight posterior portal is about 2–3 cm proximal to the tip of the olecranon. Careful attention to the location of the ulnar nerve must always be observed, because with swelling the nerve may not be palpable. The spinal needle is used to see if the portal location will allow débridement of the osteophyte.

Once the correct portal site is selected, a vertical triceps splitting incision is made, and the débrider is introduced under direct visualization. This portal can be difficult to make, and it is useful to place a cannula into the portal that the instruments can then be placed through in order to maintain the portal. With swelling and fluid extravasation the olecranon bursa can become distended, resulting in a shift in the fascial planes and difficulty in regaining the original portal.

There is usually abundant synovitis posteriorly, and after débridement of this tissue visualization is improved to allow for removal of the osteophyte. Again, care must be taken not to débride soft tissue from the medial wall of the joint, where the ulnar nerve is just external to the capsule. The posterior tip of the olecranon is then removed, using a motorized bur or a small osteotome. It is important to completely remove the posteromedial corner of the olecranon to prevent further impingement. Once the posterior osteophyte is removed, a kissing lesion is often visualized on the trochlea (Figs. 16–3 to 16–5), which can then

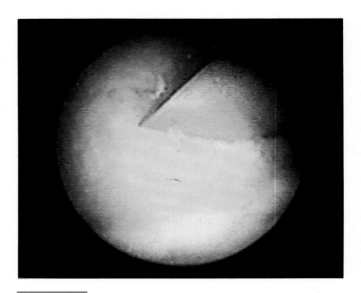

Figure 16–4 • Arthroscopic view from the posterolateral portal. The spur has been débrided, and an osteotome is in place to remove more of the spur. The osteotome is placed through the straight posterior portal.

be débrided to stimulate bleeding and fibrocartilage formation.

When the portals are healed, range of motion followed by a strengthening program for the elbow can be started. Athletes are usually able to return to an early throwing program at approximately 6–8 weeks after surgery.

In the previously mentioned study on professional baseball players, a reoperating rate of 33% in this group of

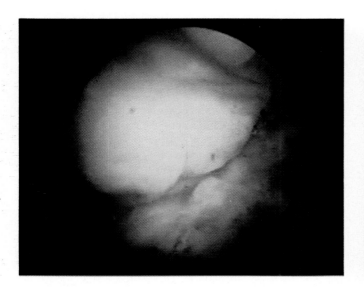

Figure 16–3 • Arthroscopic view of the posterior compartment of the elbow (in the supine position). The camera is in the posterolateral portal, and the ulna is superior, with a large posterior osteophyte on the tip.

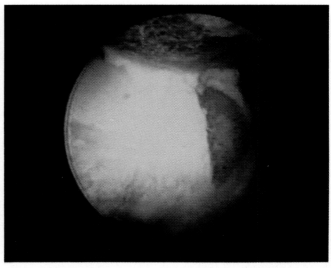

Figure 16–5 • Once the spur is removed, the area of corresponding chondromalacia of the trochlea, or the "kissing lesion," is seen.

high demand athletes was reported.[8] The most common diagnosis requiring a second procedure was posterior olecranon osteophytes. In addition, 25% of the patients who initially had débridement of a posterior osteophyte required an ulnar collateral ligament reconstruction. The osteophyte has a tendency to recur, which is not surprising since throwing creates repetitive microtrauma. This procedure is not curative; instead, it should be considered a palliative measure, and the player should be counseled regarding this prior to surgery. Also, with the presence of a posterior osteophyte, the integrity of the ulnar collateral ligament should be carefully assessed.

Instability

The medial soft tissues of the elbow are subject to tremendous tension with throwing.[14, 15] The ulnar collateral ligament is the primary stabilizer of the elbow joint to valgus stress from 20 to 120 degrees of flexion.[16-18] A sudden severe acute trauma to the elbow can result in an acute tear of the ligament,[19] but more commonly the repeated forces of throwing cause the ligament to become attenuated and lax and sometimes eventually tear.[14]

The greatest degree of instability after sectioning the ulnar collateral ligament is seen at 70 degrees of flexion, which corresponds with the degree of elbow flexion seen during the acceleration phase of throwing motion where the greatest stress is placed across the medial tissues.[17] The detection of this medial instability is often difficult clinically.[14] The instability may be dynamic in that the high forces that occur with throwing are necessary to cause the painful symptoms.

The ulnar collateral ligament complex is difficult to visualize arthroscopically.[20] Only the anterior 20–30% of the anterior bundle and the posterior 30–50% of the posterior bundle are seen during an arthroscopic examination of the elbow, using both anterior and posterior portals (Figs. 16–6 and 16–7). A complete tear of the anterior bundle of the ulnar collateral ligament can be missed at arthroscopy. However, a tear or laxity in the ligament can be diagnosed at arthroscopy by visualizing the resultant increased joint space between the ulna and the humerus to valgus stress testing.[20]

Timmerman and Andrews[21] reported on an undersurface tear of the ulnar collateral ligament seen in baseball players that may be difficult to diagnose. In a previous study,[20] they demonstrated that the anterior bundle of the ulnar collateral ligament has two layers—a thick inner layer within the capsular walls and a thinner external superficial layer. The patients presented with persistent medial elbow pain and had failed conservative treatment. In these patients the preoperative CT arthrogram demonstrated a consistent finding of contrast leakage distally, along the ulnar attachment, without extravasation outside the joint.[21] At surgery all of the patients demonstrated valgus instability under arthroscopic examination, and all of the patients demonstrated an intact external layer, with a defect in the inner layer of the ulnar collateral ligament.

When an arthroscopic examination of the elbow is performed on throwing athletes, the integrity of the ulnar collateral ligament should be evaluated. As soon as the

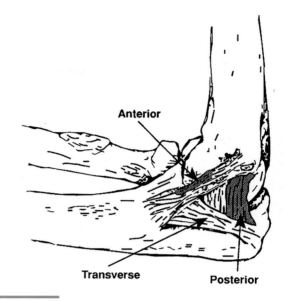

Figure 16–6 • The portion of the ulnar collateral ligament that is visualized arthroscopically. (From Timmerman LA and Andrews JR: The histologic and arthroscopic anatomy of the ulnar collateral ligament of the elbow. Am J Sports Med 22:670, 1994.)

elbow is introduced into the joint, the first structures visualized are the coronoid and the humerus (Fig. 16–8). The technique used to inspect the ligament consists of placing the elbow in about 70 degrees of flexion. This reproduces the position where the greatest stress is placed across the ligament with valgus stressing[17] and also allows room for the arthroscope to be placed in the front of the joint. The humerus is then stabilized, and a valgus stress is placed across the joint. Normally, there is no or minimal opening (<1 mm) in the ulnohumeral joint. With an injury to

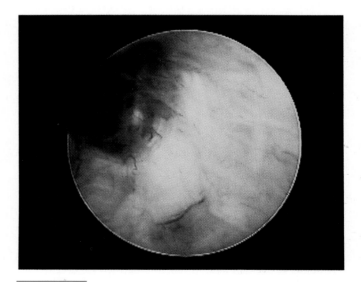

Figure 16–7 • Arthroscopic view from the posterior compartment of the posterior bundle of the ulnar collateral ligament.

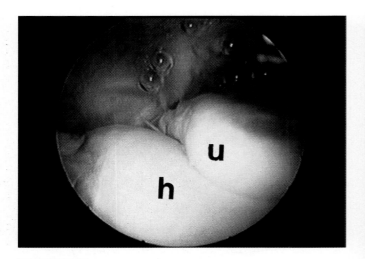

Figure 16–8 • Arthroscopic view of the coronoid process of the ulna (u) and the humerus (h) in the anterior compartment.

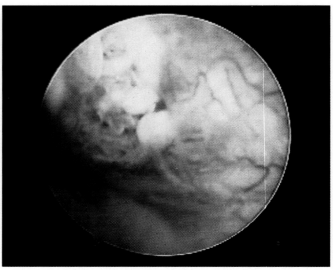

Figure 16–10 • Arthroscopic view of the medial capsule of the elbow from the anterolateral portal. Inflammatory changes are seen.

the ulnar collateral ligament, an increase in the opening between the two bones is detected (Fig. 16–9). With a large complete tear, the arthroscope may be placed in the opening between the two bones, and the tear is then visualized directly.

In addition, the nature of the medial wall can be assessed at arthroscopy; for example, the presence of inflammation and synovitis may indicate a recent injury (Fig. 16–10). The view of the medial wall from the anterolateral portal is improved with the 70 degree arthroscope.[20] Posteriorly inflammation can be noted, but the anterior bundle of the ulnar collateral ligament (the main stabilizer) is not seen. In fact, only the posterior 30–50% of the posterior bundle is seen arthroscopically and only from the posterior portal (see Fig. 16–7). The posterior bundle is not seen from the anterior portals. Despite these limitations, the arthroscope is a useful adjuvant in an evaluation of medial instability.

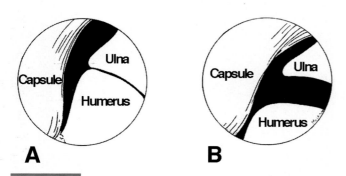

Figure 16–9 • The valgus stress test. *A*, Without stress. *B*, With stress, demonstrating the increased joint space between the humerus and the ulna. (From Timmerman LA and Andrews JR: Undersurface tear of the ulnar collateral ligament in baseball players: a newly recognized lesion. Am J Sports Med 22:34, 1994.)

Posterolateral instability has been described previously,[22] although the clinical examination can be difficult to interpret. A stress examination at the time of arthroscopy can be helpful because the intra-articular movement can be assessed (Fig. 16–11). The operative treatment involves a posterolateral stabilization procedure either with capsular reefing or an autograft.

Osteochondritis Dissecans

During the throwing, the valgus movement about the elbow results in compression of the radial head and capitellum.[10, 11] The skeletally immature are subject to osteochondritic dissecans of the capitellum, which is more common in throwing athletes and gymnasts.[23–25] This may also be associated with chondromalacia of the radial head. The indications for surgery include persistent loss of motion, which presents as a flexion contracture of the elbow, loose bodies and locking episodes, pain, and inability to participate in activities.

During arthroscopy the lateral compartment is best assessed from the anteromedial portal initially. The radial head is not well visualized from the anterolateral portal; thus, if radial head disease is suspected, an anteromedial portal is required for evaluation. The direct lateral, or soft spot, portal is also used to visualize the radial head and capitellar articulation. This space is difficult to work in because it is quite small. A second working portal is established just distal to the soft spot portal after a spinal needle is used for localization. It is useful to offset the initial soft spot portal from the exact center of the soft spot. If the portal is made at the proximal portion of the soft spot, this allows a second working portal to be made as the distal border, and the instrumentation and triangulation is much easier. The small, 2.7 mm arthroscope and small-sized

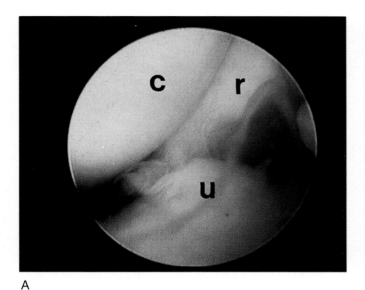
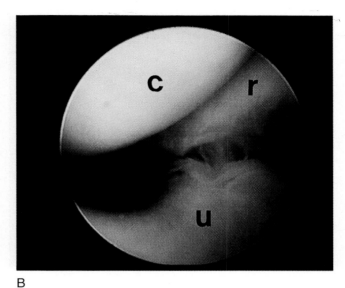

A

B

Figure 16–11 • Arthroscopic view of the lateral compartment from the direct lateral (soft spot) portal. *A*, c: capitellum; r: radial head; u: ulna. *B*, Posterolateral stress is applied. Note the increase in the joint space.

débriders are helpful. The larger size instruments can result in iatrogenic chondral damage. If the larger instruments are introduced into the joint at an angle parallel with the shafts of the radius and ulna, this avoids chondral damage and allows for easier entry into the joint. Once the capsule is entered, then the instrument can be brought up and the bony structures can be visualized. Arthroscopic technique is difficult to accomplish in the tight lateral compartment, and it is helpful for the surgeon to position himself or herself comfortably, to have his or her arms tucked to the side of the body to avoid excessive arm movement, and to prevent inadvertent pull out of the joint. The instruments will be almost parallel to the camera, and the light cord can be frequently rotated while maintaining position of the arthroscope in order to improve visualization.

Initially the synovial tissue can be débrided, and often an underlying chondral defect will then be seen. Working through the two portals in the straight lateral position is the preferred technique for evaluation of the radial head and capitellum. The lesion should be carefully inspected. A small (3.5 mm) shaver is ideal to gently probe the cartilaginous flap and to determine the extent of the lesion. A shaver, forceps, or small knife can be used to excise the free fragments and create a stable rim to the crater lesion.

Arthroscopic débridement of osteochondrotic lesions have been described previously.[23, 24] The younger athlete is often able to completely heal the lesion and return to full activity.[9] The older patients who have entered the early adolescence period have less success with the procedure.

Synovitis

Synovitis is a common finding in the painful elbow (Fig. 16–12). Thickened synovial bands can lead to popping and catching in the elbow. Synovial chondromatosis can occur in the elbow, which is associated with loose body formation. The inflammatory synovitis that is associated with rheumatoid arthritis can be treated arthroscopically, and actually the elbow joint in these patients may be easier to enter with the arthroscope because it tends to have a lax capsule and is enlarged. Arthroscopic synovectomy is performed using the standard arthroscopic portals. The entire joint may be evaluated, and a complete synovectomy is performed with a motorized débrider.

A lateral synovial band or plica can form in the elbow (Fig. 16–13).[26] This band can cause impingement on the

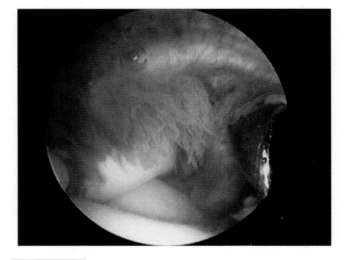

Figure 16–12 • Arthroscopic view of the anterior compartment from the anteromedial portal, demonstrating inflammatory synovitis.

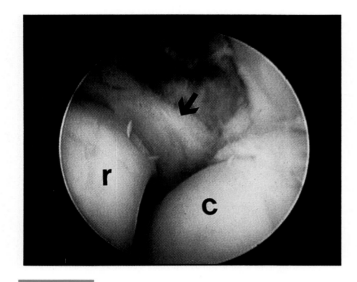

Figure 16–13 • Arthroscopic view from the anteromedial portal demonstrating a large lateral band (*arrow*) overlying the radial head (r: radial head; c: capitellum).

radial head and the capitellum, resulting in persistent pain in the lateral elbow. This lesion can be débrided arthroscopically. The arthroscope is placed through the anteromedial portal with the débrider in the anterolateral portal, or both the arthroscope and the débrider are placed through the straight lateral portals. Care must be taken not to débride too extensively, including the annular ligament and lateral collateral ligament structure. This can result in varus instability.

Anterior Lesions

Hypertrophy of the coronoid process can occur in response to distraction forces from throwing or other repetitive activities.[13] Coronoid fractures may also result in deformity in the coronoid and anterior impingement. A prominent coronoid results in a loss of flexion as the bony prominence can impinge in the coronoid fossa anteriorly, resulting in scar tissue in the fossa. This is also associated with loose body formation.[10] With trauma to the elbow joint, anterior capsular contracture can form, and both the coronoid fossa and radial fossa of the humerus can fill in with scar tissue, limiting full extension.[27, 28]

Via the anterolateral and anteromedial portal, the anterior compartment of the elbow is easily visualized. The scar tissue can then be resected using a motorized débrider, and care is taken anteriorly to avoid the nearby neurovascular structures. It is best to débride off the humerus and release the scar tissue off the bony surface, as opposed to placing the débrider in the midportion of the anterior scar tissue. An osteotome or bur can be used to remove the hypertrophied portion of the coronoid. A bur can be used to reform both the coronoid and the radial fossa.

Arthrofibrosis

Post-traumatic arthrofibrosis is common in the elbow joint, and it can be difficult to treat. It is especially common after an elbow dislocation or a radial head fracture. The elbow is frequently immobilized in 90 degrees of flexion, allowing fibrous adhesions to form in the anterior region of the elbow (Fig. 16–14). For some movements, in particular athletic movements, a limitation in flexion or extension of 20 degrees or more may be symptomatic, even though it has been reported to be acceptable for the activities of daily living.[29] Reports indicate that arthroscopic débridement of scarring in the anterior elbow joint offers promising results.[27, 28]

Byrd described a series of five patients who developed arthrofibrosis after type 1 (nondisplaced) radial head fractures.[30] He found that arthroscopic débridement of the joint, performed an average of 6 months after an injury, resulted in improvement in range of motion and crepitation.

Timmerman and Andrews reported on the outcome following arthroscopic débridement of post-traumatic elbow arthrofibrosis in 19 consecutive patients.[31] All of the patients had failed a conservative treatment course. The preoperative range of motion was an average of 29 to 123 degrees of flexion. An extensive arthroscopic débridement of the joint was performed, followed by manipulation under anesthesia and extensive postoperative rehabilitation. The motion postoperatively improved to an average of 11 to 134 degrees of flexion. Long-term follow-up showed that 84% of the patients had good-to-excellent results, and although complete return of preinjury motion was not obtained, each patient showed an improvement in motion and subjective symptoms. Fourteen patients had limitation of their sports activities before surgery, and 11

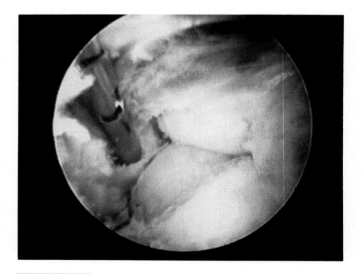

Figure 16–14 • Arthroscopic view of the anterior compartment from the anterolateral portal demonstrating extensive arthrofibrosis, after partial débridement. The cannula is in the anteromedial portal, and the humerus and coronoid process are seen.

of these patients were able to return to their preinjury level of activity.

Degenerative Arthritis

Degenerative arthritis of the elbow is usually the result of a previous trauma or is secondary to years of repetitive motion. The patients usually present with pain and loss of motion and may have catching or locking symptoms. Radiographs show degenerative changes, including loss of joint spaces and formation of osteophytes. Large osteophytes on the coronoid or tip of the olecranon can result in a bony block and loss of motion in the joint.

As with other arthroscopic procedures in other joints, the results of débridement of arthritic joints are somewhat limited. The range of motion may be improved, but pain relief is less satisfactory. Loose bodies, synovitis, arthrofibrosis, and impinging osteophytes may be removed arthroscopically. The patient should be aware that the procedure is palliative and that his or her symptoms tend to recur.

Redden and Stanley reported on a series of 12 patients with osteoarthritis who underwent arthroscopic débridement of the elbow joint using a technique involving penetration of the olecranon fossa posteriorly with a drill bit and then débridement of the anterior joint through this foramen created in the olecranon fossa.[32] They found that the thin bony membrane that normally separates the olecranon and coronoid fossa was frequently thickened in these patients and contributed to a limitation in motion. In their group of patients, they found that elbow pain was reduced, and the incidence of locking of the joint was improved postoperatively.

CONCLUSION

The developments during the last decade in operative elbow arthroscopy have proved to be advantageous in the treatment of elbow disorders. However, elbow arthroscopy requires complex technical skills, and serious complications may result if a careful operative technique is not observed.[33–35] With proper training, the arthroscopist can successfully treat many disorders of the elbow with the advantages of vastly improved intra-articular pathology and the ability to start early range of motion.

References

1. Andrews JR and Carson WG: Arthroscopy of the elbow. Arthroscopy 1:97–107, 1985.
2. Andrews JR, St. Pierre RK, and Carson WG: Arthroscopy of the elbow. Clin Sports Med 5:653–662, 1986.
3. Guhl JF: Arthroscopy and arthroscopic surgery of the elbow. Orthop 8:1290–1296, 1985.
4. O'Driscoll SW and Morrey BF: Arthroscopy of the elbow. J Bone Joint Surg Am 74:84–94, 1992.
5. Boe S: Arthroscopy of the elbow: Diagnosis and extraction of loose bodies. Acta Orthop Scand 57:52–53, 1986.
6. Ogilvie-Harris DJ and Schemitsch E: Arthroscopy of the elbow for removal of loose bodies. Arthroscopy 9:5–8, 1993.
7. Timmerman LA, Schwartz ML, and Andrews JR: Preoperative evaluation of the ulnar collateral ligament by magnetic resonance imaging and computed tomography arthrography: evaluation in 25 baseball players with surgical confirmation. Am J Sports Med 22:26–32, 1994.
8. Andrews JR and Timmerman LA: Outcome of elbow surgery in professional baseball players. Am J Sports Med 23:407–413, 1995.
9. Timmerman LA and Andrews JR: Clinical experience. In JR Andrews and SR Soffer (eds.): Elbow Arthroscopy. St. Louis, CV Mosby, 1994, pp 131–140.
10. Andrews JR: Bony injuries about the elbow in the throwing athlete. In Instructional Course Lecture No. 34. St. Louis, CV Mosby, 1985.
11. Slocum DB: Classification of elbow injuries from baseball pitching. Tex Med 64:48–53, 1968.
12. Wilson FD, Andrews JR, Blackburn TA, et al.: Valgus extension overload in the pitching elbow. Am J Sports Med 11:83, 1983.
13. Andrews JR, Schemmel SP, and Whiteside JA: Evaluation, treatment, and prevention of elbow injuries in throwing athletes. In JA Nichols and EB Hershman (eds.): The Upper Extremity in Sports Medicine. St. Louis, CV Mosby, 1990, pp 781–826.
14. Conway JE, Jobe FW, Glousman RE, et al.: Medial instability of the elbow in throwing athletes. J Bone Joint Surg Am 74:67–83, 1992.
15. Hotchkiss RN and Weiland AJ: Valgus stability of the elbow. J Orthop Res 5:372, 1987.
16. Morrey BF and An KN: Articular and ligamentous contributions to the stability of the elbow joint. Am J Sports Med 11:315–319, 1983.
17. Sojbjerg JO, Ovensen J, and Neilsen S: Experimental elbow instability after transection of the medial collateral ligament. Clin Orthop 218:186, 1987.
18. Jobe FW, Stark A, and Lombardo SJ: Reconstruction of the ulnar collateral ligament in athletes. J Bone Joint Surg Am 68:1158, 1986.
19. Norwood LA, Shook JA, and Andrews JR: Acute medial elbow ruptures. Am J Sports Med 9:16, 1981.
20. Timmerman LA and Andrews JR: The histologic and arthroscopic anatomy of the ulnar collateral ligament of the elbow. Am J Sports Med 22:667–673, 1994.
21. Timmerman LA and Andrews JR: Undersurface tear of the ulnar collateral ligament in baseball players: A newly recognized lesion. Am J Sports Med 22:33–36, 1994.
22. O'Driscoll SW, Bell DF, and Morrey BF: Posterolateral rotatory instability of the elbow. J Bone Joint Surg Am 73:440–446, 1991.
23. Jackson DW, Silvino N, and Reiman P: Osteochondritis in the female gymnast's elbow. Arthroscopy 5:129–136, 1989.
24. Ruch DS and Poehling GG: Arthroscopic treatment of Panner's disease. Clin Sports Med 10:629–636, 1991.
25. Ireland ML and Andrews JA: Shoulder and elbow injuries in the young athlete. Clin Sports Med 7:473–493, 1988.
26. Clarke RP: Symptomatic lateral synovial fringe (plica) of the elbow joint. Arthroscopy 4:112–116, 1988.
27. Jones GS and Savoie III FH: Arthroscopic capsular release of flexion contractures (arthrofibrosis) of the elbow. Arthroscopy 9:277–283, 1993.
28. Nowicki KD and Shall LM: Arthroscopic release of a posttraumatic flexion contracture in the elbow: A case report and review of the literature. Arthroscopy 8:544–547, 1992.
29. Morrey BF, Askew LJ, and An KN: A biomechanical study of normal functional elbow motion. J Bone Joint Surg Am 63:872–877, 1981.
30. Byrd JWT: Elbow arthroscopy for arthrofibrosis after type I radial head fractures. Arthroscopy 10:162–165, 1994.
31. Timmerman LA and Andrews JR: Arthroscopic treatment of posttraumatic elbow pain and stiffness. Am J Sports Med 22:230–235, 1994.
32. Redden JF and Stanley D: Arthroscopic fenestration of the olecranon fossa in the treatment of osteoarthritis of the elbow. Arthroscopy 9:14–16, 1993.
33. Lynch GJ, Meyers JF, Whipple TL, et al.: Neurovascular anatomy and elbow arthroscopy: inherent risks. Arthroscopy 2:190–197, 1986.
34. Papillion JD, Neff RS, and Shall LM: Compression neuropathy of the radial nerve as a complication of elbow arthroscopy: a case report and review of the literature. Arthroscopy 4:284–286, 1988.
35. Thomas AM and Fast A, and Shapiro D: Radial nerve damage as a complication of elbow arthroscopy. Clin Orthop 215:130–131, 1987.

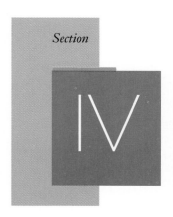

Section

IV

The Wrist

Diagnostic Arthroscopy of the Wrist

David S. Ruch • *Gary G. Poehling*

Arthroscopy of the wrist provides an unparalleled opportunity to diagnose and treat a wide variety of wrist lesions. The complex articulations and numerous ligaments make the wrist a very mobile joint, yet they also make it susceptible to a variety of bony soft-tissue trauma.[7] In addition, inflammatory diseases, arthritides, infections, ganglia, and avascular necrosis may affect this very complex joint, often creating diagnostic dilemmas.[5] Although there is a wide variety of available imaging modalities, including conventional radiographs, fluoroscopy, computed tomography (CT) scan, bone scan, and magnetic resonance imaging, none has been entirely satisfactory for evaluating the multitude of pathologic processes that may arise in the wrist joint. In contrast, wrist arthroscopy allows direct visualization of all of these lesions and provides an opportunity to evaluate dynamic problems, such as instability.[3, 4, 6] Arthroscopy provides an unparalleled view of the extrinsic and intrinsic ligaments as well as the bony anatomy, including osteochondral lesions and defects of the articular cartilage.[2, 6, 8] The use of arthroscopy as a diagnostic tool is discussed in this chapter. Specific techniques are discussed in Chapter 18.

RADIOCARPAL JOINT ARTHROSCOPY

Wrist arthroscopy may be performed under general or Bier-block anesthesia, depending on the surgeon's preference. We routinely use Bier-block anesthesia with the tourniquet placed above the elbow and exsanguination of the upper extremity, with a long-acting agent used for the Bier block.

The patient is placed supine with the upper extremity on an armboard. Traction may be applied also to the end of the table or through the use of a tower distractor, which is the technique we currently employ. Some distraction of the radiocarpal joint is helpful in allowing passage of the trocars and the arthroscope without damaging the articular surface. Approximately 5–7 lb of distraction is applied through the use of finger traps on the patient's index and long fingers (Fig. 17–1).

Portal Anatomy

The portals used in wrist arthroscopy are based on the extrinsic extensor tendons and the superficial branches of the radial and ulnar nerves (Fig. 17–2).[1] The 3-4 portal is located 1 cm distal to the Lister tubercle and may be palpated between the extensor pollicis longus (EPL) tendon (third compartment) and the extensor digitoris communis (EDC) tendon (fourth compartment) (Fig. 17–3). The 4-5 portal is located immediately ulnar to the EDC (see Fig. 17–3). The 6-R portal is located between the extensor digiti minimi and the extensor carpi ulnaris (ECU) at the distal margin of the triangular fibrocartilage (Fig. 17–4). The 6-U portal is located immediately distal to the tip of the ulnar styloid just at the ulnar margin of the ECU (see Fig. 17–4). The 1-2 portal lies immediately distal to the tip of the radial artery (Fig. 17–5). By staying proximally and dorsally within this portal, the surgeon can avoid the radial artery in the anatomic snuff box. Both the 1-2 portal and the 6-U portal place the ulnar and radial cutaneous nerves at risk and should be used cautiously.

Technique

The arthroscopic procedure is initiated by placing an 18 gauge needle into the 3-4 portal and distending the joint fully until it is under moderate pressure. The needle and subsequent instruments should be directed in a dorsal-distal to proximal-volar direction in line with the 12 degree tilt of the distal radius. Normal joints hold 5–7 mL of fluid. If there is a triangular fibrocartilage (TFC) tear, an additional 4–7 mL will be accepted, and a bulge will appear over the distal radioulnar joint. Similarly, if there is a mid-

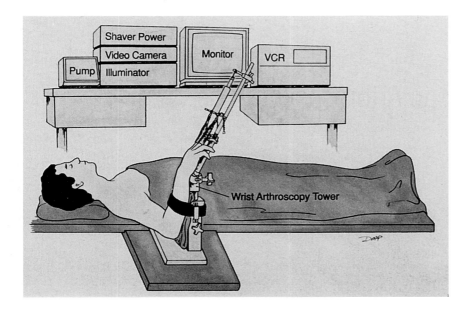

Figure 17–1 • Operating room set-up for wrist arthroscopy. The use of a tourniquet is optional; however, we prefer to use Bier-block anesthesia with the tourniquet placed above the elbow. The arthroscopy tower allows variable distraction as well as palmar flexion and radial or ulnar deviation.

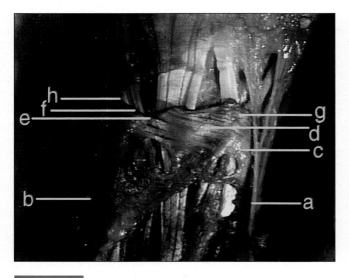

Figure 17–2 • Overview of a cadaveric wrist specimen with the extensor retinaculum in place: (*a*) superficial radial nerve. Note the proximity of the S3 branch to the 2-3 portal; (*b*) superficial (dorsal) branch of the ulnar nerve passing 1 cm distal to the ulnar styloid; (*c*) 1-2 portal; (*d*) 3-4 portal; (*e*) 4-5 portal; (*f*) 6-R portal; (*g*) anatomic snuff box; and (*h*) ECU tendon. The 6-U portal is immediately ulnar to the ECU. Note its proximity to the dorsal cutaneous branch of the ulnar nerve.

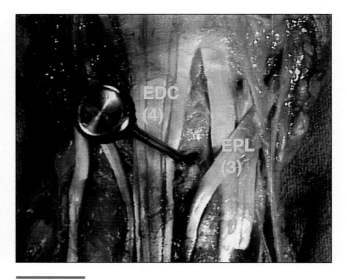

Figure 17–3 • The gross anatomy of the 3-4 portal. The trocar is inserted at a 10 degree radial inclination parallel to the articular surface of the distal radius.

carpal leak, an additional 5–7 mL of fluid will easily enter the joint with diffuse distention over the midcarpal region.

A No. 11 blade is used to make a skin incision. Care should be used to incise the skin only 2–3 mm in length. A blunt trocar and cannula are inserted through the incision. The scaphoid is palpated above and the radius below; the bulging capsule should be palpable in the center. Pressure is applied with a twisting motion above the blunt trocar to pass it through the tissues harmlessly and to penetrate the capsule, resulting in a tight seal. The trocar is removed, and the arthroscope with the video camera is inserted through the cannula. Inflow tubing from the pump is activated, and viewing is initiated (Fig. 17–6).

In order to have clear visualization, there must be circulation of fluid; therefore, an outflow portal should be established. This can vary from an 18 gauge needle in the

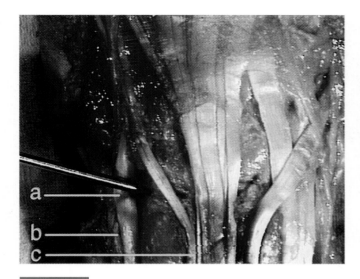

Figure 17–4 • Position of the 6-R portal: (*a*) extensor carpi ulnaris; (*b*) dorsal sensory branch of the ulnar nerve; and (*c*) extensor digiti quinti.

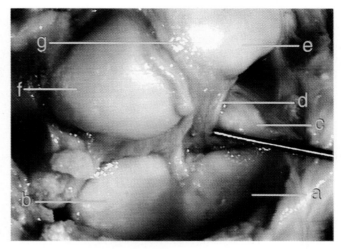

Figure 17–6 • Intra-articular anatomy as viewed from the dorsum of the wrist: (*a*) the scaphoid facet of the distal radius; (*b*) the lunate facet of the distal radius; (*c*) the radioscaphocapitate ligament; and (*d*) the probe demonstrates the radioscapholunate ligament, or the ligament of Testu. This is continuous with the membraneous portion of the scapholunate ligament; (*e*) the scaphoid; (*f*) the lunate; and (*g*) the scapholunate interosseous ligament.

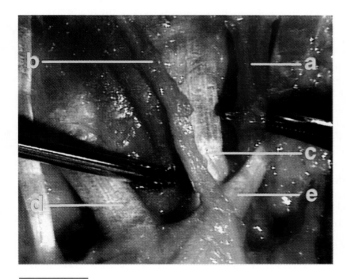

Figure 17–5 • Close-up view of the radial side of the wrist: (*a*) radial artery in the snuff box; (*b*) sensory branch radial nerve; (*c*) extensor carpi radialis longus tendon; (*d*) extensor carpi radialis brevis tendon; and (*e*) extensor pollicis longus tendon. The hemostat is under the radial artery. The nerve hook points to the location of the scaphotrapeziotrapezoid joint.

6-R portal to an outflow pressure monitoring portal or a shaver inserted through an ulnar portal. If a TFC tear is suspected, then the 4-5 portal is best. This portal is located between the EDC and the fifth extensor digiti quinti. The arthroscope is pointed to the ulnar side of the wrist. An 18 gauge needle is inserted and visualized from inside the joint to ensure entrance over the dorsal margin of the distal radius at the junction with the TFC. After verification

of the proper portal position with the needle, a No. 11 blade is inserted longitudinally until its tip is seen within the joint. This portal is used primarily for instrumentation, and it is useful to insert a blunt trocar to enlarge the portal. Instrumentation and outflow may be provided by placing a full radius shaver in the joint. Once the joint is débrided, it can be systematically evaluated.

The arthroscope is advanced under the scapholunate ligament and then moved radially to visualize the palmar ligaments. The radioscaphocapitate is the most radial structure seen (see Fig. 17–6). Moving ulnarward, there is a large ulnar angulating ligament, which is the long radiolunate ligament, formerly known as the radiolunotriquetral ligament. Centrally, at the base of the scapholunate ligament, a fat pad covers the radioscapholunate ligament. Next, the scapholunate interosseus ligament and the lunate articular surface may be visualized as the arthroscope is withdrawn to the dorsal aspect of the joint and directed upward. Evaluation of the radial aspect of the wrist is completed by examining the scaphoid fossa, radial styloid, and dorsal capsular attachment of the lunate. The arthroscope can then be rotated palmarly for inspection of the lunate fossa and the short radiolunate ligaments (Fig. 17–7).

Continuing in the ulnar direction, the TFC attachment to the ulnar border of the radius over the sigmoid notch is normally smooth and nearly imperceptible visually but is easily palpated with a probe. Inspection of the peripheral margins of the TFC can be hindered by the meniscal homolog attaching dorsally at the level of the sigmoid notch. If the entire TFC cannot be visualized, a shaver or suction basket forceps should be used to resect part of the meniscus homolog.

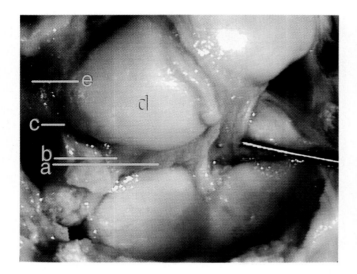

Figure 17–7 • Cadaver specimen showing ulnar-sided ligaments including: (*a*) the long radiolunate ligament; (*b*) the ulnolunate ligament; (*c*) the ulnotriquetral ligament; (*d*) the lunate; and (*e*) the triquetrum.

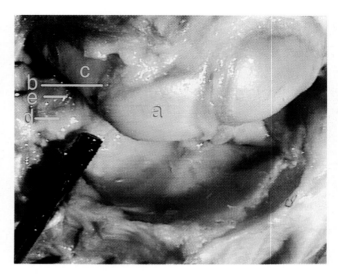

Figure 17–9 • View obtained with the arthroscope in the 6-R portal: (*a*) the lunate; (*b*) the lunotriquetral ligament; (*c*) the triquetrum; (*d*) the triangular fibrocartilage; and (*e*) the ulnotriquetral ligament. Note the superior view of the lunotriquetral ligament from this portal.

The ulnar margins of the TFC should have two perforations. The prestyloid recess is straight lateral, and the pisotriquetral space is palmar. The TFC should be resilient throughout. Loss of the "trampoline" nature of the TFC should warn the surgeon of a traumatic tear.

Visual verification of intact ulnolunate and ulnotriquetral ligaments can be accomplished by directing the arthroscope ulnarly and by using the 30 degree inclination to examine the origin of these ligaments at the base of the ulnar styloid (Fig. 17–8). Occasionally, a glimpse of the triquetrum and the lunotriquetral ligament is possible, but the 3-4 portal view of the superior lateral wrist should never be considered adequate. An ulnar portal is necessary

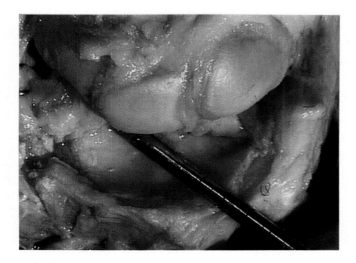

Figure 17–8 • View obtained with the arthroscope in the 3-4 portal with the goal of viewing the lunotriquetral ligament and the triquetrum.

to gain an adequate appreciation of the lunotriquetral ligament and the articular surface of the triquetrum. The lunotriquetral joint is vertical. In the case of a lunotriquetral ligament injury, the ligament avulses from the triquetrum and is suspended from the lunate, making visualization from the 3-4 portal impossible (see Fig. 17–8; Fig. 17–9).

The arthroscope is then moved to the 6-R portal to complete the diagnostic portion of the radiocarpal joint. Visualization of the triquetrum and the lunotriquetral is paramount. This can be challenging because these structures extend dorsally and superiorly and are located immediately behind the meniscus homolog. The arthroscope must be withdrawn almost out of the joint before it can show the most dorsal portion of the lunotriquetral ligament, which is a frequent area of tear. In addition, the distance from the tip of the arthroscope to the lunotriquetral ligament in this area is only 1–2 mm, and the great magnification factor present at this short distance complicates visual interpretation.

These complicating factors may be diminished by constant, adequate distention, which is best accomplished by a mechanical pump, and by the use of a probe through the 4-5 portal to retract the remnant of the meniscus homolog and to palpate the lunotriquetral ligament.

Verification of the findings from the 3-4 portal of the remainder of the joint completes the diagnostic arthroscopy of the radiocarpal joint.

MIDCARPAL JOINT ARTHROSCOPY

The midcarpal joint is approached through the midcarpal ulnar (MCU) and midcarpal radial (MCR) portals. The MCU portal is found approximately 1 cm distal to the 4-5 portal (Fig. 17–10*A*). As is the case with radiocarpal por-

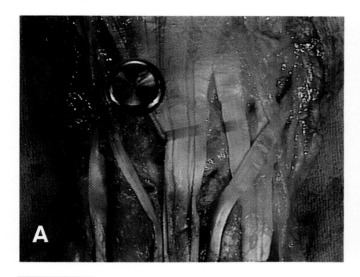
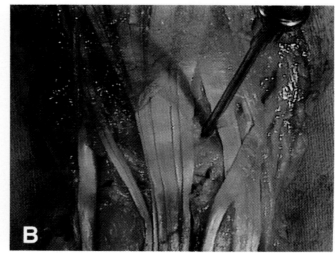

Figure 17–10 • Cadaveric specimen demonstrating: (*A*) the position of the midcarpal ulnar portal lying approximately 1 cm distal to the 4-5 portal, and (*B*) the position of the midcarpal radial portal.

tals, attention should be paid to avoiding injury to cutaneous nerves by cutting only the skin and then using gentle blunt dissection down to the level of the capsule. Entry into this portal is not as pronounced as is entry into the radial carpal portal and care must be taken to avoid injury to the articular cartilage. Use of the MCU portal allows excellent visualization of the lunate and triquetrum as well as the hamate (Fig. 17–11). This is exceptionally valuable for an evaluation of the congruity of the lunotriquetral joint. It may be necessary to establish an outflow portal for

this midcarpal joint. We routinely insert an 18 gauge needle into the MCR portal to allow for temporary outflow. If a detailed arthroscopy of the midcarpal joint is required, then the MCR portal is established.

The MCR portal is located 1 cm distal to the 3-4 portal. We find this helpful to localize this portal using the 18 gauge needle prior to making a skin incision. Once a skin incision is made using a No. 11 blade, a blunt trocar is used to introduce the sheath into the MCR portal. It is often helpful to add an additional pound of distraction at this point to facilitate entry into this joint (see Fig. 17–10*B*).

The MCR portal allows for excellent visualization of the scapholunate interval as well as the capitate (see Fig. 17–11). If the patient has relative ligamentous laxity, it is often possible to direct the arthroscope radially and to make use of the 30 degree tilt of the arthroscope in order to visualize the scaphotrapeziotrapezoid joint located immediately radial to this portal.

Again, outflow may be established using the MCU portal as previously described. Often, with appropriation of the scapholunate ligament or the lunotriquetral ligament, outflow may be maintained through the radiocarpal joint.

Postoperatively, the portals are covered with a Xeroform gauze and dressing sponges. A wrist splint is used for the immediate postoperative period and removed after 3 to 4 days. The patient is encouraged to start gentle active and passive motion of the wrist at about the 5th postoperative day and encouraged to return to routine activities by 3 weeks postoperatively.

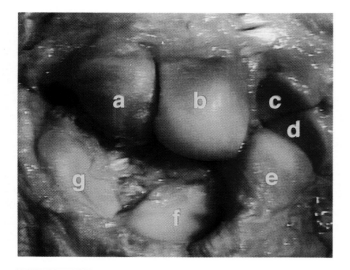

Figure 17–11 • Anatomy of the midcarpal joint: (*a*) proximal pole of the hamate; (*b*) proximal pole of the capitate; (*c*) trapezoid; (*d*) trapezium; (*e*) scaphoid; (*f*) lunate; and (*g*) triquetrum.

References

1. Abrams RA, Petersen M, and Botte MJ: Arthroscopic portals of the wrist: an anatomic study. J Hand Surg Am 19:940–944, 1994.

2. Botte MJ, Cooney WP, and Linscheid RL: Arthroscopy of the wrist: anatomy and technique. J Hand Surg Am 14:313–316, 1989.
3. Cooney WP, Dobyns JH, and Linscheid RL: Arthroscopy of the wrist: anatomy and classification of carpal instability. Arthroscopy 6:133–140, 1990.
4. Hanker GJ: Diagnostic and operative arthroscopy of the wrist. Clin Orthop 263:165–174, 1991.
5. Kelley EP and Stanley JK: Arthroscopy of the wrist. J Hand Surg Br 15:236–242, 1990.

6. North ER, Thomas S: An anatomic guide for arthroscopic visualization of the wrist capsular ligaments. J Hand Surg Am 13:815–822, 1988.
7. Roth JH, Poehling GG, and Whipple TL: Arthroscopic surgery of the wrist. Instr Course Lect 37:183–194, 1988.
8. Yung-Cheng C: Arthroscopy of the wrist and finger joints. Orthop Clin North Am 10:723–733, 1979.

Chapter

18

Operative Arthroscopy of the Wrist

David S. Ruch • Gary G. Poehling

Operative arthroscopy of the wrist has advanced dramatically during the last 10 years. Interest centered initially on the region of the triangular fibrocartilage (TFC) and débridement of injuries to that structure.[5] More recently, techniques for repair of peripheral detachments of the TFC have been described,[2, 11] and arthroscopy has proved useful for assistance in the reduction and pinning of acute ligamentous tears, wrist fractures, and ganglion resections,[8] as well as radial styloidectomies for the treatment of radiocarpal arthritis.[9, 10, 11]

DISORDERS OF THE TRIANGULAR FIBROCARTILAGE

Lesions of TFC generally can be divided into traumatic and nontraumatic tears. Traumatic tears usually occur following impaction of the ulnar-sided carpus on the distal ulna with the wrist in the flexed and supinated position and deviated toward the ulna. Degenerative TFC tears usually result from chronic ulnocarpal impingement. Degenerative lesions may or may not be associated with a full spectrum of ulnar-sided disease, as is shown in Table 18–1. Traumatic TFC lesions are classified as either central or peripheral and may have an associated avulsion fracture.

Current treatment of these lesions is based on the relative avascularity of the articular disk and radial margin compared with the attachment on the ulnar side and calls for: (1) repair of ulnar-sided lesions and lesions associated with avulsion fractures, and (2) débridement of the remainder of these lesions.[12]

CENTRAL TRIANGULAR FIBROCARTILAGE TEARS

Most lesions of the TFC occur in the central articular disk region (Fig. 18–1*A* and *B*). Traumatic lesions may be distinguished from degenerative perforation by the vertical nature of the injury and the lack of associated thinning of the articular disk and underlying chondromalacia of the ulna. Both degenerative and traumatic central tears may be treated satisfactorily with débridement.[7] However, degenerative lesions that are associated with ulnocarpal impingement may require an ulnar shortening procedure to prevent exacerbation of the symptoms.

Technique. For débridement of the ulnar portion of the flap, the arthroscope is introduced into the 4-5 portal and the suction basket is put into the 3-4 portal. This allows the arthroscopist to visualize the tear from the 4-5 portal and to pass the suction basket across the field to débride the ulnar side of the TFC. The radial side of the lesion, although usually smaller, may best be débrided by transferring the suction basket to the 6-R portal and again passing it across the field to the radial cartilage (Fig. 18–2). The edges of the torn fragments may then be débrided using the full-radius synovial resector. When débriding the ulnar side of the wrist, it is important to evaluate carefully the entire portion of the triquetrum and the lunotriquetral ligament by placing the arthroscope in the 6-R portal.

Postoperative Course. The forearm is placed in a bulky dressing for 48 hours, and then gentle active wrist motion is started. Increased activity is permitted as the swelling and pain subside.

PERIPHERAL TRIANGULAR FIBROCARTILAGE DETACHMENTS

Peripheral detachments of the TFC usually occur on the radial side. Although arthroscopic techniques for repair of this avascular portion of the TFC have been proposed,[11] we routinely débride these lesions.

Technique. The arthroscope is introduced through the 4-5 portal and the suction basket through the 6-R portal. The flaps of loose cartilage of the distal radius are re-

Table 18–1	Lesions of the Triangular Fibrocartilage (TFC) Complex[6]

Class I—Traumatic

A. Central perforation
B. Ulnar-sided avulsion with or without fracture
C. Distal (carpus) avulsion
D. Radial-sided avulsion with or without fracture

Class II—Degenerative

Stage 1—TFC wear
Stage 2—TFC wear plus lunate or ulnar chondromalacia
Stage 3—TFC perforation plus lunate or ulnar chondromalacia
Stage 4—TFC perforation plus chondromalacia and lunotriquetral ligament perforation
Stage 5—TFC perforation plus chondromalacia plus lunotriquetral perforation plus ulnocarpal arthritis

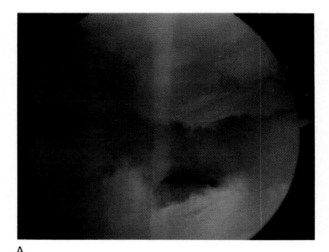

A

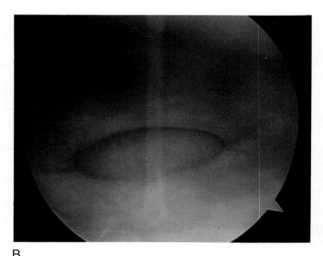

B

Figure 18–1 • *A,* Preoperative view of a central degenerative lesion of the TFC. Note the associated chondromalacia of the lunate. *B,* A TFC complex tear following débridement. Note the lack of associated chondromalacia of the ulnar head.

moved, and the surface is débrided using a full-radius synovial resector. The attached loose portions of the articular disk may also require removal. The suction basket may then be transferred to the 3-4 portal for visualization and débridement of the articular disk, as previously described.

Ulnar-sided peripheral detachments may be repaired with excellent results.[2] These lesions may best be appreciated with the arthroscope in the 4-5 portal and the 30-degree inclination of the scope being angled toward the dorsal ulnar aspect of the TFC. The diagnosis is suggested by the absence of tautness of the TFC. Synovitis is often present at the dorsal aspect of the TFC and may obscure the peripheral detachment. It is important, therefore, to initially débride these lesions by introducing the arthroscope through the 4-5 portal and the full radius synovial resector through the 6-R portal so that débridement of the synovium covering the peripheral detachment is complete. A probe may then be inserted to demonstrate the size and thickness of the traumatic lesion. This lesion must be distinguished from the normal prestyloid recess. If the prestyloid recess passes dorsally between the capsule and the peripheral margin and if the TFC has lost its usual trampoline appearance, then that lesion should be addressed.

We currently utilize the Touhy needle technique of repair of these dorsal ulnar peripheral detachments. This technique requires only a needle (which may be obtained from the anesthesiologist at the start of the case) and some 2-0 polydioxanone (PDS) sutures. It is relatively simple; it is not technically demanding; and it yields good results.[2]

Technique. The arthroscope is introduced through the 4-5 portal, and the lesion is débrided using the full-radius synovial resector inserted through the 6-R portal. For repair of the lesion, the Touhy needle is introduced through the 1-2 portal on the radial aspect of the wrist, passed across the field of the arthroscope, and inserted into the edge of the articular disk of the TFC. Once the needle has perforated the TFC, it is guided out the dorsal ulnar aspect of the capsule and through the skin. A 2-0 PDS

suture is passed through the needle from radial to ulnar, and a hemostat is placed on each end of the suture on both sides to prevent it from being pulled out. The Touhy needle is then pulled back into the wrist until it can be visualized by the arthroscope in the 4-5 portal. The needle is then advanced through the articular disk of the TFC adjacent to the first perforation. The oblique tip of the Touhy needle prevents it from cutting the suture when it is passed back through the articular disk and capsule. The needle is then directed out 3 mm adjacent to the first perforation and emerges from the dorsal ulnar aspect approximately 8 mm ulnad to the previous suture. A probe is then used to loop the suture from the end of the Touhy needle so that both ends of the suture emerge from the dorsal ulnar aspect of the wrist. The Touhy needle may then be withdrawn (Fig. 18–3).

With care being taken not to cut too deeply, a No. 15 blade is used to make a 1 cm incision in the skin directly

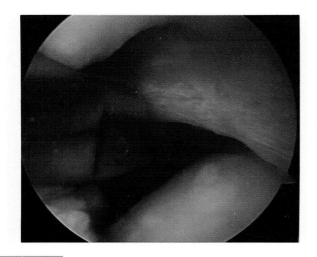

Figure 18–2 • Débridement of the TFC complex back to a stable rim of tissue.

between the two sutures. A hemostat is used to free up the underlying soft tissue, to protect the dorsal branches of the ulnar nerve, and to spread gently down to the capsule so that the capsule is preserved. Next, a nerve hook is used from the incision in the dorsal aspect of the ulna to bring the suture out through the skin incision. The other suture is hooked as well and brought out through the small skin incision. After verifying that there are no cutaneous nerves in this interval, tension is placed on the sutures and the TFC is reduced to the dorsal ulnar capsule under direct visualization through the 4-5 portal. The sutures are then tied down over the dorsal ulnar capsule. This may be sufficient for very small lesions, but for most lesions it will have to be repeated three to four times.

Postoperative Course. The wrist is then placed in a removable splint in ulnar deviation. The wounds are checked at 10 days. The wrist is then immobilized in ulnar deviation for approximately 1 month, after which gentle active flexion and extension exercises are initiated.

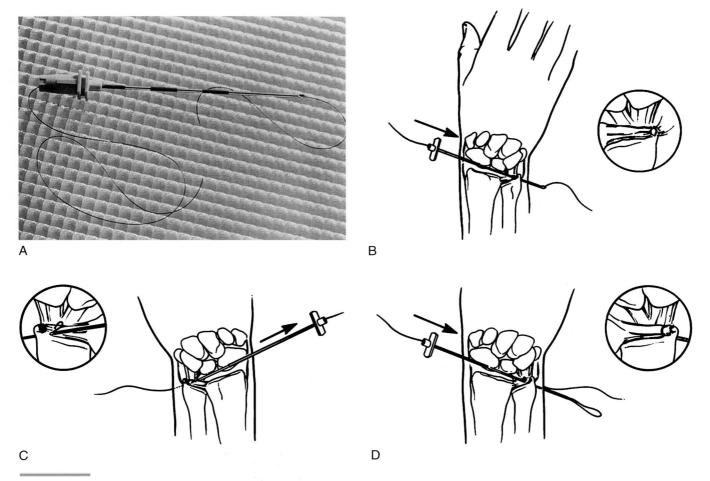

A

B

C

D

Figure 18–3 • *A–D*, The technique of repair of the TFC complex using the Touhy needle.

LIGAMENTOUS INJURIES

Incomplete lesions of the lunotriquetral and scapholunate ligaments are a relatively common source of mechanical wrist pain. Patients complain of mechanical symptoms such as locking, popping, and catching. There is usually a history of trauma involving a fall on the outstretched hand with the wrist in radial deviation. A preoperative physical examination yields point tenderness at the scapholunate interval, which can be relieved with an injection. The relief is diagnostic, whereas imaging studies are not particularly useful for that purpose. Recent evidence on both magnetic resonance imaging and arthrography demonstrates that many patients with asymptomatic wrists may in fact have perforations of the lunotriquetral and scapholunate ligaments.[3, 4] It is, therefore, imperative to distinguish between asymptomatic perforation and a traumatic tear, and we believe that this may only be accomplished by carefully taking a history and doing a physical examination.

The lunotriquetral complex and the scapholunate ligament complex have three major components, as has been elucidated by Berger and Garcia-Elias.[1] Both ligaments consist of strong volar and dorsal ligaments with transversely and horizontally oriented collagen fibers. Arthroscopy shows that the central portion of the ligament consists primarily of fibrocartilage with little mechanical strength. Lesions in this region, although they may cause mechanical symptoms similar to those of a loose body, are not a source of instability. If there is any question of instability after identification of these lesions, then a fluoroscopic examination may be performed preoperatively or intraoperatively.

These lesions appear as large patulous flaps of fibrocartilage suspended from the scapholunate or lunotriquetral interval. Often, there is a great deal of synovium in this region as well as accompanying chrondromalacia, which may obscure visualization of the interval.

Operative Technique. The arthroscope is placed in the 3-4 portal, as for a diagnostic arthroscopy. Outflow is established via the 6-R portal. For débridement of the scapholunate interval, the arthroscope is directed upward at that interval. Visualization from the 3-4 portal to the ulnar side of the wrist may be obscured by this flap of articular cartilage and ligament suspended from the scapholunate joint (Fig. 18–4A and B). A 4-5 portal must then be created, and a suction basket is used to remove this flap. Because the flap consists primarily of fibrocartilage and is not easily débrided using a full-radius synovial resector, we utilize the suction basket for our initial débridement and then introduce a synovial resector for débridement of the remaining loose portions of the ligament. The scapholunate interval is then stress-tested with a probe to detect any displacement between the scaphoid and the lunate. If there is any question of displacement, the arthroscope is withdrawn from the radiocarpal joint and placed in the ulnar midcarpal joint so that congruity of the scapholunate joint can be assessed more thoroughly.

The technique for resection of partial tears of the lunotriquetral ligament is very similar to the aforementioned technique. It is imperative that the arthroscope be placed in one of the ulnar portals for adequate visualization of the triquetrum and the entire portion of the

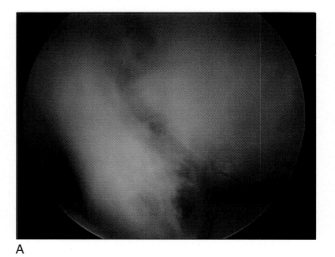

A

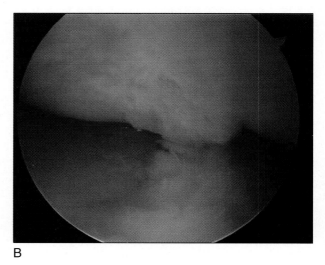

B

Figure 18–4 • *A*, A partial tear of the scapholunate ligament. *B*, A lesion after débridement with a suction punch.

lunotriquetral ligament to assess for both instability and chondromalacia secondary to ulnocarpal abutment.

In cases of a partial tear of the lunotriquetral ligament, we insert the arthroscope through the 4-5 portal and the suction basket through the 6-R portal. The flap of fibrocartilage is resected using a suction basket (see Fig. 18–4B). Again, a full-radius synovial resector may be used to débride the inflamed synovium in this area and to provide further visualization of the ligament. Chondromalacia of the triquetrum may also be débrided at this time.

Pinning these joints is somewhat controversial, and we currently reserve it for cases of true instability. We believe that the best method for evaluating instability is two-fold: (1) we use a probe to stress the ligamentous stability and to assess whether the two bones can be separated for more than 4 mm; and (2) we place the arthroscope in the ulnar midcarpal portal and a probe in the 4-5 portal and stress the junction between the two bones. Gross instability is evident when there is either incongruity in the midcarpal joint or when there is obvious gapping of the interval when viewed from either the radiocarpal joint or the midcarpal joint.

COMPLETE INTRINSIC LIGAMENT INJURIES

If instability is evident either preoperatively or following débridement, a decision regarding open or arthroscopic treatment must be made. In general, we reserve arthroscopically assisted reduction and pinning for acute lesions, and we usually perform open ligament reconstructions for chronic tears.

Technique. Once acute instability has been demonstrated, the interval is débrided of the ligament remnants to allow for visualization of the joint.

First, the full-radius synovial resector is used to débride the interval of all soft tissue and articular cartilage. Débridement must be back to bleeding subchondral bone, and all debris that might block reduction must be removed between the two bones.

Next, 0.45 Kirschner wires are used to fix the interval. Scapholunate tears are pinned through the 1-2 portal immediately distal to the radial styloid and dorsal to the first dorsal compartment. A 14 gauge Gelco needle is used as a soft-tissue protector. Alternatively, a small stab wound may be made, and the S_2 branch of the radial nerve may be found and protected. The arthroscope is then placed in the radial midcarpal joint, and the scapholunate interval is reduced. Often the first pin may be advanced 1 cm into the scaphoid and used as a joystick to bring the scaphoid up out of its volar flexed position. A second 0.45 Kirschner wire is then placed across the interval. Marrow droplets may be seen emerging from the interval, ensuring that the wire is in the proper position. This procedure is repeated until four pins are placed across the interval. Their positions should be confirmed by direct visualization through the midcarpal and radiocarpal joints and also by fluoroscopy (Fig. 18–5). Lunotriquetral tears are approached through the dorsoulnar aspect of the wrist with the arthroscope in the ulnar midcarpal portal. A 14 gauge Gelco needle may be introduced from the ulnar side of the wrist, and careful attention should be paid to avoid the dorsal sensory branch of the ulnar nerve. This requires use of a No. 11 blade to make an incision through the skin, using hemostats to spread down to the level of the capsule, and then inserting the Gelco needle to act as a soft-tissue protector. Wires (0.45) are then passed across the lunotriquetral interval. We have found that three pins are usually sufficient to achieve stability in this interval.

Like the scapholunate interval, in which the scaphoid is on the relatively long fulcrum, the lunotriquetral interval must be controlled with three-point fixation. Reduction should be assessed through the midcarpal portal, and placement of a pin in the dorsal aspect of the lunate is often advantageous in controlling that structure during the pinning. With complete disruption of the lunotriquetral ligament the lunate has the tendency to fall into palmar flexion, and placement of the pin in the dorsal aspect of the lunate, followed by depression of the joystick, usually allows the volar-flexed lunate to be brought back into its anatomic position. Arthroscopic-assisted reduction with pinning of these injuries is designed to create a pseudarthrosis of the interval, and a formal ligament reconstruction is not performed. When the instability pattern is longstanding, open reduction is required. In most cases, we currently attempt ligament reconstruction by reinforcing the ligament with a capsulodesis. Once degenerative changes have occurred, we routinely perform a limited intercarpal fusion or a complete wrist fusion.

INTRA-ARTICULAR DISTAL RADIUS FRACTURES

Wrist arthroscopy is an excellent adjunct for evaluating the articular surface of the distal radius. This technique has been previously employed in the treatment of tibial plateau fractures and has gained acceptance in the treatment of wrist fractures. Its indications include comminuted intra-articular fractures with impacted intra-articular segments.

Theoretical advantages of using this technique are: (1) it allows direct anatomic visualization of articular surface congruity; (2) it permits visualization of the intrinsic and extrinsic ligamentous structures, which are commonly injured in displaced intra-articular distal radius fractures; and (3) it allows for evaluation of the TFC, which may also be torn in these injuries, particularly with disruption of the distal radioulnar joint.

Technique. The majority of these fractures represent high-energy injuries with marked comminution of the dorsal cortex and are thus considered to be unstable. We routinely place the upper extremity in an external fixator device before performing arthroscopy, and the tower distractor is then not necessary, because distraction can be applied by the fixator itself. In addition, we routinely utilize an iliac crest bone graft because: (1) it allows for buttressing of the subchondral bone following elevation and pinning of the surface; and (2) it encourages rapid union and therefore allows the fixator to be removed earlier than would otherwise be possible.

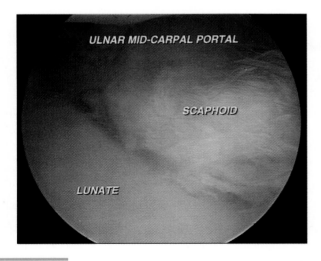

Figure 18–5 • A view from the ulnar midcarpal portal permits an accurate assessment of the congruity of the scapholunate interval.

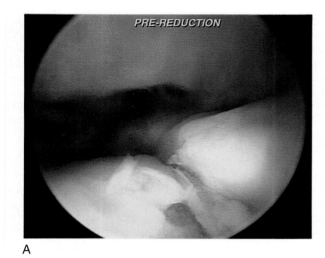

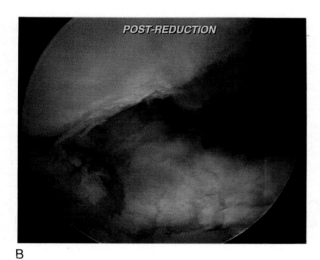

Figure 18–6 • *A* and *B*, Preoperative and postoperative views of a comminuted lunate impaction fracture. *A*, The articular surface following closed manipulation and application of the external fixator. *B*, The same joint following arthroscopic-assisted reduction and percutaneous pinning.

Once the external fixator device is placed, distraction is applied across the radiocarpal joint; the arthroscope is introduced to the 3-4 portal; and outflow is established via the 6-R portal. Approximately 5 minutes of gentle irrigation and débridement of the clot may be required for good visualization of the wrist. Once the clot is removed, the large fracture fragments can be identified and any chondral debris can be removed. At this point, we utilize a small, dorsal, longitudinal incision placed approximately 3 cm proximal to the 3-4 portal. Through this incision, we are then able to identify the break in the dorsal cortex of the distal radius and to place a Freer elevator into this fracture for gentle elevation of the lunate facets of the distal radius. The resultant vacuum in the metaphysis is filled with the iliac crest bone graft. Once the articular surface is evaluated, percutaneous wires can be applied in the stan-

dard fashion. We routinely use a transverse buttressing wire from the radius to the ulna at the level of the radiocarpal joint. A second wire is then placed through the tip of the radial styloid and directed approximately through the ulnar cortex of the radial metaphyseal-diaphyseal junction. These two pins buttress the articular surface and hold the radial styloid portion of the fracture out to length. Additional smaller wires may be added when needed to reduce the distal radioulnar joint.

The articular surface can be visualized through the radiocarpal joint while the fracture is being reduced (Fig. 18–6). We often find tenaculum forceps helpful in holding this reduction until the wires have been placed. At this point, the external fixator may be tightened, the wires cut back, and pinballs applied.

Postoperative Course. The patient is followed aggressively in occupational therapy to prevent contractures of the extrinsic and intrinsic finger extensors. Radiographic healing is usually evident at 4–6 weeks, and most fixators are removed by 6 weeks.

It is noteworthy that often partial ligamentous injuries are observed. Although we do not have any evidence to suggest that early treatment of these ligaments is necessary, it seems intuitively apparent that débridement of the fibrocartilaginous portion of the lunotriquetral and scapholunate ligaments would be helpful. In addition, we direct the arthroscope in an ulnar direction and débride the acute TFC injuries, particularly those injuries noted in the central portion of the articular disc. The peripheral lesions may heal and, therefore, are not débrided at this time.

SUMMARY

In conclusion, operative arthroscopy of the wrist is an excellent diagnostic and interventional technique. It provides an unparalleled view of the complex array of volar extrinsic and intrinsic ligaments, and it facilitates a multitude of surgical procedures without the postoperative stiffness inherent in a capsulotomy.

References

1. Berger RA and Garcia-Elias M: General anatomy of the wrist. In Cooney WP (ed.): Biomechanics of the Wrist Joint. New York, Springer-Verlag, 1991, pp 1–23.
2. deAraujo W, Poehling GG, Kuzma GR, et al.: Touhy needle technique for peripheral triangular fibrocartilage complex repair. Presented at the American Society for Surgery of the Hand 49th Annual Meeting, Cincinnati, Ohio, October 26, 1994.
3. Gropper PT, Brown JA, and Janzen DL: Positive wrist arthrography in the asymptomatic wrist. Presented at the American Society for Surgery of the Hand 49th Annual Meeting, Cincinnati, Ohio, October 26, 1994.
4. Kinschenbaum D, Loeb D, Sieler S, et al.: Wrist arthrography and MRI: association of ligament integrity.
5. Koman LA, Poehling GG, Toby EB, et al.: Chronic wrist pain: indications for wrist arthroscopy. Arthroscopy 6:116–119, 1990.
6. Palmer AK: Triangular fibrocartilage complex lesions: a classification. J Hand Surg Am 14:594–606, 1989.
7. Palmer AK: Triangular fibrocartilage disorders: injury patterns and treatment. Arthroscopy 6:125–132, 1990.

8. Poehling GG and Van Huys J: The arthroscopic treatment of the dorsal wrist ganglions. Presented at the American Society for Surgery of the Hand 46th Annual Meeting, Orlando, Fla., October 5, 1991.
9. Richards RS, Roth JH, and Bennett JD: Arthroscopy in distal radial fractures. Presented at the American Society for Surgery of the Hand 49th Annual Meeting, Cincinnati, Ohio, October 26, 1994.
10. Ruch DS, Chabon SJ, and Poehling GG: The role of arthroscopy in the treatment of scapholunate dissociation. Techn Orthop 7:42–48, 1992.

11. Sagerman SD and Short WH: Arthroscopic repair of radial-sided TFCC tears: a follow-up study. Presented at the American Society for Surgery of the Hand 49th Annual Meeting, Cincinnati, Ohio, October 26, 1994.
12. Thiru RG, Ferlic DC, Layton ML, et al.: Arterial anatomy of the triangular fibrocartilage of the wrist and its surgical significance. J Hand Surg Am 11:258–263, 1986.

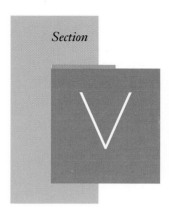

V

The Hip

Diagnostic and Operative Arthroscopy of the Hip

J. W. Thomas Byrd

INTRODUCTION

The first reported attempt at arthroscopic visualization of the hip is attributed to the cadaveric studies of Burman[1] in 1931. In 1939, Takagi[2] reported on the application of the arthroscope in four cases of Charcot and infected hip joints. Following this report, it was not until the 1970s that literature reappeared on the clinical usefulness of this procedure. There were two series on hip arthroscopy in children and two case reports of arthroscopy following total hip replacements.[3–6] In 1986, Eriksson, Arvidsson, and Arvidsson[7] reported on the forces necessary to distract the hip adequately for arthroscopy, and Johnson[8] defined the techniques for carrying out arthroscopy of the hip. Glick and colleagues have popularized the lateral position, and several authors, including those from Europe and Japan, have introduced useful concepts in both technique and indications.[9–30] Most reports of operative arthroscopy of the hip have presented data for relatively small numbers of cases. These reflect the limited present indications for the technique.

PATIENT SELECTION

Indications

The indications for hip arthroscopy are still evolving. Even in this evolutionary process, successful results depend on proper patient selection. There have been many reported indications for the technique, but there are few patients who adequately fit these indications (Table 19–1).

Retrieval of symptomatic **loose bodies** represents perhaps the most gratifying indication for this procedure.[8, 10, 12, 20] The diagnosis is usually clear. If not apparent on plain radiographs, double-contrast arthrography followed by computed tomography predictably shows both cartilaginous and bony fragments. In addition to results with post-traumatic loose bodies and foreign bodies, successful results have been reported with synovial osteo-

chondromatosis and free fragments associated with Legg-Calvé-Perthes disease.[22–24]

Débridement of symptomatic **labral tears** may produce equally gratifying results.[8, 10, 11, 20, 21] These tears may be acute or degenerative. However, the diagnosis is often elusive. Both double-contrast arthrography followed by computed tomography as well as magnetic resonance imaging are presently not dependable in defining labral lesions.

Fluoroscopically guided intra-articular injection of the joint is often a useful maneuver in differentiating symptomatic labral lesions from potential extracapsular sources of disease, such as an iliopsoas-snapping hip syndrome. Temporary relief by an injection is not specific for labral disease, but the injection may define an intracapsular source of the symptoms, suggesting the potential role for arthroscopic intervention.

Débridement of labral lesions should be addressed in a conservative and thoughtful fashion. We are still learning about normal variants, and undoubtedly there are as yet unknown long-term ramifications of labral débridement. Resection of symptomatic tears results in significant pain relief and short-term benefit. The long-term repercussions are unknown. Although magnetic resonance imaging is unpredictable in defining labral lesions, it is often an important aspect of the clinical evaluation of recent-onset hip pain to avoid potentially missing a preradiographic stage (stage I) of avascular necrosis of the femoral head.

Arthroscopic débridement has been proposed for intermediate stages of **degenerative hip disease**.[10, 11, 25] Short-term benefits and symptomatic improvement have been modestly successful in select patients. The parameters used in determining whether a patient with degenerative disease is a candidate for arthroscopic intervention include: (1) relatively young age, (2) less advanced radiographic evidence of disease, (3) relatively recent onset of symptoms, and (4) failure of response to conservative treatment (including activity modification, physical therapy, and nonsteroidal anti-inflammatory drugs). There is

Table 19–1	Indications for Hip Arthroscopy

Loose bodies
Labral tears
Degenerative hip disease
Avascular necrosis
Chondral injuries
Synovial disease
Septic hip
Total hip arthroplasty
Unresolved hip pain

no evidence that there are any preventive or arresting benefits of this procedure. It is purely a palliative procedure and indicated only as an alternative for potential pain relief when symptoms are severe enough to possibly warrant a total hip arthroplasty.

The role of arthroscopic débridement in **avascular necrosis** of the femoral head is limited.[10, 11] Again, it is a palliative procedure and is not a substitute for attempted revascularization of the femoral head. Consequently, it is usually reserved for end-stage disease (stage IV), and the results are almost uniformly poor.

Isolated **chondral injuries** are an excellent indication for arthroscopy. However, these types of lesions of the hip are rare. With the constrained bony architecture of the joint, the articular surfaces are not subjected to the types of shear forces that are present in the shoulder or knee. Consequently, these types of isolated lesions are less common and are more commonly associated with multiple loose bodies or degenerative disease.

Arthroscopy has been indicated for select cases of **synovial disease**, although a complete synovectomy cannot be performed. We have also had several cases of a symptomatic proliferative inflammatory synovial process emanating from the pulvinar in the acetabular fossa that have responded to arthroscopic débridement.

Arthroscopic débridement and lavage have been reported in the management of the **septic hip**.[16, 26, 27] Appropriate patient selection is important to avoid an increased risk of surgical failure.

There have been several case reports of debris removal following **total hip arthroplasty**.[5, 6, 30] However, be aware that there are few causes of a painful total hip that are amenable to any type of arthroscopic intervention.

Unresolved hip pain remains an indication for arthroscopy. One must be careful not to overinterpret this indication. Temporary relief from a fluoroscopically guided injection of the joint is probably the single best test to assess that the source of the hip symptoms is intra-articular and potentially amenable to arthroscopic intervention. Extravasation of anesthetic or possible communication with an extracapsular bursa precludes this being completely reliable, but it can be a very useful provocative test. Unresolved hip pain as an indication for arthroscopy should become more of historic interest as we learn to equate arthroscopic findings with the clinical presentation of these patients and as various imaging techniques improve.

Contraindications

The clearest contraindication to hip arthroscopy is ankylosis of the joint characterized by a fixed position on attempted range of motion. Lesser degrees of arthrofibrosis or capsular constriction may, similarly, preclude arthroscopy when the joint cannot be adequately distracted or distended for introduction of the instruments. Marked limitation of rotational motion is often a harbinger of this type of process.

Open wounds, ulcerative lesions, superficial infection, and other sources of soft-tissue compromise contraindicate the passage of arthroscopic instruments into the joint. Appreciation of the bony architecture and neurovascular anatomy about the hip is critical to safe arthroscopy; thus, any significant alteration in the normal anatomy of the bones or soft tissues, whether from previous trauma or surgery, may contraindicate arthroscopy.

Arthroscopy is also contraindicated in the presence of stable, nonprogressing osteonecrosis of the femoral head. There have been several reported cases of progression of the disease state following arthroscopy.

One must also keep in mind potential stress risers in the bone, whether from disease, trauma, or previous surgery. A significant stress riser that could propagate a fracture may contraindicate the use of distraction forces that are often necessary for arthroscopy.

More than for any other joint, severe obesity may be a relative contraindication to hip arthroscopy. Extra-length instruments are routinely needed, even for moderate-size patients, and extremely dense soft tissues may overcome the effective operating length of currently available instruments.

Advanced disease states with destruction of the hip joint are also a contraindication to arthroscopy; they reflect poor patient selection and emphasize the importance of proper indications.

OPERATING ROOM SET-UP

Hip arthroscopy has been described with and without distraction. By far, the most popular technique utilizes distraction. With the distraction method, the patient can be placed either supine or in the lateral decubitus position. The lateral position was principally pioneered by Glick, and a custom distractor has been developed for this approach.[9, 10] Both the supine and lateral positions utilize similar arthroscopy portals.[11] One potential advantage of the lateral position may be in the arthroscopic approach to the severely obese patient. In the supine position, excess adipose tissue tends to fall away posteriorly and is not a major hindrance. However, in the morbidly obese patient, this excess tissue may be more easily managed in the lateral decubitus position.

Arthroscopy without distraction is an attractive concept because it eliminates the potential concerns and technical considerations of the traction forces necessary for adequate hip distraction. Despite this potential advantage, it has not gained much popularity in most centers where the techniques of hip arthroscopy have been developed. There are few articles on this technique, and the overall experience has been limited.[28, 29] Visualization is limited mostly to the anterior recesses but, through various range-of-motion maneuvers, a large portion of the femoral head can be visualized as well as the peripheral rim of the acetabular labrum. Synovial disease and loose bodies that can be manipulated into this area can be addressed. Acetabular lesions and pathology within the fossa cannot be visualized.

The author presents his experience with the supine position, which is effective and reproducible. It utilizes existing operating room equipment, including a standard fracture table with only minor modifications. Orientation is eased by using a position that is familiar to all orthopaedic surgeons who have dealt with fracture management of the proximal femur and hip. Additionally, the layout of the operating room is user-friendly to both the surgeon and the staff. This includes an unobstructed ability to pass instruments into the hip joint while having the C-arm in position and visualizing the fluoroscopic and arthroscopic monitors.

Anesthesia

The procedure is performed on an outpatient basis and usually under a general anesthetic. Epidural anesthesia is an appropriate alternative but depends upon an adequate block to ensure muscle relaxation.

Patient Positioning

The patient is positioned supine on the fracture table. An oversized (12 cm outside diameter) formed urethane perineal post is used and lateralized to the operative side (Fig. 19–1). Lateralizing the perineal post adds a slight transverse component to the direction of the traction vector (Fig. 19–2).

The operative hip is positioned in extension and approximately 25 degrees of abduction. Slight flexion might relax the capsule and facilitate distraction but draws the sciatic nerve closer to the joint, making it more vulnerable to injury; thus, flexion during arthroscopy is avoided. It is important that the extremity be in neutral rotation during portal placement, but freedom of rotation of the footplate during arthroscopy facilitates visualization of the femoral head.

The contralateral extremity is abducted as necessary to accommodate the image intensifier being positioned between the legs. The contralateral foot is anchored with slight traction to provide a counterforce that keeps the pelvis from shifting during distraction of the operative hip.

Traction is then applied to the operative extremity, and distraction of the hip joint is confirmed by fluoroscopic examination. Approximately 1 cm of distraction is necessary for arthroscopy, and typically 25–50 lb of traction is required. More force may be necessary for an exceptionally tight hip but should be undertaken with some caution.

If adequate distraction is not readily achieved, allowing a few minutes for the capsule to accommodate to the tensile forces often results in relaxation of the capsule and

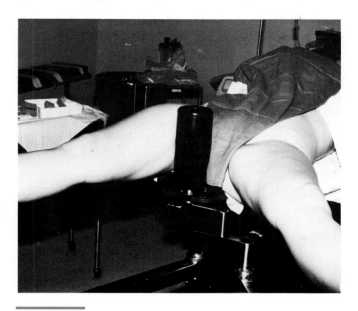

Figure 19–1 • The patient is positioned on the fracture table so that the perineal post is placed as far laterally as possible toward the operative hip resting against the medial thigh. (From Byrd JWT: Hip arthroscopy utilizing the supine position. Arthroscopy 10:275–280, 1994.)

adequate distraction without excessive force. Also, a vacuum phenomenon is apparent fluoroscopically. This is created by the negative intracapsular pressure caused by distraction. This seal is released when the joint is distended with fluid at the time of surgery and may further facilitate distraction. However, the effect is variable and should not be depended on to overcome inadequate traction.[14]

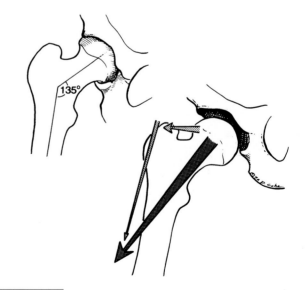

Figure 19–2 • The optimal vector for distraction is oblique relative to the axis of the body and more closely coincides with the axis of the femoral neck than the femoral shaft. This oblique vector is partially created by abduction of the hip and partially accentuated by a small transverse component to the vector. (From Byrd JWT: Hip arthroscopy utilizing the supine position. Arthroscopy 10:275–280, 1994.)

Once the ability to distract the hip joint has been confirmed, the traction is released. The hip is then prepared and draped and traction is reapplied when the surgeon is ready to begin arthroscopy (Fig. 19–3). The surgeon, assistant, and scrub nurse are positioned on the operative side of the patient. The television monitor and arthroscopy cart with an attached sterile Mayo stand to contain the videoarticulated arthroscopes and power shaver are positioned on the contralateral side (Fig. 19–4).

Equipment

A modified fracture table (Skytron model 1100) facilitates the safety and applicability of arthroscopy. A tensiometer built into the footplate allows constant intraoperative monitoring of traction forces necessary to maintain distraction. The oversized perineal post provides extra padding and distribution of pressure on the perineum and facilitates lateralization of the operative hip.

Both the 30 degree and 70 degree videoarticulated arthroscopes are used routinely to optimize visualization. Interchanging the two arthroscopes allows excellent visualization despite the limited maneuverability caused by the bony architecture of the hip and its dense soft-tissue envelope. The 70 degree arthroscope often enhances visualization of worrisome areas; perhaps more importantly, it occasionally allows the surgeon to identify lesions that could have been missed with the 30 degree arthroscope.

A mechanical pump is advantageous for maintaining flow through the hip joint and aids in visualization. Use of a high-flow-rate pump system best allows for adequate flow without having to use excessive pressure, which can lead to inordinate extravasation of fluid.

Assorted 4.5, 5.0, and 5.5 mm extra-length cannulae are used to accommodate the dense soft-tissue envelope

that surrounds the hip. A shortened bridge allows use of these cannulae with a standard arthroscope (Fig. 19–5). Special 17 gauge 6 in spinal needles allow passage of a guide wire into the joint. Special cannulated obturators then allow for passage of the cannula/obturator assembly over the guide wire (Fig. 19–6). Also, for free hand placement, a custom sharp obturator is available (Fig. 19–7). The sharp obturator facilitates penetration of the hip capsule, which is more difficult with a blunt obturator. Although a sharp trocar also easily penetrates the capsule, the configuration of the tip of the trocar is more likely to create inadvertent articular damage, especially to the head of the femur.

Extra-length curved shaver blades have been designed to allow for operative arthroscopy around the convex surface of the femoral head. Extra-length flexible cannulae allow for passage of these curved blades (Fig. 19–8).

Currently, only a few specially designed hand instruments are available specifically for hip arthroscopy (Fig. 19–9). Often, instruments designed for other purposes may be adapted to the hip. However, the surgeon must be careful to avoid using potentially fragile instruments that may not withstand the manipulation and torque potentially created by the dense soft-tissue envelope and bony architecture of the hip joint.

The scrub nurse's Mayo stand accommodates those instruments routinely needed for each case (Fig. 19–10). The 5.0 mm cannula is used for initial introduction of the arthroscope. The diameter allows adequate inflow of the fluid management system through the bridge. Once all three portals have been established, the inflow can be switched to one of the other cannulae, and the 5.0 mm cannula can be replaced with a 4.5 mm cannula. The routine use of three 4.5 mm cannulae allows complete interchangeability of the arthroscope, instruments, and inflow. The 5.5 mm cannula is also available for larger shaver blades.

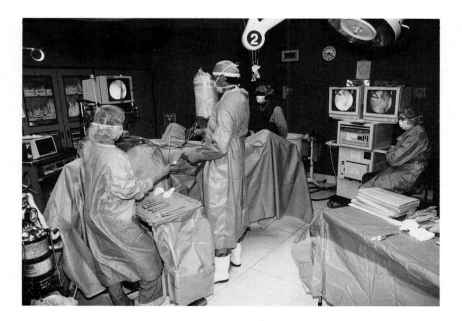

Figure 19–3 • The surgeon and scrub nurse are positioned on the operative side. The arthroscopy cart with monitor is on the nonoperative side. The C-arm, covered in a sterile drape, is positioned between the legs, with the fluoroscopic monitor at the foot. (From Byrd JWT: Hip arthroscopy utilizing the supine position. Arthroscopy 10:275–280, 1994.)

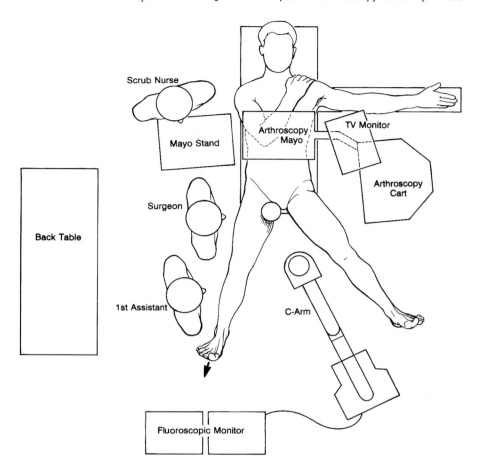

Figure 19–4 • Schematic of the operating room layout showing the position of the surgeon, assistant, scrub nurse, arthroscopy cart, monitor and Mayo stand, scrub nurse's Mayo stand, C-arm, and back table.

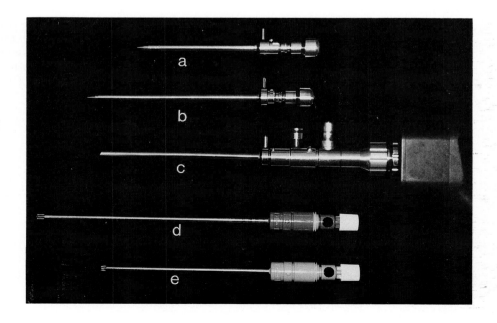

Figure 19–5 • A standard arthroscopic cannula (*a*) is compared with the extra-length cannula (*b*). A modified bridge (*c*) has been shortened to accommodate the extra-length cannula with a standard-length arthroscope. Extra-length blades (*d*) are also available as well as the standard-length blades (*e*).

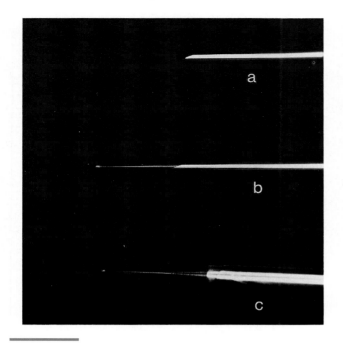

Figure 19–6 • The cannulated obturator system allows for greater ease in reliably establishing the portals after proper positioning has been achieved with the spinal needle. The 17 gauge 6 in spinal needle (*a* and *b*) accommodates passage of a Nitanol wire (*b* and *c*). Specially treated, the wire is resistant to kinking. The cannulated obturator allows for passage of the obturator/cannula assembly over the guide wire (*c*).

GENERAL TECHNIQUE

Portals

Three portals (Table 19–2) are utilized (Figs. 19–11 and 19–12): the anterior, anterolateral, and posterolateral.[13]

Anterior Portal

The anterior portal lies an average of 6.3 cm distal to the anterior superior iliac spine. It penetrates the muscle belly of the sartorius and the rectus femoris before entering through the anterior capsule.

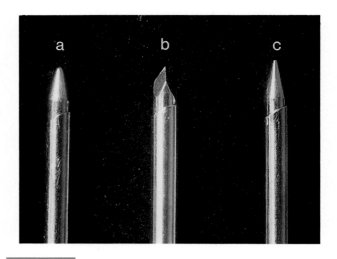

Figure 19–7 • Close-up view comparing the standard blunt obturator (*a*), sharp trocar (*b*), and the custom sharp obturator (*c*). The sharp obturator is better designed to penetrate the capsule while lessening the likelihood of inadvertent articular damage, occasionally attributed to the sharp trocar.

Typically, the lateral femoral cutaneous nerve is divided into three or more branches at the level of the anterior portal. The portal usually passes within several millimeters of one of these branches (Fig. 19–13). Because of the multiple branches, the nerve is not easily avoided by altering the portal position, but it is protected by the use of meticulous technique in portal placement. Specifically, it is most vulnerable to a skin incision placed too deeply, lacerating one of the branches.

Passing from the skin to the capsule, the anterior portal runs almost tangential to the axis of the femoral nerve and lies only slightly closer at the level of the capsule, with an average minimum distance of 3.2 cm (Fig. 19–14).

Although variable in its relationship, the ascending branch of the lateral circumflex femoral artery is usually approximately 3.7 cm inferior to the anterior portal (Fig. 19–15). In some cadaver specimens, a small terminal branch of this vessel has been identified lying within millimeters of the portal at the level of the capsule. The clinical significance of this is uncertain, and there have been

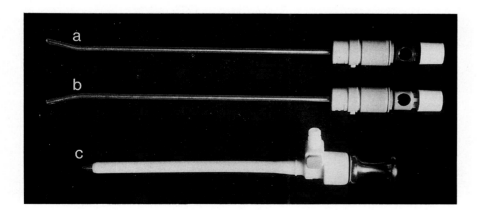

Figure 19–8 • Extra-length curved blades, with a convex (*a*) and a concave (*b*) shaver face, facilitate instrumentation around the femoral head. Extra-length disposable cannulae (*c*) accommodate these curved blades.

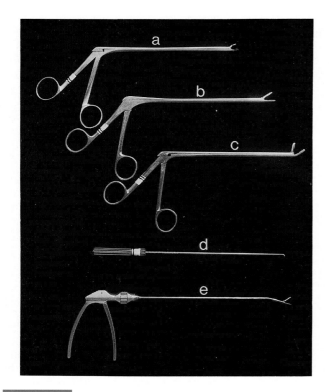

Figure 19–9 • Extra-length instruments selected for use in hip arthroscopy, such as varied-angle rongeurs (*a, b, c*), should be sturdy to lessen the likelihood of instrument breakage. A standard probe (*d*) has been modified for passage through an extra-length 4.5 mm cannula. The grip has been shortened to allow added working length of the probe, and the tip has been honed down to pass through the cannula. Custom hip instruments such as this prototype (*e*) have a rotating head to navigate around the bony contour of the joint.

no reported cases of excessive bleeding from the anterior position.

Anterolateral Portal

The anterolateral portal lies most centrally in the "safe zone" for arthroscopy and thus is the portal established first for introduction of the arthroscope. It penetrates the gluteus medius before entering the lateral aspect of the capsule at its anterior margin.

The only structure of significance relative to the anterolateral portal is the superior gluteal nerve (Fig. 19–16). After exiting the sciatic notch, it courses transversely, posterior to anterior, across the deep surface of the gluteus medius. Its relationship is the same with both of the lateral portals, with an average distance of 4.4 cm.

Posterolateral Portal

The posterolateral portal penetrates both the gluteus medius and the gluteus minimus before entering the lateral capsule at its posterior margin. Its course is superior and anterior to the piriformis tendon (Fig. 19–17). It lies closest to the sciatic nerve at the level of the capsule. The distance to the lateral edge of the nerve averages 2.9 cm.

Surgical Procedure for Normal Arthroscopic Examination

The anterolateral portal is placed first because it lies most centrally in the safe zone for arthroscopy. Subsequent portals are then placed, utilizing direct arthroscopic visualization.

Figure 19–10 • The nurse's Mayo stand contains basic instruments necessary for initiating the arthroscopic procedure: a marking pen; No. 11 blade scalpel; 18 gauge 6 in spinal needles; 60 mL syringe of saline with extension tubing; a Nitanol guide wire; three 4.5, two 5.0, and one 5.5 mm cannulae with cannulated and solid obturators; a switching stick; a separate inflow adapter; and modified probe.

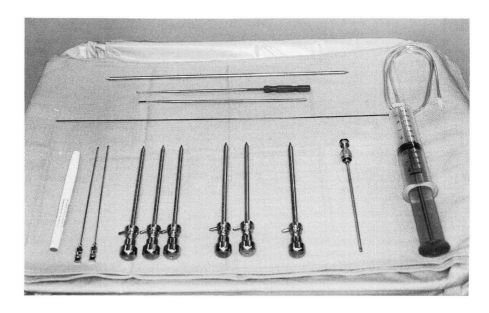

Portals	Anatomic Structure	Average (cm)	Range (cm)
Anterior	Anterior superior iliac spine	6.3	6.0–7.0
	Lateral femoral cutaneous nerve[†]	0.3	0.2–1.0
	Femoral nerve[††]		
	(level of sartorius)	4.3	3.8–5.0
	(level of rectus femoris)	3.8	2.7–5.0
	(level of capsule)	3.7	2.9–5.0
	Ascending branch of lateral circumflex femoral artery	3.7	1.0–6.0
	Terminal branch[†††]	0.3	0.2–0.4
Anterolateral	Superior gluteal nerve	4.4	3.2–5.5
Posterolateral	Sciatic nerve	2.9	2.0–4.3

*Based on an anatomic dissection of portal placements in eight fresh cadaver specimens.
[†]Nerve had divided into three or more branches, and measurement was made to the closest branch.
[††]Measurement made at superficial surface of sartorius, rectus femoris, and capsule.
[†††]Small terminal branch of ascending branch of lateral circumflex femoral artery identified in three specimens.
From Byrd JWT, Pappas JN, and Pedley MJ: Hip arthroscopy: an anatomic study of portal placement and relationship to the extra-articular structures. Arthroscopy 11:418–423, 1995.

Prepositioning is performed with the 17 gauge 6 in spinal needle under fluoroscopic control (Fig. 19–18A). The hip joint is then distended with approximately 40 mL of fluid, and the intracapsular position of the needle is confirmed by backflow of fluid.

A stab wound is made through the skin at the entrance site of the needle. The switching wire is placed through the needle. The needle is then removed, leaving the switching wire in place. The cannula/obturator assembly with the 5.0 mm arthroscopy cannula is passed over the wire into the joint (Fig. 19–18B).

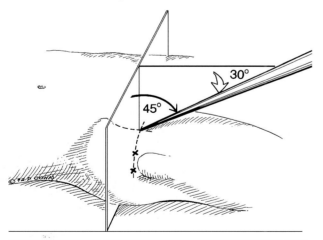

Figure 19–11 • The site of the anterior portal coincides with the intersection of a sagittal line drawn distally from the anterior superior iliac spine and a transverse line across the superior margin of the greater trochanter. The direction of this portal courses approximately 45 degrees cephalad and 30 degrees toward the midline. The anterolateral and posterolateral portals are positioned directly over the superior aspect of the trochanter at its anterior and posterior borders. (From Byrd JWT: Hip arthroscopy utilizing the supine position. Arthroscopy 10:275–280, 1994.)

While the portal is established, the cannula/obturator assembly should pass close to the superior tip of the greater trochanter and then directly above the convex surface of the femoral head. It is important to keep the assembly off the femoral head to avoid inadvertent articular surface scuffing. However, it is also important to stay below the lateral lip of the acetabulum. If the capsule is entered more cephalad to avoid the femoral head, the assembly could penetrate and damage the labrum.

Once the arthroscope has been introduced, the anterior portal is then positioned, facilitated by direct visualization through the arthroscope as well as fluoroscopy. Whereas initial orientation is easier with the 30 degree arthroscope, placement of the other cannulae is better facilitated by the 70 degree arthroscope for directly visualizing where the cannulae penetrate the capsule. Prepositioning again is performed with the 17 gauge spinal needle. Positioning is most dependent on the triangulation technique with the arthroscope. Fluoroscopy is used more to ensure that the needle is not grossly misguided.

If proper attention is given to the topographic anatomy in positioning the anterior portal, the femoral nerve lies well medial to the approach.[13] However, the lateral femoral cutaneous nerve lies quite close to this portal. It is best avoided by utilizing proper technique in portal placement. It is most vulnerable to a skin incision placed too deeply, lacerating the nerve.

The posterolateral portal is then introduced. The fluoroscopic guidelines are similar to those for the anterolateral portal, but positioning is now facilitated by direct arthroscopic visualization. This is especially important to ensure that the cannula does not stray posteriorly, potentially placing the sciatic nerve at risk. It is also important that the hip be positioned in neutral rotation during placement of the posterolateral portal. External rotation of the hip moves the greater trochanter more posteriorly. The trochanter is the main topographic landmark, and this mistake can place the sciatic nerve more at risk for injury.

Figure 19–12 • The relationship of the major neurovascular structures to the three standard portals is demonstrated. The femoral artery and nerve lie well medial to the anterior portal. The sciatic nerve lies posterior to the posterolateral portal. The lateral femoral cutaneous nerve lies close to the anterior portal. Injury to these structures is avoided by utilizing proper technique in portal placement. The anterolateral portal is established first because it lies most centrally in the safe zone for arthroscopy. (From Byrd JWT: Hip arthroscopy utilizing the supine position. Arthroscopy 10:275–280, 1994.)

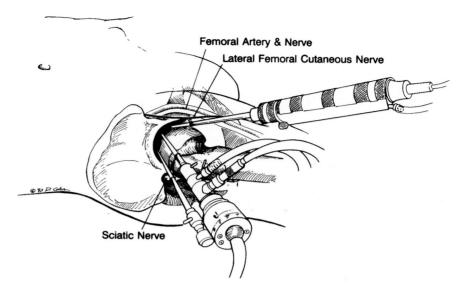

Systematic examination and operative arthroscopy about the hip are facilitated by interchanging the instruments and arthroscope between the three established portals. Releasing the capsule around the portal sites with an arthroscopic knife passed through the cannula improves maneuverability within the joint.

By utilizing both the 30 degree and 70 degree videoarticulated arthroscopes, the structures that can dependably be visualized include the superior weight-bearing portion of the acetabulum; the fossa; the ligamentum teres; and the anterior, posterior, and lateral aspects of the acetabular labrum. Most of the weight-bearing articular portion of the femoral head can be visualized; that is facilitated by internally and externally rotating the hip intraoperatively.

The anterior wall and anterior labrum are best visualized through the anterolateral portal (Fig. 19–19). The posterior wall and posterior labrum are best visualized through the posterolateral portal (Fig. 19–20). The lateral labrum and its capsular reflection are best visualized through the anterior portal (Fig. 19–21). The fossa and ligamentum teres (Fig. 19–22) can usually be visualized

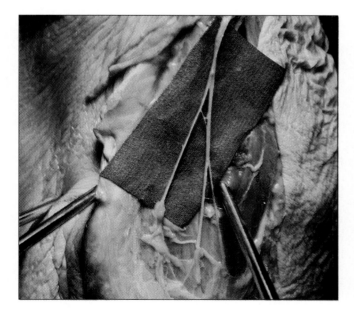

Figure 19–13 • The relationship of the anterior portal to the multiple branches of the lateral femoral cutaneous nerve is shown. Multiple branches at the level of this portal are characteristic, and the branches usually extend laterally to the portal. (From Byrd JWT, Pappas JN, and Pedley MJ: Hip arthroscopy: an anatomic study of portal placement and relationship to the extra-articular structures. Arthroscopy 11:418–423, 1995.)

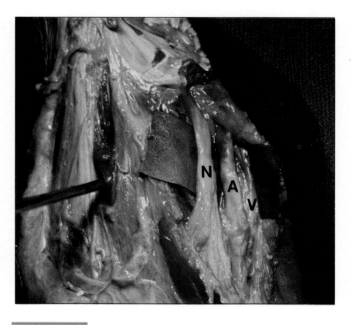

Figure 19–14 • The femoral nerve (*N*) lies lateral to the femoral artery (*A*) and vein (*V*). The relationship of the anterior portal as it pierces the sartorius muscle is shown. (From Byrd JWT, Pappas JN, and Pedley MJ: Hip arthroscopy: an anatomic study of portal placement and relationship to the extra-articular structures. Arthroscopy 11:418–423, 1995.)

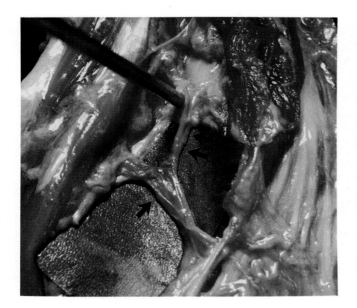

Figure 19–15 • The ascending branch of the lateral circum-flex femoral artery (*arrow*) has an oblique course distal to the anterior portal seen here at the level of the capsule. This specimen demonstrates a terminal branch (*double arrow*) coursing vertically adjacent to the pin. (From Byrd JWT, Pappas JN, and Pedley MJ: Hip arthroscopy: an anatomic study of portal placement and relationship to the extra-articular structures. Arthroscopy 11:418–423, 1995.)

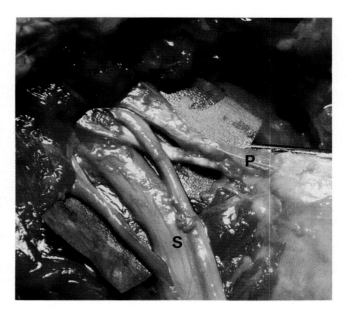

Figure 19–17 • The relationship of the posterolateral portal is shown with the piriformis tendon (*P*) and the sciatic nerve (*S*). Note the anomaly where the sciatic nerve is formed from three divisions distal to the sciatic notch and the lateral-most division passes through a split muscle belly of the piriformis. (From Byrd JWT, Pappas JN, and Pedley MJ: Hip arthroscopy: an anatomic study of portal placement and relationship to the extra-articular structures. Arthroscopy 11:418–423, 1995.)

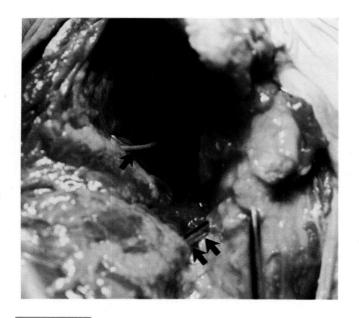

Figure 19–16 • The superior gluteal nerve (*arrow*) is shown coursing transversely on the deep surface of the gluteus medius. It passes above the anterolateral portal (*double arrow*), which is seen between the deep surface of the gluteus medius and the capsule. (From Byrd JWT, Pappas JN, and Pedley MJ: Hip arthroscopy: an anatomic study of portal placement and relationship to the extra-articular structures. Arthroscopy 11:418–423, 1995.)

from all three portals, with a different perspective from each.

Less predictably, the inferior aspect of the acetabulum and femoral head below the ligamentum teres, the inferior capsule, and the transverse acetabular ligament can occasionally be visualized.

At the completion of the procedure, the traction is immediately released. The portals are reapproximated with nylon sutures, and a sterile dressing is applied.

OPERATIVE ARTHROSCOPY

Loose Bodies

Visualization and retrieval of loose bodies can usually be effectively accomplished through the three established portals (Fig. 19–23). Fragments too large to be débrided with a motorized shaver can occasionally be flushed through an oversized cannula, such as those available for arthroscopic shoulder capsulorrhaphy. Especially large fragments can be retrieved with hand instruments, including a variety of extra-length angled rongeurs. Once the portals have been established, directing these hand instruments along the tract initially established by the cannula can be accomplished, and the joint can be effectively entered. Through combinations of inflow and suction and instrument manipulation, loose bodies can usually be positioned into an area where they can be retrieved.

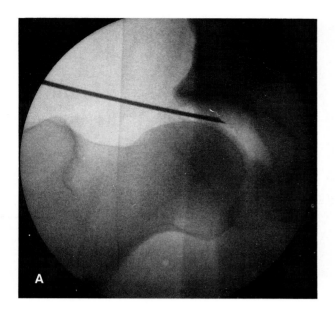

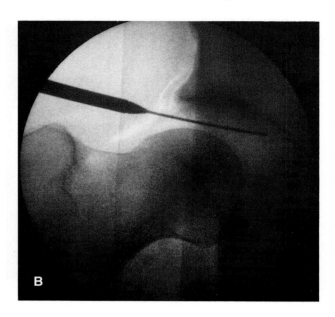

Figure 19–18 • Anteroposterior fluoroscopic view of a right hip. *A,* A spinal needle is used in prepositioning for the anterolateral portal. The needle courses above the superior tip of the trochanter and then passes under the lateral lip of the acetabulum entering the hip joint. *B,* The obturator/cannula assembly is being passed over the Nitanol wire that had been placed through the spinal needle.

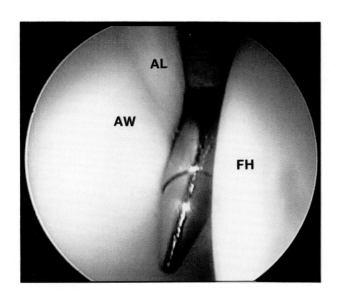

Figure 19–19 • Arthroscopic view of a right hip from the anterolateral portal showing the anterior acetabular wall (*AW*) and the anterior labrum (*AL*). The anterior cannula is seen entering underneath the labrum, and the femoral head (*FH*) is on the right. (From Byrd JWT: Hip arthroscopy: The supine position. In McGinty JB, Caspari RB, Jackson RW, et al.: Operative Arthroscopy, 2nd ed. Raven, 1996, 1091–1099.)

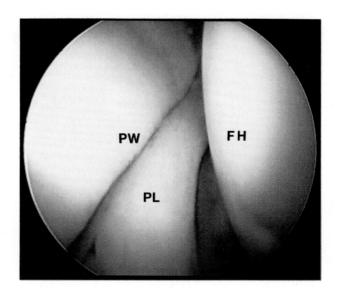

Figure 19–20 • Arthroscopic view from the posterolateral portal showing the posterior acetabular wall (*PW*), posterior labrum (*PL*), and femoral head (*FH*). (From Byrd JWT: Hip arthroscopy: The supine position. In McGinty JB, Caspari RB, Jackson RW, et al.: Operative Arthroscopy, 2nd ed. Raven, 1996, 1091–1099.)

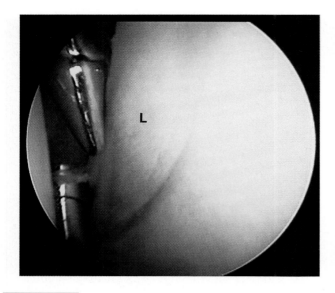

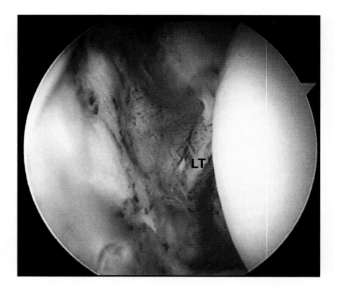

Figure 19–21 • Arthroscopic view from the anterior portal showing the lateral aspect of the labrum (*L*) and its relationship to the lateral two portals. (From Byrd JWT: Hip arthroscopy: The supine position. In McGinty JB, Caspari RB, Jackson RW, et al.: Operative Arthroscopy, 2nd ed. Raven, 1996, 1091–1099.)

Figure 19–22 • Arthroscopic view of the ligamentum teres (*LT*). It is encased in well-vascularized synovium and has a serpentine course from its acetabular to femoral attachments. (From Byrd JWT: Hip arthroscopy: The supine position. In McGinty JB, Caspari RB, Jackson RW, et al.: Operative Arthroscopy, 2nd ed. Raven, 1996, 1091–1099.)

Labral Lesions

The entire anterior, posterior, and lateral aspect of the acetabular labrum can be visualized with combinations of the 30 degree and 70 degree arthroscopes. Unstable tears are resected (Fig. 19–24). As with meniscal lesions, the principle is to débride the torn portion, preserving as

much of the healthy labrum as possible and balancing the resection site to avoid any unstable edges that may propagate further tearing.

The presence of a chronically inverted acetabular labrum has been associated with the subsequent development of osteoarthritis (Fig. 19–25) and has an increased incidence in association with acetabular dysplasia.[31–33]

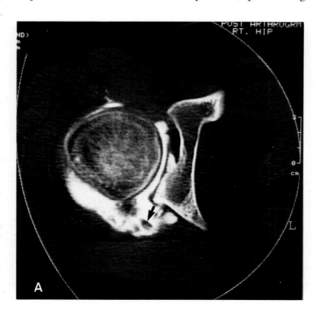

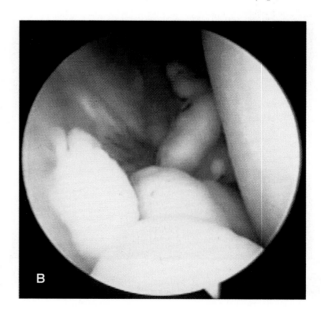

Figure 19–23 • A 16-year-old boy with mechanical right hip pain 2 years following closed treatment of an acetabular fracture. *A,* Double-contrast arthrography followed by computed tomography reveals evidence of multiple loose bodies characterized by filling defects seen posteriorly in this image (*arrow*). *B,* Arthroscopic view of the hip shows multiple loose bodies. Approximately 25 were removed. (*A* and *B* from Byrd JWT: Hip arthroscopy for post-traumatic loose fragments in the young active adult: three case reports. Clin J Sports Med 6:129–134, 1996.)

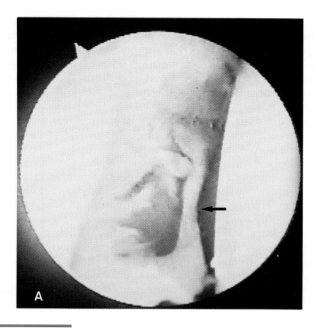

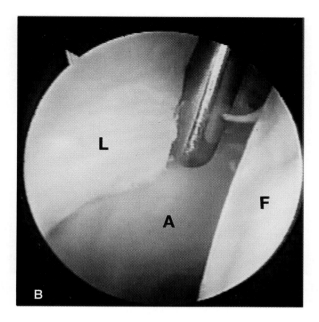

Figure 19–24 • A 35-year-old man with a 14-year history of intermittent pain, catching, and giving way of the right hip following an accident. *A,* Arthroscopic view reveals a complex tear of the anterior labrum displaced into the joint (*arrow*). (From Byrd JWT: Labral lesions: an elusive source of hip pain: case reports and literature review. Arthroscopy 12:603–612, 1996.) *B,* Débridement is carried back to healthy labrum (*L*), allowing better visualization of the acetabulum (*A*) and femoral head (*F*). This resulted in marked symptomatic improvement.

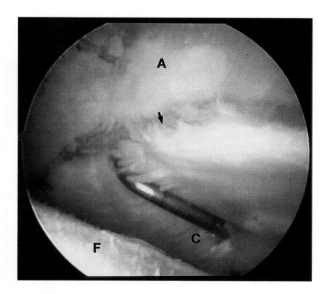

Figure 19–25 • Arthroscopic view of the left hip from the anterior portal in a 56-year-old man with radiographic evidence of mild degenerative arthritis. Articular surface erosions are present on the femoral head (*F*) and acetabulum (*A*). The probe has been introduced through the lateral aspect of the capsule (*C*), defining the presence of an inverted acetabular labrum with its deteriorating free edge (*arrow*) lying within the weight-bearing portion of the acetabulum. (From Byrd JWT: Labral lesions: an elusive source of hip pain: case reports and literature review. Arthroscopy 12:603–612, 1996.)

There is no evidence that prophylactic removal is beneficial, but an inverted labrum may be more susceptible to acute or degenerative tearing and subsequently may be a candidate for partial débridement.

We are still learning much about the normal anatomic variations of the acetabular labrum, including partial separation from the bony rim, which is often a normal finding (Fig. 19–26) that can be potentially misdiagnosed as an acute detachment.[34, 35]

Chondral Injury

Careful inspection of both the acetabular and femoral articular surfaces is necessary with the 30 degree and 70 degree arthroscopes in order to fully assess the presence of a chondral injury (Fig. 19–27). When chondral injury is present, excision and chondroplasty of unstable portions of the articular surface can be beneficial.

POSTOPERATIVE CARE

Immediate ambulation is allowed. Protected weight-bearing status with crutches or a walker is variable, depending on the disease addressed and procedure performed.

The dressing is reduced to small adhesive bandages on postoperative day 1. Sutures are removed between days 3 and 5 and replaced with Steri-Strips.

Rehabilitation actually begins with a preoperative assessment and an educational program by a physical ther-

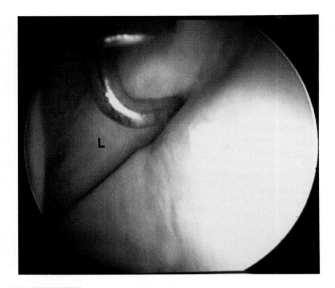

Figure 19–26 • Arthroscopic view of a right hip from the anterior portal showing the lateral aspect of the labrum (*L*), with a probe positioned within a normal separation of the labrum from the lateral aspect of the bony acetabulum. This is an incidental finding and normal variant that could be misinterpreted as an acute detachment by arthrography. (From Byrd JWT: Labral lesions: an elusive source of hip pain: case reports and literature review. Arthroscopy 12:603–612, 1996.)

apist experienced in rehabilitative techniques for hip disease and arthroscopy.[15] The specifics of the rehabilitation process vary, depending on the pathological process and the type of procedure performed. However, in all cases, the goal is to return the patient to **optimal function** with **minimal discomfort**. With the exception of occasional diagnostic procedures or combined arthroscopic and open procedures, the indications for hip arthroscopy are commonly mechanical hip pain; thus, the goals of rehabilitation are common as well.

Manual distraction mobilization techniques can be very beneficial in reducing discomfort, mobilizing the hip, and improving function. However, a therapist skilled in these techniques is required. Maximal range of motion is pushed only to tolerance. A unique feature of the hip joint, as contrasted with the shoulder or knee, is that limitation of motion is rarely a functional problem. Again, the indication for surgery is usually pain, and pushing motion to the point of discomfort may be counterproductive.

Cocontractions and isometric exercises are begun early to initiate muscle toning. Closed chain exercises such as single-leg stance may also facilitate muscle toning, proprioception, and functional return while attempting to minimize the forces across the hip joint.

Functional exercises and stationary bicycle are introduced as the patient progresses and symptoms allow. The final stage of open chain exercises and isokinetic strengthening may never be reached in some patients, depending on the functional goals and hip disease.

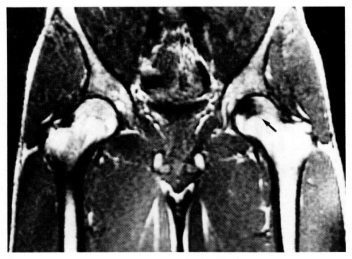

A

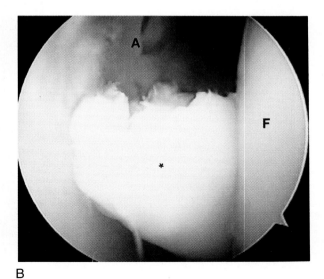

B

Figure 19–27 • A 21-year-old collegiate basketball player with persistent left hip pain following a fall with lateral impaction injury to the joint. *A,* Magnetic resonance imaging reveals signal changes in the medial aspect of the left femoral head (*arrow*) consistent with a subchondral injury and bone bruise. *B,* Arthroscopy revealed the femoral head (*F*) with its large associated unstable flap lesion of articular surface (*) impinging under the acetabulum (*A*). (From Byrd JWT: Labral lesions: an elusive source of hip pain: case reports and literature review. Arthroscopy 12:603–612, 1996.)

COMPLICATIONS

The reported complications associated with hip arthroscopy are rare. However, there are several significant sources of concern. Distraction of the hip for arthroscopy necessitates countertraction provided by a perineal post. This introduces the potential for compression injury to the perineum and especially transient neurapraxia of the pudendal nerve. This concern can be lessened by using a heavily padded post lateralized to the operative side; it is always important to use the minimal amount of traction force necessary to distract the hip and keep the traction time to a minimum.

Early in the author's experience before use of the modified fracture table, there were two cases of transient neurapraxia of the pudendal nerve, both of which resolved within a week or so. Similarly, Glick[36] reported this occurrence in his early experience as well as cases of transient neurapraxia of the sciatic nerve, which he thought was due to traction. Eriksson, Arvidsson, and Arvidsson[7] also reported a case of pressure necrosis of the scrotum. The common denominator in all these cases was that they occurred early in the surgeon's experience, reflecting both the learning curve associated with this technique and the importance of a properly adapted fracture table or device for achieving distraction.

When adhering to proper technique, the femoral neurovascular structures and the sciatic nerve should be safely away from the operative field. However, the lateral femoral cutaneous nerve is always vulnerable to injury from the anterior portal. One of its branches always lies close to the portal. It cannot be predictably avoided by significantly altering the position of the anterior portal. However, it can be avoided by utilizing meticulous technique in portal placement. The nerve is especially vulnerable to laceration by a skin incision placed too deeply through the subcutaneous tissue; this has been reported.[7] Neurapraxia has also occurred when vigorous instrumentation of the joint from the anterior position has been necessary, such as when removing loose bodies too large to be brought out through a cannula.

The single most common complication that is probably under-reported is "scope trauma." The dense soft-tissue envelope about the hip limits the maneuverability of instruments, and the hip is a tightly contained joint. The convex articular surface of the femoral head is especially vulnerable to injury. This may occur either during portal placement or subsequent instrumentation and requires a very thoughtful approach when carrying out operative arthroscopy of the hip.

The labrum is also susceptible to damage during portal placement. This is most likely to occur when trying to use a more cephalad position for penetrating the capsule, attempting to avoid the articular surface of the femoral head. The labrum may be penetrated inadvertently, resulting potentially in significant damage and uncertain long-term consequences.

During portal placement, it is best to try to come in low under the labrum but then direct upward or lift up to stay off the articular surface of the femoral head.

The risk of instrument breakage is also greater than with other joints. The dense soft-tissue envelope again limits the maneuverability of the instruments, increasing the potential for breakage. Additionally, the extra-length instruments used in hip arthroscopy create a longer lever arm and more potential for excessive torque or bending moments. Also, the variety of extra-length instruments available for arthroscopy is limited. There is a tendency to simply use extra-length instruments available for other endoscopic needs such as abdominal or gynecologic procedures. Be wary that these instruments are usually designed for more delicate soft-tissue uses, and improper application in hip arthroscopy makes them especially susceptible to breakage.

Infection following arthroscopic surgery of the hip has not been reported. The dense soft-tissue envelope may lessen the risk of its occurrence in the hip compared with other joints with only subcutaneous soft-tissue coverage such as the elbow or ankle. However, the arthroscopic portals are in relatively close to the perineal region, which emphasizes the importance of meticulous sterile technique in preparation and draping. Similarly, deep vein thrombosis and complications of anesthesia have not been reported in hip arthroscopy, but they are recognized complications associated with arthroscopic procedures.

Finally, a theoretical concern is the potential for ischemic insult to the femoral head due to its tenuous vascular supply. There have been no reported cases of avascular necrosis developing as a consequence of arthroscopy. However, the author has observed a case of previously documented avascular necrosis that progressed following arthroscopy. This observation has been made by Villar[37] as well. It is unclear whether this was a consequence of the natural course of the disease or possibly precipitated by the arthroscopic procedure.

References

1. Burman M: Arthroscopy or the direct visualization of joints. J Bone Joint Surg 13:669–694, 1931.
2. Takagi K: The arthroscope: the second report. J Jpn Orthop Assn 14:441–466, 1939.
3. Gross R: Arthroscopy in hip disorders in children. Orthop Rev 6:43–49, 1977.
4. Holgersson S, Brattström H, Mogensen B, et al.: Arthroscopy of the hip in juvenile chronic arthritis. J Pediatr Orthop 1:273–278, 1981.
5. Shifrin L and Reis N: Arthroscopy of a dislocated hip replacement: a case report. Clin Orthop 146:213–214, 1980.
6. Vakili F, Salvati E, and Warren R: Entrapped foreign body within the acetabular cup in total hip replacement. Clin Orthop 150:159–162, 1980.
7. Eriksson E, Arvidsson I, and Arvidsson H: Diagnostic and operative arthroscopy of the hip. Orthopaedics 9:169–176, 1986.
8. Johnson L: Diagnostic and Surgical Arthroscopy, 3rd ed. St. Louis, C.V. Mosby, 1986, pp 1491–1519.
9. Glick J, Sampson T, Gordon R, et al.: Hip arthroscopy by the lateral approach. Arthroscopy 3:4–12, 1987.
10. Glick J: Hip arthroscopy using the lateral approach. Instr Course Lect 37:223–231, 1988.
11. Byrd JWT: Hip arthroscopy utilizing the supine position. Arthroscopy 10:275–280, 1994.
12. Byrd JWT: Hip arthroscopy for post-traumatic loose fragments in the young active adult. Clin Sports Med 6:129–134, 1996.
13. Byrd JWT, Pappas JN, and Pedley MJ: Hip arthroscopy: an anatomic study of portal placement and relationship to the extra-articular structures. Arthroscopy 11:418–423, 1995.

14. Byrd JWT: Traction vs. distension for distraction of the hip joint during arthroscopy. In press.
15. Henry C, Middleton K, Byrd JWT: Hip rehabilitation following arthroscopy. Individual Orthopaedic Instruction Theater, American Academy of Orthopaedic Surgeons Annual Meeting, Orlando, Fla., Feb., 1995.
16. Bould M, Edwards D, and Villar RN: Arthroscopic diagnosis and treatment of septic arthritis of the hip joint. Arthroscopy 9:707–708, 1993.
17. Dvorak M, Duncan C, and Day B: Arthroscopic anatomy of the hip. Arthroscopy 6:264–273, 1990.
18. Frich L, Lauritzen J, and Juhl M: Arthroscopy in diagnosis and treatment of hip disorders. Orthopaedics 12:389–391, 1989.
19. Hawkins R: Arthroscopy of the hip. Clin Orthop 249:44–47, 1989.
20. Ide T, Akamatsu N, and Nakajima I: Arthroscopic surgery of the hip joint. Arthroscopy 7:204–211, 1991.
21. Ikeda T, Awaya G, Suzuki S, et al.: Torn acetabular labrum in young patients: arthroscopic diagnosis and management. J Bone Joint Surg Br 70:13–16, 1988.
22. Okada Y, Awaya G, Ikeda T, et al.: Arthroscopic surgery for synovial chondromatosis of the hip. J Bone Joint Surg Br 71:198–199, 1989.
23. Witwity T, Uhlmann R, and Fischer J: Arthroscopic management of chondromatosis of the hip joint. Arthroscopy 4:55–56, 1988.
24. Bowen JR, Kumar VP, Joyce JJ, et al.: Osteochondritis dissecans following Perthes' disease: arthroscopic-operative treatment. Clin Orthop 209:49–56, 1986.
25. Villar RN: Arthroscopic debridement of the hip: a minimally invasive approach to osteoarthritis. J Bone Joint Surg Br 73:170–171, 1991.
26. Blitzer C: Arthroscopic management of septic arthritis of the hip. Arthroscopy 9:414–416, 1993.
27. Chung W, Slater G, and Bates E: Treatment of septic arthritis of the hip by arthroscopic lavage. J Pediatr Orthop 13:444–446, 1993.
28. Dorfmann H, Boyer T, Henry P, De Bie B: A simple approach to hip arthroscopy. Arthroscopy 4:141–142, 1988.
29. Klapper R and Silver D: Hip arthroscopy without traction. Contemp Orthop 18:687–693, 1989.
30. Nordt W, Giangarra C, Levy I, et al.: Arthroscopic removal of entrapped debris following dislocation of a total hip arthroplasty. Arthroscopy 3:196–198, 1987.
31. Harris W, Bourne R, and Oh I: Intra-articular acetabular labrum: a possible etiological factor in certain cases of osteoarthritis of the hip. J Bone Joint Surg Am 61:510–514, 1979.
32. Kim YH: Acetabular dysplasia and osteoarthritis developed by an eversion of the acetabular labrum. Clin Orthop 215:289–295, 1987.
33. Dorrell J and Catterall A: The torn acetabular labrum. J Bone Joint Surg Br 68:400–403, 1986.
34. Nishina T, Saito S, Ohzono K, et al.: Chiari pelvic osteotomy for osteoarthritis: the influence of the torn and detached acetabular labrum. J Bone Joint Surg Br 72:765–769, 1990.
35. Klaue K, Durnin C, and Ganz R: The acetabular rim syndrome. J Bone Joint Surg Br 73B:423–429, 1991.
36. Glick JM: Complications of hip arthroscopy by the lateral approach. In Sherman OH and Minkoff J (eds.): Current Management of Complications in Orthopaedics: Arthroscopic Surgery. Baltimore, Williams & Wilkins, 1990, pp 193–201.
37. Villar RN: Hip Arthroscopy. Oxford, Butterworth-Heinemann, 1992.

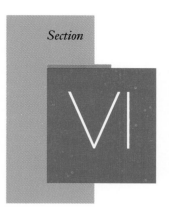

Section

VI

The Knee

Chapter 20

Diagnostic Arthroscopy of the Knee

Frederick M. Azar • *James R. Andrews*

Arthroscopy of the knee was pioneered by Takagi in 1918 in Japan.[1] Based on his initial experiments with a cystoscope in a gas medium in cadavers, he eventually designed an arthroscope and reported his early experiences with its use in 1931. During that same year, Burman[2] reported his experiences with endoscopic examination of all major joints in cadavers. Watanabe, Takeda, and Ikeuchi rekindled interest with the first atlas of arthroscopy in 1957.[3] In 1940, Macnab was the first in North America to attempt arthroscopy of the knee.[4] Jackson is credited with reintroducing the technique to North America in 1965.[5] In 1975 O'Connor designed the first operating arthroscope and was the first to describe its use in operative techniques.[6] A number of studies emerged in the 1970s, reporting successful results with arthroscopy of the knee.[7–15]

PATIENT SELECTION

Indications and Contraindications

Indications for arthroscopy of the knee include those that are diagnostic and those that are therapeutic. A careful and thorough history and physical examination are mandatory and should be followed by evaluation of imaging and laboratory data when indicated. Indications for arthroscopy include the following:[16–19]

Synovitis[20]

Lateral release[21]

Discoid meniscus[22]

Meniscal tear

Torn anterior cruciate ligament

Torn posterior cruciate ligament

Chondral lesion[23]

Chondromalacia

Loose body

Foreign body[24]

Fat pad impingement[25]

Degenerative joint disease

Infection

Symptomatic plica

Painful total knee[26, 27]

Unexplained knee pain and swelling refractory to a standard course of conservative treatment

Contraindications include local or systemic infection. Severe degenerative joint disease is a relative contraindication because it makes knee arthroscopy technically difficult.

Advantages and Disadvantages

The advantages of arthroscopy far outweigh the disadvantages. Arthroscopy provides an accurate evaluation of the entire knee with minimal soft-tissue trauma, less morbidity, fewer postoperative complications, and faster rehabilitation than do open procedures.

Disadvantages include the need for specialized equipment and the steep learning curve necessary to become proficient at arthroscopic techniques.

Conservative Treatment

Conservative treatment should be directed toward modification of activities that increase symptoms. With acute injuries this may include limitation of weight-bearing with the use of crutches. Application of ice for 15–20 minutes every hour, elevation, and compression with an elastic bandage may be helpful in controlling swelling. Immobilization is occasionally needed for control of pain and swelling; however, this should be minimized because motion is usually encouraged to prevent joint stiffness.

A supervised or home rehabilitation program that emphasizes strengthening and flexibility should be initiated. Strengthening exercises should include straight leg raises, quadriceps sets, and ankle pump, progressing to the use of weights with minisquats, leg presses, knee extensions, hamstring curls, and calf raises. Achilles tendon, hamstring, and quadriceps stretching should be included, with each stretch held for a 10-second count. Patellar mobilization and passive and active-assisted knee flexion exercises are also initiated. The number of repetitions and sets varies depending on the patient and the underlying disease. A stationary cycle may also be of benefit. The resistance can be adjusted to increase endurance, and the seat height can be lowered to increase knee flexion.

If NSAIDs are to be prescribed, the patient should be questioned about drug allergies and intolerance. A history of gastritis or peptic ulcer disease is a contraindication to the use of NSAIDs. The patient may need to consult with his or her physician before using them, especially if long-term use is anticipated, because close monitoring for the systemic side effects of these drugs is necessary.

Preoperative Evaluation

Preoperative evaluation should include a thorough history and physical examination. The history of present illness should include the chief complaint and how, when, and where the injury occurred. The medical history should include details of any previous orthopaedic injuries or procedures. As with any history, any medications or drug allergies should be noted. The patient should be questioned regarding any history of gastritis or peptic ulcer disease to determine if nonsteroidal anti-inflammatory drugs (NSAIDs) can be safely prescribed. The family history should include any anesthesia complications on prior surgeries. This last point is important because, in approximately 40% of patients with malignant hyperthermia, this complication was first recognized at the time they sought orthopaedic treatment.[28]

The physical examination should include documentation of knee effusion, range of motion, tenderness, deformity, quadriceps tone and girth, and a thorough ligament examination. The opposite knee should be examined in a similar manner for comparison. The spine and ipsilateral hip should be examined for abnormalities and causes of possible referred pain to the knee. This is especially true for adolescents and elderly patients. Lower extremity alignment and gait should be evaluated. A thorough neurovascular examination should be documented.

Treatment risks, benefits, and alternatives should be discussed with the patient before surgery, and this discussion should be documented in the outpatient notes and on the admission history and physical examination forms.

Patient Education

Patient education plays a vital role in the outcome of arthroscopic surgery, as it does with any operative procedure. This is accomplished by maintaining open lines of communication with both the patient and the family. The preoperative evaluation should include a clear description and documentation of the risks, benefits, and complications of arthroscopic surgery. The expectations of the patient and surgeon should be clearly defined. The postoperative rehabilitation plan and its significance to the overall outcome should be emphasized. Illustrations, knee models, pamphlets, radiographs, and magnetic resonance imaging scans can be used. After surgery, the pathologic condition found and the procedure performed can be demonstrated via photographs and videotapes obtained during the arthroscopic procedure. A timetable for recovery should be outlined. Common concerns about pain management, wound care, and return to activities should be discussed, with emphasis on postoperative rehabilitation.

OPERATING ROOM SET-UP

Anesthesia

Anesthesia for arthroscopy of the knee consists of a preoperative period, an operative period, and a postoperative period. The postoperative period is discussed in the section titled "Postoperative Care."

The patient should not eat or drink anything for 6–8 hours before the procedure to allow gastric content emptying, which decreases the risk of aspiration. This is aided by administration of Reglan and histamine H_2 blockers. NSAIDs should be reduced 1 week before surgery,[29] and monoamine oxidase inhibitors should be discontinued 2 weeks before surgery. Aspirin, warfarin (Coumadin), and other anticoagulants should be discontinued at least 3 days before surgery. Medications taken routinely can be given the morning of surgery unless contraindicated. Questions regarding specific medications should be addressed to the anesthesiologist or physician if present. Patients who smoke should discontinue smoking a minimum of 12 hours before surgery.

Diagnostic arthroscopy of the knee can be carried out with the use of local, regional, or general anesthesia. The type selected depends on the indication for the procedure, the patient's medical history, and the preferences of the patient, anesthesiologist, and surgeon.

Local anesthesia has gained popularity in recent years, especially for office arthroscopy. This involves the injection of portal sites, followed by intra-articular injection of a local anesthetic. Successful use of this technique with arthroscopy was first reported in the 1970s,[30–32] and subsequent studies confirmed favorable results.[33–42] Early failures with the use of local anesthesia were due to the low amounts and low concentrations of lidocaine and bupivacaine. More recent use of 30–50 mL or 20–30 mL of 0.5% bupivacaine (Marcaine) has been more effective. [Editor's note: 1 mL of 1% lidocaine has 10 mg of lidocaine.]

Local anesthesia is indicated in procedures that involve diagnostic arthroscopy, removal of loose bodies, meniscectomy, plical excision, lateral release, or chondroplasty. It is not indicated in procedures that require the prolonged use of a tourniquet or for repair or reconstruction of internal derangement of the knee in which drilling of bone is required. In one study, awake volunteers were able to tolerate pneumatic tourniquet inflation for up to 30 minutes.[43] The use of local anesthesia also requires a patient who is cooperative.

Lidocaine, bupivacaine, or combinations of both are most commonly used for local anesthesia during knee arthroscopy. A combination of 0.25% bupivacaine and 1.0% lidocaine with epinephrine, totaling 30–50 mL for intra-articular injection, has been successful.[36, 38] An additional 5–7 mL is used for portal injection. A total dosage of no more than 3 mg/kg of bupivacaine with epinephrine is recommended.[44, 45] A waiting period of up to 20 minutes may be required after intra-articular injection of a local anesthetic for maximal effect.[37] Because local and regional anesthetic agents are cumulative in their toxic effects,[46–48] the surgeon should communicate with the anesthesiologist regarding the total dosage of local anesthetic agents used. However, as much as 50% of intra-articular anesthetic can be irrigated out within the first 10 minutes,[49] so larger doses may be safe. The maximal recommended doses of the most commonly used local anesthetics are shown in Table 20–1. Supplemental intravenous sedation is used to assist in pain control and to relieve apprehension. If for some reason local anesthesia proves not to be effective during the arthroscopy, general anesthesia should be initiated; this occurs in as many as 14% of patients.[50, 51]

No significant complications during knee arthroscopy with local anesthesia have been reported; however, this depends on how much supplemental intravenous sedation is used. Patients undergoing knee arthroscopy with local anesthesia generally require a shorter postoperative observation time than those in whom general or regional anesthetic is used.

Regional anesthesia in the form of spinal or epidural anesthesia with supplemental intravenous sedation is indicated for patients who are not safe candidates for general anesthesia. Contraindications to regional anesthesia include allergic reactions, coagulopathies, local or systemic infection, and pre-existing neurologic abnormalities.[52]

Continuous epidural anesthetic through a catheter can also be used immediately after general anesthesia when prolonged postoperative pain is anticipated. This may aid in a quicker return of knee motion. Continuous spinal anesthesia is now used less frequently because of reports of cauda equina syndrome. Compared with general anesthesia, regional anesthesia has a lower incidence of deep vein thrombosis, pulmonary thromboembolism, myocardial infarction, cardiac arrhythmia, congestive heart failure, and respiratory failure.[53–55] Complications of regional anesthesia include infection, neurologic sequelae, intravascular injection, and central nervous system or cardiovascular toxicity.[56]

Epidural anesthesia involves the placement of a local anesthetic through the ligamentum flavum into the epidural space, and spinal anesthesia requires the placement of anesthetic through the dura into the subarachnoid space. The patient is positioned in the sitting or lateral position, and the needle is usually placed in the L2-L3 intervertebral space, which is where the spinal cord ends. Lidocaine, bupivacaine, and tetracaine are commonly used for spinal anesthesia, and lidocaine, bupivacaine, chloroprocaine, and etidocaine are usually used for epidural anesthesia. Of the two techniques, spinal anesthesia causes a better motor block and is less likely to cause tourniquet pain.[57] Spinal anesthesia, however, has a higher incidence of spinal headaches (approximately 1%), which tend to be more prevalent in females and young patients and when larger spinal needles are used.[57] These forms of anesthesia allow the patient to be awake during the procedure and result in fewer systemic complications than does general anesthesia.

General anesthesia is safe and effective for any arthroscopic procedure of the knee. However, it is most often indicated for procedures that involve the prolonged use of a tourniquet, require the drilling of bone, or involve the repair or reconstruction of internal derangement of the knee. General anesthesia relaxes the muscles, which allows the knee compartments to be more easily viewed with arthroscopy. It is also indicated for patients who are allergic to local anesthetics. Developments in general anesthesia have decreased postoperative side effects, minimizing discomfort with outpatient surgery. One example of this is the use of propofol for induction instead of the barbiturate thiopental. Propofol has an elimination half-life of 55 min-

Table 20–1 | **Recommended Doses of Local Anesthetic Agents**

Agent	Concentration %	Plain solutions		Epinephrine-containing solutions	
		Maximum adult dose (mg)	*Maximum dose (mg/kg)*	*Maximum adult dose (mg)*	*Maximum dose (mg/kg)*
Short duration					
Chloroprocaine	1–2	800	11	1,000	14
Moderate duration					
Lidocaine	0.5–1	300	4	500	7
Mepivacaine	0.5–1	300	4	500	7
Prilocaine	0.5–1	500	7	600	8
Long duration					
Bupivacaine	0.25–0.5	175	2.5	225	3

From White PF: Outpatient Anesthesia. Churchill Livingstone, New York, 1990, p 264.

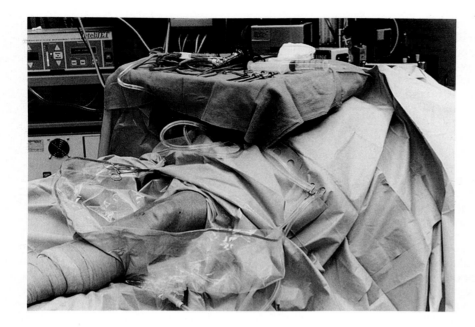

Figure 20–1 • The patient is positioned in the supine position with the knee extended.

utes, compared with the 5–12-hour elimination time of thiopental.[58, 59] This more rapid clearance leaves the patient with few, if any, side effects.

Peripheral nerve blocks of the femoral nerve, obturator nerve, lateral femoral cutaneous nerve, sciatic nerve, and lumbar plexus may be used for knee arthroscopy, but regional or local anesthesia is generally more feasible.

Many arthroscopic procedures are performed in offices, and standards for patient monitoring during anesthesia have been outlined.[60–62]

When left up to the patient, most choose general anesthesia, followed by regional anesthesia and then local anesthesia.[63] Patients undergoing general anesthesia typically have the highest level of satisfaction.[64] The author gives patients the options of regional or general anesthesia, and most select the latter.

Patient Positioning

Positioning of the patient for arthroscopic surgery of the knee depends on the preference and comfort of the surgeon. For all arthroscopic knee procedures, the patient is placed in the supine position, and the affected extremity is manipulated with or without the use of a leg holder or a lateral post. The affected extremity may be maintained in extension or flexed to 90 degrees (Figs. 20–1 and 20–2). The contralateral limb may rest on the operating table, hang off the end of the table next to the operative limb, or be abducted and elevated. Hanging the unaffected limb off the operating table increases venous stasis and subsequent risk of development of deep vein thrombosis and may also limit access to the medial and posteromedial structures of the operative knee. The surgeon may also choose to stand or sit during the arthroscopic procedure.

A well-padded tourniquet of sufficient length is usually placed around the proximal or mid thigh, no more than 4–5 fingerbreadths above the superior pole of the patella. If a leg holder is used, the device should be se-

curely placed around the tourniquet. A lateral post provides greater mobility of the hip and knee than does a leg holder. If a leg holder is used with the lower extremities extended, the leg holder should slightly flex and abduct the ipsilateral hip to allow easier manipulation during the procedure. If the leg holder is placed too proximal on the thigh, varus and valgus manipulation of the knee during arthroscopy can be difficult. Placement of the leg holder too distal on the thigh may limit access to portals and approaches to the knee during meniscal repair or ligament reconstruction. The author prefers to place the tourniquet

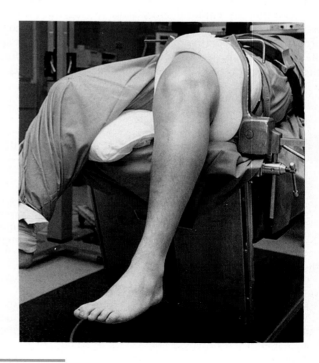

Figure 20–2 • The patient is positioned in the supine position with knees extended or flexed.

and leg holder approximately 4 fingerbreadths above the superior pole of the patella after the operative extremity has been prepared and draped.

If the arthroscopy is performed with the lower extremities flexed, the knees should lie just distal to the break in the operating table to allow flexion past 90 degrees, which is necessary for most arthroscopic procedures. The leg holder should be attached to the siderail and positioned adjacent to the break in the table. The popliteal regions of both knees, including the peroneal nerve, and the heel of the contralateral lower extremity should be well padded. The peroneal nerve is the most commonly injured nerve in the lower extremity during anesthesia.[65] A sheet can be used to hold the contralateral lower extremity in the flexed position. A thigh-length support hose or elastic wrap can be placed on the contralateral lower extremity to minimize venous pooling. In this position, the hips should be slightly flexed to relieve tension on the femoral nerves. This position also reduces tension on the posterior neurovascular structures at the knee and displaces them more posteriorly to a safer location. Elevating and abducting the uninvolved leg in a thigh holder provide an alternative position that also decreases stress on the low back and femoral nerve (Fig. 20–3). This helps prevent venous stasis and permits easier access to the medial and posteromedial compartments of the knee.

If the surgeon chooses to sit, an extra-length sterile gown or an additional gown tied around the surgeon's waist should be used to extend the sterile field and prevent contamination of the draped extremity. A stool with freely rolling wheels allows better mobilization of the surgeon and better manipulation of the extremity. With this tech-

nique, the tourniquet is placed on the proximal thigh. The operating table and rolling stool are adjusted to a comfortable height. Knee flexion can be controlled by moving the rolling stool forward or backward. The anterior compartment and intercondylar notch can be viewed by placing the sterile draped foot in the lap of the surgeon and adjusting flexion and extension as needed. The medial compartment is best viewed by placing the externally rotated foot on the outside hip of the surgeon, with the patient's hip abducted and internally rotated (Fig. 20–4). Additional valgus stress can be applied by placing the surgeon's outside forearm along the patient's lateral leg. The lateral compartment is viewed by placing the lower extremity in the figure-four position on the operating table (Fig. 20–5).

Regardless of the position used, the affected lower extremity is prepared from the upper thigh to the lower leg or to and including the foot. If the foot is not prepared, an impermeable drape must be used. A povidone-iodine (Betadine) or iodine solution is typically used. Hibiclens solution can be used for patients with iodine allergies. Commercially available impermeable drapes are then placed, a waterproof stockinette is rolled from the foot to the upper leg, and an impermeable drape with a sealed hole is placed over the thigh.

Equipment

Even with the presence of properly trained operating room personnel, responsibility for knowledge of instrumentation and use of equipment belongs to the surgeon. This is especially true in arthroscopic surgery, for which

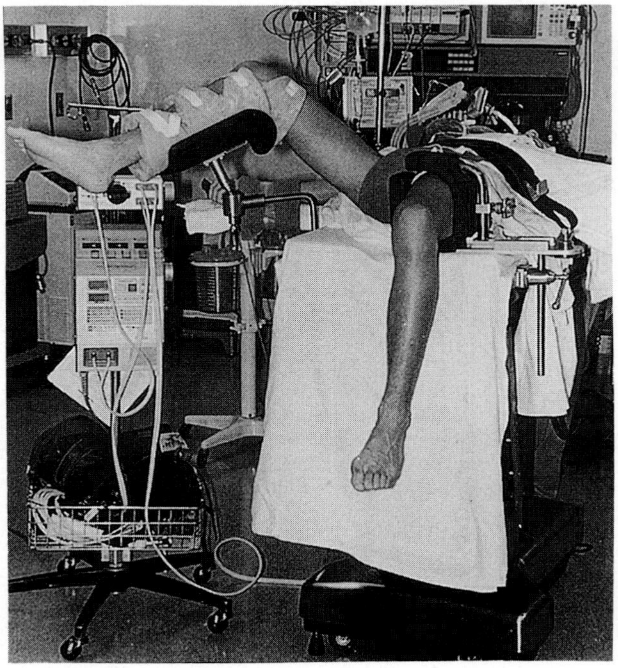

Figure 20–3 • The uninvolved leg can be flexed and abducted with the use of a well-padded gynecologic leg holder. (From Fu FH, Harner CD, and Vince KG [eds.]: Knee Surgery. Baltimore, Williams & Wilkins, 1994, p 549.)

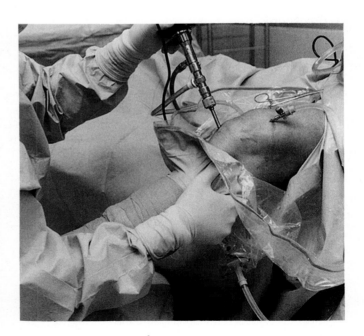

Figure 20–4 • With the surgeon sitting, the medial compartment can be viewed by applying a valgus stress across the knee. This is accomplished by an inward force of the surgeon's hand against the patient's knee and an outward force of the surgeon's hip against the patient's foot.

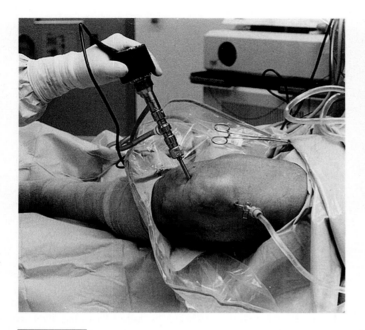

Figure 20–5 • With the surgeon sitting, the lateral compartment can be viewed by placing the leg in the figure-four position.

keeping up with rapid advances in technology can be challenging. A thorough understanding of the maintenance, set-up, and use of arthroscopic equipment is mandatory. This is best gained through in-service sessions with equipment representatives and repetitive use of the devices.

Arthroscope

The arthroscope is composed of a fiberoptic cable encased in metal with a lens at one end. Arthroscopes are available in a number of sizes and viewing angles, with diameters varying 1.7–7.5 mm. The angle of inclination (viewing angle) may be 0 degree, 15 degrees, 25 degrees, 30 degrees, or 70 degrees. The 4.0 mm arthroscopes with 0 degree, 30 degree, and 70 degree viewing angles are the most commonly used in arthroscopy of the knee (Fig. 20–6). A 4.5–5.5 mm cannula or sheath is used with the 4.0 mm arthroscope (Fig. 20–7). The cannulae for knee arthroscopy typically have side holes near the tip to allow a broader dispersion of fluid inflow. Rotation of the 30 degree and 70 degree arthroscopes provides larger areas of viewing (Fig. 20–8). With rotation of a 30 degree arthroscope, the field of view is increased nearly threefold over that provided by a 0 degree arthroscope (Fig. 20–9). A central blind spot is present immediately anterior to the 70 degree arthroscope when it is rotated (Fig. 20–10).

Fiberoptic Light Sources

The technology of fiberoptics has played an integral role in the development of arthroscopic surgery. Bundles of glass fibers are enclosed within a flexible cord to form the fiberoptic cable. Care must be taken when handling these

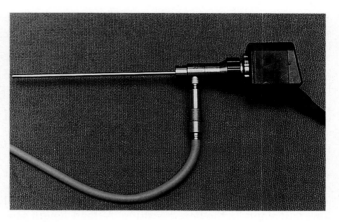

Figure 20–6 • The most commonly used arthroscope for the knee is 4 mm in diameter, with a 30 degree viewing angle.

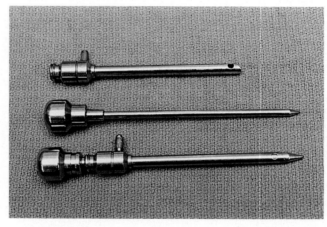

Figure 20–7 • Cannula sheaths for the arthroscope have blunt or sharp trocars. Side holes in the sheath allow better inflow of fluid.

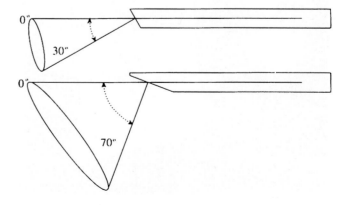

Figure 20–8 • Increasing the viewing angle of the arthroscope (degree of inclination) increases the viewing area. (From McGinty JB [ed.]: Operative Arthroscopy. New York, Raven Press, 1991, p 5.)

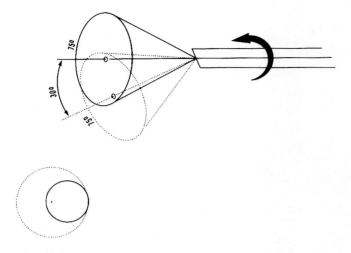

Figure 20–9 • Rotation of the 30 degree arthroscope gives three times the viewing area (large dotted circle) compared with that of the 0 degree arthroscope (small solid circle). (From Shahriaree H [ed.]: O'Connor's Textbook of Arthroscopic Surgery, 2nd ed. Philadelphia, J.B. Lippincott Co., 1992, p 230.)

cables because placing heavy objects on them or tightly bending them causes fractures of the glass fibers and compromises light transmission. The length of the cable used should be minimized because approximately 8% of light intensity is dissipated for every foot of fiberoptic cable. The fiberoptic cable connects the light source to the arthroscope. The light source consists of a high-intensity arc lamp. An automatic light control adjusts light to maintain brightness on the monitor as the arthroscope is moved

from lighter to darker areas within the knee. A manual control is present on the monitor as well as on some camera heads to allow the surgeon to change the lighting when needed.

Television Monitors and Cameras

The modern camera head is sleek and easy to hold and manipulate. Current features include buttons that allow the surgeon to control photographic prints, videocassette recording, and camera gain settings. Video monitors for arthroscopy come in an array of sizes, commonly ranging 13–20 in (Fig. 20–11). The monitors can provide up to 700 lines of resolution for excellent detail of arthroscopic anatomy. All models are required to meet certain leakage and safety standards to be considered medical-grade equipment.

Documentation and Recording Equipment

Documentation of the arthroscopic procedure can be accomplished by various techniques. In addition to a thorough description of the findings in the operative report, a standardized form that includes graphic illustrations is useful for many reasons, including research. Color prints are an effective and efficient means of recording arthroscopic problems. Still images can be recorded on disk storage for playback and for making permanent prints. Recording can be carried out within the sterile field by means of a manual control on the camera head in addition to the controls on the base unit (Fig. 20–12). Multiple images can be recorded on a single page. It is helpful to make two copies of each print, one for the patient and one for the permanent records. Videocassette recording of the pathologic condition and arthroscopic procedure is an excellent form of documentation (Fig. 20–13). The video camera can also be operated by a control on the camera head or by adjustment of the base unit by operating room personnel. Many editing features are available with these devices. Overhead cameras are helpful for recording open procedures (Fig. 20–14).

Documentation of intra-articular disease is an integral part of the procedure for many reasons. Patient education is enhanced by the use of color prints and videocassette recordings of the arthroscopic procedure. A better understanding of what was seen and what was done may aid the patient with postoperative rehabilitation. Photographs and videocassette recordings also provide the surgeon with a visual recollection of the arthroscopy. The videotapes can be valuable tools for teaching and research, and it is helpful to keep a library of these tapes for these purposes.

Accessory Instruments

The typical arthroscopic procedure cart consists of a 30 degree arthroscope, motorized shaver, probe, No. 11 scalpel, scissors, cannulae, trocars, and an assortment of basket and grasping forceps. The cart should also include

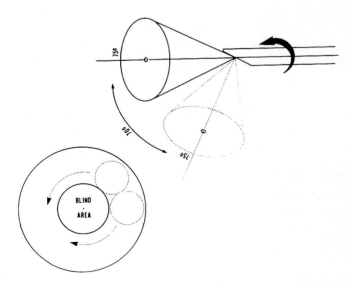

Figure 20–10 • Rotation of the 70 degree arthroscope produces a central blind spot directly in line with the tip of the scope. (From Shahriaree H [ed.]: O'Connor's Textbook of Arthroscopic Surgery, 2nd ed. Philadelphia, J.B. Lippincott Co., 1992, p 230.)

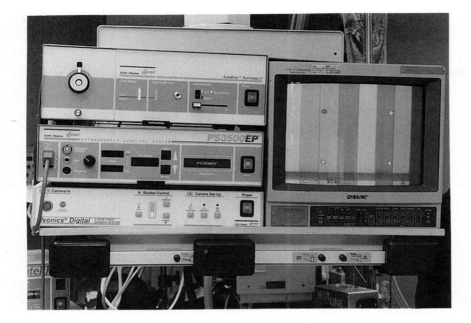

Figure 20–11 • Video monitors come in various sizes. The monitor should be placed in a position that allows clear viewing by the surgeon throughout the procedure.

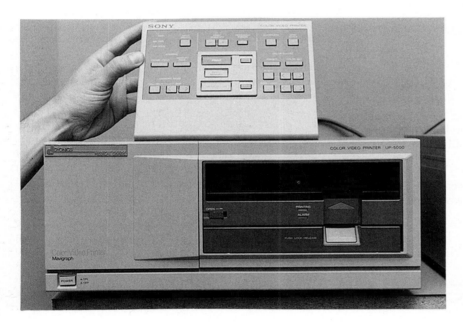

Figure 20–12 • A color video printer is the best method for documentation of intra-articular disease.

Figure 20–13 • A videocassette recorder can be used to document intra-articular disease. Still images can be produced from these recordings.

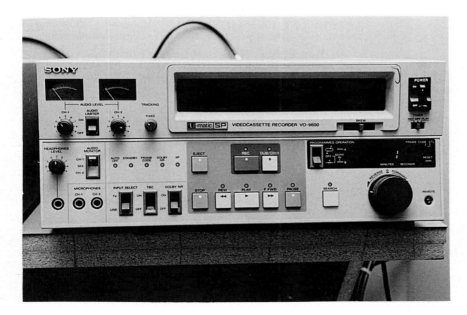

minimize scuffing of articular cartilage. The size of the tip serves as a reference when estimating the size of intra-articular structures or lesions. The probe is useful for determining and defining the extent of a meniscal tear, for evaluating the tautness of the anterior and posterior cruciate ligaments, and for evaluating the firmness or softness of the articular cartilage and the extent of chondromalacia present. This is done most safely by using the angled portion or elbow of the probe.

Scissors

Several types of scissors are available for arthroscopy of the knee (Fig. 20–16). The scissors may be small or large, left-curved or right-curved, straight, hooked, or rotary-angled. The shaft of the scissors should be no more than 4–5 mm in diameter. Hooked scissors are the ones most commonly used because of their ability to capture tissue and pull it toward the cutting edges.

Basket Forceps

Basket forceps or "biters" are used primarily for resection of meniscal tissue (Figs. 20–17 and 20–18). The basket may be flat, 15 degree up-biting, or 15 degree down-biting. Forceps are available in 0 degree, 30 degree, 45 degree, and 90 degree angles in the side-to-side plane (Fig. 20–19). The shaft of the basket forceps may be straight or curved and is usually no more than 5 mm in diameter. The width of the tissue being resected can be estimated by knowing the size of the basket forceps and how wide the jaw opens. The typical configuration of a basket forceps includes a straight or hooked upper jaw with a lower open base. This punch mechanism allows resection of tissue by an action similar to that of a puncher device used for making holes in paper. When the basket is closed, the tissue drops below the base and free within the

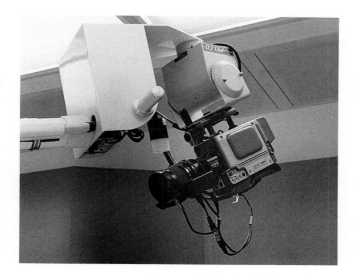

Figure 20–14 • An overhead camera can be used to record surgical technique, and it produces recordings that are useful for teaching.

instruments for which the surgeon has a personal preference. Instruments are available in a variety of shapes, sizes, and angles to allow placement in most areas of the joint with minimal damage to surrounding structures.

Probe

The probe is probably the most valuable tool used in arthroscopy of the knee.[66] As an extension of the hand, it allows the surgeon to feel as well as see the structures of the knee and provides information about the size and consistency of a lesion. The typical probe is angled 90 degrees and has a tip that measures approximately 4 mm (Fig. 20–15). The tip of the probe is smooth and round to

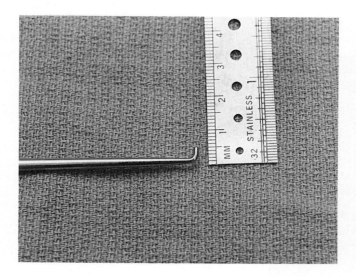

Figure 20–15 • The arthroscopic probe is basic to all arthroscopic procedures. The typical probe is angled 90 degrees and has a tip that measures 3–4 mm.

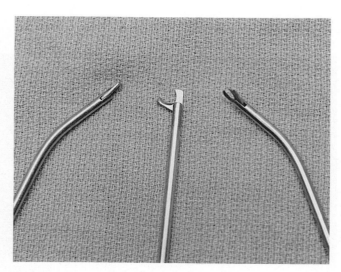

Figure 20–16 • Arthroscopic scissors come in various sizes and angles to allow proper excision of meniscal or plical tissue.

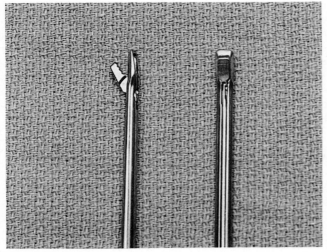

Figure 20–17 • Basket forceps are configured in a low-profile design for ease of passage between the articular surfaces.

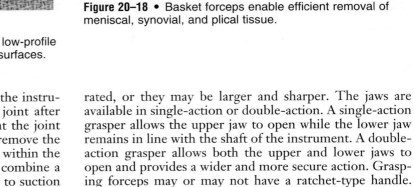

Figure 20–18 • Basket forceps enable efficient removal of meniscal, synovial, and plical tissue.

joint. The advantage of this mechanism is that the instrument does not have to be removed from the joint after each punch maneuver. The disadvantage is that the joint must be irrigated and suctioned thoroughly to remove the resected tissue to prevent loose body formation within the joint. Suction punch devices are available that combine a basket forceps with a cannulated shaft attached to suction tubing to allow simultaneous resection and removal of tissue (Fig. 20–20).

Grasping Forceps

Grasping forceps are used for the removal of tissue, such as loose bodies, meniscal tissue, and cartilage, from the joint (Fig. 20–21). The forceps can be used to apply tension to the meniscus while another instrument is used to resect it. The teeth of the jaws may be multiple and ser-

rated, or they may be larger and sharper. The jaws are available in single-action or double-action. A single-action grasper allows the upper jaw to open while the lower jaw remains in line with the shaft of the instrument. A double-action grasper allows both the upper and lower jaws to open and provides a wider and more secure action. Grasping forceps may or may not have a ratchet-type handle. The ratchet provides a firmer grasp of tissue and decreases the chances of losing the material in the joint or in the soft tissues surrounding the portal.

Knife Blades

Knife blades are used for cutting meniscal tissue before they are removed (Fig. 20–22). The knives come in an assortment of styles, with straight, curved, hooked, or end-cutting blades. Knives are either reusable or disposable.

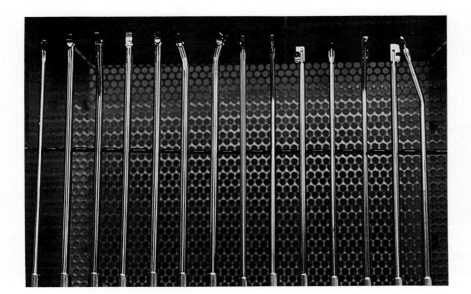

Figure 20–19 • Basket forceps come in various sizes and configurations for ease of manipulation within the knee joint.

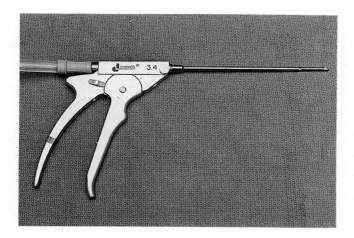

Figure 20–20 • The suction punch allows simultaneous resection and suction removal of meniscal tissue; this dual action requires fewer passages into the knee joint, decreasing the risk of incidental articular damage.

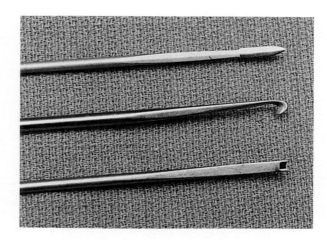

Figure 20–22 • Knife blades for meniscal excision come in various configurations.

Reusable knives have blades that are fixed to the handle, with no risk of being lost within the knee joint. The disadvantage is that they dull with use and become less effective. Disposable knives are always sharp, but older models had the disadvantage of becoming dislodged from the handle and floating free within the joint. Newer types of disposable knives are more difficult to break. The knife should always be passed through a cannula to protect the structures surrounding the portal and within the joint.

Motorized Shaving and Bur Systems

The motorized shaver is a hand-held device that powers numerous types of rotating blades or burs while simultaneously suctioning resected tissue (Fig. 20–23). This device, first described by Johnson,[67] consists of an outer sheath and an inner sheath. The inner sheath spins within the outer sheath, and both have matching openings or windows at the ends. Tissue is cut by the rotating action of the inner sheath, and suction power is generated down the center of the two sheaths. The motorized shaver is controlled by foot pedals mounted on a base (Fig. 20–24). Depressing one pedal rotates the blade in a forward or clockwise direction; depressing another pedal rotates the blade in a reverse or counterclockwise direction. Simultaneously depressing both pedals or a separate pedal oscillates the blade forward and backward. The oscillating mode allows clearance of tissue within the blade and increases the efficiency of the instrument; it is the optimal cutting mode. A sterile power cord connects the motorized shaving unit to a base unit. Sterile suction tubing attached to the base of the motorized shaver removes resected tis-

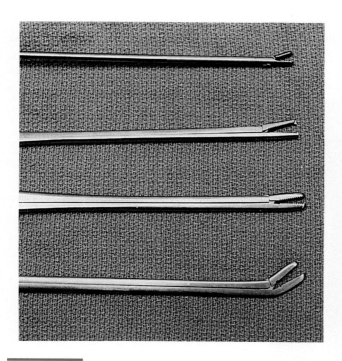

Figure 20–21 • Grasping forceps are used for retrieval of loose bodies or meniscal cartilage.

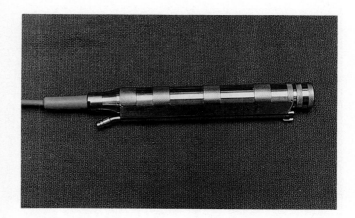

Figure 20–23 • The motorized shaver is the workhorse of knee arthroscopy; it allows simultaneous resection and suction removal of intra-articular pathologic tissue.

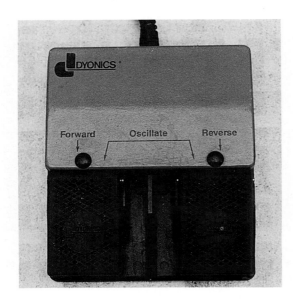

Figure 20–24 • The motorized shaver is controlled by an attached foot pedal that causes the attached blade to be rotated forward or backward or to be oscillated in both directions.

sue. The suction power can be controlled by a minimum-maximum switch, which is located near the head of the unit.

Arthroscopic blade performance with the motorized shaver is determined by proper blade selection, fluid dynamics, and controlled motor drive torque. Blade design is based on the type of tissue to be resected and size of the compartment in which the blade is to be used (Fig. 20–25). The design of the blade must also be safe for adjacent structures. Dozens of disposable arthroscopic surgery blades have been developed. These blades are color-coded,

which makes locating them easier. Once a blade is inserted into the motorized shaving unit, a predetermined initial set speed and speed range for that particular blade is locked in and is displayed on the base unit. The blades range in size from 2.0 to 5.5 mm; blades larger than 3.5 mm are typically used in the knee. Most blades are straight, although some have a slight upward curve. Specific designs are available for resecting meniscus, cartilage, and synovium and for using burs on bone for notchplasty, abrasion chondroplasty, and removal of osteophytes. The 5.5 mm full-radius resector is the most commonly used blade for routine arthroscopy of the knee. This blade has a beveled-end design that works effectively as both a side-cutter and an end-cutter. The blade or bur tip should always be viewed within the joint before use. The blades can be inserted in the knee directly through a portal or through a cannula placed within the portal.

Laser Instruments

Laser is the acronym for Light Amplification by the Stimulated Emission of Radiation. A laser beam can be formed by any wavelength within the electromagnetic spectrum, including infrared, ultraviolet, and visible light. Ultraviolet lasers use the ionizing portion of the electromagnetic spectrum. Infrared or near-infrared lasers use the nonionizing portion of the electromagnetic spectrum and are most commonly used in arthroscopic procedures.[68, 69] Lasers that function in this capacity include the Ho:YAG laser, the Nd:YAG laser, and the CO_2 laser. Because these lasers fall within the invisible portion of the electromagnetic spectrum, a visible laser, such as a red helium-neon laser, is needed as a targeting device.

A laser consists of a medium, a resonator, and an excitation source. The laser medium produces the photons that are converted to energy; the medium may be solid, liquid, or gas. This medium is contained in the laser tube.

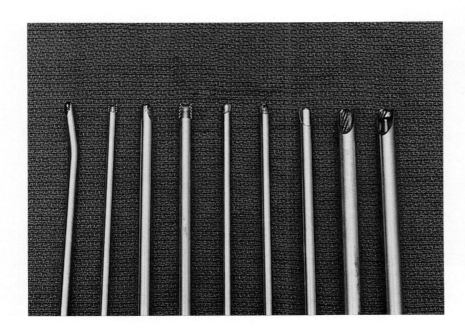

Figure 20–25 • Blades for the motorized shaver come in different designs for varying tissues and compartment sizes. The blades are color-coded for easier location.

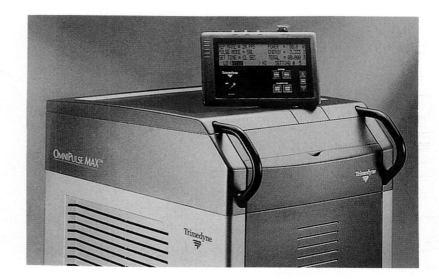

Figure 20–26 • A base unit for the laser allows adjustment of the delivery of the laser beam, depending on the type of procedure.

The excitation source stimulates the electrons contained within the medium into an excited state that causes photons to be emitted once the electrons return to their original state. Laser light can be delivered in continuous or pulsed beams. Operation modes may be contact, noncontact, or near-contact. The latter two operate at variable distances from the target tissue.

The Ho:YAG laser currently is the one most commonly used in arthroscopic procedures of the knee.[70] It is derived from the near-infrared portion of the electromagnetic spectrum and can be used in a standard fluid medium. A reusable fiberoptic cable connects the laser from the base machine to the sterile, operative field (Fig. 20–26). Disposable fiberoptic probes with varying degrees of angulation, including 0 degree, 15 degrees, 30 degrees, 70 degrees, and 90 degrees, can be used for the arthroscopic procedure (Fig. 20–27). The laser's ability to simultaneously cut, coagulate, and ablate allow it to be used in place of a number of arthroscopic instruments, including those used for meniscal ablation and cutting, chondroplasty, removal of synovial plica, lateral release, synovectomy, notchplasty, and débridement of arthrofibrotic scar tissue and osteophytes.[71–75] The laser is especially advantageous in tight knees and for resection of anterior horn meniscal tears, bucket-handle tears, and discoid menisci.[70] Because the laser requires fewer passes within the joint, articular scuffing and operative time are decreased. Its ability to simultaneously cut and coagulate obviates the need for a tourniquet.[76–80] The laser also can be used to contour areas of grades II and III chondromalacia and to congeal small tears, although this welded portion of tissue probably is not as strong as repaired tissue. The laser may, however, stimulate a healing response. The precision of the laser is compromised by a procedure that requires removal of a large amount of material. The time needed to remove a large amount of material with a laser might be better spent by using mechanical instrumentation. In this situation, the laser best serves as a supplemental tool after the bulk of material has been removed by mechanical instrumentation.

A number of safeguards must be observed with the use of lasers in arthroscopy. The eye is the organ most vulnerable to damage by the laser. To prevent damage to the cornea or retina, protective eyewear that is specific to the wavelength of the laser must be worn by the surgeon, the patient, and all operating room personnel while the laser is in use. A sign stating that a laser is in use should be posted on all entrances to the operating room. Although laser

Figure 20–27 • Fiberoptic probes come in various sizes and angles for contouring or ablating soft tissues and bone.

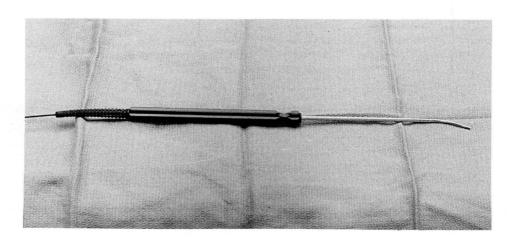

energy is dissipated within several millimeters of the hand-piece tip and is turned on only in the fluid medium contained within the knee joint, the laser can be accidentally engaged when the device is removed from the knee joint. It is important that the surgeon and the operating room personnel be familiar with all aspects of laser use.

Experimental applications of lasers in arthroscopy include cartilage sculpting, meniscal welding, bone drilling, and cement removal.[81, 82] Selective tissue ablation also is a possibility.[76] Research involving the transmission of low levels of laser energy into human chondrocytes for induction of DNA stimulation[83, 84] could lead to potential cartilage repair and regeneration. The use of photoradiation to control certain cellular functions could make possible the biomodulation of various pathologic conditions, such as arthritis, osteonecrosis, and inflammatory states.

Miscellaneous Equipment

The arthroscope is protected by a metal sheath, or cannula, that is slightly larger in diameter; for example, a 4.0 mm arthroscope is placed within a 4.5–5.5 mm cannula. The sheath is placed in the knee joint with a blunt or sharp trocar or obturator. If a sharp trocar is used, the tip should not be placed beyond the capsule to avoid damaging the intra-articular structures. When placing the sheath and obturator through the anterior portals, it is best to direct them toward the intercondylar notch or into the suprapatellar pouch.

An intra-articular electrocautery is available with both cutting and coagulation modes. The plastic tip is insulated and longer than conventional cautery tips. This device can be used safely with physiologic saline solutions. A cannula may be needed to pass the device into the joint to prevent breakage.

Care and Sterilization of Instruments

Although the steam autoclave (Fig. 20–28) is the mainstay of sterilization for most surgical instrumentation, it is not safe for arthroscopic equipment because the high temperatures generated by steam cause deterioration of the sealants. Arthroscopes, cameras, fiberoptic cables, and motorized shavers are quite heat-sensitive. Ethylene oxide gas sterilization is effective but not always feasible in the operating room setting. Because this method typically requires 6–8 hours, it is most useful when sterilizing instruments overnight.[85, 86] Between cases during the day the instruments can be soaked in glutaraldehyde or sterilized in peracetic acid.

Cold disinfection with activated glutaraldehyde has proved to be both safe and effective[85, 87, 88] (Fig. 20–29); however it does not kill spores. Arthroscopes, cameras, fiberoptic cables, and motorized shavers can be soaked in a 2% aqueous solution of glutaraldehyde for approximately 10 minutes after use. Cannulae, forceps, probes, and other arthroscopic instrumentation should be autoclaved. Contact dermatitis, respiratory irritation, and mucous membrane irritation that results in side effects such as epistaxis have been reported in patients and in operating room per-

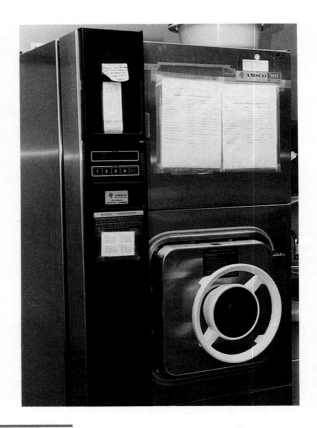

Figure 20–28 • Although arthroscopes, cameras, fiberoptic cables, and motorized shavers are quite heat-sensitive, the steam autoclave is useful for sterilization of accessory arthroscopic instruments, such as probes, cannulae, and forceps.

sonnel from the use of glutaraldehyde-sterilized instruments,[88, 89, 90] and glutaraldehyde-induced synovitis has been reported in patients after arthroscopy. Because of this risk, instruments should be double-rinsed in sterile water after glutaraldehyde soaks.

Peracetic acid sterilization, a more recent technique of disinfection[85, 91] (Fig. 20–30) is bactericidal, fungicidal, and sporicidal yet noncorrosive to instruments. The sterilizer is portable and uses tap water. It functions between 50

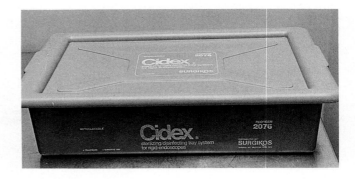

Figure 20–29 • Cold disinfection of arthroscopes, cameras, fiberoptic cables, and motorized shavers with activated glutaraldehyde is safe and effective and requires little time.

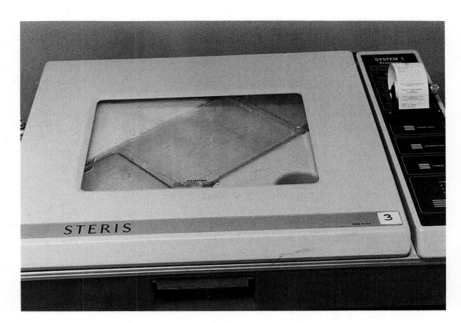

Figure 20–30 • Peracetic acid sterilization is effective and noncorrosive to instruments, which can be safely sterilized in 20–30 minutes.

and 56 degrees centigrade, making it safe for heat-sensitive instruments. Sterilization requires about 20–30 minutes, thus making it efficient for turnover time between cases.

Irrigation Systems

Irrigation systems using continuous inflow and outflow are necessary to provide joint distention and irrigation of the knee for visibility and ease of manipulation of instrumentation. Effective joint distention is essential, especially when working through posterior portals, and the use of continuous irrigation probably plays a role in limiting infection. A physiologic solution is typically recommended for arthroscopic use. Ringer lactate solution is more physiologic than normal saline, causes fewer articular and synovial changes,[92] and has a more positive effect on cartilage metabolism.

Joint distention is maintained by hydrostatic pressure, which is dependent on the rate of inflow and outflow and is accomplished by gravity or inflow-outflow pumps (Fig. 20–31). A number of different set-ups may be used.

One combination is to provide inflow through a large-bore cannula and outflow through the small-bore sheath of the arthroscope. The ingress of fluids should exceed the egress of fluids to maintain hydrostatic pressure and distention of the joint. The possible concentration of bloody fluid or debris flowing toward the arthroscope tip may compromise visibility with this technique. Another common set-up provides inflow through the arthroscope and outflow through a cannula in the suprapatellar pouch. A larger arthroscopic cannula, such as a 5.5 mm cannula, maximizes inflow in this technique. With this technique, cloudy fluid and debris can be forced away from the tip of the arthroscope, leading to a clearer view. This is quite effective when a tourniquet is not used. Another method uses the arthroscope for inflow without the use of a cannula for outflow. Instead, cloudy fluid and debris are cleared by backwashing through the arthroscope cannula

and through a motorized shaver placed in an adjacent portal. The author prefers this method.

At the start of the procedure, two or three 3 L bags of Ringer lactate solution are suspended from an intravenous pole to provide flow to the knee joint by connection with large-bore tubing. Inflow can be provided with the assistance of gravity or by use of an arthroscopic pump. If gravity is used, the fluid bags should be elevated a minimum of 3–5 feet above the level of the knee.[93] Approximately 8–10 feet may be needed for proper joint distention. Arthroscopic pumps have proved to be more effective than the gravity method. A transducer attached to the arthroscope allows a more efficient regulation of fluid to the knee joint. A constant infusion pressure of at least 35–45 mm Hg is required to maintain joint distention. Careful monitoring of fluid pressure is essential to prevent rupture of the knee joint capsule and subsequent compartment syndrome from extravasation of fluid into the surrounding tissues.[94] The pumps typically come with a safety mechanism that shuts down and reverses flow when it senses extreme pressures.

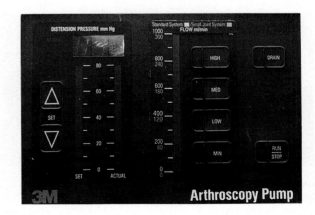

Figure 20–31 • Arthroscopic pumps are helpful in providing joint distention and maintaining hemostasis.

Tourniquet

Even if a tourniquet is not commonly used during knee arthroscopy, it is always wise to have one in place preoperatively in case it is needed. The typical adult pneumatic tourniquet comes in an assortment of lengths, depending on thigh circumference. A tourniquet of sufficient width is required to prevent damage to underlying soft tissues, especially nerves and muscles. The tourniquet width should be at least half the circumference of the limb.[95] A curved tourniquet is believed to provide a more uniform pressure than a straight one. The tourniquet is attached to a monitor that controls the amount of time the tourniquet is inflated and the pressure to which it is inflated (Fig. 20–32). The unit of time is minutes, and the unit of pressure is millimeters of mercury. An alarm on the monitor can be preset to notify the surgeon of a specific tourniquet time.

The maximum tourniquet time and tourniquet pressure are controversial. Muscle necrosis has been reported in animals with a minimum tourniquet time of 120 minutes.[96] Larger-diameter nerves are more susceptible to ischemia than are smaller nerves.[97] Abnormal electromyogram findings have been reported from 6 weeks to 5 months after arthroscopy of the knee involving tourniquet use,[30, 57] especially if tourniquet time exceeded 60 minutes. The use of a tourniquet for more than 30 minutes has been shown to decrease the ability for speedy rehabilitation.[98, 99]

Tourniquet time for procedures of the lower extremity generally should not exceed 120 consecutive minutes because ischemia of nerves and muscle develops at this point. Thus, 90 minutes has been recommended as a safe tourniquet time, although 60 minutes also has been suggested.[100, 101] Other suggestions for preventing nerve or muscle ischemia include deflating the tourniquet for 5 minutes for every hour of inflation to re-establish equilibrium, deflating the tourniquet for 5 minutes after 90 minutes of use before reinflating for an additional 90 minutes, and reperfusion for 10 minutes after 60 minutes of tourniquet time.[102] Other researchers, however, maintain that reperfusion after 120 minutes of tourniquet time could exacerbate muscle and nerve damage and that up to 40 minutes is required for tissues to return to normal after prolonged tourniquet inflation.[103]

The risk of muscle or nerve ischemia can be decreased by the use of lower tourniquet pressures. Tourniquet pressures of up to 350 mm Hg have been recommended for the lower extremity. Some advocate pressures of 100–150 mmHg above the preoperative systolic arm blood pressure. The author routinely uses a tourniquet pressure of 300 mm Hg for arthroscopy of the knee. An Esmarch bandage 4–6 in wide is used to exsanguinate the limb before inflation of the tourniquet.

Leg Holder

A leg holder or lateral post is commonly used during arthroscopy of the knee (Figs. 20–33 and 20–34). Most leg holders allow a pneumatic tourniquet to be placed within them. A leg holder may restrict manipulation of instrumentation in the superior portals and, in some situations, the lateral portals. Although rare, iatrogenic ligament injuries and fractures about the knee may occur with the use of the leg holder, and care must be taken when using this device. The leg holder may be placed proximally or distally on the thigh. Placing it distally allows easier varus and valgus stressing for opening of the lateral and medial compartments, respectively. This may, however, limit

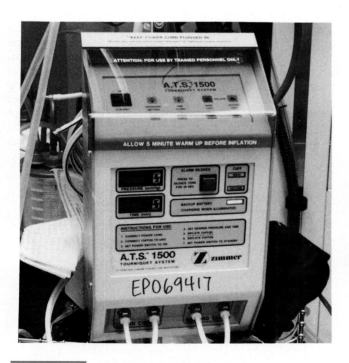

Figure 20–32 • The tourniquet, usually inflated to 300–350 mm Hg for knee arthroscopy, should be left in place no longer than 120 consecutive minutes. The tourniquet should always be placed on the thigh, even though it may not be used routinely during knee arthroscopy.

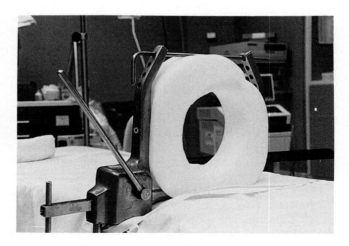

Figure 20–33 • The leg holder should be positioned approximately 8–10 cm above the superior pole of the patella for maximal effectiveness.

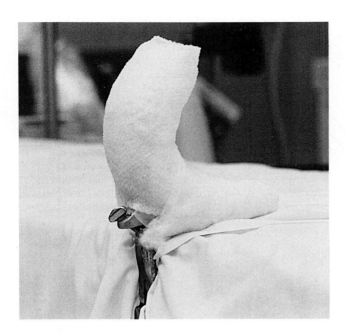

Figure 20–34 • A lateral post allows better access to the superior portals and easier manipulation of the knee during arthroscopy than does a leg holder.

access to the anterior compartment. A more proximal placement provides more space for superior portals and the passing of pins during endoscopic reconstruction of the anterior cruciate ligament. A lateral post is less restrictive, more readily allows the knee to be flexed or placed in the figure-four position, and allows valgus stress to be applied to the knee for better access to the medial compartment.

Regardless of the device used, the extremity should be placed in the various anticipated positions before preparation and draping to ensure proper maneuverability. Abduction of the hip with a valgus external rotation force on the knee allows viewing of the medial compartment, and placing the knee in the figure-of-four position with a downward pressure applied to produce a varus internal rotation force allows viewing of the lateral compartment. The lateral compartment of the knee is usually looser than the medial compartment.[104] With the knee flexed, access to the posterior compartment is easier, whereas with the table flat and the knee extended, access to the anterior compartment is easier.

GENERAL TECHNIQUE

Portals

Portal sites for diagnostic arthroscopy may be either standard or optional (Figs. 20–35 to 20–37). The standard portals generally consist of the anteromedial, anterolateral, posteromedial, and superolateral sites. In the early development of knee arthroscopy, investigators recognized the need for additional portals to carry out a thorough examination of the knee.[105–107] These optional portals include the posterolateral, superomedial, medial parapatellar ten-

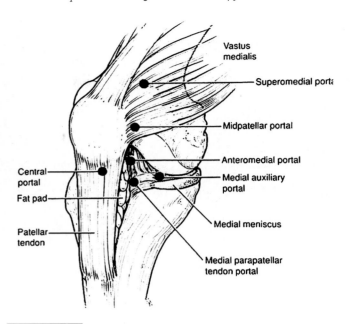

Figure 20–35 • The medial portals. The anteromedial portal is the most commonly used medial portal. (From Scott WN, Insall JN, and Kelly MA: Arthroscopy and meniscectomy: surgical approaches, anatomy, and techniques. In Insall JN [ed.]: Surgery of the Knee, 2nd ed. New York, Churchill Livingstone, 1993, p 166. Copyright by Elizabeth Roselius.)

don, lateral parapatellar tendon, medial auxiliary, lateral auxiliary, medial utility, proximal superomedial, medial midpatellar, lateral midpatellar, and central midpatellar portals.

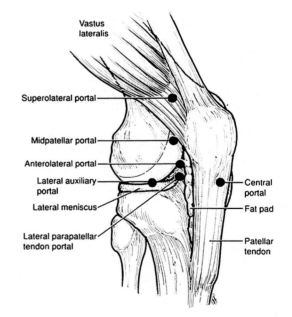

Figure 20–36 • The lateral portals. The anterolateral portal is the most commonly used lateral portal. (From Scott WN, Insall JN, and Kelly MA: Arthroscopy and meniscectomy: surgical approaches, anatomy, and techniques. In Insall JN [ed.]: Surgery of the Knee, 2nd ed. New York, Churchill Livingstone, 1993, p 167. Copyright by Elizabeth Roselius.)

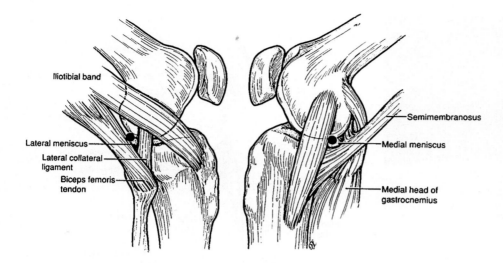

Iliotibial band

Lateral meniscus

Lateral collateral ligament

Biceps femoris tendon

Semimembranosus

Medial meniscus

Medial head of gastrocnemius

Figure 20–37 • The posterolateral and posteromedial portals are useful for lateral and medial meniscal repairs, respectively. (From Scott WN, Insall JN, and Kelly MA: Arthroscopy and meniscectomy: surgical approaches, anatomy, and techniques. In Insall JN [ed.]: Surgery of the Knee, 2nd ed. New York, Churchill Livingstone, 1993, p 168. Copyright by Elizabeth Roselius.)

Knowledge of surface anatomy is essential to safe and successful arthroscopy of the knee. Accurate portal placement minimizes the risk of operative morbidity and allows effective viewing of intra-articular anatomy and efficient manipulation of instruments. When first learning arthroscopy of the knee, it is helpful to mark the anatomic landmarks of the knee before portal placement. These should include the patella, patellar tendon, tibial tubercle, joint line, fibular head, and femoral condyles. The portal sites can then be marked with respect to these structures. This is best accomplished with the knee in about 90 degrees of flexion.

An 18 gauge spinal needle is helpful in locating an initial portal site or subsequent portal sites under direct vision. A No. 11 blade is used to make an incision in the skin and capsule. Because the knife blade is tapered, it should be directed up to extend the capsular incision as it is being withdrawn. The anterior portals may be established before joint distention, once the surgeon is comfortable with the technique. The capsular portal incision may be extended within the skin incision to accommodate larger instrumentation. This results in a more cosmetic incision. When placing the trocar and cannula, the trocar should remain unlocked within the cannula to prevent articular damage in the event of slippage.

Anterolateral Portal

The anterolateral portal is located no more than 1 cm lateral to the edge of the patellar tendon to prevent penetration of the fat pad and approximately 1 cm superior to the lateral joint line to prevent injury to the anterior horn of the lateral meniscus (Fig. 20–38). Penetration and damage to the fat pad can occur if the portal is placed too close to the patellar tendon. With the knee flexed to 90 degrees, this portal is located just distal to the inferior tip of the patella; the presence of the patella alta or patella baja may alter this location. The portal is made by making a vertical or horizontal incision with a No. 11 blade. The incision need be no more than 6–8 mm wide. When using a horizontal incision, the sharp edge of the scalpel should be directed away from the patellar tendon. The horizontal incision is more aesthetically pleasing and minimizes the risk of cutting the meniscus, but portal placement is more critical with this incision than with a vertical incision because improper placement makes manipulation of instruments more difficult. When making a vertical incision, the scalpel should be directed superiorly to minimize the risk of cutting the meniscus. Regardless of the incision made, the knife blade should be directed toward the intercondylar notch to avoid injury to the lateral femoral condyle. The anterolateral portal alone allows viewing of nearly all the structures within the knee and is the principal viewing portal for knee arthroscopy.[108] The posteromedial compartment can also be viewed through the intercondylar notch using this portal.[109, 110]

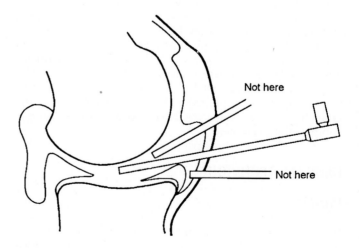

Not here

Not here

Figure 20–38 • The anterior portals should be made just above the superior aspects of the medial and lateral menisci to prevent articular or meniscal damage. (From Johnson LL: Diagnostic and Surgical Arthroscopy of the Knee and Other Joints, 2nd ed. St. Louis, Mosby, 1981.)

Anteromedial Portal

The anteromedial portal is located no more than 1 cm medial to the edge of the patellar tendon and approximately 1 cm superior to the medial joint line in a manner similar to that for the anterolateral portal. Again, this position is optimal for preventing entrapment of the fat pad and damage to the anterior horn of the medial meniscus. The portal is best made under direct vision by first placing an 18 gauge needle into the medial compartment followed by a No. 11 blade. To enter the medial compartment, the needle should be directed in the anterior-to-posterior plane and not toward the intercondylar notch. The anteromedial portal is the main operative instrument portal for knee arthroscopy.

Posteromedial Portal

The posteromedial portal is located posterior to the superficial medial collateral ligament in the soft spot, which is located adjacent to the posteromedial femoral condyle and approximately 1 cm superior to the posteromedial tibial plateau. The portal site is best palpated before distention of the joint and can be marked with a skin marker before beginning the procedure. This portal should not be attempted without proper distention of the joint and without the knee flexed to 90 degrees to protect the posterior neurovascular structures. By placing the arthroscope in the anterolateral portal and through the intercondylar notch, and by looking posteromedially, the skin can be transilluminated with the arthroscope, and the posteromedial corner can be palpated.[111–113] An 18 gauge needle is then directed toward the joint before making an incision and placing a trocar and cannula. The needle can be used as a probe. This portal allows viewing of the posterior horn of the medial meniscus and the posterior cruciate ligament, in addition to removal of loose bodies and synovectomy.[114] The saphenous nerve and vein can be injured during placement of this portal. The vein can be transilluminated to protect it from injury during portal placement.

Posterolateral Portal

The posterolateral portal is located posterior to the iliotibial band and the lateral collateral ligament and anterior to the biceps femoris tendon, lateral head of the gastrocnemius, and peroneal nerve. This is 1–2 cm above the joint line, along the posterolateral edge of the femoral condyle. This portal is best palpated with the joint maximally distended and with the knee flexed to 90 degrees in the figure-four position to protect the posterior neurovascular structures. A stab incision is made in the skin over the portal site. A cannula and trocar are then used to puncture the capsule, using the posterior edge of the lateral femoral condyle as a guide to enter the posterolateral compartment. The cannula and trocar should be directed toward the joint and away from the neurovascular structures posteriorly. This portal can be used for repairs of the posterior horn of the lateral meniscus.

Superomedial and Superolateral Portals

The superomedial and superolateral portals are located at the superior border of the patella. The portals have been described 0.5–4.0 cm superior to the patella and slightly medial or lateral to the respective border of the quadriceps tendon.[115] The portals should be made with the knee held in extension to increase the space in the anterior compartment. If placed improperly, a subsynovial location may be entered. If placed too distally, the cannula may become bound in the patellofemoral joint with flexion past 90 degrees. With the knee in extension, the extensor mechanism is sufficiently relaxed to allow passage of the arthroscope beyond the patella.[104] These portals are commonly used for inflow or outflow. If used for inflow, an extrasynovial placement of fluid and subsequent collapse of the joint may occur, which would inhibit arthroscopy of the joint. There should be free movement of the cannula within the joint before initiating inflow. In addition to inflow of fluids, these portals can be used for evaluation of patellofemoral tracking, synovectomy, removal of loose bodies, excision of a pathologic medial plica, and arthroscopic lateral reiease. The portals are made by a stab incision in the skin with a No. 11 blade. The superolateral portal is made by subluxing the patella laterally to provide better identification of the extensor mechanism. The superomedial portal is made by displacing the patella medially. A cannula with a blunt trocar should be used to prevent damage to the cartilage. The cannula and trocar should be directed horizontally or perpendicularly to the patella to prevent damage to the articular cartilage. Some authors have suggested that in making a superomedial portal, the medial retinaculum is partially released, increasing the risk of lateral subluxation. Injury to the anterior branches of the femoral cutaneous nerve and the anterior branches of the saphenous nerve can occur with use of the superomedial portal. Postoperative numbness due to injury to the lateral femoral cutaneous nerve is possible with use of the superolateral portal.[116] Use of the superolateral portal with the two-incision anterior cruciate ligament reconstruction technique may be cumbersome.

Proximal Superomedial Portal

The proximal superomedial portal is located 4 cm superior to the patella and in line with the medial border of the patella. This portal is useful in evaluating the anterior compartment, especially the patellofemoral joint.[117]

Medial and Lateral Auxiliary Portals

The medial auxiliary portal is located approximately 2–3 cm medial to the anteromedial portal, immediately anterior to the medial collateral ligament. The lateral auxiliary portal is located approximately 2–3 cm lateral to the anterolateral portal, well anterior to the lateral collateral ligament. Both are placed 1 cm above the joint line. These supplemental portals provide sites for additional instruments required for certain procedures. These portals are best made under direct vision by first placing an 18 gauge spinal needle because the risk of damage to the respective femoral condyle or meniscus is increased in such a tight area.

Medial and Lateral Midpatellar Portals

The medial and lateral midpatellar portals are located adjacent to their respective medial and lateral borders of the patella at its widest point.[118] These portals are useful when viewing of the anterior compartment is desired while other anterior portals are being used. Use of one of these portals for viewing frees the remaining anterior portals for instrumentation[119] and allows thorough inspection of most of the anterior and some of the posterior intra-articular knee structures.

Medial Utility Portal

The medial utility portal is located approximately 1–2 cm proximal to the standard anteromedial portal.[120] This portal is immediately bounded by the contour of the medial femoral condyle, the medial tibial plateau, and the medial edge of the patella and proximal patella tendon. It allows viewing of the anterior horn of the lateral meniscus, intercondylar notch, and medial compartment.

Central Transpatellar Tendon Portal

The central transpatellar tendon portal is located in the midline of the patellar tendon, approximately 1 cm inferior to the patella. It has also been described at the halfway point between the medial and lateral femoral condyles, which is slightly medial to the midline of the patellar tendon.[121, 122] With the knee flexed 90 degrees, a vertical incision is made through the skin and in line with the fibers of the patellar tendon. A blunt trocar and cannula are placed, followed by insertion of the arthroscope directed superiorly to the fat pad. This portal allows viewing of the posterior compartment and frees the anterior portals for additional instrumentation.[123, 124] A 70 degree arthroscope placed through the intercondylar notch may be used for viewing the posterior compartment, including the posterior cruciate ligament.[125, 126] Care must be taken not to damage fibers of the patellar tendon. Triangulation with instruments in the adjacent anteromedial or anterolateral portals may be difficult because of their proximity. Postoperative pain and stiffness have been reported after the use of the central transpatellar tendon portal,[67] and isokinetic testing of the extensor mechanism performed 2 weeks postoperatively revealed a 9% decrease in strength.[127] This portal can also be used after harvest of the central third of the patellar tendon.

Triangulation

Triangulation involves the use of the arthroscope with at least one other instrument. The separate instrument or instruments form the apex of a triangle with the arthroscope. Triangulation requires a minimum of two portals, usually the anterolateral and anteromedial portals. A minimum distance of 2–3 cm between the portals is required for effective triangulation. Three basic principles apply:[128] the pathologic condition should be defined, the steps required to accomplish the procedure should be conceptualized, and the appropriate portals and instrumentation should be selected. When first learning to triangulate, it is helpful to use a probe with the arthroscope. Other types of instrumentation can be added once skill is gained. There is a learning curve associated with mastery of this procedure.

AUTHOR'S METHOD FOR STANDARD ARTHROSCOPIC EXAMINATION

With the patient supine and with satisfactory anesthesia initiated, knee examination is carried out and documented. This includes measurement of the range of motion from extension to flexion, patellar mobility, tibial stepoff, and a thorough ligament examination. Results of anterior and posterior drawer, Lachman, pivot-shift, reverse pivot-shift, and McMurray tests and evaluation of varus and valgus stability at 0 degree and 30 degrees of flexion are recorded. External rotation is checked at 30 degrees and 90 degrees of flexion. These findings are compared with those of the uninvolved extremity. A well-padded tourniquet is placed on the mid-to-distal thigh, which is placed within a leg holder 4–5 fingerbreadths above the superior pole of the patella. The operating table is then adjusted to allow both knees to flex to 90 degrees. The popliteal regions of both knees are protected with eggshell pads, as is the heel of the nonoperative extremity. The nonoperative extremity is secured to the flexed portion of the operating table with a sheet. An Esmarch bandage is used to exsanguinate the limb, and the tourniquet is inflated to 300 mm Hg. The lower extremity is then prepared and draped (Fig. 20–39).

The anterolateral portal is made by palpating the lateral joint line and making a horizontal incision no more than 1 cm lateral to the patellar tendon and just inferior to the patella. The sharp edge of the blade should be directed away from the patellar tendon to prevent incidental damage to this structure. Inflow is provided through the arthroscope by using a pump set at 55–65 mm Hg. [Editor's note: 35–40 mm Hg is often sufficient for the knee.] With the medial compartment viewed through the arthroscope, an anteromedial portal is made under direct vision. This is accomplished by first placing an 18 gauge needle into the medial compartment to locate the proper portal site. The needle is then removed, and a horizontal portal is made with a No. 11 blade, again with the sharp edge of the blade pointed away from the patellar tendon. A probe is placed in this portal, and a systematic diagnostic arthroscopic examination is performed.

With the knee held in extension and the foot supported by the waist of the surgeon, the anterior compartment is viewed by directing the arthroscope up toward the patella and down toward the trochlear groove of the femur. Patellar tracking is then evaluated by flexing the knee. The presence of a plica is noted. The knee is then

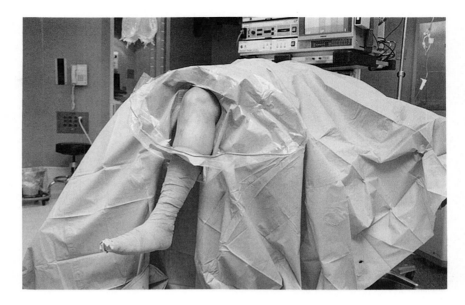

Figure 20–39 • For diagnostic knee arthroscopy, the patient is placed in the supine position with both knees flexed just beyond the break in the operating table.

allowed to flex approximately 30 degrees, and the medial compartment is viewed by applying a valgus stress, with the heel supported on the outside waist of the surgeon (Fig. 20–40). Better leverage can be obtained by lowering the table. The medial gutter is checked for disease when moving the arthroscope from the anterior compartment to the medial compartment. The articular surfaces of the medial compartment are examined and probed with the angled part of the probe. The knee is flexed to allow a better view of the posterior portion of the medial femoral condyle. The medial meniscus is probed on its superior and inferior surfaces. The posterior horn of the medial meniscus is viewed through the intercondylar notch medial to the posterior cruciate ligament. This is accomplished by directing the arthroscope to this position or by first placing a blunt trocar and cannula blindly along the lateral border of the medial femoral condyle, then remov-

ing the trocar and placing the arthroscope. Again, the top surfaces and undersurfaces of the medial meniscus are probed. The capsule adjacent to the posterior horn is probed with an 18 gauge needle placed in the site of the posteromedial portal. The notch is then viewed, and the anterior and posterior cruciate ligaments are probed. The extremity is then placed in the figure-four position, and the lateral compartment is examined in a manner similar to that of the medial compartment (Fig. 20–41). The lateral gutter is also examined for disease. At the completion of the procedure, a drain is placed through a cannula into one of the portals. The portals are not closed. A sterile, compressive dressing is applied, and the tourniquet is deflated.

If ligament reconstruction is anticipated, the knee is kept in extension, and the full operating table with a lateral post is used (Fig. 20–42). A bean bag is secured to the end of the table before preparing and draping. With the pa-

Figure 20–40 • The medial compartment is viewed by applying a valgus stress to the knee with the hip of the surgeon.

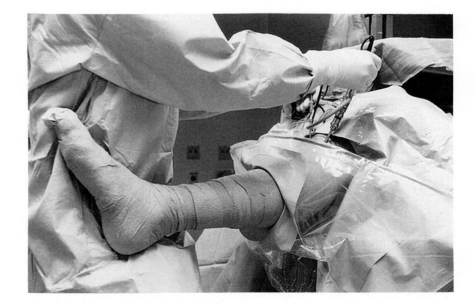

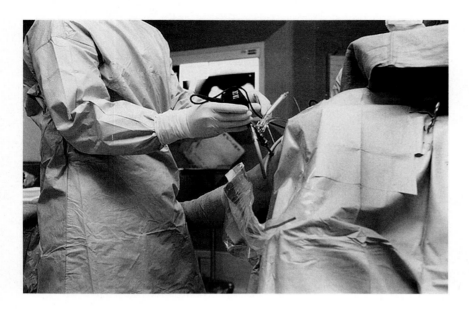

Figure 20–41 • The lateral compartment is viewed by applying a varus stress; the patient's leg is held in a figure-four position against the surgeon's hip.

tient's toes placed on the bean bag, the knee should be flexed to 90 degrees (Fig. 20–43). With the heel placed on the bean bag, the knee should be flexed to 60 degrees. The medial compartment is viewed with valgus stress applied to the knee at the lateral post (Fig. 20–44). The lateral compartment is viewed by placing the knee in the figure-four position (Fig. 20–45).

POSTOPERATIVE CARE

An intra-articular drain should be placed if postoperative bleeding is anticipated. The drain should be brought out through a separate incision and can be removed before the patient is discharged from the outpatient unit or at 1–2 days postoperatively, depending on the procedure performed. Prophylactic antibiotics, intravenous or by mouth,

typically are not indicated after surgery unless an open procedure has been performed, in which case they are given for 24–48 hours.

A postoperative intra-articular injection of bupivacaine has been shown to be useful for postoperative pain control.[129–134] The dosage required is controversial. Thirty milliliters of 0.50% bupivacaine has been found to be effective in reducing opioid use in the recovery room, improving early mobility, and allowing earlier discharge from the hospital.[135] Thirty milliliters of 0.25% bupivacaine injected intra-articularly has not been shown to have any apparent benefit, although this is controversial.[35] Bupivacaine has been shown not to damage articular cartilage, and serum levels of bupivacaine have been observed to remain below toxic levels even after intra-articular injection of up to 150 mg.[136–141] Morphine, alone or with bupivacaine, has not been found to significantly affect

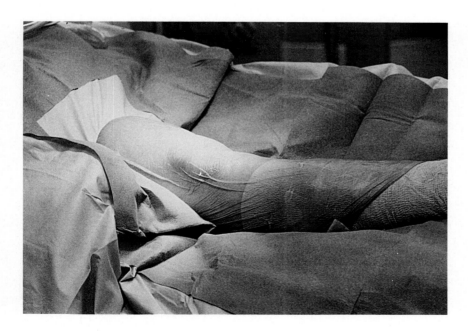

Figure 20–42 • If ligament reconstruction is planned, the patient is placed in the supine position with both lower extremities supported on the operating table.

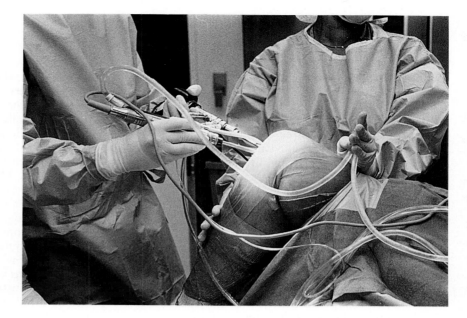

Figure 20–43 • A sand bag or large intravenous bag is secured to the foot of the bed preoperatively to allow the knee to be held flexed with minimal support.

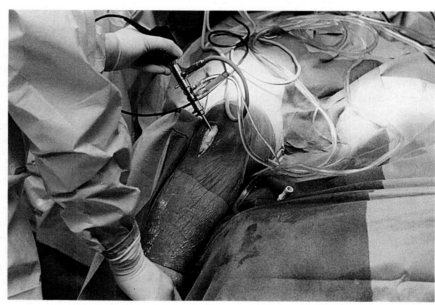

Figure 20–44 • Using the lateral post to apply a valgus stress across the knee allows viewing of the medial compartment.

Figure 20–45 • Placing the lower extremity in the figure-four position allows viewing of the lateral compartment.

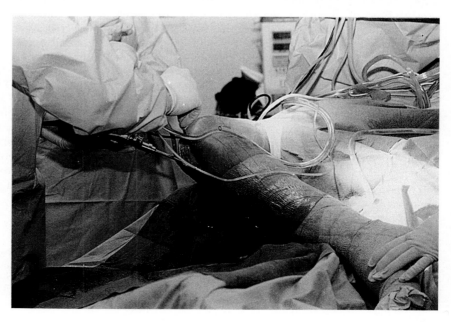

postoperative pain, need for supplemental anesthesia, or weight-bearing status.[142] Preoperative pain has been found to be an important predictor of postoperative pain.

The portal sites can be closed with an interrupted 2-0 or 3-0 nylon suture or with adhesive strips or can be left open to heal primarily. A sterile, compressive dressing and a knee immobilizer or brace, when indicated, are placed, followed by immediate icing and elevation of the extremity. A predetermined limit of flexion or extension may be selected for the brace. Elevation of the affected limb with icing of the knee for 10–15 minutes every 1–2 hours minimizes postoperative pain and swelling. Crutches are used after treatment of chondral defects or osteochondritis dissecans or other procedures that require protected weight-bearing.

Oral narcotic analgesia is usually sufficient for 4–5 days following surgery. Oral or intramuscular NSAIDs may be indicated, especially when synovectomy or lysis of adhesions has been performed, provided there are no contraindications to the use of these medications.

An organized approach to outpatient arthroscopic surgery is required to allow early return to function.[143, 144] Sedentary activities can usually be resumed within the first few days after surgery,[145] but this is relative, and factors that influence return include the procedure performed, level of pain, wound status, range of motion, strength, and type of activity, job, or sport the patient is returning to.

Postoperative rehabilitation depends on the procedure performed. The typical postoperative rehabilitation program after partial meniscectomy consists of stretching and strengthening exercises. Isometrics should be begun in the immediate postoperative period. Strengthening exercises should include quadriceps sets, ankle pumps, 90–45-degree knee extensions, minisquats, and abduction and adduction straight leg raises. Stretching to maintain or improve range of motion should include hamstring, quadriceps, and heel cord stretches. Stationary cycling, in addition to passive and active-assisted knee flexion, may also be included. More progressive lower extremity weight exercises are sometimes indicated. Supervised rehabilitation should progress to a home program when deemed appropriate by the physician and therapist.

At time of discharge, whether from the outpatient unit or after a brief hospital stay, an instruction sheet should be provided to the patient. It should reiterate what the physician should have already explained to the patient regarding potential postoperative complications. A follow-up phone call by the physician, nurse, or other qualified personnel can be quite helpful to the patient after surgery and before the initial postoperative visit.

COMPLICATIONS

Potential complications after arthroscopic surgery of the knee are numerous but, fortunately, uncommon. Complications can occur at the time of surgery or during the postoperative period. Compications at the time of surgery include problems with anesthesia, instrumentation, and surgical technique.

Most arthroscopic procedures are performed on an outpatient basis. An unusual set of problems with anesthe-

sia may occur as a result of this. As with any procedure, careful preoperative assessment by the surgeon and anesthesiologist should be performed. Even though the patient has been instructed not to eat or drink anything for 6–8 hours before the procedure, problems with communication or compliance may lead to aspiration of gastric contents. Drug allergies and idiosyncratic reactions may occur with regional anesthesia, especially spinal anesthesia. Spinal headaches may also develop as a result of this form of anesthesia. The patient should be carefully monitored for an appropriate amount of time after the procedure, and certain criteria must be met after outpatient surgery and before the patient is discharged.

Arthroscopy of the knee requires the use of numerous pieces of equipment. It is the responsibility of the surgeon to be familiar with all instruments used during the procedure. Problems with the tourniquet, leg holder, pump, and arthroscopic instruments may occur during the procedure. Specific problems with and suggested guidelines for the use of a tourniquet are discussed earlier.

Injuries to the medial collateral ligament with the use of a leg holder have been reported to occur in 0.04% of arthroscopic knee procedures and account for 4.4% of all complications.[146] For this reason, the surgeon must use great care when manipulating the knee with a leg holder.

If a pump is used during arthroscopy, it must be carefully monitored, especially when the medial or lateral collateral ligaments and their respective adjacent capsules have been disrupted. Rupture of the capsules and compartment syndrome have been reported.[147, 148]

The arthroscope and various instruments used during the procedure all have potential for breakage within the joint. If this occurs, the position of the knee must be maintained, and the inflow should be directed away from the broken piece to prevent movement away from the field of view. Fluoroscopy may be needed to locate a fragment of instrumentation that can no longer be seen within the joint. Magnetic retrieval devices have been designed for such situations.

Complications as a result of surgical technique are usually related to the experience and skill of the surgeon. Hemarthrosis is common after arthroscopy of the knee, especially after arthroscopic lateral release.[32, 149, 150] An electrocautery can be used on the anterior branch of the lateral geniculate artery and can reduce the risk of this problem. The incidence of infection after arthroscopic knee surgery has been reported to range from 0.04 to 0.8%.[87, 146] Thrombophlebitis has been reported after 0.1–1.6% of arthroscopic procedures,[146, 151] with pulmonary emboli occurring in up to 25% of those patients. Arterial injury can occur by accidental penetration of the posterior capsule and should be treated immediately by a vascular surgeon. Complications can be minimized by paying attention to detail and by using the correct instruments designed for a particular situation.

References

1. Takagi N: Practical experiences using Takagi's arthroscope. J Jpn Orthop Assoc 8:132–139, 1933.
2. Burman MS: Arthroscopy of the direct visualization of joints. J Bone Joint Surg 13:669–695, 1931.

3. Watanabe M, Takeda S, and Ikeuchi H: Atlas of Arthroscopy. Tokyo, Igaku Shoin, Ltd., 1957.

4. Jackson RW: The scope of arthroscopy. Clin Orthop 208:69–71, 1986.

5. Joyce JJ and Jackson RW: History of arthroscopy. In American Academy of Orthopaedic Surgery Symposium of Arthroscopy and Arthrography of the Knee. St. Louis, C.V. Mosby Co.:1978, 1–8.

6. O'Connor RL: Arthroscopy. Philadelphia, J.B. Lippincott Co., 1977.

7. Casscells SW: Arthroscopy of the knee joint. J Bone Joint Surg Am 53:287–298, 1971.

8. Jackson RW and Abe I: The role of arthroscopy in the management of disorders of the knee. J Bone Joint Surg Br 57:310–322, 1972.

9. O'Connor RL: Arthroscopy in the diagnosis and treatment of acute ligament injuries of the knee. J Bone Joint Surg Am 56:333–337, 1974.

10. Dandy DJ and Jackson RW: The impact of arthroscopy in the management of disorders of the knee. J Bone Joint Surg Br 57:346–348, 1975.

11. DeHaven KE and Collins HR: Diagnosis of internal derangement of the knee: the role of arthroscopy. J Bone Joint Surg Am 57:802–810, 1975.

12. McGinty JB and Freedman PA: Arthroscopy of the knee. Clin Orthop 121:173–180, 1976.

13. Jackson RW: Current concepts review: arthroscopic surgery. J Bone Joint Surg Am 65:416–420, 1983.

14. Ikeuchi H: Surgery under arthroscopic control. Rheumatologie 33:57–64, 1976.

15. Casscells SW: Arthroscopy: Diagnostic and Surgical Practice. Philadelphia, Lea & Febiger, 1984.

16. Dandy DJ: The impact of arthroscopic surgery on the management of disorders of the knee. Arthroscopy 6:96–99, 1990.

17. Jackson RW: The scope of arthroscopy. Clin Orthop 208:69–71, 1986.

18. Dandy DJ: Arthroscopy in the treatment of young patients with anterior knee pain. Orthop Clin North Am 17:221–229, 1986.

19. Drez D: Arthroscopic evaluation of the injured athlete's knee. Clin Sports Med 4:275–278, 1985.

20. Kurosaka M, Ohno O, and Hirohata K: Arthroscopic evaluation of synovitis in the knee joints. Arthroscopy 7:162–170, 1991.

21. Dzioba RB, Stroken A, and Mulbry L: Diagnostic arthroscopy and longitudinal open lateral release: a safe and effective treatment for "chondromalacia patella." Arthroscopy 1:131–135, 1985.

22. Sugawara O, Miyatsu M, Yamashita I, et al.: Problems with repeated arthroscopic surgery in the discoid meniscus. Arthroscopy 7:68–71, 1991.

23. Dzioba RB: The classification and treatment of acute articular cartilage lesions. Arthroscopy 4:72–80, 1988.

24. Chapple CR and Porter KM: An unusual use for the arthroscope. Injury 15:351–352, 1984.

25. Zarins B: Arthroscopic surgery in a sports medicine practice. Orthop Clin North Am 13:415–421, 1982.

26. Wasilewski SA and Frankl U: Arthroscopy of the painful dysfunctional total knee replacement. Arthroscopy 5:294–297, 1989.

27. Wasilewski SA and Frankl U: Fracture of polyethylene of patellar component in total knee arthroscopy, diagnosed by arthroscopy. J Arthroplasty 4(suppl):19–22, 1989.

28. Jardon OM, Huurman WW, and Barak AJ: Malignant hyperthermia: avoiding a lethal complication. Contemp Orthop 7:77–84, 1983.

29. Lidge RT: Environment in operative arthroscopy. In McGinty JB et al. (eds.): Operative Arthroscopy. New York, Raven Press, 1991.

30. Johnson LL and Becker RL: Arthroscopy, technique, and the role of the assistant. Orthop Rev 5:31–43, 1976.

31. Pevey JK: Outpatient arthroscopy of the knee under local anesthesia. Am J Sports Med 6:122–127, 1978.

32. McGinty JB and Matza RA: Arthroscopy of the knee: evaluation of an outpatient procedure under local anesthesia. J Bone Joint Surg Am 60:787–789, 1978.

33. Chirwa SS, Macleod BA, and Day B: Intraarticular bupivacaine (Marcaine) after arthroscopic meniscectomy: a randomized double-blind controlled study. Arthroscopy 5:33–35, 1989.

34. Gerber H, Censier K, Gachter A, et al.: Intraarticular absorption of bupivacaine during arthroscopy—comparison of 0.25%, 0.5% and 0.75% solution (abstract). Anesthesiology 61A:217, 1985.

35. Henderson RC, Campion ER, DeMasi RA, et al.: Postarthroscopy analgesia with bupivacaine. Am J Sports Med 18:614–617, 1990.

36. Martin RC, Brow DE, Zell BK, et al.: Diagnostic and operative arthroscopy of the knee under local anesthesia with parenteral medication. Am J Sports Med 17:436–439, 1988.

37. Hultin J, Hambert P, and Stenstrom A: Knee arthroscopy using local anesthesia. Arthroscopy 8:239–241, 1992.

38. Yoshiya S, Kurosaka M, Hirohata K, et al.: Knee arthroscopy using local anesthetic. Arthroscopy 4:86–89, 1988.

39. Kirkeby OJ and Aase S: Knee arthroscopy and arthrotomy under local anesthesia. Acta Orthop Scand 58:133–134, 1987.

40. Ngo IU, Hamilton WG, Wichern WA, et al.: Local anesthesia with sedation for arthroscopic surgery of the knee: a report of 100 consecutive cases. Arthroscopy 1:237–241, 1985.

41. Shapiro MS, Safran MR, Crockett H, et al.: Local anesthesia for knee arthroscopy: efficacy and cost benefits. Am J Sports Med 23:50–53, 1995.

42. Halperin N, Axer A, Hirschberg E, et al.: Arthroscopy of the knee under local anesthesia and controlled pressure irrigation. Clin Orthop 134:176–179, 1978.

43. Hagenouw R, Bridenbaugh PO, van Egmond J, et al.: Tourniquet pain: a volunteer study. Anesth Analg 65:1171–1180, 1986.

44. Gerber H, Censier K, Gachter A, et al.: Intraarticular absorption of bupivacaine during arthroscopy: a comparison of 0.25%, 0.5% and 0.75% solution. Anesthesiology 63A:217, 1985.

45. Meining RB, Holtgrewe JL, Weidel JD, et al.: Plasma bupivacaine levels following single dose intraarticular instillation for arthroscopy. Am J Sports Med 16:295–300, 1988.

46. Carnes RS, Butterworth JF, Poehling GG, et al.: Safety and efficacy of intraarticular bupivacaine and epinephrine anesthesia for knee arthroscopy. Anesthesiology 71A:729, 1989.

47. Yoshiya S, Kurosaka M, Hirohita K, et al.: Knee arthroscopy using local anesthetic. Arthroscopy 4:86–89, 1988.

48. Weiker GG, Kuivila TE, and Pippingen CE: Serum lidocaine and bupivacaine levels in local technique knee arthroscopy. Am J Sports Med 19: 499–502, 1991.

49. Saunders B and Wing PC: Washout of local anesthetic during arthroscopy. Arthroscopy 4:90–92, 1988.

50. Erikson E, Haggmark T, Saartok T, et al.: Knee arthroscopy with local anesthesia in ambulatory patients. Orthopedics 9:186–188, 1986.

51. Hultin J, Hamberg P, and Stenstiom A: Knee arthroscopy under local anesthesia. Arthroscopy 8:239–241, 1992.

52. Raj PP: Rationale and choice for surgical procedures. In Raj PP (ed.): Clinical Practice of Regional Anesthesia. New York, Churchill Livingstone, 1990.

53. Modig J, Borg T, Karlstrom G, et al.: Thromboembolism after total hip replacement: role of epidural and general anesthesia. Anesth Analg 62:174–180, 1983.

54. Modig J, Maripuu E, and Sahlstedt B: Thromboembolism following total hip replacement: a prospective investigation of 94 patients with emphasis on the efficacy of lumbar epidural anesthesia in prophylaxis. Reg Anesth 11:72–79, 1986.

55. Yeager MP, Glass DD, Neff RK, et al.: Epidural anesthesia and analgesia in high-risk surgical patients. Anesthesiology 66:729–736, 1987.

56. DeJong RH and Heavner JE: Diazepam prevents and aborts lidocaine convulsions in monkeys. Anesthesiology 41:226–230, 1974.

57. Abbott PJ and Shiffrin J: Anesthesia and postoperative pain management for knee surgery. In Fu FH, Harner CD, and Vince KG (eds.): Knee Surgery. Baltimore, Williams & Wilkins, 1994, pp 557–581.

58. Adam HK, Briggs LP, Bahar M, et al.: Pharmacokinetic evaluation of ICI 35 868 in man: single induction doses with different rates of injection. Br J Anaesth 55:97–103, 1983.

59. Way WL and Trevor AJ: Pharmacology of intravenous nonnarcotic anesthetics. In Miller RD (ed.): Anesthesia, 2nd ed. New York, Churchill Livingstone, 1986, pp 779–883.

60. Wetchler BV: Anesthesia for Ambulatory Surgery. Philadelphia, J.B. Lippincott Co., 1985.

61. American Board of Anesthesiology, Inc.: Book of Information. Office of the Board, 1985.

62. Eichhorn JH, Cooper JB, Cullen DJ, et al.: Standards for patient monitoring during anesthesia at Harvard Medical School. JAMA 256:1017–1020, 1986.

63. Shevde K and Panagopoulos G: A survey of 800 patients' knowl-

edge, attitudes and concerns regarding anesthesia. Anesth Analg 73:190–198, 1991.

64. Eriksson E, Haggmark T, Saartok T, et al.: Knee arthroscopy with local anesthesia in ambulatory patients: methods, results and patient compliance. Orthopedics 9:186–188, 1986.

65. Hall BA: Nerve injury during anesthesia. In: Faust RJ (ed.): Anesthesiology Review. New York, Churchill Livingstone, 1991, pp 477–478.

66. Metcalf RW: Instr Course Lect 30. C.V. Mosby Co., St. Louis, 1981.

67. Johnson LL: Diagnostic and Surgical Arthroscopy of the Knee and Other Joints, 2nd ed. St. Louis, C.V. Mosby Co., 1981, p 128.

68. Dew DK: Laser biophysics for the orthopaedic surgeon. Clin Orthop 310:6–13, 1995.

69. Glossop ND, Jackson RW, Koort HJ, et al.: The excimer laser in orthopaedics. Clin Orthop 310:72–81, 1995.

70. Dillingham MF, Fanton GS, and Thabit G: Laser-assisted arthroscopic meniscal surgery of the knee. Oper Tech Orthop 5:39–45, 1995.

71. Sherk HH, Black JD, Prodoehl JA, et al.: The effects of lasers and electrosurgical devices on human meniscal tissue. Clin Orthop 310:14–20, 1995.

72. Vangsness CT, Akl Y, Nelson SJ, et al.: In vitro analysis of laser meniscectomy. Clin Orthop 310:21–26, 1995.

73. Schaffer JL, Dark M, Itzkan I, et al.: Mechanisms of meniscal ablation by short pulse laser irradiation. Clin Orthop 310:30–36, 1995.

74. Forman SK, Oz MC, Lontz JF, et al.: Laser-assisted fibrin clot soldering of human menisci. Clin Orthop 310:37–41, 1995.

75. Shapiro GS, Fanton GS, Dillingham MF, et al.: Lateral retinacular release: the holmium: YAG laser versus electrocautery. Clin Orthop 310:42–47, 1995.

76. O'Brien SJ, Garrick JG, Jackson RW, et al.: Lasers in orthopaedic surgery. Contemp Orthop 22:61–91, 1991.

77. O'Brien SJ and Miller DV: The contact Nd:YAG laser: a new approach to arthroscopic laser surgery. Clin Orthop 252:95–100, 1990.

78. Smith CF, Johansen WE, Vangsness CT, et al.: The carbon dioxide laser: a potential tool for orthopaedic surgery. Clin Orthop 242:43–50, 1985.

79. Whipple TL, Caspari RB, and Meyers JF: Laser energy in arthroscopic meniscectomy. Orthopedics 6:1165–1169, 1983.

80. Whipple TL, Caspari RB, and Meyers JF: Arthroscopic meniscectomy by CO2 laser vaporization in a gas medium. Arthroscopy 1:2–7, 1985.

81. Forman SK, Oz MC, Lontz JF, et al.: Laser-assisted fibrin clot soldering of human menisci. Clin Orthop 310: 37–41, 1995.

82. Trauner KB, Nishioka NS, Flotte T, et al.: Acute and chronic response of articular cartilage to holmium:YAG laser irradiation. Clin Orthop 310:52–57, 1995.

83. Ohta A, Abergel RP, and Uitto J: Laser modulation of human immune system: inhibition of lymphocyte proliferation by gallium-arsenide laser at low energy. Lasers Surg Med 7:199–201, 1987.

84. Whipple TL: The future of lasers in orthopaedic surgery. Semin Orthop 7:131–133, 1992.

85. Johnson GM, Mancuso R, and Whitbook C: Sterilization methods: keeping up with health trends. Med Rev Outlook 3:1, 1992.

86. Johnson LL, Schneider D, Goodman FG, et al.: A cold sterilization method for arthroscopes using activated dialdehyde. Orthop Rev 6:75–77, 1977.

87. Johnson LL, Shneider DA, Austin MD, et al.: Two percent glutaraldehyde: a disinfectant in arthroscopy and arthroscopic surgery. J Bone Joint Surg Am 64:237–239, 1982.

88. Harner CD, Fu FH, Mason GC, et al.: Cidex-induced synovitis. Am J Sports Med 17:96–102, 1989.

89. Fowler JF Jr: Allergic contact dermatitis from glutaraldehyde exposure. J Occup Med 31:852–853, 1989.

90. Wiggins P, McCurdy SA, and Zeidenberg W: Epistaxis due to glutaraldehyde exposure. J Occup Med 31:854–856, 1989.

91. Crow S: Peracetic acid sterilization: a timely development for a busy healthcare industry. Infect Control Hosp Epidemiol 13:111–113, 1992.

92. Reagan BF, McInery VK, Treadwell BZ, et al.: Irrigating solutions for arthroscopy: a metabolic study. J Bone Joint Surg Am 65:629–631, 1983.

93. Rosenberg TD, Paulos LE, Parker RD, et al.: Arthroscopic surgery of the knee. In: Chapman MW (ed.): Operative Orthopaedics. Philadelphia, J.B. Lippincott Co., 1988, pp 1585–1604.

94. Noyes FR and Spievack ES: Extraarticular fluid dissection in tissues during arthroscopy: a report of clinical cases and a study of intraarticular and thigh pressures in cadavers. Am J Sports Med 10:346–351, 1982.

95. Graham B, Breault MJ, McEwen JA, et al.: Occlusion of arterial flow in the extremities at subsystolic pressures through the use of wide tourniquet cuffs. Clin Orthop 266:257–261, 1993.

96. Pedowitz RA, Gershuni DH, Schmidt AH, et al.: Muscle induced beneath and distal to a pneumatic tourniquet: a quantitative animal study of the effects of tourniquet pressure and duration. J Hand Surg Am 16:610–621, 1991.

97. Nitz A, Dobner J, and Matulionis D: Pneumatic tourniquet application and nerve integrity: motor function and electrophysiology. Exp Neurol 94:264–279, 1986.

98. Thorblad J, Ekstrand J, Hamberg P, et al.: Muscle rehabilitation after arthroscopic meniscectomy with or without tourniquet control. Am J Sports Med 13:133–135, 1985.

99. Dobner JJ and Nitz AJ: Postmeniscectomy tourniquet palsy and functional sequela. Am J Sports Med 10:211–214, 1982.

100. Sapega AA, Heppenstall RD, Chance B, et al.: Optimizing tourniquet application and release times in extremity surgery: a biomechanical and ultrastructural study. J Bone Joint Surg Am 67:303–314, 1985.

101. Shaw J and Murray D: The relationship between tourniquet pressure and underlying soft-tissue pressure in the thigh. J Bone Joint Surg Am 64:1148–1152, 1982.

102. Pedowitz RA, Gershuni DH, Friden J, et al.: Effects of reperfusion intervals on skeletal muscle injury beneath and distal to a pneumatic tourniquet. J Hand Surg Am 17:245–255, 1992.

103. Jacobson MD, Pedowitz RA, Oyama BK, et al.: Muscle functional deficits after tourniquet ischemia. Am J Sports Med 22:372–377, 1994.

104. Joyce JJ: Arthroscopic anatomy. Orthopedics 6:1115–1118, 1983.

105. Whipple TL and Bassett FH III: Arthroscopic examination of the knee: polypuncture technique with percutaneous intra-articular manipulation. J Bone Joint Surg Am 60:444–453, 1978.

106. Johnson L: Comprehensive arthroscopic examination of the knees. St. Louis, C.V. Mosby Co., 1977.

107. Kuhlman JR and Sapega AA: Complete arthroscopic visualization of the menisci. Oper Tech Orthop 5:20–27, 1995.

108. Tolin BS and Sapega AA: Arthroscopic visual field mapping at the periphery of the medial meniscus: a comparison of different portal approaches. Arthroscopy 9:265–271, 1993.

109. Morin WD and Steadman JR: Arthroscopic assessment of the posterior compartments of the knee via the intercondylar notch: the arthroscopist's field of view. Arthroscopy 9:284–290, 1993.

110. Boytim MJ, Smith JP, Fischer DA, and Quick DC: Arthroscopic posteromedial visualization of the knee. Clin Orthop 310:82–86, 1995.

111. Pettrone FA: Arthroscopic examination of the posterior compartment of the knee. Orthop Rev 12:107–109, 1983.

112. Lewicky RT and Abeshaus MM: Simplified technique for posterior knee arthroscopy. Am J Sports Med 10:22–23, 1982.

113. Sapega AA: Posteromedial portal guide system for knee arthroscopy. Andover, Mass., Smith & Nephew Dyonics, 1990.

114. Sapega AA, Gold DL, Schaner PJ, et al.: The posteromedial portal in knee arthroscopy: analysis of visual fields and diagnostic utility. Scientific exhibit at the 60th annual meeting of the American Academy of Orthopaedic Surgeons, San Francisco, Calif., 1993.

115. Schreiber SN: Proximal superomedial portal in arthroscopy of the knee. Arthroscopy 7:246–251, 1991.

116. Muller W: The Knee: Form, Function and Ligament Reconstruction. Berlin, Springer-Verlag, 1983.

117. Schreiber SN: Proximal superomedial portal in arthroscopy of the knee. Arthroscopy 7:246–251, 1991.

118. Patel D: Proximal approaches to arthroscopic surgery of the knee. Am J Sports Med 9:296–303, 1981.

119. Patel D: Superior medial-lateral approach to arthroscopic meniscectomy. Orthop Clin North Am 13: 299–305, 1982.

120. Lehman RC: The utility medial portal: a new arthroscopic approach to the knee. Contemp Orthop 21:142–148, 1990.

121. Gillquist J and Hagburg G: A new modification of the technique

of arthroscopy of the knee joint. Acta Chir Scand 142:123–130, 1976.

122. Mulhollan JS: Swedish arthroscopic system. Orthop Clin North Am 13:349–362, 1982.

123. Erikisson E and Sebik A: A comparison between the transpatellar tendon and lateral approach to the knee during arthroscopy. Am J Sports Med 8:103–105, 1980.

124. Gillquist J and Oretorp N: Different techniques for diagnostic arthroscopy: a randomized comparative study. Acta Orthop Scand 52:353–356, 1981.

125. Gillquist J, Hagberg G, and Oretorp N: Arthroscopic visualization of the posteromedial compartment of the knee joint. Orthop Clin North Am 10:545–547, 1979.

126. Lysholm J and Gillquist J: Arthroscopic examination of the posterior cruciate ligament. J Bone Joint Surg Am 63:363–366, 1981.

127. Mariani PP, Ferretti A, Gigli C, et al.: Isokinetic evaluation of the knee after arthroscopic meniscectomy: comparison between anterolateral and central approaches. Arthroscopy 3:123–126, 1987.

128. DeHaven KE: Principles of triangulation for arthroscopic surgery. Orthop Clin North Am 13:329–336, 1982.

129. Chirwa SS, MacLeod BA, and Day B: Intraarticular bupivacaine (Marcaine) after arthroscopic meniscectomy: a randomized double-blind controlled study. Arthroscopy 5:33–35, 1989.

130. Henderson RC, Campion ER, DeMasi RA, et al.: Postarthroscopy analgesia with bupivacaine. Am J Sports Med 18:614–617, 1990.

131. Kaeding CC, Hill JA, Katz J, et al.: Bupivacaine use after knee arthroscopy: pharmacokinetics and pain control study. Arthroscopy 6:33–39, 1990.

132. Milligan KA, Mowbray MJ, Mulrooney L, et al.: Intraarticular bupivacaine for pain relief after arthroscopic surgery of the knee joint in daycase patients. Anaesthesia 43:563–564, 1988.

133. Smith I, Van Hamelnijck J, White PF, et al.: Effects of local anesthesia on recovery after outpatient arthroscopy. Anesthesiology 73:536–539, 1991.

134. Sørensen TS, Sørensen AI, and Strange K: The effect of intraarticular instillation of bupivacaine on postarthroscopic morbidity: a placebo-controlled double-blind trial. Arthroscopy 7:364–367, 1991.

135. Smith I, Van Hemelrijck J, White PF, et al.: Effects of local anesthesia on recovery after outpatient arthroscopy. Anesth Analg 73:536–539, 1991.

136. Gerber H, Censier K, Gachter A, et al.: Intra-articular absorption of bupivacaine during arthroscopy: comparison of 0.25%, 0.5% and 0.75% solution. Anesthesiology Am 63:217, 1985.

137. Meinig RP, Holtgrewe JL, Wiedel JD, et al.: Plasma bupivacaine levels following single dose intraarticular instillation for arthroscopy. Am J Sports Med 16:295–300, 1988.

138. Nole R, Munson NML, and Fulkerson JP: Bupivacaine and saline effects on articular cartilage. Arthroscopy 1:123–127, 1985.

139. Wasudev G, Smith BE, and Limbird TJ: Blood levels of bupivacaine after arthroscopy of the knee joint. Arthroscopy 6:40–42, 1990.

140. Weiker GG, Kuivila TE, and Pippinger CE: Serum lidocaine and bupivacaine levels in local technique knee arthroscopy. Am J Sports Med 19:499–502, 1991.

141. Yoshiya S, Kurasaka M, Hirohata K, et al.: Knee arthroscopy using local anesthetic. Arthroscopy 4:86–89, 1988.

142. Ruwe PA, Klein I, and Shields CL: The effect of intraarticular injection of morphine and bupivacaine on postarthroscopic pain control. Am J Sports Med 23:59–64, 1995.

143. Zarins B, Boyle J, and Harris BA: Knee rehabilitation following arthroscopic meniscectomy. Clin Orthop 198:36–42, 1985.

144. Paulos LE, Rosenberg TD, and Beck CL: Postsurgical care for arthroscopic surgery of the knee and shoulder. Orthop Clin North Am 19:715–723, 1988.

145. Dandy DJ and Hodge GJ: Closed partial meniscectomy. Physiotherapy 64:367–368, 1978.

146. DeLee JC: Complications of arthroscopy and arthroscopic surgery: results of a national survey. Arthroscopy 1:204–220, 1985.

147. Metcalf RW: An arthroscopic procedure for lateral release of the subluxing or dislocating patella. Clin Orthop 167:9–18, 1982.

148. Noyes FR and Spievack ES: Extraarticular fluid dissection in tissues during arthroscopy. Am J Sports Med 10:346–351, 1982.

149. McGinty JB and McCartay JC: Endoscopic lateral retinacular release: a preliminary report. Clin Orthop 158:120–125, 1981.

150. Sherman OH, Fox JM, Snyder SJ, et al.: Arthroscopy—"No problem surgery": an analysis of complications in 2640 cases. J Bone Joint Surg 68A:256–265, 1986.

151. Dunn PM, Post RH, and Jones SR: Thromboembolic complications of knee arthroscopy (letter). West J Med 140:291, 1984.

Chapter

21

Normal and Pathologic Arthroscopic Anatomy of the Knee

Michael E. Joyce • *James R. Andrews*

INTRODUCTION

Arthroscopy is clearly one of the great advancements in orthopaedic surgery of this century. Its proven ability to diagnose and treat joint diseases more specifically and with less morbidity than traditional open surgery has earned it this high status. Whereas the surgical contribution of arthroscopy is common knowledge, less recognized is its contribution to the advancement of our understanding of normal and abnormal anatomy. The purpose of this chapter is to provide an in-depth understanding of the normal and pathologic anatomy of the knee as seen and understood with an arthroscope.

Arthroscopy is the gold standard for the diagnosis of intra-articular knee disorders.[1] Diagnostic arthroscopy of the knee has both a higher sensitivity and specificity than clinical examination and radiographic and arthrographic studies.[2, 3] In the evaluation of sport knee injuries, clinical examination in conjunction with diagnostic arthroscopy has been found to be more sensitive, specific, and cost-effective than magnetic resonance imaging (MRI).[4] Furthermore, MRI is far more prone than arthroscopy to false-positive findings.[5] Using either the anterolateral or the central approach, good arthroscopic technique dictates that a systematic examination[6, 7] of the knee be completed with each procedure. This chapter provides an anatomic foundation for a complete arthroscopic knee evaluation.

SUPRAPATELLAR POUCH

Normal Anatomy

The arthroscopic examination of the knee routinely begins in the suprapatellar pouch, also known as the stratum proper. Four types of plicae have been described: suprapatellar, infrapatellar, lateral, and medial. At the apex of the pouch is the deep reddish muscle that is the attachment of the articularis genu to the synovial membrane.

The absence of this finding suggests the presence of a complete suprapatellar plical membrane. More often, the suprapatellar membrane is incomplete, and only a superomedial or superolateral plica is identified (Fig. 21–1). These medial and lateral bands, along the proximal border of the patella in the horizontal plane, should be distinguished from the medial and lateral synovial shelves. Running from the anterior fat pad to the side of the patellar retinaculum in the coronal plane, the medial and lateral synovial shelves often converge on or pass through the suprapatellar plica.

A well-distended suprapatellar pouch offers the best opportunity to closely examine the synovial membranes that line the knee joint. Abnormalities of the synovial membrane arise as either primary, as in rheumatoid arthritis, or secondary, as in reactive synovitis. With careful examination of the characteristics of the synovial villi—their vascularity and signs of inflammation—these two conditions should be easily distinguished.

Finally, any evidence of crystalline deposition or the presence of intra-articular adhesions can be documented.

Normal Variants

As many knees come to arthroscopy for treatment of a traumatic injury, it is common for the appearance of the suprapatellar pouch to vary considerably. For example, an injury hematoma can collect and organize within this space, or the suprapatellar plica could become inflamed with fibrotic thickening and tissue fraying (Fig. 21–2). In the setting of a chronic injury, a reactive synovitis can form throughout the suprapatellar pouch (Fig. 21–3). This should not be confused with synovitis seen in the setting of inflammatory disease, such as rheumatoid arthritis.

During fetal development, the knee forms from three compartments that are separated by synovial membranes. Medial and lateral plicae result from the incomplete resorption of these membranes. The suprapatellar mem-

254

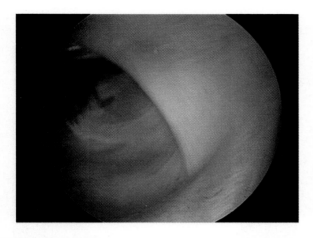

Figure 21–1 • Suprapatellar plica. Viewed through the anterolateral portal, with the knee in extension, an incomplete medial suprapatellar plica is seen.

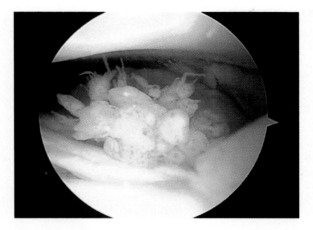

Figure 21–3 • Suprapatellar synovial hyperplasia. Viewed with the knee in extension, through an anterolateral portal, evaluation of the synovial membranes within the suprapatellar pouch reveals reactive synovitis.

brane separates the knee joint from the suprapatellar bursa. In 20% of adults this membrane is complete, but for all other adults a variably sized remnant remains.[8] Treatment depends on correctly separating symptomatic from asymptomatic plicae, a distinction that is best made preoperatively. At arthroscopy, the normal inner plica edge is smooth and rounded, with a dome or crescent shape that lacks interruptions. Following a direct injury to the knee, the plica can become thickened, inflamed, and, eventually, fibrosed. These post-traumatic changes alter the characteristic of the plica such that at arthroscopy it appears stiff and less elastic.

Common Pathologic Conditions

The arthroscope plays an important role in the diagnosis of synovial disease. In conjunction with an office arthroscopy set-up, rheumatologists advocate the use of arthroscopy for tissue resection and diagnostic biopsy.[9] In the setting of routine arthroscopy, a preoperative diagnosis is usually known; therefore, when unexpected synovial hyperplasia is encountered, biopsy should be performed (Fig. 21–4). Pigmented villonodular synovitis (PVNS) is a rare condition of the knee characterized by hypertrophic, hemosiderin-stained villi. PVNS occurs as either a discrete nodule of tissue or diffuse distribution throughout the joint.[10] Localized PVNS has also been seen in a patient presenting with signs and symptoms of a loose body.[11]

Synovial chondromatosis is a proliferative disease of the synovium characterized by the presence of cartilaginous or osteocartilaginous metaplasia and loose bodies within the joint.[12] The disease has three phases: first, chondrometaplasia without loose bodies; second, synovial hyperplasia with loose bodies; and third, loose bodies with normal synovium. Only the first and second phases are amenable to arthroscopic treatment. Lipoma arborescens is a rare intra-articular lesion consisting of a villous lipo-

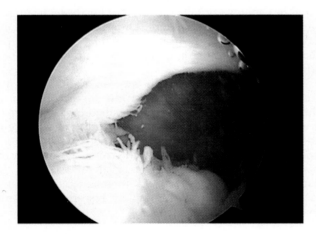

Figure 21–2 • Inflamed suprapatellar plica. Viewed with the knee in extension, through an anterolateral portal, this post-traumatic knee has a thickened and inflamed superolateral plica.

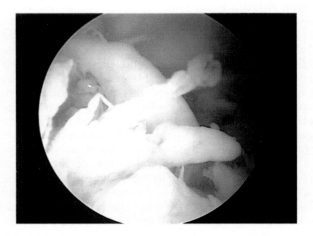

Figure 21–4 • Rheumatoid arthritis and synovial hyperplasia. Viewed with the knee in extension, through an anterolateral portal, tremendous hyperplasia of synovial tissue in the setting of rheumatoid arthritis is seen.

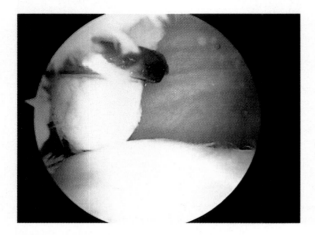

Figure 21–5 • Suprapatellar loose body. Viewed with the knee in extension, through an anterolateral portal, loose bodies are commonly found trapped in the suprapatellar pouch; they are occasionally found behind an incomplete suprapatellar plica.

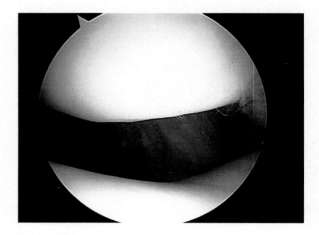

Figure 21–6 • Patellofemoral joint. View with the knee in extension, through an anterolateral portal, the arthroscope is gently withdrawn, allowing visualization of the articular surface of the patellofemoral joint.

matous proliferation of the synovial lining. Arthroscopically, the lesion appears as a synovial lesion with numerous fatty-appearing globules and villous projections.[13]

Because plicae are present in most knees, plica syndrome is diagnosed by a history and physical examination consistent with the syndrome, in the absence of other internal derangement. Suprapatellar plicae vary in size but are rarely abnormal. Infrequently, the presence of a small portal, in an otherwise nearly complete plica, can hide and trap a symptomatic free-floating loose body. This necessitates the surgical widening of the portal to complete the knee examination (Fig. 21–5).[14] Pathologic medial and lateral plica shelves are discussed in the sections on the medial and lateral gutter, respectively.

PATELLOFEMORAL JOINT

Normal Anatomy

The arthroscopic examination of the patellofemoral joint reveals only a small piece of a much larger puzzle.[15] The patella functions to improve the efficiency of the extensor mechanism of the knee when the large forces generated by the quadriceps are transferred through this fulcrum to extend the lower leg. The patella is divided into two large facets (medial and lateral) that are separated by a median ridge. An odd facet extends along the most medial portion of the medial facet and contacts the femur only in deep-knee flexion.[16, 17] The normal anatomy of the femoral trochlear groove is subject to wide variability. Femoral neck anteversion determines trochlear orientation and influences patellofemoral tracking. At 45 degrees of flexion the tangential view of the distal femur shows the lateral femoral condyle approximately 1 cm higher than the medial femoral condyle.

When it is essential for the articular surface of the patellofemoral joint to be thoroughly visualized, placement of a suprapatellar portal is required (Fig. 21–6).[18]

The location and extent of any articular cartilage damage are fully documented. A complete examination also includes an assessment of patellar tracking through the superolateral or superomedial portal. Examination of patellofemoral tracking, through a full range of motion, adds insight into the specific anatomic relationship of the joint surfaces for each patient. Normally, the patella articulates medially by 40 degrees of knee flexion. Articulation at 60 degrees or greater or lateral overhang of the patella in full extension suggests a pathologically tight lateral retinaculum.[19, 20]

Normal Variants

Variability in both the anatomy of the extensor mechanism and the articulation of the patellofemoral joint is tremendous. Care should be taken when subtle signs of patellar lateral compression and patellar instability are encountered in patients not taken to surgery for those diagnoses. In addition, mild or moderate (Outerbridge grades 1 and 2) abnormalities of the patellar articular surface, in patients without specific anterior-knee symptoms, are best left alone.

A bipartite patella is a well-known variation of normal patellar anatomy that results from the abnormal fusion of the patella ossification centers. Classified by Saupe, type I is at the inferior pole; type II is found at the lateral margin; and type III, the most common, is at the superolateral pole.[21] In the setting of acute anterior-knee injury with persistent tenderness at the superolateral aspect of the patella, excision of the accessory fragment can give satisfactory relief of pain and complete restoration of knee function.[22]

Common Pathologic Conditions

In the setting of acute high-energy trauma to the anterior knee, without radiographic evidence of a fracture, arthros-

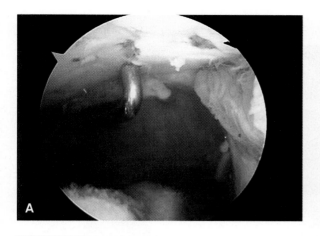
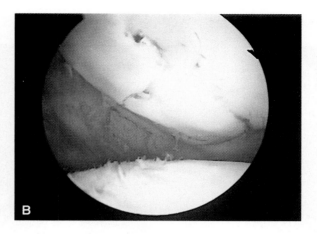

Figure 21–7 • Patellar fracture. *A,* Viewed with the knee in extension, through an antero-lateral portal, disruption of the articular surface is seen. Stability of the fracture fragments can be assessed by palpation with a probe placed through the anteromedial portal. *B,* Viewed with the knee in extension, through a superomedial portal, assessment of the lateral facet fracture is completed.

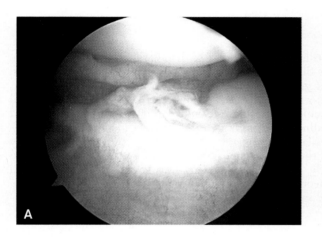
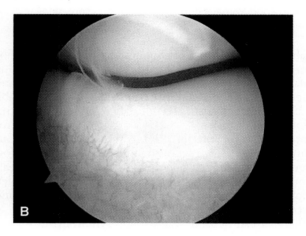

Figure 21–8 • Infrapatellar plica. *A,* Viewed with the knee in 20 degrees of flexion, through a superomedial portal, trapping of an inflamed infrapatellar plica within the patellofemoral joint is seen. *B,* Same view after débridement of the plica.

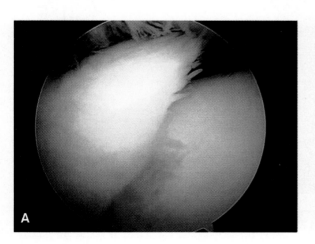
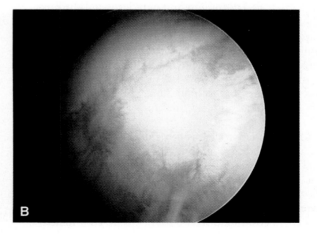

Figure 21–9 • Hypertrophic infrapatellar fat pad. *A,* Viewed with the knee in extension, through an anterolateral portal, a thickened and fibrotic infrapatellar fat pad impinging within the femoral trochlea groove is seen. *B,* Same view after débridement of the abnormal fat pad.

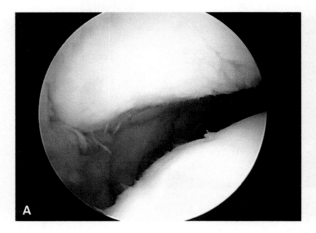
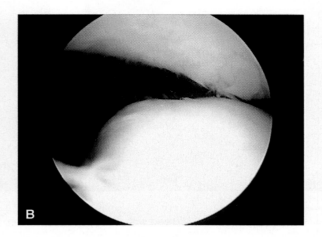

Figure 21–10 • Patellofemoral lateral subluxation with chondromalacia. *A*, Viewed with the knee in extension, through an anterolateral portal, subluxation of the lateral patellar facet lateral to the lateral femoral condyle is seen. *B*, The median ridge of the patella is seen subluxating out of the femoral trochlear groove and onto the lateral femoral condyle with noted grade II/III chondromalacia (the result of recurrent patellar dislocation).

copy is helpful in the evaluation of chondral or osteochondral injury (Fig. 21–7). Because there is no evidence of patellar malalignment or instability, débridement of damaged cartilage alone is indicated. More commonly, patellar articular cartilage damage occurs secondarily to an underlying patellofemoral disorder.

The infrapatellar or anterior plica, commonly called the ligamentum mucosum, is a synovial fold anterior to the anterior cruciate ligament.[23] It may be in continuity with the ligament, partially separated, or completely separate. This is the most common knee plica and is not considered a frequent source of knee pain.[24] However, following anterior knee injury, it can become trapped and symptomatic in the patellofemoral joint (Fig. 21–8). Hypertrophy of the infrapatellar fat pad, with impingement within the patellofemoral joint, is a potential cause of patellofemoral pain and subsequent patellofemoral chondromalacia (Fig. 21–9).

Both patellar malalignment and patellar instability are principally diagnosed with clinical examination and radiographic appearance. Arthroscopic examination demonstrates findings in patients at risk for these disorders, such as a shallow intercondylar sulcus or patellar incongruence. Similarly, arthroscopy can show lateral subluxation of the patella and secondary pathologic damage to the articular surface of the patella and lateral femoral condyle (Fig. 21–10).

Chondromalacia patellae is not a diagnosis; instead, it is a term used to describe the articular surface of the patella.[25] The location and degree of damage are documented as follows. The quadrant of articular cartilage damage is classified according to Fulkerson[26]: type I—distal midpatellar midline or medial; type II—lateral facet; types I and II—a combination of I and II; type III—medial facet shear fracture (usually secondary to forceful reduction of a dislocated patella); and type IV—superior medial and lateral facet. Documentation of the extent of articular cartilage damage is completed with the Outerbridge classification.[27] Grade 1 is cartilage softening alone; grade 2 is

fibrillation measuring less than 0.5 inch in diameter; grade 3 is fibrillation measuring more than 0.5 inch in diameter; and grade 4 is exposed bone. In addition to the patellar, abnormalities of the articular cartilage within the femoral trochlear groove are localized and graded. After damaged hyaline cartilage is débrided, the lesion heals with fibrocartilage, an inferior repair matrix with a limited capacity for the biomechanical demands of the knee and subject to early wear and degeneration (Fig. 21–11). Chondral defects treated with abrasion chondroplasty heal slowly and incompletely.[28–31]

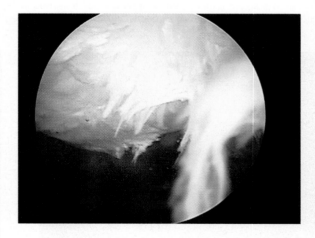

Figure 21–11 • Fibrocartilage repair of damaged articular cartilage. Viewed with the knee in extension, through an anterolateral portal, a fibrocartilaginous repair matrix is seen. This knee sustained a full-thickness articular cartilage injury and was treated with abrasion chondroplasty in 1978. The inferior repair matrix is seen with the expected fibrillation and degeneration.

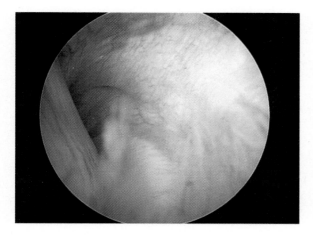

Figure 21–12 • Medial gutter–meniscal synovial junction. Viewed with slight knee flexion, through an anterolateral portal, the normal meniscal synovial junction of the medial gutter is seen.

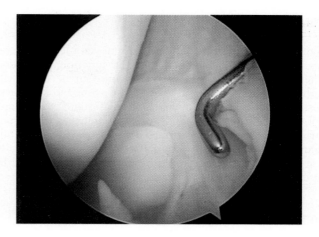

Figure 21–13 • Transverse meniscal ligament–anteromedial gutter. Viewed with slight knee flexion, through an anterolateral portal, the normal meniscal synovial junction is seen from the attachment of the transverse meniscal ligament, across the anterior meniscus, to the anteromedial wall.

MEDIAL GUTTER

Normal Anatomy

In the routine examination of the knee, the arthroscope is rotated from the suprapatellar pouch, over the medial femoral condyle, into the medial gutter. The femur is then inspected. A synovial membrane covers the femoral condyle up to the articular cartilage border. The opposing wall of the gutter extends to the meniscal synovial border (Fig. 21–12). The inspection is begun in the most posterior aspect of the gutter, and then the scope is slowly withdrawn to allow visualization of the entire gutter. Here, the anterior medial synovial meniscal junction is visualized (Fig. 21–13).

Moving the arthroscope from the suprapatellar pouch to the medial gutter allows visualization of the medial plica shelf, which is present in about 30% of knees.[32] When this plica is large it may prevent the arthroscope from moving easily into the medial compartment without the knee being fully extended. The mere presence of this plica shelf is not necessarily abnormal. Asymptomatic plicae have a smooth border, are thin, and lack inflammation or thickening (Fig. 21–14*A*). While under direct visualization the knee is slowly brought into flexion, and the plica shelf tightens and bowstrings across the femoral condyle (Fig. 21–14*B*).

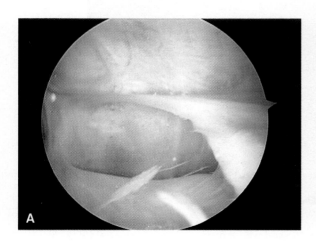

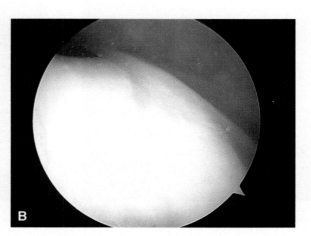

Figure 21–14 • Medial plica shelf. *A*, Viewed with the knee in extension, through an anterolateral portal, a large medial plical shelf above the medial femoral condyle is seen. *B*, As the knee is brought into 30–40 degrees of flexion, the plica band pulls over the top of the femoral condyle.

Normal Variants

Significant variation is found at the synovial meniscal border. Unless adequate probing of the junction is undertaken, deep folds within the synovium can be confused with a peripheral meniscal tear. In the acute and subacute post-traumatic knee, synovial hyperplasia and inflammation extend into the medial gutter. Finally, as discussed earlier, plica bands demonstrate wide variation in size and characteristics. The site on the medial femoral condyle that contacts the plica should be normal in patients with asymptomatic plicae.

Common Pathologic Conditions

When treating a complete tear of the medial collateral ligament (MCL) (grade III—MCL tear), arthroscopy is used to rule out other intra-articular damage and assess the torn ligament. Injury to the medial meniscus or the meniscal synovial junction is treated with resection or arthroscopic repair. Severe injuries result in the disruption of the MCL as well as of the medial capsule. In this setting, displacement of a torn MCL can occasionally be seen in the medial gutter.[33] Complete MCL tears without ligament displacement are treated nonoperatively.

Loose bodies are commonly found trapped in the medial gutter. Both in patients with known loose bodies and in those in whom loose bodies are found incidentally, examination of the medial gutter is essential. As the arthroscope is passed from the suprapatellar pouch to the medial gutter, the medial femoral condyle is inspected. Degenerative spurs of the condyle are easily identified (Fig. 21–15). A medial plica shelf that snaps over a condyle spur results in obvious damage to the articular surface.

Pathologic medial plica bands can be found during examination of the medial gutter (Fig. 21–16). Although a

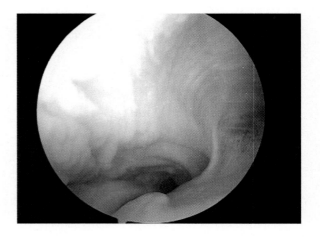

Figure 21–15 • Degenerative medial condylar spur. Viewed with the knee in full extension, through an anterolateral portal, the arthroscope is directed inferiorly, and the medial condyle border with a small-to-moderate degenerative spur is seen.

plica can become symptomatic for several reasons, most often a discrete injury initiates the onset of medial pain.[34] In addition, the elasticity of a plica diminishes with age, thereby changing the relationship of the plica to the medial condyle.[35] Sherman and Jackson[36] proposed that the plica develops an avascular fibrotic edge that impinges on the medial femoral condyle during knee flexion. A localized area of chondromalacia at the site of impingement may also cause symptoms. At 2 years' follow-up in a prospective randomized trial, 83% had good and excellent results in the arthroscopic plica resection group compared with 29% in the arthroscopic nonresected group.[37]

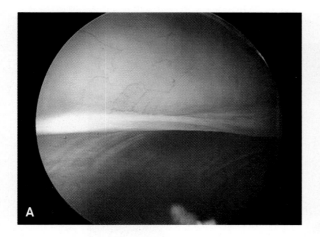

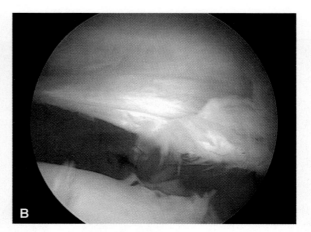

Figure 21–16 • Abnormal plica band with associated chondromalacia. *A,* Viewed with the knee in full extension, through an anterolateral portal, the proximal aspect of a medial plica band is seen. *B,* As the arthroscope is withdrawn, the plica appears fibrotic, frayed, and thickened with associated destruction of the articular surface of the corresponding aspect of the medial femoral condyle.

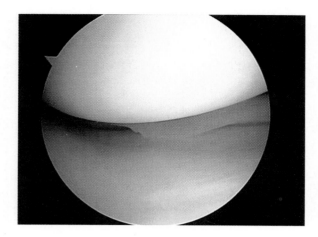

Figure 21–17 • Medial meniscus. Viewed with the knee in 10–30 degrees of flexion with a valgus stress, through an anterolateral portal, the body and posterior horn of the medial meniscus, with its normal flounce on its free margin, are seen.

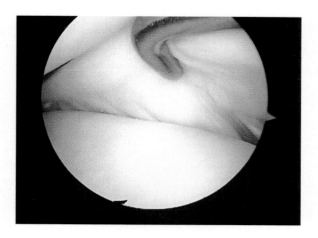

Figure 21–18 • Undersurface of medial meniscus. Viewed with the knee in slight flexion with a valgus stress, through an anterolateral portal, the meniscus is elevated with a probe, allowing visualization of the undersurface and the attachment of the coronary ligament.

MEDIAL COMPARTMENT

Normal Anatomy

The arthroscope is moved from the medial gutter into the medial compartment, with the knee in 10–30 degrees of flexion, the tibia externally rotated, and with placement of a valgus stress on the knee. The normal medial meniscus has a small flounce on its free margin. Viewing from the anterolateral portal, the meniscus is divided into thirds: anterior (see Fig. 21–13), body, and posterior horn (Fig. 21–17). The anteromedial portal is established after spinal needle localization places the portal above the superior meniscal edge; a probe is then inserted and the examination continues. The probe gently elevates the meniscus to expose its undersurface and the coronary ligament that comprises the meniscal tibia junction (Fig. 21–18). Probing and tugging the meniscus is necessary to reveal any reduced- or partial-thickness meniscal tears. With a combination of probing and direct visualization during knee flexion and extension, the mobility of the meniscus is assessed dynamically. The attachment of the posterior horn onto the tibia is visualized as the arthroscope is passed into the posterior medial compartment. The peripheral attachment of the posterior horn of the medial meniscus is seen here (Fig. 21–19). The transverse ligament connects the anterior aspect of the medial and lateral menisci.

A systematic examination of the articular surfaces of the femoral condyle and tibia plateau is necessary to detect chondromalacia or osteochondral injury. Beginning with the knee in extension, the femoral condyle is visualized as the knee is flexed to 90 degrees; the most common site of wear is seen at 30–45 degrees of flexion. Examination is not complete until the articular surface is gently probed to establish that the articular cartilage is firmly affixed to subchondral bone.

Normal Variants

When a valgus stress is placed at the knee, the free meniscal border normally shows a small ruffle or flounce, which should not be confused with a meniscal tear (see Fig. 21–17). Whereas limited amount of meniscal motion is normal, abnormal motion is indicative of a peripheral tear. On average, the meniscus can move 5 mm in the anteroposterior plane, with relatively more motion in the anterior horn.[38] Finally, the appearance of the meniscus and the femoral condyle changes with age. The free edge of the meniscus becomes frayed; unless there are nearly

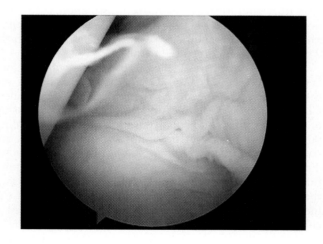

Figure 21–19 • Posterior horn of medial meniscus. Viewed with the knee in slight flexion, through an anterolateral portal, with the arthroscope passed through the notch into the posteromedial compartment, the peripheral attachment of the posterior horn of the medial meniscus is seen. Notice the normal fold in the synovial tissue.

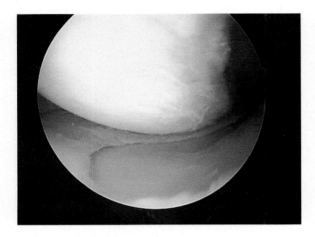

Figure 21–20 • Articular cartilage fraying. Viewed with the knee in 40 degrees of flexion, through an anterolateral portal, fraying of the articular cartilage of the femoral condyle, at the border of the intercondylar notch, is frequently seen in aging knees.

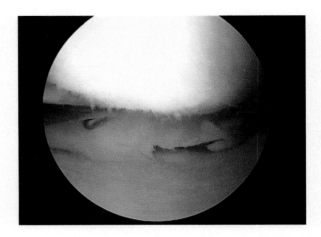

Figure 21–21 • Degenerative meniscal tear. Viewed with the knee in 10 degrees of flexion, through an anterior lateral portal, a degenerative tear of the medial meniscus is seen.

detached fragments, this is not necessarily abnormal. Likewise, the medial femoral condyle shows age-related changes. Fraying of the articular cartilage on the border of the intercondylar notch is frequently encountered and is not abnormal (Fig. 21–20).

Common Pathologic Conditions

A complete discussion on meniscal tears is the focus of the following chapter. Arthroscopy is the gold standard in the diagnosis of a meniscal tear.[39–41] Because the majority of patients coming to surgery for treatment of a suspected meniscal tear have met the indications for surgery, MRI adds little additional preoperative information.[42] In addition, arthroscopy is necessary to adequately assess meniscal healing as MRI shows persistent grade 3 or 4 lesions in 96% of successfully repaired menisci.[43]

Meniscal tears are divided into traumatic and degenerative types (Fig. 21–21). Traumatic meniscal tears are then classified by location, orientation, and appearance. Classification based on location describes the relationship of the tear to its blood supply and is predictive of healing potential.[44, 45] Tears of the inner and middle thirds are seen with the arthroscope in the medial compartment. Tears in the peripheral third of the meniscus require reflection with a probe (Fig. 21–22) or visualization from the posteromedial compartment (see Fig. 21–43). At the meniscal body, a tear of the oblique fibers of the medial collateral ligament can be confused with a peripheral meniscal tear (Fig. 21–23). The tear length, pattern, and one of the many commonly used descriptive terms (such as longitudinal, radial, bucket-handle, horizontal, or flap tear) should be documented.

Noninflammatory damage to the articular surface arises from three different mechanisms: (1) osteoarthritis, (2) osteochondral and chondral fracture, and (3) osteo-

chondritis dissecans. Osteoarthritis, or degenerative arthritis, is the most common form of joint destruction in elderly people. Accelerated osteoarthritis can also be seen in much younger patients who have chronic knee instability. For example, young patients with chronic anterior cruciate ligament (ACL) tears can have a posteromedial tibial condyle worn down to bone (Fig. 21–24). Osteochondral and chondral injuries are caused by impaction, avulsion, or shearing forces and most often involve the patella (see Fig. 21–7) or femoral condyle.[46, 47] Classification according to Bauer and Jackson[48] has been accepted. Probing of the articular surface is as important as visualization, especially

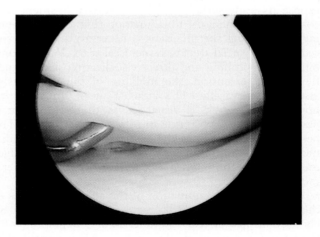

Figure 21–22 • Medial meniscal tear. Viewed with the knee in 10 degrees of flexion with a strong valgus stress, through an anterolateral portal, a peripheral tear of the medial meniscus is seen after elevation of the free margin with a probe placed through the anteromedial portal.

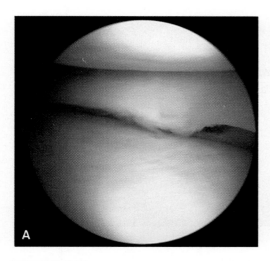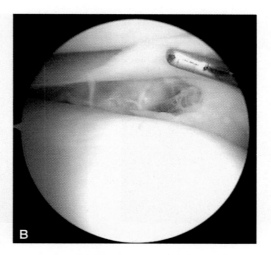

Figure 21–23 • Tear of oblique fibers of medial collateral ligament. *A,* Viewed with the knee in slight flexion with a valgus stress, through an anterolateral portal, a normal medial meniscus is seen. *B,* After elevation of the free margin with a probe, a tear of the oblique fibers of the medial collateral ligament with extension into the coronary ligament is seen. This injury required open repair.

if symptoms are longstanding, because healing with an inferior fibrous surface can mask the underlying abnormality (Fig. 21–25). Osteochondritis dissecans is a localized chondral or osteochondral separation, with or without necrosis of the bony fragment.[49, 50] The lateral aspect of the medial femoral condyle is the most common site of the lesion, and children with an open physis, regardless of treatment, have a better prognosis.[51] Understanding of the variability of

Figure 21–24 • Medial compartment wear in chronic anterior cruciate ligament–deficient knee. Medial compartment viewed, with slight knee flexion and a valgus stress, through an anterolateral portal. This knee has fraying of the posteromedial condylar articular cartilage and of the medial meniscus and complete loss of articular cartilage on the posterior aspect of the medial tibial plateau. This wear pattern is commonly seen in knees with chronic anterior cruciate ligament tears.

the arthroscopic appearance is important because patients can present with mechanical symptoms when radiographic studies are normal (Fig. 21–26).

INTERCONDYLAR NOTCH

Normal Anatomy

The arthroscope is moved from the medial compartment to the intercondylar notch with a sweeping motion to keep the fat pad anterior to the arthroscope. While the knee is flexed 45–90 degrees, the arthroscope is slowly withdrawn, thereby allowing the ACL to come into view. The anteromedial bundle of the ACL is tight in flexion, whereas the posterolateral bundle is tight in extension. The ACL's varies with age, and it is often hidden by the infrapatellar plica (ligamentum mucosum), which can be resected for full visualization of the notch (Fig. 21–27). The femoral insertion of the posterior cruciate ligament (PCL) is seen posteromedial to the ACL, most often covered with synovium. With the arthroscope high in the notch, visualization anterior to the ACL shows the transverse meniscal ligament.

In conjunction with clinical examination, arthroscopy is the most accurate method for diagnosing a torn ACL.[52] While the ACL is under direct visualization an anterior drawer is placed on the knee, forcing the ACL fibers to become taut. The ACL is also probed from its femoral insertion to the tibia, on both the medial and lateral sides. This tension test permits detection of a rare partial rupture of the ligament. Passing the arthroscope deep between the lateral femoral condyle and the ACL allows visualization of the femoral ACL insertion, the most frequent site of rupture. Finally, any hemorrhage with the ligament suggests a tear.

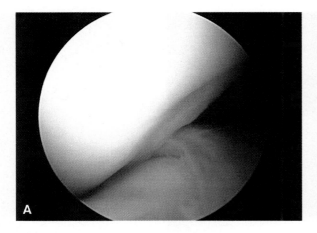
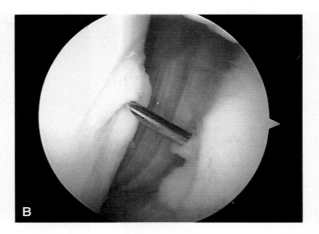

Figure 21–25 • Articular cartilage injury. *A*, Medial compartment viewed, with 50 degrees of knee flexion and a slight valgus stress, through an anterolateral portal. The medial aspect of the medial femoral condyle appears with a slightly irregular contour. *B*, Probing with a spinal needle shows that the tissue, overlying this irregular surface, is not articular cartilage but instead an abnormal fibrous tissue.

Normal Variants

The femoral insertion of the ACL is a semicircular area on the most posteromedial aspect of the lateral femoral condyle. Its long axis is tilted slightly forward, and the posterior convexity is parallel to the posterior articular margin of the femoral condyle.[53, 54] Identification of this precise location is important in ACL reconstruction of isometric placement of the graft. Anatomic variation of the lateral condyle within the notch can lead to misplacement of the graft. "Residents ridge" is the name given to an elevation in the condylar wall that arthroscopically appears initially as the most posterior margin of the condyle. However, once this is removed, during notchplasty, the true posterior margin is found (Fig. 21–28).

Rarely can intraligament cysts of the ACL cause knee pain. In one series this diagnosis was made by MRI in 3 of 681 studies. Arthroscopic visualization can be accom-

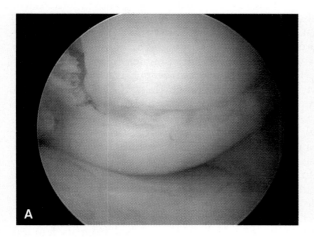
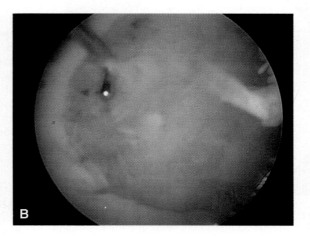

Figure 21–26 • Osteochondritis dissecans (OCD). *A*, Medial compartment viewed, with 50 degrees of knee flexion, through an anterolateral portal. A large OCD lesion on the lateral aspect of the medial femoral condyle is seen. A raised appearance and the junction between normal and abnormal articular cartilage are helpful in the diagnosis. *B*, This type III lesion was probed and found to be loose. The fibrocartilaginous interface, formed between the fragment and its bed, is seen after the fragment was removed for subsequent repair.

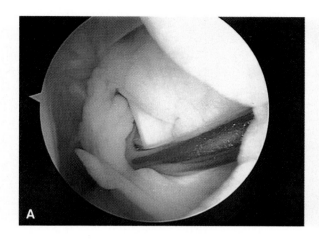

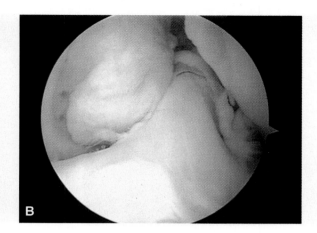

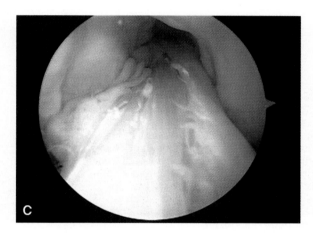

Figure 21–27 • Normal anterior cruciate ligament (ACL). *A,* With the knee flexed 45–90 degrees, the arthroscope is slowly withdrawn from the medial compartment, and the ACL comes into view. Here, the ACL is found beneath the infrapatellar plica (ligamentum mucosum) that is retracted with a probe. *B,* The ACL is often seen without manipulation or resection of the ligamentum mucosum. Here, the fibrous tissue lateral (left) to the ACL should be appreciated as a normal variant of the infrapatellar plica. *C,* Often, as seen here, the ligamentum mucosum is resected to fully visualize the ACL.

plished with the use of a 70 degree arthroscope and additional portals.[55] Guidance from preoperative MRI is necessary for localization with the probe.

Common Pathologic Conditions

The most common abnormality seen within the intercondylar notch is rupture of the ACL, PCL, or both. With an acute rupture of the ACL, hemorrhage with the synovial tissue and between the individual ACL fibers is evident. Probing the ACL reveals fibers with complete disruption, stretched fibers that are still attached, and some normal-appearing fibers. In adults ACL rupture is more common at the proximal femoral insertion. Unless the torn ligament can be displaced into the anterior joint, débridement of the intercondylar synovium is necessary to assess the injury.

The appearance of a chronic ACL tear is different from and possibly more confusing than an acute injury. The most straightforward case is a complete disruption in which the remaining ACL fibers atrophy and are covered with a thin synovial membrane (Fig. 21–29). With some proximal ruptures, the ACL is displaced from its femoral insertion, but scars to the PCL occur deep within the notch (Fig. 21–30). This can present a confusing physical

and arthroscopic examination. On Lachman testing the knee comes to a firm endpoint, but with increased displacement. However, the pivot shift remains abnormal. Arthroscopically, the anterior aspect of the ligament can appear normal, with fibers expanding toward their insertion on the tibia. These fibers become taut with an anterior drawer maneuver. Only with probing and visualization deep along the lateral femoral condylar wall can the correct diagnosis be made when the ligament is found not to have any attachment to the femur.

Ruptures of the isolated PCL are better visualized through a posterior medial or posterior lateral portal because the intact ACL hides the majority of the injury. This is especially true with chronic and partial PCL tears. Combined ACL and PCL ruptures appear as complete destruction within the intercondylar notch. Débridement of hematoma, scar tissue, and synovium reveals the extent of the injury.

Hoffa[56] first described impingement and subsequent fibrosis of the infrapatellar fat pad as a cause of anterior knee pain. Arthroscopically, this is seen as a white fibrotic piece of synovium that impinges within the joint on flexion and extension, best visualized via the suprapatellar portal. When diagnostic lidocaine injection relieves symptoms, arthroscopic resection of the fibrotic fat pad usually leads to good-to-excellent results.[57]

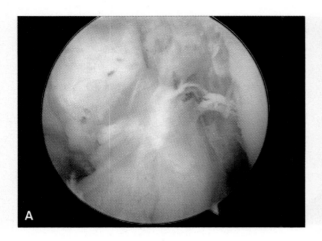

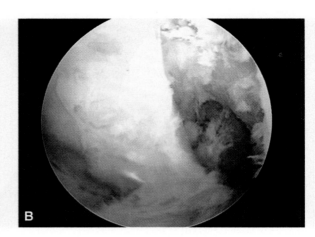

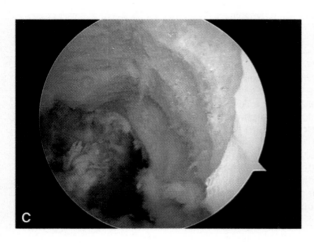

Figure 21–28 • Torn anterior cruciate ligament (ACL) and "residents ridge." *A,* A subacute tear of an ACL is seen through an anterolateral portal. *B,* After the ACL was resected, in preparation for ligament reconstruction, the normal posterior cruciate ligament is seen. The lateral condylar wall with a ridge suggestive of the most posterior aspect of the notch is seen. *C,* After a notchplasty was performed, the true posterior aspect of the notch is seen nearly 1.5 cm more posterior than the original "residents ridge" suggests.

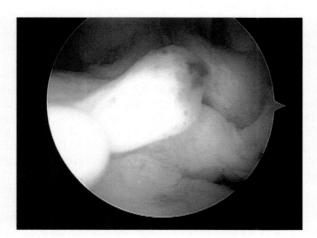

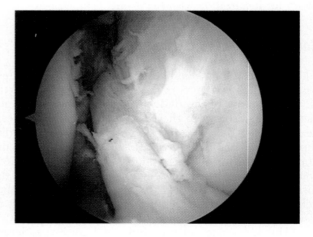

Figure 21–29 • Chronic anterior cruciate ligament (ACL) tear. Viewed through an anterolateral portal, a chronic ACL tear with its characteristic synovial membrane is seen.

Figure 21–30 • Chronic anterior cruciate ligament (ACL) tear with healing to posterior cruciate ligament (PCL). Viewed through an anterolateral portal, this chronic ACL tear is seen without attachment on the lateral femoral condyle but healed to the anterior surface of the PCL. Before synovial tissue is resected from the posterior intercondylar notch, this tissue can appear as a normal ACL.

LATERAL COMPARTMENT

Normal Anatomy

The lateral compartment is entered from the intercondylar notch either above or below the ligamentum mucosum. As soon as the arthroscope reaches the most medial edge of the lateral meniscus, the knee is flexed and a varus force is applied (figure-four position). This should open the lateral compartment and allow the arthroscope to pass over the anterior horn of the lateral meniscus and pass gently between the articular surfaces. Because the lateral meniscus is more circular than the medial meniscus, it is often visualized in its entirety (Fig. 21–31). A probe is used to inspect the undersurface of the meniscus and to examine the popliteal hiatus (Fig. 21–32). With the knee in deep flexion, load is transferred to the posterior horn.[58] The anterior horn of the lateral meniscus is attached to the tibia in front of the intercondylar eminence and behind the attachment of the ACL, with which its fibers partially blend.

The articular surface of the tibial plateau and lateral condyle are inspected as the knee is brought through a full arch of motion. A probe is used to test the firmness of the articular surface.

Normal Variants

Because the lateral meniscus is not attached to the lateral collateral ligament, it is more mobile than the medial meniscus and translates on the tibial plateau 9–11 mm during flexion and extension. In addition, the probe can easily be placed into the popliteal hiatus, and the meniscus can be pulled forward; an inexperienced surgeon can mistake this

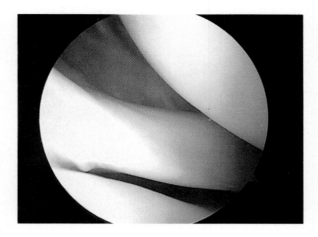

Figure 21–32 • Popliteal hiatus. Viewed through an anterolateral portal, with the knee in the figure-four position, the arthroscope is advanced into the lateral compartment until the popliteal hiatus is seen.

pulled meniscus for a meniscal tear, although it is actually normal. As part of the aging process the lateral meniscus undergoes some degree of calcification, and the inner edge often frays (Fig. 21–33). These conditions alone are not a common cause of knee pain, but they do make the meniscus susceptible to degenerative tearing. A fissure of the articular cartilage, parallel to the lateral meniscal rim, can be found in up to 17% of knees. As clinically significant degeneration of this joint surface has not been documented, this is likely to be a normal variation of the lateral tibial plateau.[59]

Discoid lateral menisci are classified as one of three types: (1) incomplete, (2) complete, and (3) Wrisberg.[60]

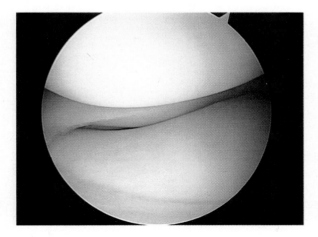

Figure 21–31 • Normal lateral meniscus. Viewed through an anterolateral portal, the knee is manipulated into the figure-four position (flexed 90 degrees with a varus force), and the arthroscope is advanced over the medial edge of the lateral meniscus so that the lateral compartment is seen.

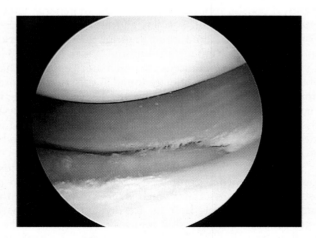

Figure 21–33 • Calcification and fraying of lateral meniscus. Viewed through an anterolateral portal, this aging lateral meniscus has a normal amount of calcification and fraying of the inner margin.

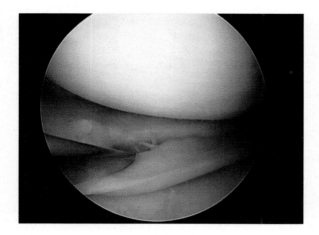

Figure 21–34 • Lateral meniscus tear. Viewed from an anterolateral portal, with the knee in the figure-four position, a probe is used to expose a tear of the lateral meniscus.

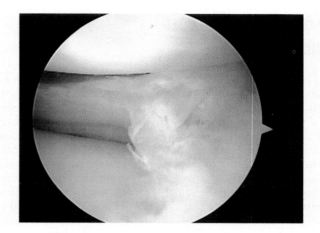

Figure 21–35 • Degenerative lateral meniscal tear with meniscal cyst. Viewed from an anterolateral portal, with the knee in the figure-four position, a degenerative tear of the body of the lateral meniscus is seen in a patient with a large lateral meniscal cyst that was resected by means of separate incision.

The classic description of "snapping knee syndrome" is most closely related to the hypermobile Wrisberg type, in which the meniscus has lost its peripheral attachment except for the posterior meniscofemoral ligament. Asymptomatic types 1 and 2 discoid meniscus should be left alone. The arthroscopic treatment of symptomatic discoid meniscus is a complex problem beyond the scope of this chapter. However, a frequent reason for repeat arthroscopy is found in patients who underwent arthroscopic resection of a discoid meniscus only to be found later to have a horizontal tear on the remnant meniscus.[61]

Common Pathologic Conditions

The same method used to describe and classify medial meniscal tears is applied to lateral tears. In general, lateral tears are less frequent, smaller, and more easily reduced. For this reason, it is important to probe the entire superior and inferior surface before ruling out a tear (Fig. 21–34). Cysts of the lateral meniscus are much more common than of the medial meniscus and are found at the joint line anterior to the lateral collateral ligament. They are palpable in knee extension but less so in knee flexion. Meniscal cysts arise in conjunction with either traumatic or degenerative meniscal tears with a horizontal cleavage plane that can be probed deep into the joint capsule (Fig. 21–35).[62]

Lesions of the articular cartilage are similar to those found in the medial compartment, with the exception of osteochondritis dissecans, which is rarely found within the lateral compartment. Lesions are divided into traumatic osteochondral and chondral injuries or articular cartilage degeneration (Fig. 21–36). Probing of the joint surface is essential to a complete examination. Soft articular cartilage is abnormal and, in the presence of normal radiographs and MRI, represents a subchondral separation of the cartilage from the underlying bone (Fig. 21–37).

LATERAL GUTTER

Normal Anatomy

The lateral gutter is entered by passing the arthroscope from the lateral compartment over the lateral edge of the meniscus, with a varus stress on the knee. The lateral patellofemoral ligament is attached to the lateral condyle and is of variable size and tightness (Fig. 21–38). The superior meniscosynovial junction is best visualized from the gutter by directing the arthroscope to view in an infe-

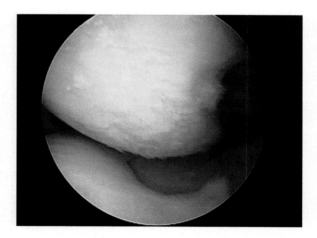

Figure 21–36 • Early degenerative arthritis of lateral femoral condyle. Viewed from an anterolateral portal, with the knee in 45 degrees of flexion, the irregular surface of a knee with early degenerative arthritis is seen. On palpation, the surface was soft and easily damaged.

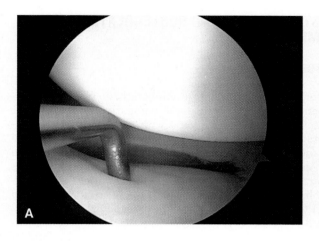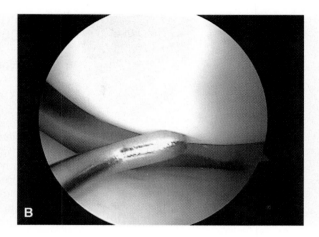

Figure 21–37 • Separation of articular cartilage from subchondral bone. *A*, Viewed from an anterolateral portal, with the knee in the figure-four position, a probe finds soft cartilage on the posterior aspect of the lateral tibial plateau. *B*, In comparison, the articular cartilage on the lateral femoral condyle is firm on palpation.

rior direction (Fig. 21–39). A wide cleft along this junction is often found as a normal variant. Moving the arthroscope deeper into the knee allows visualization of the popliteus tendon and a defect in the inferior meniscal synovial junction known as the popliteal hiatus (Fig. 21–40).

Normal Variants

Minor variations exist within the lateral gutter. Deep folds within the meniscal synovial border can be probed to ensure that there are no peripheral meniscal tears. Synovial hyperplasia is often found in the post-traumatic knee.

Plica bands within the lateral compartment, while less common than in the medial gutter, are considered abnormal only if they coincide with specific symptoms and demonstrate arthroscopic evidence of inflammation and fibrosis.

Common Pathologic Conditions

Pathologic plicae within the lateral gutter are diagnosed in the same manner as those in the medial compartment. Hemorrhage seen within the lateral wall of the lateral gutter is suggestive of a lateral collateral ligament tear. With

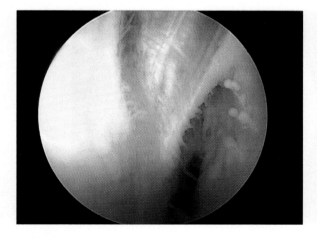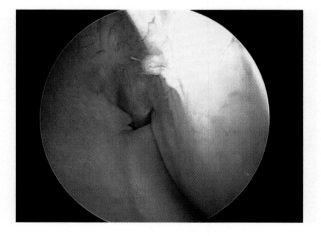

Figure 21–38 • Patellofemoral ligament. The lateral gutter is viewed from the anterolateral compartment, with the knee in extension. A firm band of tissue arises from the lateral condyle and becomes confluent with the lateral capsule as it attaches to the patella.

Figure 21–39 • Lateral gutter. Viewed from an anterolateral compartment, with the knee in extension, the normal meniscal synovial junction of the lateral meniscus is seen. The lateral opening of the popliteal hiatus is at the most posterior aspect.

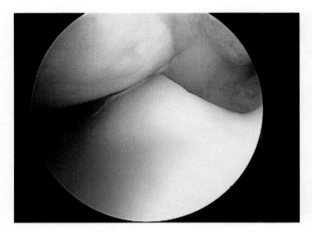

Figure 21–40 • Popliteal hiatus. View from an anterolateral compartment, with the knee in extension, the arthroscope is advanced deep into the knee, allowing visualization of the popliteal tendon and hiatus.

a grade III tear of this ligament, disruption of the lateral capsule can also be found. A rare vascular abnormality, consisting of a venous aneurysm–like tumor, has been described adjacent to the lateral meniscus in a patient thought to have a meniscal tear.[63] Finally, the compartment must be thoroughly inspected for loose bodies that hide within the synovial fold, anterior to the femoral attachment of the popliteus tendon.

POSTEROMEDIAL AND POSTEROLATERAL COMPARTMENTS

Normal Anatomy

A complete arthroscopic examination includes the posteromedial and posterolateral compartments. With the knee flexed at 30 degrees and with the use of the anterolateral portal, the tip of the arthroscope is placed between the medial femoral condyle and the cruciate ligaments and advanced until a soft "pop" is felt as the compartment is entered. The posterior medial femoral condyle, the posterior horn of the medial meniscus, the posterior portion of the PCL, and the posterior meniscal synovial fold are visualized (Fig. 21–41).[64] Exchanging the 30 degree arthroscope for a 70 degree arthroscope increases the field of view. Similarly, under direct visualization, a spinal needle is used to establish a posteromedial portal.

The posterolateral portal is visualized from an anterolateral portal by advancing the arthroscope to the posterior horn of the lateral meniscus, with a varus stress placed on the knee. If the view is directed superiorly, as the arthroscope is moved between the lateral meniscus and the lateral condyle, the inferior aspect of the ACL origin is seen. With the arthroscope advanced past the rim of the meniscus, the posterolateral compartment is entered. The meniscal synovial fold is seen, but the popliteus tendon is not normally visualized through this portal.

The anatomy of the posterolateral corner of the knee is complex. Just below the joint capsular tissue and lateral meniscus border, the popliteal tendon divides into two fascicles of equal size. One fascicle attaches to the popliteal muscle belly and the other inserts directly onto the most proximal and posterior projection of the fibular head.[65]

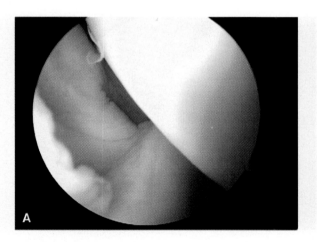 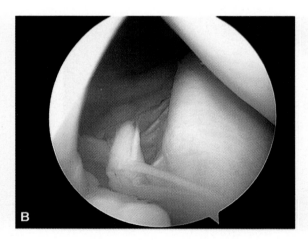

Figure 21–41 • Posteromedial and posterolateral compartments. *A*, Viewed from an anterolateral portal, with the knee in slight flexion, the arthroscope is advanced through the intercondylar notch into the posterolateral compartment. A normal lateral meniscal synovial junction is seen. *B*, Viewed from an anteromedial portal, with the knee in slight flexion, the arthroscope is advanced through the intercondylar notch into the posteromedial compartment. A normal medial meniscal synovial junction is seen.

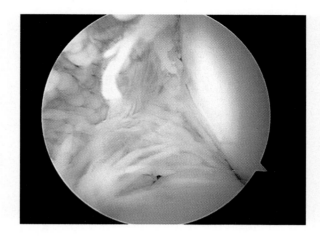

Figure 21–42 • Synovial hyperplasia in rheumatoid arthritis: posterolateral compartment. Viewed from an anterolateral compartment, with the knee in slight flexion, the arthroscope is advanced into the posterolateral compartment. Synovial hyperplasia hinders visualization until the knee is flexed to 90 degrees and the pump pressure is increased.

During flexion the meniscofemoral ligament pulls the posterior horn of the lateral meniscus anteriorly. This structure extends from the posterior horn of the lateral meniscus to the lateral aspect of the medial femoral condyle. This ligament is divided into two bundles and passes anteriorly (ligament of Humphrey) and posteriorly (ligament of Wrisberg) to the PCL.[66, 67] There is considerable variation in size of these ligaments, often approaching one-third the diameter of the PCL.

Normal Variants

Normal variation with the posteromedial and posterolateral compartments is limited. Often the meniscal synovial fold is deep and, on inspection, may appear as a peripheral meniscal tear. However, either by pulling on the meniscus with a probe or by placing a spinal needle through a posterior accessory portal, a tear is easily ruled out. In the post-traumatic knee a hematoma collects in the posterior; prolonged irrigation improves visualization. In a knee with chronic inflammation, hyperplasia of the synovium hinders visualization within the posterior compartments (Fig. 21–42), a problem corrected by flexing the knee to 90 degrees and increasing the pump pressure or by establishing an accessory portal.

Common Pathologic Conditions

Visualization of the posterior meniscal attachment is especially important in the diagnosis of medial meniscal tears because they commonly arise at the meniscal synovial junction. This is especially true in the setting of an ACL tear, where this is a frequent concomitant injury. In one

study, this lesion was missed in 63% of the cases when routine anterior portal viewing was used alone.[68] Once the posterior compartment is entered, the arthroscope is directed inferiorly and a tear will come into view (Fig. 21–43). Tearing of the posterior capsule can be seen in patients with hyperextension injuries in conjunction with multiple intra-articular abnormalities.

Gillquiest, Hagberg, and Oretorp[69] have emphasized the importance of posterior visualization in the evaluation of the PCL, even in the setting of a negative clinical examination.[70] Complete visualization from the anterolateral portal is achieved by a combination of medial and lateral views obtained with the arthroscope passed through the notch medially and laterally to the cruciate ligaments. A separate posterolateral accessory portal also allows good visualization of the torn PCL (Fig. 21–44). In the evaluation of trauma patients with acute hemarthrosis, diagnostic arthroscopy found a 44% prevalence of PCL tears, much higher than reported in sport-related traumatic hemarthrosis.[71] The broader use of diagnostic arthroscopy, in the setting of an acute knee hematoma, found a 71% prevalence of ACL rupture and an 18% prevalence of osteochondral fracture or patellar dislocation.[72]

CONCLUSIONS

The understanding of knee anatomy has advanced with the use of arthroscopy. Understanding the complexity of normal anatomy, as well as normal variations of that anatomy, is essential to the proper diagnosis and treatment of knee injuries. Furthermore, the ability of arthroscopy to dynamically examine the relationship between anatomic structures adds a final element of importance to the role of this technique.

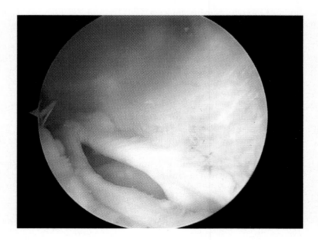

Figure 21–43 • Posterior medial meniscal tear. Viewed from an anteromedial portal, with the knee in slight flexion, the arthroscope is advanced through the intercondylar notch into the posteromedial compartment, allowing visualization of a peripheral medial meniscal tear.

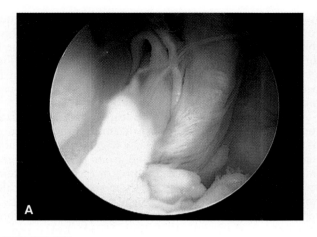
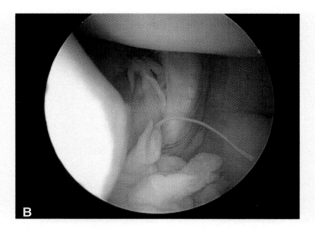

Figure 21–44 • Partial posterior cruciate ligament (PCL) tear. *A,* Under direct visualization, a posterolateral portal is established. Viewed through a 30 degree arthroscope, a tear of the anterolateral bundle of the PCL is seen. *B,* Slowly withdrawing the arthroscope allows for a wider field of view.

References

1. Dandy DJ: The impact of arthroscopic surgery on the management of disorders of the knee. Arthroscopy 6:96–99, 1990.
2. Clevers GJ, deVries LS, and Haarman HJ: Diagnostic arthroscopy of the knee joint: comparison of the accuracy to physical examination, contract arthrography and arthroscopy. Neth J Surg 40:104–107, 1988.
3. Guercio H and Solini A: Arthrography in the study of extra-meniscal pathology of the knee. Ital J Orthop Traumatol 14:257–265, 1988.
4. Gelb HJ, Glasgow SG, Sapega AA, et al.: Magnetic resonance imaging of knee disorders: clinical value and cost-effectiveness in a sports medicine practice. Am J Sports Med 24:99–103, 1996.
5. Boden SD, Davis DO, Dina TS, et al.: A prospective and blinded investigation of magnetic resonance imaging of the knee: abnormal findings in asymptomatic subjects. Clin Orthop 282:177–185, 1992.
6. Watanabe I, Takeda S, and Ikeuchi H: Atlas of Arthroscopy, 2nd ed. Tokyo, Igaku Shoin Ltd., 1969.
7. Gillquist J and Hagberg G: A new modification of the technique of arthroscopy of the knee joint. Acta Chir Scand 142:123–130, 1976.
8. Pipdin G: Knee injuries: the role of suprapatellar plica and suprapatellar bursa in stimulating internal derangement. Clin Orthop 74:161–175, 1971.
9. O'Rourke KS and Ike RW: Diagnostic anthroscopy in the arthritis patient. Rheum Dis Clin North Am 20:321–342, 1994.
10. Byers PD, Cotton RE, Deacon OW, et al.: The diagnosis and treatment of pigmented villonodular synovitis. J Bone Joint Surg Br 50:290, 1968.
11. Bronstein RD, Sebastianelli WJ, and DeHaven KE: Localized pigmented villonodular synovitis presenting as a loose body in a knee. Arthroscopy 9:596–598, 1993.
12. Milgram JW: Synovial osteochondromatosis: a histopathologic study of thirty-one cases. J Bone Joint Surg Am 59:792, 1977.
13. Blais RE, LaPrade RF, Chaljub G, et al.: The arthroscopic appearance of lipoma arborescens of the knee. Arthroscopy 11:623–627, 1995.
14. Joyce JJ III and Harty M: Surgery of the synovial fold: arthroscopy. In Casscells W (ed.): Diagnosis and Surgical Procedures. Philadelphia, Lea & Febiger, 1984, pp 201–209.
15. Lindberg U, Hamberg P, Lysholm J, et al.: Arthroscopic examination of the patellofemoral joint. Orthop Clin North Am 17:263–268, 1986.
16. Ficat RP and Hungerford DS: Disorders of the Patellofemoral Joint. Baltimore, Williams & Wilkins, 1977.
17. Ficat RP, Philippe J, and Hungerford DS: Chondromalacia patellae: a system of classification. Clin Orthop 144:55–62, 1979.
18. Schreiber SN: Technical note: proximal superomedial portal in arthroscopy of the knee. Arthroscopy 7:246–251, 1991.
19. Hughston JC, Walsh WM, and Puddu G: Patellar Subluxation and Dislocation. Philadelphia, W.B. Saunders Co., 1984.
20. Hughston JC: Subluxation of the patella. J Bone Joint Surg Am 50:1003–1026, 1968.
21. Green WT Jr: Painful bipartite patellae: a report of three cases. Clin Orthop 110:197–200, 1975.
22. Iossifidis A and Brueton RN: Painful bipartite patella following injury. Injury 26:175–176, 1995.
23. Johnson LL: Diagnostic and Surgical Arthroscopy: The Knee and Other Joints. St. Louis, C.V. Mosby, 1981.
24. Hardaker WT, Whipple TL, and Basset RH III: Diagnosis and treatment of the plica syndrome of the knee. J Bone Joint Surg Am 62:221–225, 1980.
25. Goodfellow J: Chondromalacia of the patella. In Pickett J and Radin EL (eds.): Chondromalacia of the Patella. Baltimore, Williams and Wilkins, 1977, p 120.
26. Fulkerson JP: Patellofemoral pain disorders: evaluation and management. Instr Course Lect 2:124–132, 1994.
27. Outerbridge RE: The etiology of chondromalacia patellae. J Bone Joint Surg Br 43:752–757, 1961.
28. Mitchell N and Shepherd N: The resurfacing of adult rabbit cartilage following multiple drill holes through the subchondral bone. J Bone Joint Surg Am 58:230, 1976.
29. Mankin HJ: The reaction of articular cartilage to injury and osteoarthritis: part I. N Engl J Med 291:1285, 1974.
30. Mankin HJ: The reaction of articular cartilage to injury and osteoarthritis: part II. N Engl J Med 291:1335, 1974.
31. Mankin HJ and Lippiello L: Biochemical and metabolic abnormalities in articular cartilage from osteoarthritic human hips. J Bone Joint Surg Am 52:424, 1970.
32. Patel D: Arthroscopy of the plica-synovial folds and their significance. Am J Sports Med 6:217–225, 1978.
33. Indelicato PA: Nonoperative management of complete tears of the medial collateral ligament. Orthop Rev 18:947–952, 1989.
34. Hansen H and Boe S: The pathological plica in the knee: results after arthroscopic resection. Arch Orthop Trauma Surg 108:282–284, 1989.

35. Broom HJ and Fulkerson JP: The plica syndrome: a new perspective. Orthop Clin North Am 17:279–281, 1986.
36. Sherman RMP and Jackson RW: The pathological medial plica: criteria for diagnosis and prognosis. J Bone Joint Surg Br 71:351, 1989.
37. Johnson DP, Eastwood DM, and Witherow PJ: Symptomatic synovial plicae of the knee. J Bone Joint Surg Am 75:1485–1496, 1993.
38. Thompson WO, Thaete FL, Fu FH, et al.: Tibial meniscal dynamics using 3D reconstruction of MR images. In Proceedings of the Orthopaedic Research Society 389, Chicago, Ill., 1990.
39. Jackson DW, Jennings LD, and Maywood RM: Magnetic resonance imaging of the knee. Am J Sports Med 16:29–38, 1988.
40. Barronian AD, Zoltan JD, and Bucon KA: Magnetic resonance imaging of the knee: correlation with arthroscopy. Arthroscopy 5:184–186, 1989.
41. Bellon EM, Keith MW, Coleman PE, et al.: Magnetic resonance imaging of internal derangement of the knee. Radiographics 8:95–118, 1988.
42. Herman LJ and Beltran J: Pitfalls in MR imaging of the knee. Radiology 167:775–781, 1988.
43. Eggli S, Wegmuller H, Kosina J, et al.: Long-term results of arthroscopic meniscal repair: an analysis of isolated tears. Am J Sports Med 23:715–720, 1995.
44. Arnoczky SP and Warren RF: The microvasculature of the meniscus and its response to injury: an experimental study in the dog. Am J Sports Med 11:131–141, 1983.
45. Arnoczky SP and Warren RF: Microvasculature of the human meniscus. Am J Sports Med 10:90–95, 1982.
46. Matthewson MH and Dandy J: Osteochondral fractures of the lateral femoral condyle. J Bone Joint Surg Br 48:436–440, 1978.
47. Johnson-Nurse C and Dandy DJ: Fracture-separation of articular cartilage in the adult knee. J Bone Joint Surg Br 67:42–43, 1985.
48. Bauer J and Jackson RW: Chondral lesions of the femoral condyles: a system of arthroscopic classification. Arthroscopy 4:97–102, 1988.
49. Aichroth P: Osteochondritis dissecans of the knee: a clinical survey. J Bone Joint Surg Br 53:440, 1971.
50. Hughston JC, Hergenroeder PT, and Courtenay BG: Osteochondritis dissecans of the femoral condyles. J Bone Joint Surg Am 66:1340, 1984.
51. Pappas A: Osteochondritis dissecans. Clin Orthop 158:59–68, 1981.
52. Oberlander MA, Shalvoy RM, and Hughston JC: The accuracy of the clinical knee examination documented by arthroscopy: a prospective study. Am J Sports Med 21:773–778, 1993.
53. Arnoczky SP: Anatomy of the anterior cruciate ligament. Clin Orthop 172:19, 1983.
54. Arnoczky SP and Warren RF: Anatomy of the cruciate ligaments. In Feagin JA (ed.): The Cruciate Ligaments. New York, Churchill Livingstone, 1988, pp 179–195.
55. Do-Dai DD, Youngberg RA, Lanchbury FD, et al.: Intraligamentous ganglion cysts of the anterior cruciate ligaments: MR findings with clinical and arthroscopic correlations. J Comput Assist Tomogr 20:80–84, 1996.
56. Hoffa A: The influence of the adipose tissue with regard to the pathology of the knee joint. JAMA 43:795, 1904.
57. Ogilvie-Harris DJ and Giddens J: Hoffa's disease: arthroscopic resection of the infrapatellar fat pad. Arthroscopy 10:184–187, 1994.
58. Shoemaker SC and Markolf KL: The role of the meniscus in the anterior-posterior stability of the loaded anterior cruciate deficient knee. J Bone Joint Surg Am 68:71–79, 1986.
59. Fine KM, Glasgow SG, and Torg JS: Tibial chondral fissures associated with the lateral meniscus. Arthroscopy 11:292–295, 1995.
60. Dickhaut SC and DeLee JC: The discoid lateral meniscus syndrome. J Bone Joint Surg Am 64:1068–1073, 1982.
61. Sugaqara O, Miyatsu M, Yamashita I, et al.: Problems with repeated arthroscopic surgery in the discoid meniscus. Arthroscopy 7:68–71, 1991.
62. Seger BM and Woods WG: Arthroscopic management of lateral meniscal cysts. Am J Sports Med 14:105–112, 1986.
63. Vergis A, Maletius W, and Messner K: An unusual case of vascular abnormality mimicking a lateral meniscal cyst. Arthroscopy 11:616–619, 1995.
64. Gillquist J, Hagberg G, and Oretorp N: Arthroscopic examination of the posteromedial compartment of the knee joint. Int Orthop 3:13–18, 1979.
65. Maynard MJ, Deng X, Wickiewicz TL, et al.: The popliteofibular ligament: rediscovery of a key element in posterolateral stability. Am J Sports Med 24:311–316, 1996.
66. Brantigan OC and Voshell AF: Ligaments of the knee joint: the relationship of the ligament of Wrisberg. J Bone Joint Surg Am 28:66–72, 1946.
67. Heller L and Langman J: The meniscofemoral ligaments of the human knee. J Bone Joint Surg Br 46:307–314, 1964.
68. Gold DL, Schaner PJ, and Sapega AA: The posteromedial portal in knee arthroscopy: an analysis of diagnostic and surgical utility. Arthroscopy 11:139–145, 1995.
69. Gillquiest J, Hagberg G, and Oretorp N: Arthroscopy in acute injuries of the knee joint. Acta Orthop Scand 48:190–204, 1977.
70. DeHaven KE: Diagnosis of acute knee injuries with hemarthrosis. Am J Sports Med 8:9–15, 1980.
71. Fanelli GC: Posterior cruciate ligament injuries in trauma patients. Arthroscopy 9:291–294, 1993.
72. Bomberg BC and McGinty JB: Acute hemarthrosis of the knee: indications for diagnostic arthroscopy. Arthroscopy 6:221–225, 1990.

22 Meniscus Tears/Repair

Daniel G. McBride • *William G. Clancy, Jr*

Only in the last 15–20 years has the importance of the menisci to knee function been fully appreciated. With this appreciation has come an intense effort to define ways of either successfully preserving or replacing injured menisci. The menisci were initially presumed to be inconsequential and functionless, evolutionary remnants of leg muscle that could be removed without causing dysfunction to the knee.[1] Annandale[2] in 1885 first described meniscal repair and noted that the procedure was quite tedious. King[3] first described the harmful effects of meniscal excision, later popularized by Fairbank,[4] and showed that menisci were capable of healing if the tear had access to a synovial blood supply. The concept of the need for meniscal preservation was slow to gain acceptance, and even as recently as 1970 Smilie[1] advocated meniscectomy if damage to the posterior horn was suspected. Subsequent studies have confirmed the detrimental effects of meniscectomy, and intensive basic science studies have documented the structure and function of the meniscus.[5–11] Ikeuchi[12] first reported meniscal repair using arthroscopic technique, and DeHaven[13] first reported meniscal repair using open technique. Since 1980 there has been significant advance in meniscal repair technique and understanding of meniscal healing. However, efforts to stimulate meniscal healing have met with only limited success to date.

MENISCAL FUNCTION

The various functions of the menisci include load transmission, shock absorption, joint stabilization, cartilage nutrition, and joint lubrication.[5, 6, 9, 14–16] They transmit approximately 50% of the weight-bearing forces in extension and 85% in flexion.[9] Their role in shock absorption in the gait cycle occurs via viscoelastic deformation. The shape of the menisci contributes to synovial fluid distribution throughout the joint, joint lubrication, and cartilage nutrition.[16] The medial meniscus also contributes to joint stability in the absence of the anterior cruciate ligament (ACL).[6] Meniscectomy would be expected to disrupt all of

these functions and result in knee dysfunction. Studies have shown significant (up to 300%) increases in articular cartilage contact stresses with meniscal excision.[5, 9, 16] Partial meniscectomy results in similar, although less dramatic, increases.[9] The principal orientation of collagen fibers within the meniscus is circumferential, which is critical to the ability of the menisci to withstand "hoop stresses" created when compressive loads are applied. Complete transverse meniscal tears, or even "small" resections incorporating the entire transverse thickness, can nearly result in complete compromise of function. These data, along with studies that document the presence of premature degenerative changes after meniscectomy, have resulted in attempts to preserve the menisci and promote their healing.[4, 8, 11]

BASIC SCIENCE

The major goal of current research is to understand and promote meniscal healing. In 1936 King[3] first demonstrated meniscal healing in the canine stifle. He concluded that this occurs only if the tear is accessible to the synovial blood supply, limiting healing to the periphery of the meniscus. Almost 50 years later Arnoczky and Warren[7] first demonstrated the microvasculature of the human meniscus. They showed that only the peripheral 10–25% of the menisci are vascularized, supplied by a perimeniscal capillary plexus originating in the capsular and synovial tissues (Fig. 22–1). Only this vascular portion of the meniscus can mount a healing response, and this concept had led to the delineation of "reparable" regions of menisci (Fig. 22–2).

Efforts have been directed toward finding ways of stimulating meniscal healing in regions with poor or no blood supply. Arnoczky, Warren, and Spivak[17] first demonstrated in dogs that insertion of fibrin clot in a tear can promote healing. Since that time, others[14, 18–22] have used this technique in humans and have documented improved healing rates of their meniscal repairs compared

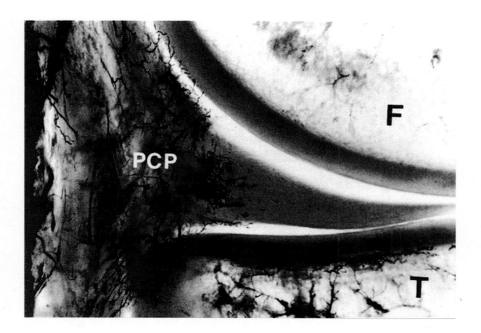

Figure 22–1 • Frontal section 5 mm thick of the medial compartment of the knee (Spalteholz ×3). Branching radial vessels from the perimeniscal capillary plexus (*PCP*) can be seen penetrating the peripheral border of the medial meniscus (*F*: femur, *T*: tibia). (From Arnoczky SP and Warren RF: Microvasculature of the human meniscus. Am J Sports Med 10:91, 1982.)

with prior results in which no clot was used. In 1988 Zhang[23] introduced the concept of trephination as a means of promoting vascular ingrowth to an avascular region of the meniscus to stimulate healing in these regions. This technique has had only limited success in clinical studies, with contradictory reports on results and concerns regarding injury to remaining intact meniscal

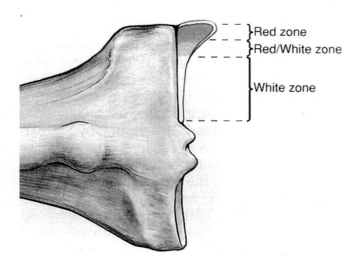

Figure 22–2 • Schematic drawing indicating the various zones of the meniscus. Note the red and red/white zones are capable of healing, and repair is recommended. The red zone, 0–2 mm from the periphery, has an excellent propensity to heal; the red/white zone, 2–5 mm from the periphery, has a good-to-excellent propensity to heal; the white zone, more than 5 mm from the periphery, has a fair-to-poor propensity to heal. (From Miller MD, Warner JJP, and Harner CD: Meniscal repair. In Fu FH, Harner CD, and Vince KG [eds.]: Knee Surgery. Baltimore, Williams & Wilkins, 1994, p 616.)

architecture by the trephination technique.[14, 24–26] Henning et al.[20] reported limited success using fascial sheath coverage and fibrin clot along with suture repair of complex, traditionally irreparable, tears of menisci in the avascular zones. This method is technically demanding, time-consuming, and not likely to become routine practice for meniscal repair.

For healing of the meniscus, in addition to an adequate vascular supply, tissue stability is critical, and this can be determined only at arthroscopy. If the tear is stable, repair is not necessary. Stability has been defined as a tear 10 mm or less in length and displaced less than 3 mm into the joint with probing.[14, 15, 27–29] A less precise but clinically relevant definition of stability is a tear that cannot be displaced so as to be caught between femoral and tibial articular surfaces. It is recommended that efforts be made to stimulate vascular response to these stable tears, including freshening of tear edges, synovial abrasion, and, if no procedure such as ACL reconstruction is being performed concomitantly, fibrin clot placement.[14, 15, 18, 20, 22, 30–32] If the tear is judged unstable, but reparable, suture repair is performed using the techniques described in this chapter.

A number of studies have shown conclusively that a stable knee is important for success of meniscal repair and healing.[20, 22, 26, 30, 33, 34] Many reports have shown superior healing rates, 90–100%, in knees that have undergone concomitant ligament, principally ACL, reconstruction. This has been attributed both to restored joint stability and to the liberation of factors important to tissue healing by the reconstructive procedure, factors not present in abundance in isolated meniscal repair. Healing rates have uniformly been significantly less at 30–70% in unstable joints. In a well-documented study with strict criteria for assessment of healing, Scott, Jolly, and Henning[35] showed that healing rates of repairs of isolated tears in stable, ACL-intact knees were significantly less than those in stable ACL-reconstructed knees; however, both rates were higher than those observed in unstable knees. They attrib-

Table 22–1	Healing Criteria
Healed	Healed over entire tear length and residual cleft at tear site of <10% meniscal thickness
Partially healed	Healed over entire tear length and residual cleft at tear site of <50% meniscal thickness
Not healed	Residual cleft of >50% of full thickness at any location along tear site

Adapted from Scott GA, Jolly BL, and Henning CE: Combined posterior incision and arthroscopic intra-articular repair of the meniscus. J Bone Joint Surg Am 68:847, 1986.

uted this to the lack of tissue-healing factors in the unstable knees that are liberated in the reconstructed knees. Others have not reported this difference but their criteria for defining a repair were less stringent than those of Scott, Jolly, and Henning. These data have led to the general consensus that a meniscal repair in an ACL-deficient knee should be performed in concert with ACL reconstruction. Of note, Shelbourne and Johnson[36] recommended that meniscal repair and ACL reconstruction be performed in two stages in patients presenting with an ACL tear and a locked bucket-handle meniscal tear with flexion contractures in the 20 degree range. Their study showed that these patients had significantly greater motion loss (lack of full extension) when the procedures were combined.

Studies reporting meniscal repair and healing must be carefully assessed for means of defining "healed." The strictest criteria to date are those of Scott, Jolly, and Henning,[35] determined by arthroscopy and arthrography (Table 22–1). Many studies determine healing as having occurred when the patient is asymptomatic. However, Henning and others have shown by arthrography or arthroscopy that a significant number of clinically healed tears are partially healed or not healed.[19, 32, 35] Magnetic resonance imaging has not yet proved reliable in assessing meniscal healing.

INDICATIONS FOR REPAIR

There are many factors to consider regarding meniscal repair. Selecting the appropriate patient before observing the meniscus is critical to clinical success of the procedure. Although there is no particular age cutoff, younger patients are better served with meniscal repair than are older patients. Studies have shown that in older patients, tears heal as well as in younger patients; however, in older patients complications such as deep venous thrombosis and postoperative stiffness occur more frequently, and the long-term benefit of meniscal preservation owing to fewer remaining years of knee use decreases.[18, 35] Patients including professional athletes and laborers who require a rapid return to work may not be able to comply with the downtime required for meniscal repair, especially compared with the relatively short period of recovery for meniscal resection. Finally, a noncompliant patient in any category is probably best served with a meniscal resection.

Each patient should be informed of the benefits and risks of the procedures in addition to the required postoperative regimens and should contribute to the decision for repair or resection.

Newman, Daniels, and Burks[15] detailed three important issues to be considered when assessing a meniscus and whether to repair it. First, the tear must be technically reparable. Factors important in this regard include surgeon proficiency with meniscal repair, tissue quality, location of the tear, and tear pattern. Those surgeons dealing with meniscal disease should be technically proficient in one of the standard techniques of repair, either open or arthroscopic. Degenerated tissue, or menisci with multiple or complex tears, is generally not reparable, even in experienced hands. A vertical longitudinal tear at the periphery is an indication for repair, whereas radial, flap, and horizontal cleavage–type tears are not. Very long tears generally do not heal quite as well as shorter ones, but if the tear is "good" and is peripheral, it still should be repaired. Old, chronic tears are less reparable than acute tears. Finally, chronically displaced bucket-handle tears may be deformed to the extent that they cannot be adequately reapproximated to the rim bed and are not good candidates for repair.

Healing potential is the second important issue in assessing repair. In order for the tear to heal, it must have a vascular supply or be provided with an environment that stimulates a repair response. Presently, tears in the red or red/white zone are considered good candidates for healing as they have access to a blood supply. Meniscal tears performed in concert with an ACL reconstruction are provided with a stimulus for healing even if they are in the white zone, and thus indication for repair should be liberalized in these cases. In addition, fibrin clot, vascularized synovial flaps and, possibly, trephination can provide an appropriate healing environment.

Functional restoration is the third issue to consider in making a decision about repair. If a meniscus can be technically repaired, but will not retain function, then repair is not productive. A complete radial tear and repair of a central fragment to a capsular bed without the peripheral rim are examples of cases in which function will not be restored. Finally, not all tears need repair. Partial tears and stable tears less than 10 mm in length need not be repaired as they have been shown to heal and remain functional.[29]

PATIENT EDUCATION

Ideally, the patient should be educated about all the considerations in the preceding section. The patient should understand the expected postoperative course and rehabilitation time commitment of meniscal repair and resection; the patient may not wish or be able to comply with restrictions attendant on repair. The expected short-term and long-term benefits to meniscal repair of concomitant ligament reconstruction should be thoroughly understood preoperatively so that an appropriate decision can be made for or against reconstruction. The patient should be made aware of possible additional scars and potential complications, including possibility of failure and need for return to the operating room for symptomatic failure that attend meniscal repair. Despite the long-term benefits of meniscal repair, the patient may choose the easier short-term course of resection and should be allowed to do so if he or she has been properly informed.

SURGICAL TECHNIQUES

General

There are four basic techniques of meniscal repair currently performed. They are open repair and arthroscopic techniques including inside-out, outside-in, and all-inside. Each has been shown to have a high rate of success when properly applied to an appropriate tear. The arthroscopic techniques inside-out and outside-in are the ones most commonly used. The major factors to consider when deciding which to use include the surgeon's familiarity with a particular technique and the location of the meniscal tear. As outcomes are comparable with all of the techniques, the surgeon should choose the one that he or she can perform well and in a timely fashion. This caveat should be modified only if a particular tear is not amenable to repair by that procedure. For example, tears not within 1 or 2 mm from the rim are not good candidates for open repair, and only posterior horn tears are treatable by the all-inside technique.

Meniscal Preparation

The principles of meniscal preparation are applicable to all four repair techniques.[14, 22, 27] An effort should be made to place the torn surfaces in good position for healing. Débridement of old scar tissue with hand-held rasps or gently maneuvered motorized shavers should be performed. Resection of the peripheral rim of the meniscus, so that the central portion can be reattached to the vascular capsule, is not advocated as it has been shown not to be any more advantageous for healing and is detrimental to meniscal function because the remaining fragment sutured peripherally is no longer in a position to bear weight.[9, 10, 13, 37] Synovial abrasion is advocated in an attempt to stimulate vascular ingrowth to the tear site. Placement of vascular access channels, or trephination, can be performed at this time if this method is favored. After the meniscus has been prepared, the repair sutures are placed as described later. It is now generally accepted that the repair sutures should be tied directly over capsular structures instead of over the skin or subcutaneous tissues, as was performed early on. This requires a skin incision and tissue dissection down to the capsular layer. If fibrin clot is to be used, it is placed into the tear site before the sutures are tied. It can be placed into the site with a syringe or can be sutured into place as previously described.[20] The fibrin clot is prepared in the following manner: 60 mL of the patient's blood is stirred in a container with a glass rod for 5–10 minutes. The clot forms on the glass rod and can then be washed off with saline and set aside for eventual placement in the tear as described earlier.[14, 20, 22] If Henning's[20] technique of fascial sheath is to be attempted, the fascial sheath is placed but not tied down, followed by insertion of the fibrin clot, the clot being placed under the

sheath.[20] In the knee where concomitant ligament reconstruction is being performed, a fibrin clot is not necessary because the bleeding resulting from the reconstruction is thought to be sufficient. Also, the sutures should be tied down after completion of the repair and deflation of the tourniquet to allow blood to enter the tear space more easily and to avoid excess stress to the repair while the knee is being manipulated during the reconstructive procedure.

Open Repair Technique

Although first reported by Annandale[2] in 1885, not until the 1980s did DeHaven[13] report on the results of open meniscal repairs. DeHaven's technique remains the standard for open repairs and has been well described.[13, 28, 31, 37, 38] The indications for and technique of open repair are described in this section.

The general indications for meniscal repair described in the section titled Indications for Repair, apply to the open technique. DeHaven advocated initial arthroscopic examination of the menisci and knee to asses suitability for repair. The decision regarding open versus arthroscopic repair is made at the time of arthroscopic examination. He preferred to repair posterior meniscal capsular disruptions using the open technique and stated that the primary indication for open repair is a vertical tear of the posterior horn of the lateral or medial meniscus that is within 1–2 mm of the meniscosynovial junction. Tears not within 1–2 mm of the meniscosynovial junction or those extending beyond the posterior third of the meniscus into the middle and anterior thirds are better addressed using arthroscopic techniques. Those tears greater than 1–2 mm from the junction are not easily visualized using the open technique, and tears extending into the middle and anterior thirds would require extensive dissection beyond the usual open incision.

Those who advocate open repair note that injured meniscal tissue can best be reapproximated to its site of origin using this technique. This applies to both security of the repair and to accurate spatial approximation of the meniscus to its bed. Additionally, as most arthroscopic techniques require an incision down to the capsule, the traditional advantage of arthroscopic procedures over the open technique is not realized in this case. Finally, the open technique is not associated with blind needle passage in the proximity of the neurovascular structures and the possible catastrophic complications of this maneuver.

Medial Meniscal Repair

DeHaven approaches the medial meniscal repair in the following fashion (Fig. 22–3). The knee is flexed to 90 degrees, and a vertical skin incision is made posterior to the medial collateral ligament. Care is taken to avoid the saphenous nerve during the dissection. The deep fascia is incised, and the posteromedial capsule is visualized and opened vertically just posterior to the posterior oblique ligament. The meniscal rim and capsular bed are trimmed of unstable fragments and scar and freshened to ensure vascularity. Stable meniscal tissue still attached to the capsule is not excised because this tissue remains vascular;

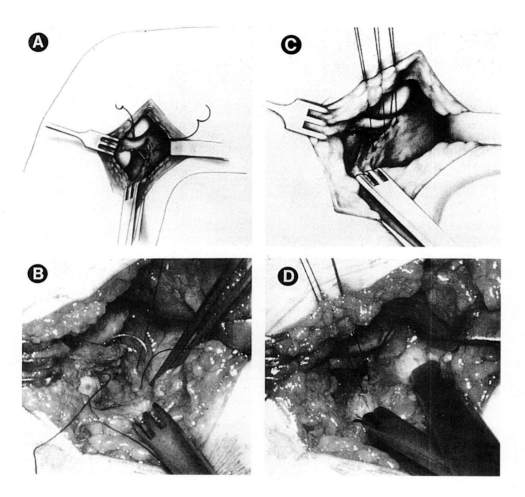

Figure 22–3 • *A* and *B,* An oblique capsular incision is made posterior to the medial collateral ligament to expose the meniscus tear. After preparation of the tear site, the meniscal rim is sutured to its capsular bed with a vertically placed 4-0 absorbable suture. A double-armed suture is used, first passing the small needle from the inferior to superior surface of the meniscus, and then the larger needle is passed, from below, upward through the capsular bed. *C* and *D,* Individual sutures are placed 3–4 mm apart and tied intracapsularly, using as many sutures as are necessary to achieve a strong repair. (From DeHaven KD and Bronstein RD: Open meniscus repair. Oper Tech Sports Med 2:173, 1994.)

excision of it would compromise function of the remaining repaired portion. Repair is then accomplished using a double-armed 4-0 absorbable suture with a smaller needle on one end. The smaller needle is passed, from below, upward through the meniscal rim while the larger needle is passed, from below, upward through the capsular bed. In this way the capsular bed is reapproximated to the entire height of the meniscal rim with vertically oriented sutures. Sutures are placed 3–4 mm apart, and the knots are tied inside the capsule. DeHaven uses a 2-0 suture to secure the meniscus to the capsule at the site of the capsular incision as well as repair the capsular incision. The subcutaneous and skin incisions are then closed in standard fashion.

Lateral Meniscal Repair

The knee is flexed at 90 degrees for lateral repairs, and a vertical skin incision is made just posterior to the lateral collateral ligament at the level of the joint line. The iliotibial band is then split in line with its fibers at the level of the joint line, and the biceps femoris tendon is retracted posteriorly, exposing the capsule and popliteus tendon. The capsule is opened obliquely along the posterior border of the popliteus tendon, exposing the meniscal tear (Fig. 22–4). The meniscus and capsular bed are prepared in the same fashion as was done on the medial side.

The presence of the popliteus tendon makes suture passage more difficult laterally than medially, and this necessitates a change in mode of throwing the sutures. In this case, the small needle of the 4-0 absorbable suture is passed, from above, downward through the meniscus rim and then, from below, upward through the capsular bed (see Fig. 22–4D and E). The sutures are again placed 3–4 mm apart and are not usually placed into the popliteus tendon itself but may be if this is necessary to achieve stability of the repair. The capsule, subcutaneous, and skin tissues are closed in the same fashion as on the medial side.

Outside-In Meniscal Repair

Advantage cited for outside-in meniscal repair include versatility, little specialized instrumentation, relatively easy access to anterior and middle thirds of the menisci, and allowance for only small incisions to protect the neurovascular structures.[21, 39–41] The technique uses small incisions placed perpendicularly to and at the level of the joint line for each pair of sutures placed. Subcutaneous tissue is spread down to the capsule and the sutures are tied at this layer. Strategies to avoid the neurovascular structures include retraction to expose the capsule, prebending the needles when working posteriorly to avoid a posterior entry site and trajectory, and proper positioning of the

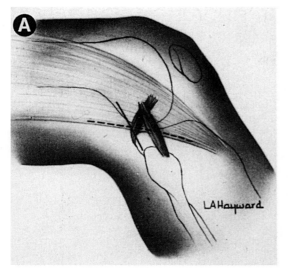

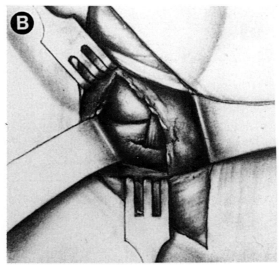

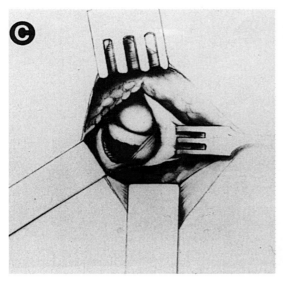

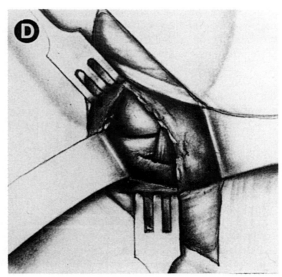

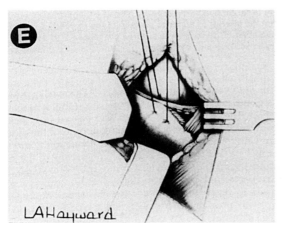

Figure 22–4 • *A,* A vertical skin incision is made in line with the posterior border of the fibula. The iliotibial band is split in line with its fibers, and the biceps muscle is retracted posteriorly. *B,* An oblique capsular incision is then made posterior to the popliteus tendon. *C,* Peripheral tear of the posterior horn of the lateral meniscus extends into the popliteal hiatus. *D* and *E,* The suture is passed first from superior to inferior through the meniscus and then through the strong fibers that run from the medial belly of the popliteus to the lateral meniscus and then through the surgical bed. (From DeHaven KD and Bronstein RD: Open meniscus repair. Oper Tech Sports Med 2:174, 1994.)

knee. The knee is placed in 90 degrees of flexion when lateral meniscal repairs are performed.[21] With the knee in this degree of flexion, all needles should enter at a point anterior to the biceps femoris tendon to aid in protecting the peroneal nerve. Cooper, Arnoczky, and Warren[21, 40] advocated 90 degrees of flexion when working medially because the saphenous nerve falls posteriorly and out of harm's way in this position. Cooper[40] noted the importance of retractor placement deep to the sartorius muscle as placement superficial to the sartorial fascia may not protect the saphenous nerve. Morgan and Casscells[41] advocated only slight flexion because they found that the saphenous nerve was drawn anteriorly by knee extension. Additionally, it has been noted that posteromedial meniscal repairs should be performed in only slight flexion to avoid obliterating the posterior capsular pouch that is formed in flexion and consequently "capturing" the knee in flexion (Fig. 22–5).

Repair is begun by preparing the meniscal surfaces as described in the preceding paragraph. The knee is positioned, and small incisions are made where necessary. An 18 gauge spinal needle is then passed across the tear from the outside in, taking care to avoid neurovascular structures. The unstable torn portion can be stabilized using a probe or grasper during needle passage. The stylet is then removed, followed by passage of an 0 or 1 polydioxanone suture. A few variations in technique have been presented for securing the tear.

Cooper, Arnoczky, and Warren[21] described delivering this suture end through an anterior portal, tying a large mulberry knot in its end, and pulling the suture and knot back into the joint so that the knot lies against the meniscal surface. Two adjacent sutures placed in this fashion are tied together over the capsule under direct visualization to secure fixation of the tear. Cooper[40] described a modification of this technique, whereby a double-throw knot is placed in one suture, and then two adjacent sutures, having been simultaneously drawn out the anterior portal, are tied together with three throws. The sutures are then pulled into the joint, the one with the double throw leading. The smaller double knot is drawn across the tear followed by the larger knot and trailing suture, followed finally by tying the external ends over capsule. This creates a horizontal mattress meniscal repair stitch (Fig. 22–6).

Johnson[39] described a technique using needles with stylets followed by wire snares. The cannulated needles are passed outside-in in the usual fashion and are placed adjacent to each other in a position to secure the tear (approximately 3 mm apart). The stylets are successively replaced by looped wire snares that are used to grasp the two ends of a free suture placed into the joint via the same anterior portal. A grasper is used to place the suture end into the snare so that it can then be pulled out of the needle into the smaller wound (Figs. 22–7 and 22–8). The suture ends are then tied snugly over the capsule, creating a horizontal mattress repair of the meniscus. This process is repeated as many times as necessary to secure the length of the tear. O'Donnell, Ruland, and Ruland[42] described a variation of this technique whereby the wire loop from one needle can be placed about the second needle to "automatically" grasp a suture directed from the outside in through the second

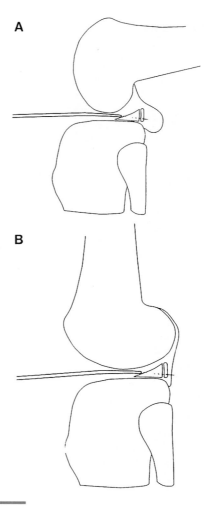

Figure 22–5 • In flexion (*A*), there is a pouch between the meniscus and the posterior capsular wall that disappears when the knee is extended (*B*). If a medial meniscal repair needle is passed with the knee in flexion, the pouch can be obliterated, thus interfering with the ability to fully extend the knee. (From Newman AP and Burks RT: Arthroscopic meniscal repair: "inside-out" technique. Oper Tech Sports Med 2:179, 1994.)

needle, thus streamlining the procedure. After securing the sutures over the capsule, the subcutaneous and skin tissues are closed in standard fashion.

Inside-Out Meniscal Repair

Inside-out meniscal repair is currently the most popular repair technique.[14, 43, 44] First popularized by Henning in the early 1980s, it involves placement of sutures across the tear from inside the knee out, using specialized cannulae for needle delivery. The primary advantage of this technique over others is accurate suture placement. Potential for neurovascular injury is greater than for outside-in techniques as needle passage is to some degree blind, although appropriately placed incisions and retractors decrease the

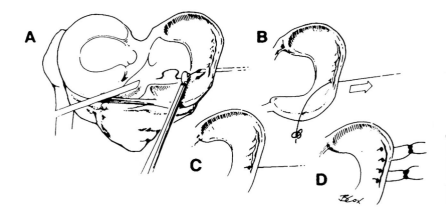

Figure 22–6 • Illustration (*A* to *D*) demonstrating outside-in technique. (From Hanks GA and Kalenak A: Alternative arthroscopic techniques for meniscal repair: a review. Orthop Rev 19:541–548, 1990.)

risk, and specialized cannulae that direct the needles away from the neurovascular structures provide an increased margin of safety. This technique uses nearly the same incisions as the open technique, making the advantage of arthroscopic repair artificial. However, significantly more tears are accessible for repair using the inside-out technique than with the open procedure.

The repair begins by first assessing the tear arthroscopically and then appropriately preparing the meniscus. For medial meniscal repairs, an approach similar to an open repair is performed. The saphenous nerve can be transilluminated in the posteromedial corner with the arthroscope facilitating its protection.[14, 32, 43, 44] The incision is carried down to the joint capsule deep to the semimembranosus and the medial half of the medial gastrocnemius. All of the medial hamstrings and the medial half of the gastrocnemius are retracted posteriorly. A popliteal retractor is placed between the capsule and these structures (Fig. 22–9). Laterally, the incision is placed just posterior to the lateral collateral ligament, and the iliotibial band is split in line of its fibers at the level of the joint line.

The biceps femoris is bluntly dissected between its anterior and middle thirds, and this is continued between the lateral half of the lateral head of the gastrocnemius and the posterior capsule–arcuate ligament complex (Fig. 22–10). The popliteal retractor is then placed in front of the gastrocnemius; the gastrocnemius, not the biceps femoris, protects the peroneal nerve as it courses along the medial side of the biceps. Figure 22–11 illustrates this concept.

Devices to assist in suture passage have proliferated since Henning used only a modified needle holder and a doubly bent Keith needle. Clancy and Graf[45] in 1983 described a double-lumen cannula system through which two small needles linked by a suture were simultaneously passed. Rosenberg[46] later described repair using malleable single-lumen cannulae with different curvatures. These provided greater versatility in suture placement because vertical and oblique sutures could more easily be placed. In 1993 Mooney and Rosenberg[43] reported their use of zone-specific cannulae; these were rigidly prebent to conform to the normal anatomy of the tibial spines and femoral condyles and also facilitated repair of the anterior, middle,

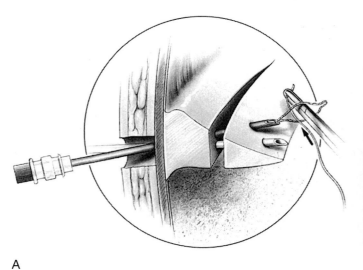

A

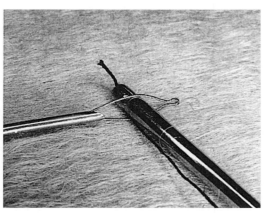

B

Figure 22–7 • *A*, A suture is placed through the cable loop with a miniature forceps. *B*, Photograph of simulation. (From Johnson LL: Meniscus repair: the outside-in technique. In Jackson DW [ed.]: Reconstructive Knee Surgery. New York, Raven Press, 1995, pp 51–68.)

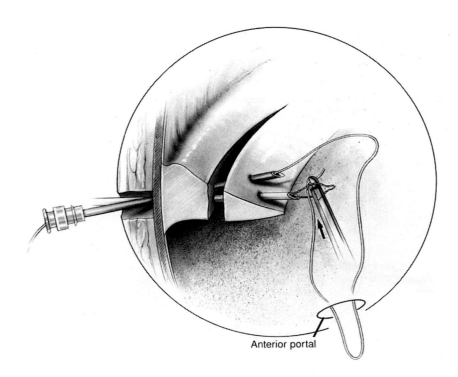

Figure 22–8 • Second suture placement in the cable loop of second needle. (From Johnson LL: Meniscus repair: the outside-in technique. In Jackson DW [eds.]: Reconstructive Knee Surgery. New York, Raven Press, 1995, pp 51–68.)

Anterior portal

or posterior third of the meniscus. The set consists of six cannulae, three for the right medial meniscus and three for the left medial meniscus (Fig. 22–12). The right and left medial cannulae allow repair of the left and right lateral menisci, respectively. In 1988 Jakob, Staubli, Zuber, et al.[47] described a set of three cannulae with various radii to be used with needles with a perforation 15 mm from the needle tip that functioned in a manner reminiscent of a sewing machine needle. These cannulae facilitated suture passage and required passage of only a small length of needle. Finally, Esser[48] in 1993 described a meniscal repair needle useful for either inside-out or outside-in repairs.

The needle has an eye 3 mm from the tip that can be opened and closed via a remote notch placed on the handle. This device allows precise suture placement and requires minimal traverse of the needle through soft tissues. Each of these devices can be safely and successfully used for inside-out meniscal repair.

The choice of portal for cannulae and suture placement is important for ease of repair, adequacy of repair, and safety. It is ideal to place sutures perpendicular to the tear as viewed from the axial plane in order that coaptation of the tear and suture resistance to shear be maximized. However, the neurovascular structures must be avoided,

Figure 22–9 • Posteromedial exposure. The posteromedial exposure requires an incision of 3 cm made posterior to the posterior oblique ligament and extended distally from the joint line. The sartorius and sartorial branch of the saphenous nerve are retracted posteriorly, along with the gracilis and semitendinosus muscles. Blunt dissection then permits palpation of the joint-line sulcus. It is not necessary to dissect deep to the semimembranosus or medial gastrocnemius tendon, because these structures are suitable for suture fixation (*MCL*: medial collateral ligament). (From Mooney MF and Rosenberg TD: Meniscus repair: the inside-out technique. In Jackson DW [ed.]: Reconstructive Knee Surgery. New York, Raven Press, 1995, pp 69–86.)

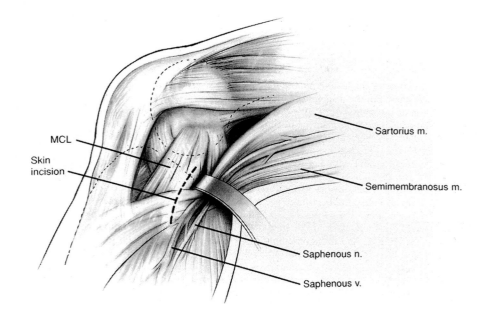

MCL

Skin incision

Sartorius m.

Semimembranosus m.

Saphenous n.

Saphenous v.

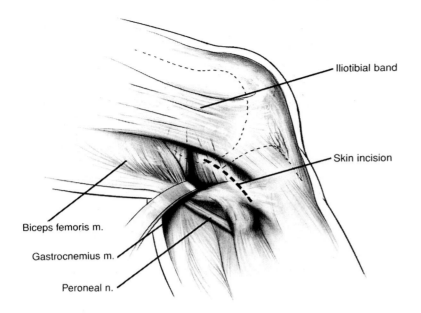

Iliotibial band

Skin incision

Biceps femoris m.

Gastrocnemius m.

Peroneal n.

Figure 22–10 • Posterolateral exposure. The posterolateral exposure for meniscal repair starts with an incision along the posterior edge of the iliotibial band and extends 3 cm distally from the joint line. Dissection is accomplished between the anterior border of the biceps and the posterior margin of the iliotibial band. Blunt dissection is completed between the arcuate complex and the capsule anteriorly and the lateral gastrocnemius tendon posteriorly. The peroneal nerve lies medial to the biceps and is not protected by retraction of the biceps alone; rather, it is the retracted gastrocnemius tendon that also protects the peroneal nerve. (From Mooney MF and Rosenberg TD: Meniscus repair: the inside-out technique. In Jackson DW [ed.]: Reconstructive Knee Surgery. New York, Raven Press, 1995, pp 69–86.)

making ideal suture placement in some cases impractical, particularly in the often-injured posterior horns. Some authors have recommended that curved cannulae should always be placed from the contralateral portal with the curve directing the needle away from the midline neurovascular structures. Scott, Jolly, and Henning[35] advocated repair of the posteromedial meniscus with a cannula in the anteromedial portal while orienting the curves in the Keith needle away from the midline and, after the needle has passed through the tear, maneuvering the cannula against the medial spine to maximize direction of the needle away from the neurovascular structures. Mooney and Rosenberg's[43] zone-specific cannulae system seeks to eliminate problems in this area. They note that all repairs are performed from the contralateral portal while viewing from the ipsilateral portal. The posterior cannulae can be positioned posterior or anterior to the tibial spines while the middle and anterior cannulae are placed anterior to the tibial spines (Fig. 22–13).

It has been shown that vertical mattress suture orientation provides the most secure repair, whereas horizontal mattress sutures involving the meniscal surface failed at a respectable 85% tearing stress of the vertical mattress.[49] Horizontal sutures should not be placed on only one surface (femoral or tibial) as eversion of the tear on the opposite surface will result (Fig. 22–14). Vertical sutures should be placed in a diverging fashion as Henning[20] described; this provides for maximal coaptation of the tear. Horizontal mattress sutures should be placed such that there is a 2–4 mm intact bridge between the two arms to prevent cutting through of the suture. Additionally, most authors advocate placement of a separate suture for every 3–5 mm of tear. Finally, sutures should not be placed so close to the tear margin that they can easily cut out nor so close to the free margin that they cause puckering of the meniscus.

It is generally accepted that either nonabsorbable or polydioxanone absorbable sutures be used for meniscal repairs because they have been shown to retain significant strength beyond 6 weeks' time while exposed to synovial fluid.[50, 51]

Meniscal repair proceeds as follows. The needle is advanced through the cannula of choice until 2–3 mm protrudes from the tip. The needle tip is used to "harpoon" and reduce the torn central portion of the meniscus to the stable rim. The needle is then advanced 1–2 cm until it is visualized through the incision; the needle can then be grasped with a needle holder and delivered with the attached suture out of the incision. The companion needle is then passed in similar fashion, placing it in either a vertical, oblique, or horizontal fashion. The needles are removed, and the two sutures are tagged with a hemostat. Placement of the remainder of necessary sutures proceeds with the same technique, adjusting cannulae or selecting appropriately designed cannulae as needed. On the lateral side, sutures are passed with the knee in 70–90 degrees of flexion, allowing the peroneal nerve to fall posteriorly; on the medial side, 10–30 degrees of flexion is required in order that the posteromedial capsular recess not be obliterated (see Fig. 22–5). After all the sutures have been placed, light tension should applied on the sutures, and the meniscus should be probed to ensure adequacy of the repair. The sutures are not tied until after all are passed and any concomitant surgery is completed. They are then tied with modest tension over the capsule, followed by subcutaneous tissue and skin closure.

All-Inside Meniscal Repair

All-inside repair of the meniscus has been described by Morgan[52, 53] and is indicated for repair of mobile, single, vertical longitudinal tears of the posterior horn of either meniscus located with 3 mm of the meniscocapsular junction. This technique utilizes specialized instrumentation that allows placement and tying of vertically oriented sutures across the meniscus tear all under arthroscopic control. It is attractive because it requires no incisions except those for portal placement, avoids neurovascular risk from suture needle passage, and can address tears far

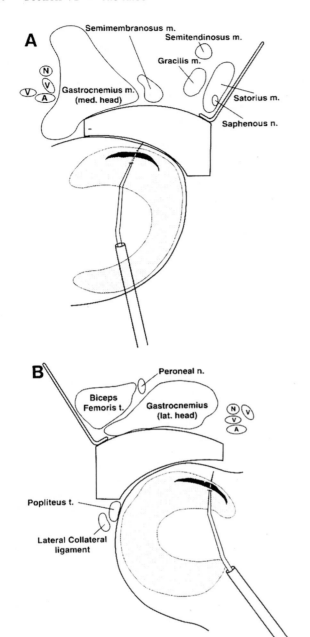

Figure 22–11 • *A* and *B*, Henning's technique improves the ability to place the repair sutures perpendicular to the tear, but the needles are closer to the neurovascular structures. With this method, it is imperative that careful posterior dissections and popliteal retractors be used. (From Newman AP and Burks RT: Arthroscopic meniscal repair: "inside-out" technique. Oper Tech Sports Med 2:181, 1994.)

posterocentrally near the root attachment not accessible with the other arthroscopic techniques.

The injured meniscus is viewed with a 70 degree arthroscope placed through the intercondylar notch from either the anteromedial or anterolateral portal. An 8 mm cannula is inserted through either posterior portal that had been created under direct visualization. Laterally, this portal is placed in the soft spot above the biceps femoris ten-

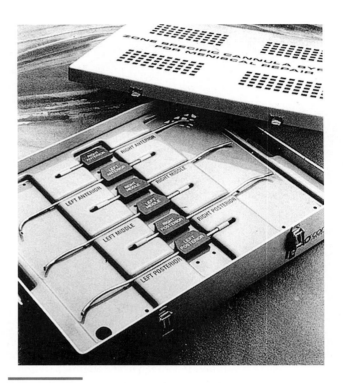

Figure 22–12 • Zone-specific repair. Zone-specific repair cannulae are specially designed for each zone of the meniscus and are rigidly prebent to conform to the normal anatomy of the tibial spines and femoral condyles. (From Mooney MF and Rosenberg TD: Meniscus repair: the inside-out technique. In Jackson DW [ed.]: Reconstructive Knee Surgery. New York, Raven Press, 1995, pp 69–86.)

don behind and above the joint line, with the knee flexed to 90 degrees (Fig. 22–15). Medially, the portal is placed through the soft spot above the medial hamstring tendons behind and above the joint line, again with the knee flexed to 90 degrees (Fig. 22–16). The meniscal tissue is then débrided to stimulate a healing response, using rasps in a manner described earlier.

Suturing of the tear is accomplished using the various suture hooks in Figure 22–17. Suture hooks are available in three types of terminal design: a straight hook, a 45 degree right and left hook, and a right and left corkscrew. They are placed through the working posterior portals and then manipulated across the tear by first penetrating the stable posterior inferior rim and then advancing across the tear into the mobile fragment in an inferior-to-superior direction (Fig. 22–18). Then, 12–14 in of suture is then advanced into the posterior compartment through the hook, followed by withdrawal of the hook, leaving the suture in place spanning the tear. The intra-articular free ends of suture are grasped and delivered up and out of the posterior cannula. Four sequential half-hitched throws are placed and advanced down the cannula with a double-holed knot pusher (Fig. 22–19), resulting in a double square knot securing the meniscal tear at the suture site (Fig. 22–20). The knot tails are cut intra-articularly, and additional sutures are placed in the same fashion until the entire tear is stabilized; this usually requires three sutures for a large tear in the posterior horn.

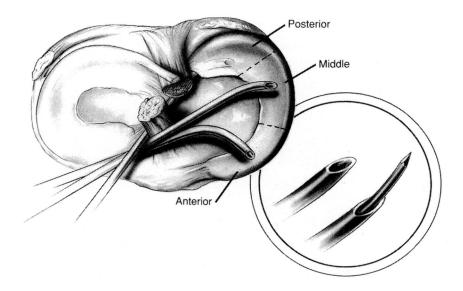

Figure 22–13 • Zone-specific repair. This is a schematic representation of the three separate zones of the medial and lateral menisci. The cannulae are designed so that there is a specific cannula for each designated zone of the meniscus. Each cannula has a 15 degree upcurve near its tip that facilitates needle passage at the joint-line level. (From Mooney MF and Rosenberg TD: Meniscus repair: the inside-out technique. In Jackson DW [ed.]: Reconstructive Knee Surgery. New York, Raven Press, 1995, pp 69–86.)

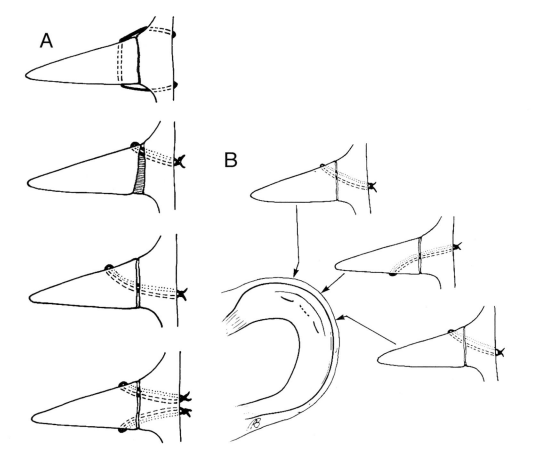

Figure 22–14 • *A*, Diagram demonstrates the possible suture placement patterns for meniscal repair. The vertical and centrally placed horizontal suture patterns adequately reapproximate the tear surfaces, whereas a suture placed off-center superiorly or inferiorly may close the tear inadequately. *B*, Diagram demonstrates "stacking" of horizontal mattress sutures on the superior and inferior surfaces of the meniscus. This optimizes reapproximation of the tear surfaces. (From Cooper DE: Arthroscopic meniscal repair: "outside-in" technique. Oper Tech Sports Med 2:193, 1994.)

Flex Knee 90°

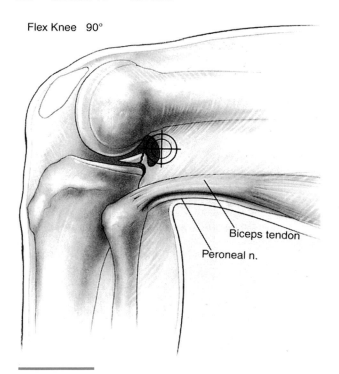

Figure 22–15 • Proper placement of the posterolateral surgical cannula begins outside and above the biceps tendon, above and behind the posterolateral joint line, and aims for the center of the joint with the knee flexed to 90 degrees. (From Morgan CD: Meniscus repair: the all-inside arthroscopic technique. In Jackson DW [ed.]: Reconstructive Knee Surgery. New York, Raven Press, 1995, pp 87–97.)

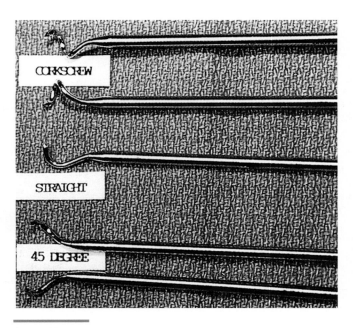

Figure 22–17 • Variable terminal hook designs of the suture hooks: corkscrew right and left, straight, and 45 degree right and left. (From Morgan CD: "All-inside" arthroscopic meniscus repair. Oper Tech Sports Med 2:203, 1994.)

Flex Knee 90°

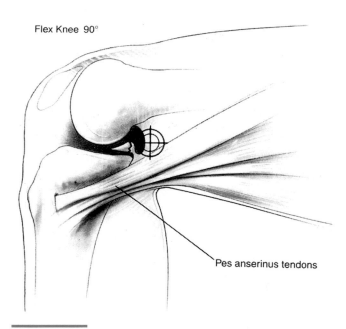

Figure 22–16 • Proper placement of the posteromedial surgical cannula begins outside and above the medial hamstring tendons, above and behind the posteromedial joint line, and aims for the center of the joint with the knee flexed to 90 degrees. (From Morgan CD: Meniscus repair: the all-inside arthroscopic technique. In Jackson DW [ed.]: Reconstructive Knee Surgery. New York, Raven Press, 1995, pp 87–97.)

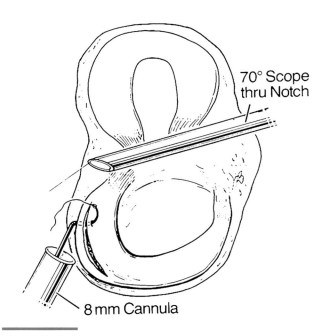

Figure 22–18 • Suture placement through a posterior operative cannula with a suture hook while viewing with a 70 degree arthroscope advanced through the intercondylar notch. (From Morgan CD: "All-inside" arthroscopic meniscus repair. Oper Tech Sports Med 2:204, 1994.)

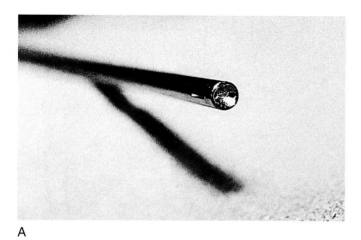

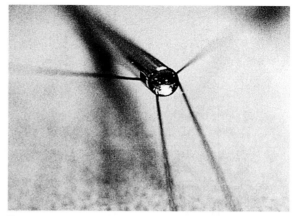

A   B

Figure 22–19 • *A*, Terminal end of the arthroscopic knot pusher (Arthrex, Inc., Naples, Fla.). *B*, Terminal end of the knot pusher advancing a surgeon's knot (Arthrex, Inc., Naples, Fla.). (From Morgan CD: Meniscus repair: the all-inside arthroscopic technique. In Jackson DW [ed.]: Reconstructive Knee Surgery. New York, Raven Press, 1995, pp 87–97.)

A recent suturing device allows performance of an all-inside type of repair performed in inside-out fashion. This device allows passage of a suture across the tear from inside-out, leaving behind a small plastic piece similar to the small piece of material behind a button stitch, anchoring the stitch to the periphery of the capsule. The needle need not penetrate further than a few millimeters beyond the capsule to allow passage of the anchoring device, thus eliminating the danger to neurovascular structures and also the need for incisions. Two successive sutures are tied together with an arthroscopic knot tier, completing a repair stitch (Fig. 22–21). This is repeated as many times as necessary to complete stabilization of the torn fragment.

POSTOPERATIVE MANAGEMENT

Literature recommendations for immobilization, allowed range of motion, and weight-bearing after isolated meniscal repairs have varied significantly over the last 15–20 years. DeHaven noted two basic principles that should guide the rehabilitation protocol: a period (6 weeks) of maximum protection to allow for initial healing followed by a period of restricted activity to allow maturation of the healing collagen tissue.[13, 14, 31, 37] DeHaven allowed only touchdown weight-bearing for the first 6 weeks. The extremity is then placed in a hinged brace locked at 0 degrees for 2 weeks. At 2 weeks the hinges are unlocked, and limited motion of 20–80 degrees is allowed for the next 4 weeks. Low-impact nonagility activities are allowed at 3 months, and not until 6 months are activities such as agility sports and squats allowed. Johnson[39] prefers 4 weeks of restrictive bracing (at 20–60 degrees of flexion) and partial weight-bearing. Full motion and full weight-bearing are initiated at 6 weeks, and patients are restricted from acceleration and deceleration sports for 6 months. Henning[18–20] was particularly restrictive, having patients use crutches with touchdown weight-bearing for 3 months. Motion was allowed early, however, beginning with continuous passive motion on the second postoperative day. Flexion progressed in a graduated fashion to 110 degrees by 4 weeks, and Henning allowed bicycling at 2 months. Lateral movement activities were not allowed until 8–9 months. Morgan,[52, 53] for his all-inside repairs, immobilizes the knee in full extension, allowing full weight-bearing immediately. He notes that in full extension the screw-home mechanism is in effect, and with full weight-bearing in this position the menisci do not move or translate. Progressive knee motion is begun at 2 weeks followed, as soon as motion allows, by bicycling and arc-thigh strengthening exercises. Recent literature advocates significant liberalization of these restrictions.[54–57]

Several reports have documented good results of meniscal repair with few or no postoperative restrictions on range of motion and weight-bearing. In 1994, Barber[55] reported no significant difference in healing rates of meniscal repairs between two groups, one treated with a standard rehabilitation protocol including immobilized brace protection for 6 weeks, non–weight-bearing for up to 12 weeks, and restriction of pivoting sports for 6 months, and the other treated with an accelerated protocol that allowed "unrestricted return to full function." The latter protocol allowed immediate full weight-bearing, no bracing, unrestricted motion, and return to all activities including pivoting sports as soon as the patient desired. Shelbourne, Adsit, and Porter[57] advocated an accelerated postoperative rehabilitation protocol allowing full weight-bearing and early motion. Finally, animal studies have supported unrestricted motion after meniscal repairs.[54]

When meniscal repairs are performed with ligament reconstructions, there is general agreement that the rehabilitation program follow the protocol used for the liga-

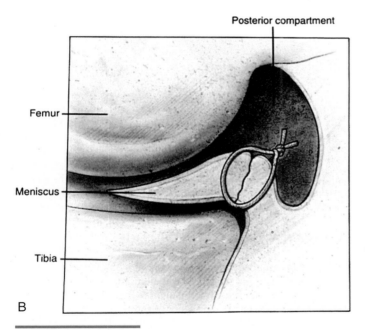

8 mm cannula

A

70° scope through notch

Posterior compartment

Femur

Meniscus

Tibia

B

Figure 22–20 • *A*, A completed all-inside repair. *B*, A completed all-inside repair produces a vertically oriented, balanced suture repair that apposes the two edges of a meniscal tear and excludes the posterior capsule from the repair. (From Morgan CD: Meniscus repair: the all-inside arthroscopic technique. In Jackson DW [ed.]: Reconstructive Knee Surgery. New York, Raven Press, 1995, pp 87–97.)

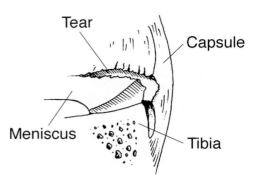

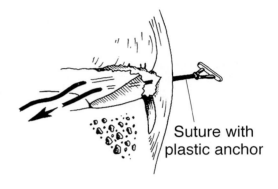

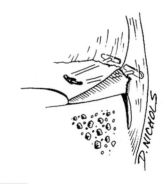

Tear

Capsule

Meniscus

Tibia

Suture with plastic anchor

Figure 22–21 • Arthroscopic view of all-inside/inside-out meniscal repair stitch. (Courtesy of Darrell Lowrey, M.D., Harbin Orthopedic Clinic, Rome, Ga.)

ment reconstruction. After ligament reconstruction the propensity for stiffness with restrictive bracing is significant, and the time restrictions on return to full activity to allow for ligament incorporation and maturation are sufficient to the meniscus.

COMPLICATIONS

Neurovascular injury represents the most significant potential complication during meniscal repair.[14, 58, 59] On the medial side the structure most at risk is the sartorial branch of the saphenous nerve, whereas on the lateral side injury can occur to the peroneal nerve and popliteal artery. Injury to the saphenous nerve is the single most common complication in meniscal repair. Careful dissection and retractor placement, as discussed earlier in this chapter, are crucial in avoiding injury to these structures. Additionally, proper positioning of the knee and extreme care in passage of arthroscopic needles, especially using the inside-out technique, minimize chance of injury.

Failure of repair has been stated to be the most common complication of meniscal repair.[14, 57, 58] Reports of rates of retearing or failure to heal have ranged from 5% to 30%.[20, 30, 31, 34, 35, 41, 46] Comparison of failure rates in the literature can be difficult because failures have been defined clinically based on imaging studies, or they have been firmly established by arthroscopic evaluation. Studies in which second-look arthroscopy was performed have shown clinical failure rates to be approximately half those shown arthroscopically[18–20, 26, 33–35, 46] Thus, only 50% of those patients who have arthroscopic evidence of complete failure to heal will be symptomatic. As noted earlier, failure of meniscal repair is least in the knee undergoing concomitant ligament reconstruction, and failure is significantly higher both in unstable knees and in isolated repairs in stable knees. The general complications of arthroscopy also apply to meniscal repair. These include hemarthrosis, thrombophlebitis, infection, reflex sympathetic dystrophy, and broken instruments.[58, 59]

RESULTS OF MENISCAL REPAIR

Follow-up studies have revealed healing rates of meniscal repair 75–96%. In general the healing rates have been higher in more recent reports. Comparison of reports is difficult for a number of reasons. Technique of repair, including type of repair (arthroscopic or open), methods for stimulating healing, and suture placement, as well as postoperative management have continued to evolve. Also, criteria for patient inclusion in these studies differ. Additionally, the means of assessing the degree of healing vary, ranging from clinical evaluation to arthroscopic second-look. Those reports attempting to follow the stringent criteria set by Henning have noted rates of complete healing of 75–80%, partial healing of approximately 15%, and failure to heal of 5–15%. Reports of meniscal repairs performed in conjunction with ligament reconstruction have uniformly high healing rates, whereas repairs done in the presence of untreated knee instability have significantly lower rates. Of note, reports reveal that isolated repairs done in a stable nonligamentously injured knee have an increased failure rate compared with those done in a reconstructed knee, lending support to the concept of hemarthrosis and fibrin clot as a stimulus to healing.[18–20, 26, 33–35, 46] Authors have advocated significantly liberalizing postoperative rehabilitation protocols, allowing immediate weight-bearing, early motion, and earlier return to sports, citing their data supporting equally good healing rates with the accelerated rehabilitation.[55, 57] However, these studies have defined healing in clinical terms instead of in the more objective imaging or arthroscopic evaluation.

Finally, DeHaven and Lohrer[38] noted that, in a group of 33 meniscal repairs with a mean follow-up of 11 years, the average time between surgery to failure or retear was 4 years. These data indicate that the majority of studies that have reported results with follow-up of 2 years or less may be inadequate in delineating the true long-term success of meniscal repair.[56]

CONCLUSION

The critical importance of the menisci for normal knee function as well as the accelerated deterioration of the knee that occurs in their injury or absence has been conclusively shown with numerous studies. Clearly, efforts to preserve the menisci should be pursued aggressively. There have been significant advances in the technique of meniscal repair during the last 15–20 years. Stabilization of meniscal tears can be performed fairly easily with reproducible results, but only when the stabilized tear actually heals is the repair successful. Some progress has been made in methods to stimulate healing of repaired menisci, but further research is required to improve rates of meniscal healing and attempt to extend the ability of avascular areas of menisci to heal. In addition, work is currently proceeding on meniscal transplantation, and this may provide a solution for meniscal-deficient knees when repair is not possible. However, preservation of the native menisci is clearly preferable to this option.

References

1. Smilie IS: Injuries of the Knee Joint, 4th ed. Edinburgh, Churchill Livingstone, 1970, p 68.
2. Annandale T: An operation for displaced semilunar cartilage. Br Med J 1:779, 1885.
3. King D: The healing of the semilunar cartilages. J Bone Joint Surg Am 18:333, 1936.
4. Fairbank TJ: Knee joint changes after meniscectomy. J Bone Joint Surg Br 30:664, 1948.
5. Shrive NG, O'Connor JJ, and Good fellow JW: Load-bearing in the knee joint. Clin Orthop 131:279, 1978.
6. Levi IM, Torzilli PA, and Warren RF: The effect of medial meniscectomy on anterior-posterior motion of the knee. J Bone Joint Surg Am 64:883, 1982.
7. Arnoczky SP and Warren RF: Microvasculature of the human meniscus. Am J Sports Med 10:90, 1982.
8. Yocum LA, Kerlan RK, Jobe FW, et al.: Isolated lateral meniscectomy: a study of twenty-six patients with isolated tears. J Bone Joint Surg Am 61:338, 1979.
9. Baratz ME, Fu FH, and Mengato R: Meniscal tears: the effect of meniscectomy and of repair on intraarticular contact areas and stress in the human knee; a preliminary report. Am J Sports Med 14:270, 1986.
10. Cabaud HE, Rodkey WG, and Fitzwater JE: Medial meniscus repairs: an experimental and morphologic study. Am J Sports Med 9:129, 1981.
11. Rangger C, Klestil T, Gloetzer W, et al.: Osteoarthritis after arthroscopic partial meniscectomy. Am J Sports Med 23:240, 1995.
12. Ikeuchi H: Surgery under arthroscopic control. Rheumatology (special issue) 57–62, 1976.
13. DeHaven KE: Peripheral meniscal repair: An alternative to meniscectomy. J Bone Joint Surg Br 63:463, 1981.
14. Miller MD, Warner JJP, and Harner CD: Meniscal repair. In Fu FH, Harner CD, and Vince KG (eds.): Knee Surgery. Baltimore, Williams & Wilkins, 1994, pp 615–630.
15. Newman AP, Daniels AU, and Burks RT: Principles and decision making in meniscal surgery. Arthroscopy 9:33, 1993.
16. Ahmed AM: The load-bearing role of the knee menisci. In Mow

VC, Arnoczky SP, and Jackson DW (eds.): Knee Meniscus: Basic and Clinical Foundations. New York, Raven Press, 1992, pp 59–74.

17. Arnoczky SP, Warren RF, and Spivak JM: Meniscal repair using an exogenous fibrin clot: an experimental study in dogs. J Bone Joint Surg Am 70:1209, 1988.
18. Henning CE, Lynch MA, Yearout KM, et al.: Arthroscopic meniscal repair using an exogenous fibrin clot. Clin Orthop 252:64, 1990.
19. Henning CE, Lynch MA, and Clark JR: Vascularity for healing of meniscus repairs. Arthroscopy 3:13, 1987.
20. Henning CE, Yearout KM, Vequist SW, et al.: Use of the fascia sheath coverage and exogenous fibrin clot in the treatment of complex meniscal tears. Am J Sports Med 19:626, 1991.
21. Cooper DE, Arnoczky SP, and Warren RF: Arthroscopic meniscal repair. Clin Sports Med 9:589, 1990.
22. Rodeo SA and Warren RF: Indications and techniques for use of a fibrin clot in meniscal repair. Oper Tech Sports Med 2:217, 1994.
23. Zhang Z, Tu KY, Xu YK, et al.: Treatment of longitudinal injuries in avascular area of meniscus in dogs by trephination. Arthroscopy 4:151, 1988.
24. Fox JM, Rintz KG, and Ferkel RD: Trephination of incomplete meniscal tears. Arthroscopy, 9:451, 1993.
25. Zhang Z, Arnold JA, Williams T, et al.: Repairs by trephination and suturing of longitudinal injuries in the avascular area of the meniscus in goats. Am J Sports Med 23:35, 1995.
26. Tenuta JJ and Arciero RA: Arthroscopic evaluation of meniscal repairs: factors that affect healing. Am J Sports Med 22:797, 1994.
27. Miller MD, Ritchie JR, and Harner CD: Meniscus surgery: indications for repair. Oper Tech Sports Med 2:164, 1994.
28. DeHaven KE and Sebastianelli WJ: Open meniscus repair: indications, technique, and results. Clin Sports Med 9:577, 1990.
29. Fitzgibbons RD and Shelbourne KD: "Aggressive" nontreatment of lateral meniscal tears seen during anterior cruciate ligament reconstruction. Am J Sports Med 23:156, 1995.
30. Cannon WD and Vittori JM: The incidence of healing in arthroscopic meniscal repairs in anterior cruciate ligament reconstructed knees versus stable knees. Am J Sports Med 20:176, 1992.
31. DeHaven KE, Black KP, and Griffiths HJ: Open meniscus repair: technique and two to nine year results. Am J Sports Med 17:788, 1989.
32. Henning CE: Current status of meniscus salvage. Clin Sports Med 9:567, 1990.
33. Morgan CD, Wojtys EM, Lasscells CD, et al.: Arthroscopic meniscal repair evaluated by second-look arthroscopy. Am J Sports Med 19:632, 1991.
34. Buseck MS and Noyes FR: Arthroscopic evaluation of meniscal repairs after anterior cruciate ligament reconstruction and immediate motion. Am J Sports Med 19:489, 1991.
35. Scott GA, Jolly BL, and Henning CE: Combined posterior incision and arthroscopic intra-articular repair of the meniscus. J Bone Joint Surg Am 68:847, 1986.
36. Shelbourne KD and Johnson GE: Locked bucket-handle meniscal tears in knees with chronic anterior cruciate ligament deficiency. Am J Sports Med 21:779, 1993.
37. DeHaven KD and Bronstein RD: Open meniscus repair. Oper Tech Sports Med 2:172, 1994.

38. DeHaven KE and Lohrer WA: Long term results of meniscus repair. Presented at the International Arthroscopy Association, Toronto, Canada, May 14, 1991.
39. Johnson LL: Meniscus repair: The outside-in technique. In Jackson DW (ed.): Reconstructive Knee Surgery. New York, Raven Press, 1995, pp 51–68.
40. Cooper DE: Arthroscopic meniscal repair: "Outside-in" technique. Oper Tech Sports Med 2:190, 1994.
41. Morgan CD and Casscells SW: Arthroscopic meniscus repair: a safe approach to the posterior horns. Arthroscopy 2:3, 1986.
42. O'Donnell JB, Ruland CM, and Ruland LJ III: Technical note: a modified outside-in meniscal repair technique. Arthroscopy 9:472, 1993.
43. Mooney MF and Rosenberg TD: Meniscus repair: the inside-out technique. In Jackson DW (ed.): Reconstructive Knee Surgery. New York, Raven Press, 1995, pp 69–86.
44. Newman AP and Burks RT: Arthroscopic meniscal repair: "inside-out" technique. Oper Tech Sports Med 2:177, 1994.
45. Clancy WG and Graf BK: Arthroscopic meniscal repair. Orthopedics 6:1125, 1983.
46. Rosenberg TD, Scott SM, Coward DB, et al.: Arthroscopic meniscal repair evaluated with repeat arthroscopy. Arthroscopy 2:14, 1986.
47. Jakob RP, Staubli HU, Zuber K, et al.: The arthroscopic meniscal repair: techniques and clinical experience. Am J Sports Med 16:137, 1988.
48. Esser RD: Technical note: arthroscopic meniscus repair: the easy way. Arthroscopy 9:231, 1993.
49. Kohn D and Siebert W: Meniscus suture techniques: a comparative biomechanical cadaver study. Arthroscopy 5:324, 1989.
50. Barber FA and Gurwitz GS: The effect of synovial fluid on suture strength. Am J Knee Surg 1:189, 1988.
51. Kawai Y, Fukubayashi T, and Nishino J: Meniscal suture: an experimental study in the dog. Clin Orthop 243:286, 1989.
52. Morgan CD: Meniscus repair: the all-inside arthroscopic technique. In Jackson DW (ed.): Reconstructive Knee Surgery. New York, Raven Press, 1995, pp 87–97.
53. Morgan CD: "All-inside" arthroscopic meniscal repair. Oper Tech Sports Med 2:201, 1994.
54. Miller MD, Ritchie JR, Gomez BA, et al.: Meniscus repair: an experimental study in the goat. Am J Sports Med 23:124, 1995.
55. Barber FA: Accelerated rehabilitation for meniscus repairs. Arthroscopy 10:206, 1994.
56. Cannon WD: Future directions in meniscal surgery. Oper Tech Sports Med 2:232, 1994.
57. Shelbourne KD, Adsit WS, and Porter DA: Accelerated rehabilitation after isolated meniscal repair. Presented at the 19th Annual meeting of the American Orthopaedic Society for Sports Medicine, Sun Valley, Idaho, July 13, 1993.
58. Small NC: Complications in arthroscopic meniscal surgery. Clin Sports Med 9:609, 1990.
59. Edelson RH, Katchis SD, and Parker RD: Complications of meniscal repair. Oper Tech Sports Med 2:208, 1994.

Chapter

23 Treatment of Articular Cartilage

Lawrence J. Lemak • Michael M. Marushack

Articular cartilage is a highly specialized tissue that allows for unique functions within synovial joints. It has been known for many years that the healing potential of articular cartilage after injury is poor if the structural integrity is disrupted.[1-5] Disruption of the cartilage framework results in alterations of its biomechanical properties. These changes, in turn, can lead to the patient's perception of pain, loss of motion, strength, or instability. Although recently a great deal of research has been performed in this area, our understanding of this tissue is far from complete, and treatment of articular cartilage injuries remains challenging and controversial.

STRUCTURE AND COMPOSITION

Articular cartilage consists of chondrocytes and an extracellular matrix with water[6-9] (Fig. 23–1). The chondrocytes are highly differentiated cells that account for only about 5% of the total volume and are quite metabolically active, despite limited ability to replicate. These cells are responsible for synthesizing and maintaining the extracellular matrix through the formation of proteoglycans, collagen, noncollagenous proteins, and glycoproteins. They also form degradative enzymes that are responsible for the normal turnover of these macromolecules.[10-12]

The extracellular matrix consists of collagen (15–20% of the wet mass), proteoglycans (10–15% of the wet mass), noncollagenous proteins, glycoproteins, and water (65–75% of the wet mass). The collagen is primarily type II and principally provides tensile strength to the articular cartilage. Proteoglycans consist of glycosaminoglycans (e.g., keratin sulfate and chondroitin sulfate), which are associated with a core protein (Fig. 23–2 and 23–3). This core protein is then linked to a long hyaluronic acid molecule.[13] Along with counterions, this matrix has a major influence on cartilage hydration and its biomechanical properties.[14, 15]

The cells in extracellular matrix are organized into four distinct zones: (1) the superficial tangential zone in which chondrocytes and collagen fibers have axes aligned parallel to the joint surface, and the matrix has less proteoglycans, (2) the middle zone with randomly aligned spherical cells, (3) the deep zone with cells forming columns perpendicular to the calcified zone, and (4) the calcified cartilage that serves to attach the articular cartilage to bone[16] (Fig. 23–4).

This specialized structure of articular cartilage results in a quite durable surface and allows it to perform two basic functions. Due to its viscoelastic properties that allow for time- and rate-dependent deformation, articular cartilage functions as a load distributor to decrease joint contact pressures. Second, articular cartilage has a low coefficient of friction and provides a smooth, efficient surface for joint motion.

Although there is good evidence that chondrocytes have the ability to respond to mechanical stresses, their capacity to synthesize new macromolecules for repair of the damaged matrix is limited. If the chondrocyte repair process cannot keep up with the degradative process, irreversible damage may occur.

Despite the wear resistance of articular cartilage, damage can occur due to repetitive and prolonged overloading, sudden impact with high compression, or high shear stresses at the subchondral junction. Buckwalter, Mow, and Ratcliffe separated articular cartilage lesions into acute injuries and degenerative processes.[17] Articular cartilage injuries are further categorized into: (1) microdamage to the cells and matrix with visible disruption of the articular cartilage surface; (2) macrodisruption of the articular cartilage alone, like that seen with chondral fractures; and (3) fracture of the articular cartilage and subchondral bone, such as that seen in osteochondral fractures. Osteochondritis dissecans represents an additional type of articular cartilage lesion.

ACUTE CHONDRAL AND OSTEOCHONDRAL LESIONS

Chondral lesions within the knee present difficult diagnostic dilemmas. The presentation and examination of the

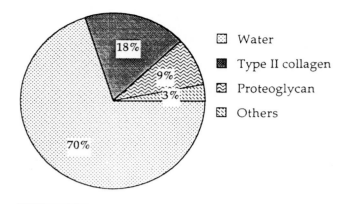

Figure 23–1 • Constituents of articular cartilage. (From Suh J-K, Scherping S, Marui T, et al.: Operative Techniques in Sports Medicine. Oper Tech Sports Med 3:78–86, 1995.)

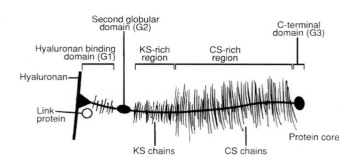

Figure 23–2 • Diagram of an aggregen molecule. The protein core has several globular domains (G1, G2, and G3). Other regions contain the keratan sulfate (KS) and chondroitin sulfate (CS) glycosaminoglycan chains. The N-terminal G1 domain is able to bind specifically to hyaluronan. This binding is stabilized by link protein. The total molecular weight of an aggregen ranges from 0.5 million to 1.0 million daltons. (From Simon SR [ed.]: Orthopaedic Basic Science. Rosemont, Ill., American Academy of Orthopaedic Surgeons, 1994, p 9.)

patient often fail to clearly elucidate the nature of the pathologic process. Diagnostic tests, although improving, do not reach the same level of sensitivity and specificity when compared with their use in the diagnosis of other intra-articular derangements of the knee. In addition, these injuries often occur with other intra-articular pathologic conditions clouding the clinical presentation.

Clinical Presentation

Several authors warn that there is no reliable method of predicting intra-articular surface integrity based only on symptoms.[18–20] Often a specific injury is recounted, although the injury may be direct or indirect, with a shear, twisting, or compression mechanism.[21] Patellar lesions can

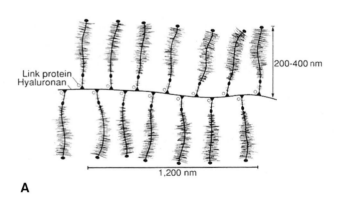

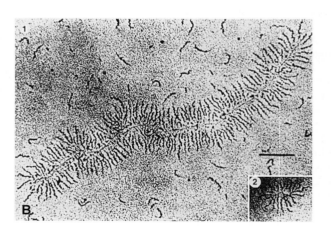

Figure 23–3 • *A*, A proteoglycan aggregate consists of a long hyaluronan chain to which many aggregens are attached, forming macromolecular complexes that are effectively immobilized within the collagen network. The length of the hyaluronan chain determines the size of the aggregate. The total molecular weight may be as high as 200 million daltons in immature cartilage; in adult and aging articular cartilage, the aggregate gradually decreases in size. (From Simon SR [eds.]: Orthopaedic Basic Science. Rosemont, Ill., American Academy of Orthopaedic Surgeons, 1994, p 10.) *B*, Electron micrographs of proteoglycan aggregates in bovine articular cartilage from a skeletally immature calf (1) and a skeletally mature steer (2). The aggregates consist of a central hyaluronan filament and multiple attached monomers. Bar represents 500 µm. (From Buckwalter JA, Kuettner KE, and Thonar EF: Age-related changes in articular cartilage proteoglycans: electron microscopic studies. J Orthop Res 3:251–257, 1985).

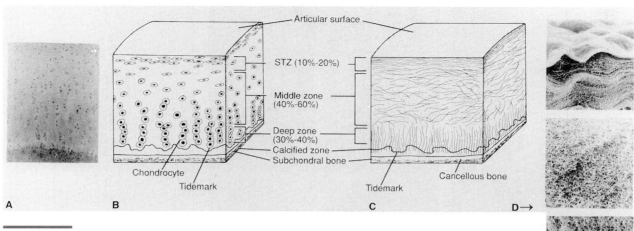

Figure 23–4 • Structure of articular cartilage. *A*, Histologic section of cartilage from a young, healthy adult shows even safranin O staining and distribution of chondrocytes. *B*, Schematic diagram of chondrocyte organization in the three main zones of the uncalcified cartilage (STZ: superficial tangential zone), the tidemark, and the subchondral bone. *C*, Sagittal cross-sectional diagram of collagen fiber architecture shows the three salient zones of articular cartilage. *D*, Scanning electron micrographs depict the arrangement of collagen in the three zones (*top*: STZ; *center*: middle zone; *bottom*: deep zone). (From Mow VC, Proctor CS, and Kelly MA: Biomechanics of articular cartilage. In Nordin M and Frankel VH [eds.]: Basic Biomechanics of the Musculoskeletal System, 2nd ed. Philadelphia, Lea & Febiger, 1989, pp 32 and 34.)

result from a variety of mechanisms, including abnormal patellar tracking,[22, 23] aberrant instant centers of motion,[24] meniscal tears, high load transmission,[24–28] and other mechanisms.

Patients with lesions on the weight-bearing surface may present with complaints of pain, swelling, popping, or decreased range of motion if significant cartilage loss has occurred. If a large enough chondral fragment breaks free, the patient may note locking or catching. The pain is often related to activity and can often be localized to a particular compartment. Patients with patellar lesions may present with anterior knee pain, complaints of anterior popping, catching, or grinding, and difficulty with stairs or sitting for long periods (Fig. 23–5).

On examination, the patient may have localized tenderness and an effusion, but often the examination is quite unremarkable. Symptoms secondary to other intra-articular pathology may dominate the clinical picture and examination, thus overshadowing any chondral lesions. The lesions encountered have some age dependence. Johnson-Nurse and Dandy[29] evaluated 76 knees with articular cartilage injuries and found that full-thickness lesions often occurred in the third decade of life, partial-thickness lesions in the fourth decade, and osteochondral fractures in adolescents or young adults.

It is also important to note the length of time since the symptoms began. Dzioba separated injuries into acute (younger than 3 weeks of age), acute or chronic (lesion treated previously now with a new injury), and chronic (older than 3 weeks of age).[30] Patients with acute symptoms were noted to have a better prognosis.

Osteochondral lesions are distinguished from chondral lesions in several ways (Table 23–1). In skeletally mature patients, the tidemark provides a relatively weak transitional zone through which forces are transferred. In the adolescent, however, no tidemark exists, and therefore stresses are transmitted to the subchondral bone. Acute osteochondral lesions may present with a hemarthrosis on evaluation and a more marked inflammatory response.

Association with Other Lesions

One of the reasons why it is difficult to diagnose patients with articular cartilage injuries is that they are frequently associated with other pathologic symptoms, and these symptoms may be the predominant complaints of the patient. Many of the mechanisms of injury that cause articular cartilage damage can also cause meniscal or ligamentous injury. In addition, the patient may have coincidental lesions in which several lesions are found at the time of arthroscopy but are unrelated with regard to their cause.

There is a large amount of information relating to meniscal pathology and articular surface defects.[24, 27, 28, 31, 32] Zamber and colleagues[18] prospectively evaluated 200 consecutive patients who were treated arthroscopically for knee symptoms. Of these patients, 61.5% had articular cartilage lesions, but only 6.5% of the 200 patients had isolated defects; 32.5% had intra-articular pathologic problems without articular cartilage lesions. Articular cartilage lesions were frequently associated with an unstable torn meniscus, especially on the medial side. Medial changes were more common than lateral or trochlear changes. Similarly, Fahmy, Williams, and Noble found articular cartilage injuries in 13 of 14 patients with ipsilateral, unstable meniscal tears that were thought to be directly related.[19]

There is evidence that chondral lesions are associated with anterior cruciate ligament injuries. It has also been noted that as the time from the ligament injury increases, the frequency of chondral lesions increases within the knee, regardless of meniscal pathologic problems.[18, 33–37]

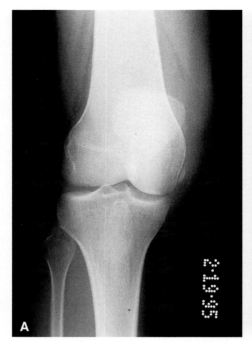

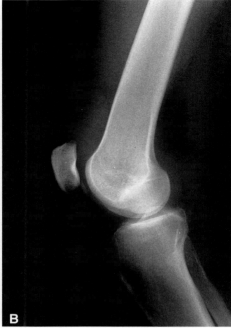

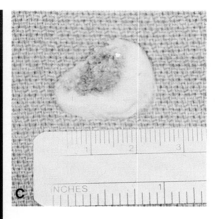

Figure 23–5 • Patient presenting with acute, traumatic injury to the right knee. *A* and *B*, Radiographs demonstrating a loose body in the medial gutter and medial to the patella. *C*, An osteochondral fragment removed at the time of arthroscopy.

Articular cartilage lesions were also noted despite anterior cruciate ligament reconstruction. However, it is difficult to determine if these lesions occurred at the initial injury or after the reconstruction.[38, 39]

Articular cartilage lesions have been associated with both acute and chronic posterior cruciate ligament injuries. These lesions were noted especially in the medial compartment and patellofemoral articulation with chronic injuries.[40–43]

Besides trauma, other conditions can be responsible for articular cartilage damage, including immobilization, aging, previous knee surgery, and some drugs such as corticosteroids.[19, 33, 44, 45]

Radiographic Evaluation

Radiographs may be quite helpful for evaluation of osteochondral lesions, but they have little or no use in the evaluation of chondral lesions alone.[21] One's level of suspicion for an osteochondral injury should increase in the skeletally immature patient, and careful evaluation of radiographs is required.

Table 23–1 Chondral Versus Osteochondral Fractures	
Osteochondral Fracture	**Chondral Fracture**
Seen on radiograph	Radiograph normal
Bloody effusion, fat droplets	May have effusion, no blood
Adolescent	Skeletally mature
Healing potential present	Large defects may not heal

From Hopkinson WJ, Mitchell WA, and Curl WW: Chondral fractures of the knee: cause for confusion. Am J Sports Med 13:311, 1985.

Many authors have investigated the use of magnetic resonance imaging (MRI) in the evaluation of the chondral lesions. Although helpful for visualizing some articular cartilage lesions, MRI cannot be used to reliably rule out these injuries.[46–52] The larger the size and the depth of the lesion, the more likely the defect can be identified by MRI. The techniques may be more sensitive after injection of the knee with gadolinium or in patients with an effusion.[49, 53]

Treatment

The treatment of acute chondral and osteochondral lesions in the literature is controversial. Several authors have attempted to classify articular cartilage injuries in order to provide treatment protocols and prognostic significance[54–59] (Table 23–2). Many of these classification schemes relate to patellar chondromalacia[54–56, 58, 59] and have been extrapolated to use within the medial and lateral compartments and other joints as well. All systems have their relative merits, but some are more cumbersome to use, and it is difficult to provide specific prognostic significance with any. Most are based on the location, size, and appearance of the lesion; but there is high variability and little consensus with regard to when the extent of these variables becomes important clinically.

The Outerbridge[54] classification was one of the first described and classifies lesions as grade I softening and swelling, grade II fissuring and fragmentation of 1/2 in or less in size, grade III same as grade II but greater than 1/2 in in size, and grade IV erosion of cartilage to bone. Although these authors make a distinction between lesions less or greater than 1/2 in in size, there is little indication that this arbitrary distinction has true clinical importance.

Table 23–2	**Review of Previous Classification Symptoms of Articular Cartilage**		
Author	**Surface Description of Articular Cartilage**	**Diameter**	**Location**
Outerbridge	I—Softening and swelling II—Fragmentation and fissuring III—Fragmentation and fissuring IV—Erosion of cartilage down to bone	I—none II—<1/2 in III—>1/2 in IV—None	Starts most frequently on the medial facet of patella; later extends to the lateral facet "mirror" lesion on the intercondylar area of the femoral condyles; upper border medial femoral condyle

Hungerford and Ficat	I—Closed chondromalacia; simple softening (small blister) macroscopically: surface intact; varying degrees of severity from simple softening to "pitting edema"; loss of elasticity
	II—Open chondromalacia
	  a. Fissures—Single or multiple, relatively superficial or extending down to subchondral bone
	  b. Ulceration—Localized loss of cartilage substance, exposes dense subchondral bone. When extensive, bone has polished appearance (eburnated).
	Chondrosclerosis—Abnormally hard, not depressible
	
	Tuft formation—Multiple deep fronds of cartilage separated from one another by deep clefts that extend to the subchondral bone
	Superficial surface changes—Surface fibrillation; longitudinal striations present in the axis of movement of the joint
		I—1 cm² and then extends progressively in all directions
		II—None
		
		Not localized but involves the entire contact zone
			Lateral facet—Secondary excessive lateral pressure
			
			Medial facet—Secondary incongruence and combination of compression and shearing forces
			
			Centered on the crest separating the medial and odd facets

Bentley	I—Fibrillation or fissuring II—Fibrillation or fissuring III—Fibrillation or fissuring IV—Fibrillation with or without exposure of subchondral bone	I—<0.5 cm II—0.5–1.0 cm III—1.0–2.0 cm IV—>2.0 cm	Most common at the junction of the medial and odd facets of patella
Casscells	I—Superficial area of erosion II—Deeper layers of cartilage involved III—Cartilage is completely eroded and bone is exposed IV—Articular cartilage completely destroyed	I—≤1 cm II—1–2 cm III—2–4 cm IV—"Wide area"	Patella and anterior femoral surfaces
Insall	I—Swelling and softening of cartilage (closed chondromalacia) II—Deep fissures extending to subchondral bone III—Fibrillation IV—Erosive changes and exposures of subchondral bone (osteoarthrosis)	None	I–IV—Midpoint of the patellar crest with extension equally onto medial and lateral patellar facets IV—Also involves the opposite or mirror surface of the femur. Upper and lower one-third nearly always spared (patella); femur never severe

Goodfellow	Surface degeneration—Surface flaking progressing to fibrillation
	Basilar degeneration—Fasciculation of collagen in the middle and deep zones, without at first affecting the surface
	  • Fasciculation—articular surface is smoothly intact; spongy consistency; exhibits "pitting edema"
	  • Blister
	  • Fasciculation—rupture of tangential surface fibers
		1 cm	"Odd" facet of the patella
			
			Inferior part of the central ridge separating the medial and lateral facets

From Noyes FR and Stabler CL: A system for grading articular cartilage lesions at arthroscopy. Am J Sports Med 17:506, 1989.

Perhaps the most comprehensive classification system of articular cartilage injuries is that of Noyes and Stabler.[60] This system grades four variables: (1) appearance of the articular cartilage, (2) depth, (3) size, and (4) location. Grade I lesions are described as closed chondromalacia. Grade II lesions have disruption of the articular cartilage without visible bone exposed. Grade III lesions have exposed bone. Within each of these grades are subcategories taking into account the size of lesion, location, and qualitative differences in the articular cartilage surface. The main limitations of this system are the somewhat subjective distinctions within subcategories, and although a point system is used for research purposes, it is difficult to use the scale for prognostic significance.

Rock, Kruger, and Fowler have suggested these classification systems based on initial size may greatly underestimate the actual lesion after appropriate treatment has been rendered.[61]

Several authors have reported their experience in the treatment of acute chondral lesions. Dzioba treated 65 patients with an initial diagnostic arthroscopy, then 53 patients were treated with open surgery, and 12 treated by arthroscopic means.[30] His overall results, as judged by clinical evaluation, revealed 69% good, 28% poor, and 3% fair knees. Forty-six knees underwent follow-up arthroscopy at 12–15 months, and many had a biopsy performed. Further analysis of these patients revealed that 81% of patients in the acute group had good results. Of note, most lesions in Dzioba's study were partial-thickness injuries. He believed that patients with the best prognosis had small-to-medium lesions that were acute, partial-thickness in depth, on the weight-bearing surface, and in healthy patients younger than 45 years of age. Osteochondral lesions also fell into the category of the best prognosis. Patients with the worst prognosis had a large, full-thickness lesion with loss of the tidemark, a chronic nature, degenerative changes, and being submeniscal on the weight-bearing surface; the patients were older than 50 years of age and in poor medical condition.

Authors' Preferred Treatment

Initially during arthroscopy, a systematic and complete inspection of the knee joint is carried out to diagnose and treat ligamentous and meniscal pathologic conditions. One must be careful when evaluating the depth of articular lesions. The tidemark represents a stress riser, and although separation through this layer may appear to be a full-thickness lesion, in fact the layer of calcified cartilage remains. Treatment of the articular cartilage injuries depends on the size, location, and depth of the lesion. Medial lesions are approximately four times as common as lateral lesions and are more common on the weight-bearing surface.[30] Small (<1 cm), superficial lesions are left alone for observation. Larger, superficial lesions with fragmentation or fissuring are débrided with a radial shaver so that a stable cartilage edge remains. Care must be taken to avoid débridement to subchondral bone. Attempts are made to remove the fragmented or loose cartilage perpendicular to the subchondral bone plate. It is important to

document the size of the lesion after débridement to a stable border.

If visible bone is exposed in the depths of the lesion, again all loose or fragmented cartilage is débrided so that a smooth, stable rim of cartilage remains. In addition, a small pick is used to create a series of microfractures[75] approximately 2–3 mm deep so that the subchondral bone is traversed. This allows for capillary bleeding and the formation of a fibrin clot. The holes are spaced approximately 3–4 mm apart. This technique is carried out on both femoral and tibial weight-bearing surfaces. The trochlear groove is treated in a similar fashion depending on the depth of involvement. Patellar injuries are débrided of the loose and fragmented cartilage as well. However, we have found that it is extremely difficult to perform a microfracture procedure on the patellar articular surface.

Postoperatively, patients are treated with aggressive physical therapy so that full range of motion is obtained within the 1st week. Icing and compressive dressings are used to minimize effusions. The patients' activities are then advanced over the next several months so that they resume full activities in 6 months' time.

The treatment of osteochondral lesions depends on the size of the lesion. If the bony fragment is less than 1 cm or is a wafer with limited depth, our experience is that it is very difficult to get adequate fixation to make repair of this fracture worthwhile. In general, these lesions are removed arthroscopically, and then the basal lesion is débrided and loose cartilaginous debris is removed.

If the osteochondral fragment is larger than 1 cm, attempts to anatomically repair the lesion are performed. It is important not to cross the physis in skeletally immature patients in order to avoid iatrogenic physeal closure. This procedure can often be done arthroscopically; however, if there is difficulty performing an anatomic reduction, we do not hesitate to perform this as an open procedure.

Postoperatively, patients are treated with aggressive physical therapy so that full range of motion is obtained within the first week, and then activities are advanced. In general, these patients are younger and can be returned to full activities at 3 months.

TREATMENT OF THE ARTHRITIC KNEE

The use of arthroscopy in the treatment of osteoarthritis of the knee has played a significantly more important role as larger numbers of people grow older. Several arthroscopic techniques have been used to provide temporary relief of arthritic symptoms.

Clinical Evaluation

The presentation, examination, and radiographic features of patients with osteoarthritis are well known to the orthopedic surgeon. Patients who have failed conservative management, including physical therapy, avoidance of aggravating activities, nonsteroidal anti-inflammatory drugs, and weight reduction, but are unwilling to undergo total

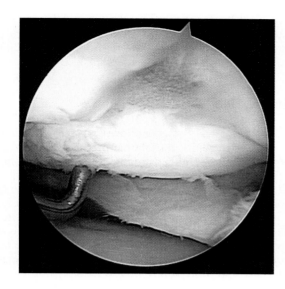

Figure 23–6 • Arthroscopic appearance of medial compartment degenerative joint disease with softening, fissuring, and progression to calcified cartilage.

knee replacement, may be candidates for arthroscopic débridement of the knee. These patients must understand that this is a temporizing procedure and is not curative. They must also agree to participate in a postoperative rehabilitation program, which may include partial weight-bearing for 6–8 weeks. Relative contraindications include joint instability, inflammatory arthritides, excessive weight, or significant malalignment problems.

The appearance of articular cartilage with osteoarthritis arthroscopically includes superficial roughening, fibrillation, fissuring, and progression deeper to the zone of calcified cartilage and subchondral bone[14, 63–65] (Fig. 23–6). Free fragments are also seen occasionally within the knee joint. The classification of these lesions is similar to that of acute chondral lesions. Some authors have attempted to place degenerative articular injuries into a separate category. Bauer and Jackson included two types that were considered to be secondary to degenerative changes.[66]

Treatment

The arthroscopic treatment options include lavage, débridement, abrasion chondroplasty, or drilling chondroplasty. The beneficial effect of knee lavage has been documented.[67–69] This technique alone theoretically results in the removal of microscopic and macroscopic debris. It has been shown that intra-articular injection of cartilage fragments can result in an inflammatory process in rabbits' knees with formation of joint effusions, increased level of synovial enzymes, and articular cartilage fissuring and discoloration.[70]

Jackson, Marans, and Silver found that 80% of patients with osteoarthritis improved after lavage alone, and 45% had long-term benefit.[71] A number of the failures reported had deterioration after an injury had occurred. In patients with articular cartilage and meniscal damage treated by partial meniscectomy and débridement, 88% improved initially, and 68% maintained a good result.

Baumgaertner and colleagues reported treatment of osteoarthritic knees with débridement, synovectomy, partial meniscectomy, excision of osteophytes, and chondroplasty as necessary.[72] They found that 52% of patients had good or excellent results initially, and 40% maintained these results at final follow-up. Preoperative factors correlating with good results included symptoms that had occurred for less than 12 months, mechanical pain rather than load-related pain, presence of chondrocalcinosis, normal alignment, and mild degenerative changes.

Other authors believe that débridement and lavage alone are inadequate treatment, and they argue that cartilage damage superficial to the subchondral bone fails to heal. Lesions penetrating cartilage undergo a vascular response with capillary bleeding, fibrin clot formation, and metaplasia of mesenchymal cells to fibrocartilage in some cases. Some authors recommend more aggressive treatment in patients with lesions with visible bone exposed.

Johnson recommended abrasion arthroplasty.[73] His technique involves abrasion of the entire surface of the exposed bone with a motorized bur. Approximately 1–2 mm of cortical bone are removed. Postoperatively, the patients are treated with non–weight-bearing and active range of motion. Johnson reports that a second-look arthroscopic examination at 8 weeks shows a soft patch of white tissue composed of avascular spindle cells. At 4–6 months there is evidence of fibrocartilage differentiation, and at 9 months there is adherence to the subchondral bone and adjacent articular cartilage. Histologically, the fibrocartilage shows cells that are smaller and more numerous, and the area is more vascular compared with hyaline cartilage. Over time, the tissue may contain type II collagen. Results of abrasion chondroplasty from this approach showed that 75% of patients improved at 2 years follow-up, with 33% reporting no pain and 44% requiring medication for their pain.

The concept of bone drilling was introduced by Pridie.[74] He recommended the performance of a synovectomy, removal of loose pieces, excision of osteophytes, meniscectomy, and drilling of eburnated bone to stimulate fibrocartilage formation.

A microfracture technique with small awls has also been used to stimulate the migration, proliferation, and differentiation of cells to a fibrocartilaginous articular surface.[75]

Although many surgeons débride frayed and fibrillated superficial cartilage with anecdotal improvement, the long-term efficacy of this procedure is poorly documented. In one series of patients, only 25% had satisfactory results.[62] Clearly, further investigation must be done to determine the optimal treatment of these lesions.

Authors' Preferred Method

In symptomatic patients with mild to moderate osteoarthritis who are not candidates or unwilling to undergo total knee arthroplasty but who are able and willing to participate in an aggressive rehabilitation program postoperatively, we recommend arthroscopic treatment. The treatment of articular cartilage changes associated with osteoarthritis depends on the depth of involvement. Osteophytes should be removed with a high-speed bur or osteotome. A synovectomy should be performed if indicated. Partial medical and lateral meniscectomies to remove degenerative menisci should be performed as necessary. All loose articular cartilage flaps, fissures, or fragmentation are débrided with a radial shaver. Margins of lesions should be removed perpendicular to the subchondral surface until a stable edge is produced. If subchondral bone is exposed, small angled, arthroscopic awls are then used to create 2 mm defects through the subchondral bone to allow capillary bleeding and fibrin clot formation.[75] The defects should be spaced 3 or 4 mm apart. The knee joint is then thoroughly irrigated with saline to remove any debris. Postoperatively, patients are encouraged to regain full range of motion within 1 week. Physical therapy is begun immediately with active and passive range of motion, quadriceps and hamstring strengthening, and partial weight-bearing. We have found that it is extremely difficult for these patients to be completely non–weight-bearing for any extended period. An icing program is used extensively, and nonsteroidal anti-inflammatory drugs are used when necessary.

With this approach we have found that a high percentage of patients improved initially by both subjective and objective criteria and that 60–70% of patients improved at 1 year follow-up.

OSTEOCHONDRITIS DISSECANS

Although the lesion itself had been previously described, König was the first person to use the term "osteochondritis dissecans" in 1887.[76]

The causes of osteochondritis dissecans are unclear, but many have been theorized. Causes include endocrine imbalances, focal ischemic infarction caused by limited anastomoses of femoral arterial branches in the subchondral bone, genetic influences, anatomic variations such that the femoral articular surface abuts the tibial spine, overuse with microtrauma, trauma, and abnormal ossification of the epiphysis.

It is important to realize that patients with osteochondritis dissecans really consist of two subsets of patients. The first subset consists of patients who are skeletally immature, and the second subset consists of patients who are skeletally mature. There is often some confusion in the literature regarding patients grouped into series who have both types of osteochondritis dissecans.

Epidemiology

Osteochondritis dissecans is most common in patients between the ages of 10 and 20 years but can occur in any age group. There is a male predominance of approximately 3:1. Bilateral involvement is noted in about 30–40% of cases.

A Swedish study showed the incidence of osteochondritis dissecans to be 150 per 250,000 population.[77] In a

follow-up study, the same author found that the incidence of osteochondritis dissecans in skeletally immature patients was 18 per 100,000 in females and 29 per 100,000 in males.[78]

Clinical Evaluation

The diagnosis of an osteochondritis dissecans lesion is made by history, physical examination, plain radiographs, and other radiographic techniques. Diagnostic arthroscopy may also aid in the evaluation of these lesions.

Patients may have a vague ache within the knee that may be poorly localized. They may complain of effusions, joint line tenderness, and possible "locking" if the fragments are loose within the knee joint. Osteochondritis dissecans is responsible for approximately 50% of loose bodies in the knee.[79] Symptoms are often initially associated with activity, but more severe involvement symptoms may occur even with routine daily activities. On physical examination patients may have tenderness over the femoral condyle with direct pressure while the knee is flexed. Because 75% of osteochondritis dissecans lesions in the knee are on the medial side, this area should be particularly well evaluated. There may also be an effusion present, quadriceps atrophy, or subtle differences in range of motion, particularly flexion if the lesion is very posterior on either condyle. On rare occasions a loose body may be palpated.

Plain radiographs should be obtained to aid in the diagnosis. Radiographic views should include anterior, posterior, lateral, and tunnel views. Osteochondritis dissecans appears as a well-circumscribed area of radiolucency above an area of subchondral bone. Again, the most common location is on the lateral aspect of the medial femoral condyle, but the lateral femoral condyle or patella may also be involved.

Bone scans are helpful if clinical suspicion is high, but routine radiographs are nondiagnostic. They may also help to rule out occult bilateral involvement; however, they are of little or no help when determining the age of the lesion or its healing potential.

MRI may help to determine the vascularity of the lesion, bilateral involvement, and small lesions especially if gadolinium is used.[53] In addition, MRI may be beneficial in determining the degree of loosening of the lesion.[80]

Classification

Pappas proposed a classification scheme based on the patient's skeletal age.[81] Category I included patients up to age 11 in girls and age 13 in boys. These patients in general have a good prognosis and are treated conservatively. Category II includes patients near skeletal maturity—girls aged 11 to 15 years and boys aged 13 to 17 years. Treatment for these patients depends on the looseness of the lesion. Category III includes patients after physeal closure and skeletal maturity. Treatment again depends on the looseness of the lesion, but the prognosis is more guarded.

Another classification system uses the looseness of the lesion as a prime determinant. Grade I lesions are lesions noted radiographically but have an intact articular surface at arthroscopy. Grade II lesions have an articular surface injury noted at arthroscopy; however, they are not mobile. Grade III lesions are mobile but sit within the bed of the lesion. Grade IV lesions are loose within the knee joint.[82]

Treatment

Arthroscopic evaluation of osteochondritis dissecans lesions was first described by Casscells.[83] O'Connor described arthroscopic treatment of osteochondritis dissecans lesions, including fragment removal and débridement of the condylar defect.[84]

Arthroscopic evaluation of the knee allows determination of the size and stability of the osteochondritis dissecans lesion. It is also beneficial when following these lesions for evidence of healing. The most important variables in the treatment of osteochondritis dissecans is the patient's age, the size of the lesion, and its stability. Treatment options include drilling, pinning with either K-wires or screws, or removal of loose bodies with débridement.

Authors' Preferred Treatment

A complete and systematic diagnostic arthroscopy is carried out to evaluate all intra-articular lesions. Evaluation of the osteochondritis dissecans lesions includes determination of the size, location, weight-bearing surface, articular cartilage status, and stability of the lesion. Stability is aided by the use of a probe to determine motion of the fragment. After these factors have been documented, treatment depends on the patient's age, the location of the lesion, and the stability of the lesion.

Lesions in skeletally immature patients that are stable can be observed with non–weight-bearing and range of motion.

Drilling

The indications for arthroscopic drilling include stable lesions in skeletally immature patients. The rationale of treatment arises from penetration of the subchondral bone, which allows capillary bleeding, fibrin clot formation, and revascularization of the fragment. Using a 0.62 K-wire, a series of holes can be made in the fragment into the subchondral bone, approximately 3 or 4 mm apart.

Pinning

The indications for pinning include partially separated lesions in younger patients or wafer thin lesions on the weight-bearing surface where screw fixation may comminute the fragment or remain above the articular surface. The rationale for treatment is that stabilization of the fragment may allow for healing and revascularization of the fragment.

Smooth K-wires, either 0.45 or 0.62, are inserted arthroscopically at different angles in the fragment to lock the piece in place. This can be facilitated with use of a guide from the anterior cruciate ligament reconstruction set used to make bone tunnels. Pins are inserted antegrade then pulled retrograde until just below the articular surface. These pins should be left in place from 3 to 6 weeks until the fragment heals. This may require immobilization of the knee until the pins are removed in order to prevent damage to the opposing articular surface.

Screw Fixation

The indications for screw fixation in the treatment of osteochondritis dissecans lesions include stable or unstable lesions in near skeletally mature or skeletally mature patients and unstable lesions in skeletally immature patients. Rigid fixation of the lesion allows for healing and revascularization to potentially occur.

For stable lesions the lesion is left in situ. Cannulated reamers, taps, and finally the screw is then placed arthroscopically over the pin. Two screws should be placed if possible to provide fixation with rotational control.

Unstable lesions may require more comprehensive treatment with removal of the lesion out of its crater, followed by curettage of the base of the lesion to provide a vascular bed. The undersurface of the lesion itself should also be freshened with a curet. The lesion can then be placed back into the crater, and treatment proceeds like that of a stable lesion. It may be necessary to bone graft these lesions if significant bone loss is noted. Care should be taken to avoid crossing the physis in skeletally immature patients with an unstable lesion. The head of the screw should be countersunk below the articular cartilage surface. Screws should be removed in 6–8 weeks or when the lesion has healed. If the removal of the screw is delayed, the result may be overgrowth of soft tissue above the screw head and difficulty with its removal later on. Postoperatively, range of motion is encouraged, but the patient should remain non–weight-bearing until healing occurs.

Removal of Loose Bodies and Débridement

Indications for removal of loose bodies and débridement include unstable, multiple fragments with poor quality bone or lesions with very thin bone that are unable to withstand fixation. Lesions that have been free for greater than 1 month should be removed because these lesions have poor healing potential, and this eliminates the possibility of a second surgery for definitive treatment (Fig. 23–7).

Removal of loose bodies may proceed in a routine manner. After the loose body has been removed, the edges of the lesion can be débrided to stable, healthy articular cartilage, and the base should be débrided of fibrous tissue followed by curettage or drilling the base in order to stimulate fibrin clot formation and fibrocartilage formation.

Regardless of the treatment chosen, our patients are begun on physical therapy to obtain full range of motion and return full strength to the quadriceps and hamstrings. Patients are kept strictly non–weight-bearing for 6 weeks.

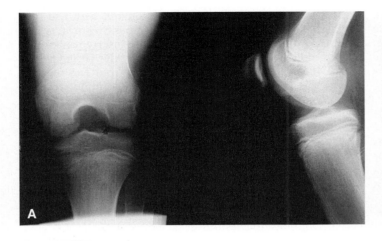

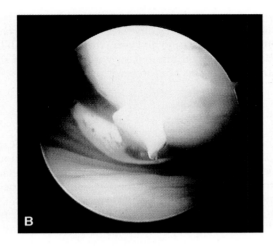

Figure 23–7 • *A*, A notch and lateral view of a skeletally immature patient who presented with pain in the left knee of several months' duration. The pain was acutely exacerbated after mild trauma to the knee. *B*, Arthroscopic appearance of a loose body that was found and removed at the time of surgery.

At that time partial weight-bearing is begun if radiographs demonstrate healing. Activities are advanced so that patients may return to full activities 3–4 months postoperatively.

References

1. Rosenberg NJ: Osteochondral fractures of the lateral femoral condyle. J Bone Joint Surg Am 45:1013, 1964.
2. Gillquist J, Hogberg G, and Oretop N: Arthroscopy in acute injuries of the knee joint. Acta Orthop Scand 48:190–196, 1977.
3. Hunter W: On the structure and diseases of articulating cartilage. Philos Trans R Soc Lond 9:267, 1743.
4. Wojtys E, Wilson M, Buckwalter K, et al.: Magnetic resonance imaging of knee hyaline cartilage and intraarticular pathology. Am J Sports Med 15:455–463, 1987.
5. Paget J: Healing of injuries in various tissues. Lect Surg Pathol T:262, 1853.
6. Buckwalter JA and Cooper RR: The cells and matrices of skeletal connective tissues. In Albright JA and Brand RA (eds.): The Scientific Basis of Orthopaedics. Norwalk, Conn., Appleton & Lange, 1987, pp 1–30.
7. Buckwalter JA, Hunziker EB, Rosenberg RC, et al.: Articular cartilage: composition and structure. In Woo SL-Y and Buckwalter JA (eds.): Injury and Repair of the Musculoskeletal Soft Tissues. Park Ridge, Ill., American Academy of Orthopaedic Surgeons, 1988, pp 405–426.
8. Buckwalter JA, Rosenberg LA, and Hunziker EB: Articular cartilage: composition, structure, response to injury, and methods of facilitation repair. In Ewing JW (ed.): Articular Cartilage and Knee Joint Function: Basic Science and Arthroscopy. New York, Raven Press, 1990, pp 19–56.
9. Mow VC, Fithian DC, and Kelly MA: Fundamentals of articular cartilage and meniscus biomechanics. In Ewing JW (ed.): Articular Cartilage and Knee Joint Function. New York, Raven Press, 1989, pp 1–18.
10. Muir H: Proteoglycans as organizers of the extracellular matrix. Biochem Soc Trans 11:613–622, 1983.
11. Nimni ME: Collagen: Structure, function and metabolism in normal and fibrotic tissues. Semin Arthritis Rheum 13:1–86, 1983.
12. Stockwell RS: Biology of Cartilage Cells. Cambridge, Cambridge University Press, 1979.
13. Orthopaedic Knowledge Update 3, Home Study Syllabus. Park Ridge, Ill., American Academy of Orthopaedic Surgeons, 1990, p 193.
14. Mankin HJ, Mow VC, Buckwalter JA, et al.: Form and function of articular cartilage. In Simon SR (ed.): Orthopaedic Basic Science. Rosemont, Ill., American Academy of Orthopaedic Surgeons, 1994, pp 1–44.
15. Mow VC, Ratcliffe A, and Poole AR: Cartilage and diarthroidial joints as paradigms for hierarchical materials and structures. Biomaterials 13:67–97, 1992.
16. Mow VC, Proctor CS, and Kelly MA: Biomechanics of articular cartilage. In Nordin M and Frankel VH (eds.): Basic Biomechanics of the Musculoskeletal System, 2nd ed. Philadelphia, Lea & Febiger, 1989, pp 32–34.
17. Buckwalter JA, Mow VC, and Ratcliffe A: Restoration of injured or degenerated articular cartilage. J Am Acad Orthop Surg 2:192–201, 1994.
18. Zamber RW, Teitz CC, McGuire DA, et al.: Articular cartilage lesions of the knee. Arthroscopy 5:258–268, 1989.
19. Fahmy NRM, Williams EA, and Noble J: Meniscal pathology and osteoarthritis of the knee. J Bone Joint Surg Br 65:24, 1983.
20. Noble J and Erat K: In defence of the meniscus. J Bone Joint Surg Br 62:7, 1980.
21. Hopkinson WJ, Mitchell WA, and Curl WW: Chondral fractures of the knee: cause for confusion. Am J Sports Med 13:309–312, 1985.
22. Goodfellow J, Hungerford DSA, and Woods C: Patello-femoral joint mechanics and pathology. 2: Chondromalacia patellae. J Bone Joint Surg Br 58:291, 1976.
23. Insall J: Patellar pain. J Bone Joint Surg Am 64:147, 1982.
24. Frankel VH, Burstein AH, and Brooks DB: Biomechanics of internal derangement of the knee. J Bone Joint Surg Am 53:945, 1971.
25. Kettlekamp DB and Jacobs AW: Tibiofemoral contact area: determination and implications. J Bone Joint Surg Am 54:349, 1972.
26. Salter RB and McNeil R: Pathological changes in articular cartilage secondary to persistent joint deformity. J Bone Joint Surg Br 47:185, 1965.
27. Tasker T and Waugh W: Articular changes associated with internal derangement of the knee. J Bone Joint Surg Br 64:486, 1982.
28. Waugh W, Newton G, and Tew M: Articular changes associated with a flexion deformity in rheumatoid and osteoarthritic knees. J Bone Joint Surg Br 62:180, 1980.
29. Johnson-Nurse C and Dandy DJ: Fracture separation of articular cartilage in the adult knee. J Bone Joint Surg Br 67:42–43, 1985.
30. Dzioba RB: The classification and treatment of acute articular cartilage lesions. Arthroscopy 4:72–80, 1988.
31. Krause WR, Pope MH, Johnson RJ, et al.: Mechanical changes in the knee after meniscectomy. J Bone Joint Surg Am 58:599, 1976.
32. Williams PL and Warwick R (eds.): Gray's Anatomy, 36th ed. Philadelphia, W.B. Saunders, 1980, pp 486–487.

33. Casscells SW: The torn meniscus, the torn anterior cruciate ligament, and their relationship to degenerative joint disease. Arthroscopy 1:28, 1985.

34. McDaniel WJ and Dameron TB: Untreated ruptures of the anterior cruciate ligament. J Bone Joint Surg Am 62:696, 1980.

35. Arnold JA, Coker TP, Heaton LM, et al.: Natural history of anterior cruciate ligament tears. Am J Sports Med 7:305, 1979.

36. Marshall JL, Rubin RM, Wang JB, et al.: The anterior cruciate ligament: the diagnosis and treatment of its injuries and their serious prognostic implications. Orthop Rev 7:35, 1978.

37. Noyes FR, Mooar PA, Matthews DS, et al.: The symptomatic anterior cruciate deficient knee (part I). J Bone Joint Surg Am 65:154, 1983.

38. Andersson C, Odenstein M, and Gillquist J: Early arthroscopic evaluation of acute repair of the anterior cruciate ligament. Arthroscopy 5:331–335, 1989.

39. Meyers JF, St Pierre RK, Sutter JS, et al.: Arthroscopic evaluation of anterior cruciate ligament reconstructions. Arthroscopy 2:155–161, 1986.

40. Geissler WB and Whipple TL: Intraarticular abnormalities in association with posterior cruciate ligament injuries. Am J Sports Med 21:846–849, 1993.

41. Clancy WG, Shelbourne KD, Zoellner GB, et al.: Treatment of knee joint instability secondary to rupture of the posterior cruciate ligament. J Bone Joint Surg Am 65:310–322, 1983.

42. Parolie JM and Bergfeld JA: Long-term results of nonoperative treatment of isolated posterior cruciate ligament injuries in the athlete. Am J Sports Med 14:35–38, 1986.

43. Fowler PJ and Messieh SS: Isolated posterior cruciate ligament injuries in athletes. Am J Sports Med 15:553–557, 1987.

44. Noyes FR, Grood ES, Nusshaum NS, et al.: Effect of intraarticular corticosteroids on ligament properties: a biomechanical and histological study in Rhesus knees. Clin Orthop 123:197–207, 1977.

45. Palmoski M, Perricone E, and Brandt KD: Development and reversal of a proteoglycan aggregation defect in normal canine knee cartilage after immobilization. Arthritis Rheum 22:508–517, 1979.

46. Spiers ASD, Meagher T, Ostlere SJ, et al.: Can MRI of the knee affect arthroscopic practice? J Bone Joint Surg Br 75:49–52, 1993.

47. Adam G, Nolte-Ernsting C, Prescher A, et al.: Experimental hyaline cartilage lesions: two-dimensional spin-echo versus three-dimensional gradient-echo MR imaging. J Magn Reson Imaging 1:665–672, 1991.

48. DeSmet AA, Mann JU, Fisher DR, et al.: Signs of patellar chondromalacia on sagittal T_2-weighted magnetic resonance imaging. Skeletal Radiol 21:103–105, 1992.

49. Speer KP, Spritzer CE, Guldner JL, et al.: Magnetic resonance imaging of traumatic knee articular cartilage injuries. Am J Sports Med 19:396–402, 1991.

50. Tervonen O, Dietz MJ, Carmichael SW, et al.: MR imaging of knee hyaline cartilage: Evaluation of two- and three-dimensional sequences. J Magn Reson Imaging 3:663–668, 1993.

51. Burk DL Jr, Kanal E, Brunberg JA, et al.: 1.5-T surface-coil MRI of the knee. Am J Roentgenol 147:293–300, 1986.

52. Wojtys E, Wilson M, Buckwalter K, et al.: Magnetic resonance imaging of knee hyaline cartilage and intraarticular pathology. Am J Sports Med 15:455–463, 1987.

53. Gylys-Morin VM, Hajek PC, Sortoris DJ, et al.: Articular cartilage defects: detectability in cadaver knees with MR. Am J Roentgenol 148:1153–1157, 1987.

54. Outerbridge RE: The etiology of chondromalacia patellae. J Bone Joint Surg Br 43:752–757, 1961.

55. Ficat RP, Philippe J, and Hungerford DS: Chondromalacia patellae: a system of classification. Clin Orthop 144:55–62, 1979.

56. Bentley G and Dowd G: Current concepts of etiology and treatment of chondromalacia patellae. Clin Orthop 189:209–228, 1984.

57. Casscells SW: Gross pathological changes in the knee joint of the aged individual: a study of 300 cases. Clin Orthop 132:225–332, 1978.

58. Aglietti P, Buzzi R, Insall JN: Disorders of the patellofemoral joint. In Insall JN (ed.): Surgery of the Knee 2nd ed. New York, Churchill Livingstone, 1993, pp. 241–385.

59. Goodfellow J, Hungerford DS, and Woods C: Patellofemoral joint mechanics and pathology—Part 2: Chondromalacia patellae. J Bone Joint Surg Br 58:291–299, 1976.

60. Noyes FR and Stabler CL: A system for grading articular cartilage lesions at arthroscopy. Am J Sports Med 17:505–513, 1989.

61. Rock MG, Kruger G, and Fowler PJ: London, Canada: Grading biomechanical characteristics of normal and degenerative articular cartilage: A correlative study. 5th Congress of the International Society of the Knee, Sydney, Australia, April 5–10, 1987.

62. Bentley G: The surgical treatment of chondromalacia patellae. J Bone Joint Surg Br 60:74–81, 1978.

63. Howell DS, Treadwell BV, and Trippel SB: Etiopathogenesis of osteoarthritis. In Moskowitz RW, Howell DS, Goldberg VM, et al. (eds.): Osteoarthritis: Diagnosis and Medical/Surgical Management, 2nd ed. Philadelphia, W.B. Saunders, 1992, pp 233–252.

64. Poole AR: Immunochemical markers of joint inflammation, skeletal damage and repair: where are we now? Ann Rheum Dis 53:3–5, 1994.

65. Lohmander LS, Dahlberg L, Ryd L, et al.: Increased levels of proteoglycan fragments in knee joint fluid after injury. Arthritis Rheum 32:1434–1442, 1989.

66. Bauer M and Jackson RW: Chondral lesions of the femoral condyles: a system of arthroscopic classification. Arthroscopy 4:97–102, 1988.

67. Bircher E: Die Arthroendoskopie. Zentralbl Chir 48:1460–1461, 1921.

68. Burman MS, Finkelstein H, and Mayer L: Arthroscopy of the knee joint. J Bone Joint Surg 16:255–268, 1934.

69. Watanabe M, Takeda S, and Ikeuchi H: Atlas of Arthroscopy. Tokyo, Igaku Shoin Ltd, 1957.

70. Evans CH, Mazzocchi RA, Nelson DD, et al.: Experimental arthritis induced by intraarticular injection of allogenic cartilaginous particles into rabbit knees. Arthritis Rheum 27:200–215, 1984.

71. Jackson RW, Marans HJ, and Silver RS: The arthroscopic treatment of degenerative arthritis of the knee. J Bone Joint Surg Br 70:332, 1988.

72. Baumgaertner MR, Cannon WD Jr, Vittori JM, et al.: Arthroscopic débridement of the arthritic knee. Clin Orthop 253:197–202, 1990.

73. Johnson LL: Arthroscopic Surgery: Principles and Practice. St. Louis, C.V. Mosby, 1986, pp 737–773.

74. Pridie KH: A method of resurfacing osteoarthritic knee joints. J Bone Joint Surg Br 41:618, 1959.

75. Rodrigo JJ, Steadman JR, and Silliman JF: Osteoarticular injuries of the knee. In Chapman MW (ed.): Operative Orthopaedics, vol 3, 2nd ed. Philadelphia, J.B. Lippincott Co., 1993, pp 2077–2082.

76. König F: Ueber freie Körper in den Gelenken. Dtsch Z Chir 27:90–109, 1887.

77. Linden B: Osteochondritis dissecans of the knee. J Bone Joint Surg Br 53:448–454, 1971.

78. Lindén B: The incidence of osteochondritis dissecans in the condyles of the femur. Acta Orthop Scand 47:664–667, 1976.

79. Luck JV, Smith HMA, Lacey HB, et al.: Orthopaedic surgery in Army Air Forces during World War II: introduction and internal derangements of the knee. Arch Surg 57:642, 1948.

80. Mesgarzadeh M, Sapega AA, Bonakdarpout A, et al.: Osteochondritis dissecans: analysis of mechanical stability with radiography, scintigraphy, and MR imaging. Radiology 165:775–778, 1987.

81. Pappas A: Osteochondritis dissecans. Clin Orthop 158:59–69, 1981.

82. Rosenberg TD, Paulos LE, Parker RD, et al.: Arthroscopic surgery of the knee. In Chapman MW (ed.): Operative Orthopaedics, 2nd ed. Philadelphia, J.B. Lippincott Co., 1993.

83. Casscells SW: Arthroscopy of the knee joint. J Bone Joint Surg Am 53:287, 1971.

84. O'Connor RL: Arthroscopy. Philadelphia, J.B. Lippincott Co., 1977.

24

Arthroscopic Techniques of Fracture Fixation of the Knee

Richard A. Marder • *Jan P. Ertl*

INTRODUCTION

Both diagnostic and operative arthroscopy can be useful in the management of intra-articular fractures. To date, most experience has been with fractures involving the knee, specifically tibial plateau and avulsion fractures of the anterior cruciate ligament.[1–5] Arthroscopic fracture stabilization has its basis in fracture treatment by closed reduction and percutaneous fixation.[6] In the knee, arthroscopy is helpful for removal of small chondral flakes and bony debris as well as assessment for meniscal and cruciate ligament injury. The major appeal of arthroscopic methods for treating amenable fractures is the minimalization of additional soft-tissue disruption, which is associated with the extensile dissection often necessary for open reduction and internal fixation. Therefore, provided that satisfactory fracture stabilization is achieved, arthroscopic techniques can facilitate improvement in regaining range of motion and functional recovery of the extremity.

ANTERIOR CRUCIATE LIGAMENT AVULSION

General Considerations

This injury is less common than midsubstance rupture and results from lower rates of loading.[7] Although generally regarded as an injury in children, one series noted a greater frequency in adults.[8] The anterior cruciate ligament (ACL) fibers may undergo plastic deformation before the avulsion fracture occurs; this deformation can result in residual laxity despite bony healing of the fracture.[9, 10] The injury typically involves a variable degree of involvement of the tibial eminence and may extend to involve the articular surface. Associated fracture of the fibular neck and injury of the collateral ligaments and menisci can occur.[8, 9, 11, 12] Significant complications of both nonoperative and surgical treatment include nonunion, malunion, and stiffness.[8, 9, 11–16]

Classification

Meyers and McKeever[11, 12] developed the most widely used classification scheme for anterior tibial eminence fractures: type I fractures are nondisplaced; type II fractures are superiorly angulated and are hinged posteriorly; and type III fractures are completely displaced from the tibia, and rotation may cause the fragment to be oriented 180 degrees from its tibial bed (Fig. 24–1).[11, 12] Subsequently, comminuted and displaced tibial eminence fractures have been referred to as type IV.[16]

Indications

Type I fractures are treated by nonoperative means; types II, III, and IV fractures require either closed reduction and immobilization or surgical reduction and fixation. In general, closed treatment can produce a satisfactory outcome in the skeletally immature knee, regardless of fracture type.

Nonoperative Treatment

If the fracture is nondisplaced (type I), maintain the knee in full extension with a cylinder cast for 4–6 weeks. If the fracture is displaced, aspiration of the joint and injection of a local anesthetic or use of a general anesthetic followed by extension of the knee may result in satisfactory reduction of the fragment. Asymmetry of knee extension is usually due to meniscal interposition or failure of the fragment to reduce. If successful, closed reduction is followed by immobilization of the knee in extension by using a well-molded cylinder cast for 4–6 weeks. At that point, joint range of motion is started aggressively. If knee flexion of more than 90 degrees is not present within 3 weeks after removing the cast, manipulation is performed. Return to activity usually occurs by 3–4 months when motion is nor-

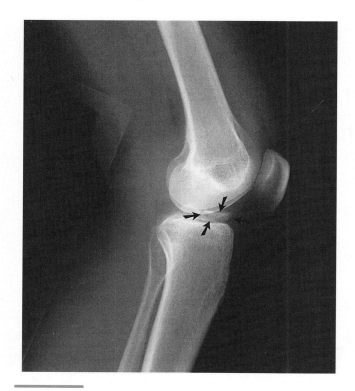

Figure 24–1 • Arthroscopic view of the anterior notch (*arrows*) demonstrates the avulsed anterior cruciate ligament (ACL) and its tibial fragment rotated 180 degrees.

mal and muscle strength approaches 90% of the normal extremity.

Operative Treatment

Open reduction alone followed by cast maintenance of extension and open reduction with internal fixation using suture, wire loops, pins, and screws have been described.[7–9, 11, 12, 16, 17] Arthroscopic treatment with reduction followed by retrograde screw insertion as well as use of suture has been used successfully.[5, 13, 18]

The authors use one of two arthroscopic methods to achieve reduction and fixation. If the avulsed fragment is small or comminuted, the authors perform arthroscopic-assisted reduction and fixation using a No. 5 Tevdek suture through the base of the ACL. A second method of arthroscopic fixation involves antegrade lag screw fixation using arthroscopic and fluoroscopic techniques. This latter method works well in adults for larger, noncomminuted fragments and in adolescents with transitional growth plates.

Techniques

With the patient under anesthesia, examine the knee to determine the degree of anterior laxity using the manual and instrumented Lachman test and whether there is associated collateral ligament injury. Aspirate the knee asepti-

cally and then determine if full extension (compared with normal) can be achieved. If so, obtain a lateral radiograph to confirm satisfactory reduction, and apply a cylinder cast. If a satisfactory reduction is not obtained, proceed with arthroscopy.

Suture Fixation. Using standard arthroscopic portals, perform routine examination of the entire joint, and treat any associated pathologic condition. Visualize the fracture from the anterolateral portal. Instrumentation is introduced through a standard anteromedial portal. After a small curet has been used to clean debris from the tibial bed, the fragment with the attached ACL is guided toward the tibial bed using a probe or grasper (Fig. 24–2A). Temporary reduction and fixation to the tibial bed are achieved by using the tibial aiming device from a standard ACL set. The tip should be alongside the lateral or medial border of the fragment, with ample margin to prevent pin cutout.

A 2–3 cm longitudinal incision is made alongside the medial border of the tibial tubercle, and a 2 mm guide pin is drilled through the bed, engaging the fragment. It may be helpful to use a probe or other instrument inserted through a second medial or transpatellar tendon portal to prevent displacement of the avulsed fragment. Drill a second smooth guide pin into position, maintaining a minimum of 8–10 mm of spacing between pins (Fig. 24–2B).

Leave one pin in place, and insert a suture passer through the reduced fragment (Fig. 24–2C). Introduce a No. 5 Tevdek suture through the medial portal using a protective cannula, and withdraw it through the track to the external opening at the tibial cortex, using the suture passer (Fig. 24–2D). Now withdraw the remaining guide pin, insert the suture passer, pass the other end of the No. 5 Tevdek suture into the joint through the medial portal into the suture passer, and withdraw it outside of the tibial cortex. This leaves a loop of suture passing through the avulsed fragment, which is seated (Fig. 24–2E) as the suture is tied.

An alternate method is to use two suture passers, with the second one inserted before passing any suture ends; this reduces the risk of fragment displacement during the process of passing the suture. The fracture is reduced by longitudinal traction on the suture ends, and a gentle range of motion of the knee is performed to note any tendency of the fragment to separate. Tie the sutures around a post and washer (6.5 mm cancellous screw and smooth washer) with the knee near extension while visualizing fracture reduction. Check that the Lachman test result is normal. In the operating room, obtain a postfixation radiograph. Apply a sterile compression dressing incorporating a cryotherapy sleeve. Position the knee in a knee immobilizer or in a hinged brace set initially in extension.

Modification of this technique may be needed in two instances: avulsion combined with plastic deformation of the ACL and comminution of the avulsion fragment. If laxity is present after the avulsed fragment is advanced back into its bed on the tibia (indicating that the ACL has undergone plastic deformation), then excavate the tibial bed before fixation in order to restore tension in the ACL. If the avulsed fragment is comminuted, arthroscopy will demonstrate if suture fixation can be performed with or without modification as described earlier or if reconstruc-

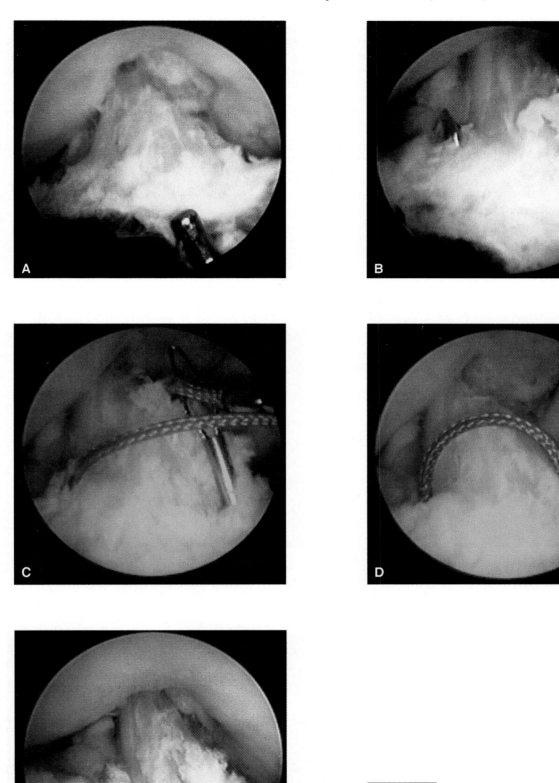

Figure 24–2 • *A*, Reduction of the avulsed ACL. *B*, Two parallel smooth guide pins passed across the avulsed ACL, achieving reduction and creating the tunnels for suture passage. *C*, Suture passer inserted through one pin track. *D*, Grasping a No. 5 Tevdek suture. *E*, After passage of both limbs of the No. 5 Tevdek suture to create a loop that will tighten with manual knot tying.

tion will be necessary in cases in which severe interligamentous disruption is present as well. If the bulk of the ligament appears intact visually and by palpation but the tibial fragment is comminuted, suture fixation through one or more of the osteoarticular fragments combined with weaving the suture through the base of the ligament may be necessary.

Lag Screw Fixation. Proceed with the previously described arthroscopic routine, including débridement and reduction (Fig. 24–3*A*). Introduce a K-wire through the anteromedial portal or a large bone-reduction forceps for temporary stabilization (Fig. 24–3*B*). Create an additional medial midpatellar portal to insert the guide wire from a 3.5 mm cannulated system. Using biplanar fluoroscopic control, insert the guide wire from an anteromedial direction into the fragment, engaging the posterolateral cortex of the proximal tibia (Fig. 24–3*C*). Measure the length of this guide wire indirectly with a second wire. When using the cannulated drill, avoid advancing the wire, checking the position with the image intensifier. When withdrawing the drill, disengage the bit from the drill as soon as its tip reaches the articular surface of the avulsed fragment. If the guide wire is retracted, insert a second wire through the back of the drill bit to push the original guide wire back into place. Insert the appropriate-length 3.5 mm screw, and achieve interfragmentary compression. Verify screw position on anteroposterior and lateral radiographs in the operating room (Fig. 24–3*D*).

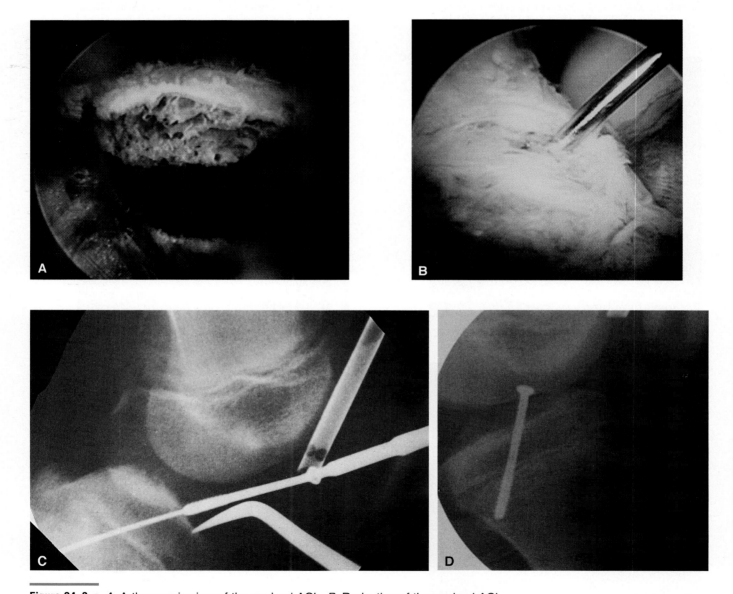

Figure 24–3 • *A*, Arthroscopic view of the avulsed ACL. *B*, Reduction of the avulsed ACL. *C*, Radiographic appearance of cannulated 3.5 mm screw fixation of avulsed ACL fragment (bone forceps maintaining reduction). *D*, Reduced ACL avulsion secured by 3.5 mm screw.

Postoperative Management

Stiffness can be a significant problem following open repair of these injuries and may be caused by immobilization superimposed on the trauma of surgery. In an effort to prevent stiffness, the authors institute early passive flexion of the knee from 0 to 90 degrees in all cases in which stable fixation is achieved. Immobilization may be necessary for 3–4 weeks if the avulsed fragment is comminuted and the repair has been secured primarily through the ligament proper.

Protected weight-bearing with the brace in extension is used for 3–4 weeks after bone-to-bone repair and for up to 6 weeks after ligament-to-bone repair. Isometric quadriceps and straight leg raise exercises are started immediately, but closed chain quadriceps resistive exercises are deferred until the fragment is thought to be healed. This period is usually 4 weeks when the avulsed fragment is intact and 6–8 weeks when the fragment is comminuted. Functional exercises are then advanced in a manner similar to that for ACL reconstruction (see Chapter 28). Many patients are able to resume sports by 4 months after repair. The authors do not routinely use derotation braces because residual anterior knee laxity is uncommon in our experience.

POSTERIOR CRUCIATE LIGAMENT AVULSION

General Considerations

Avulsion fracture of the posterior cruciate ligament (PCL) is more frequent than midsubstance rupture in isolated injury. Whereas Loos et al. noted avulsion from the tibia to be more frequent than from the femur, others have found a greater incidence of tears at the femoral origin.[19–21] Treatment of a tibial avulsion requires careful protection of the popliteal structures. For this, the authors elect to perform open repair by a direct posterior or posteromedial approach. In conjunction with a direct posterior approach, arthroscopy is useful in evaluating and treating other intra-articular injury. The authors have used arthroscopic methods to successfully repair femoral avulsions of the PCL.

Indications

In general, the indications for surgical treatment of acute, isolated PCL injuries are more controversial than for ACL injuries. The single exception is bony avulsion of the PCL from the tibia, in which repair has been shown to produce good results and failure to perform surgical repair has been shown to produce poor results.[22] It is logical to conclude that femoral avulsions should be treated similarly. When radiographs and arthroscopy indicate minimal bony attachments of the avulsed ligament that would be difficult to repair by suture or screw fixation, treatment should be undertaken based on the knowledge that joint deterioration after PCL rupture is difficult to predict on an individual basis and that functional stability can be achieved by rehabilitation alone.[23]

Nonoperative Treatment

If the knee with an isolated PCL bony avulsion is displaced less than 2 mm and the posterior drawer is less than 1+, a cylinder cast to maintain the knee in extension for 4 weeks prevents displacement. Repeat radiographs are obtained at 7 and 14 days to check for potential displacement.

Nonoperative treatment is also elected if the avulsion cannot be repaired because of minimal bony attachment, comminution, and associated interligamentous failure. Follow the protocol in Chapter 29.

Operative Treatment

Arthroscopy is performed before open repair of PCL tibial avulsions. This permits documentation and treatment of associated chondral injury and, less frequently, meniscal injury.[24]

When feasible, the authors perform arthroscopic-assisted repair of bony avulsions of the PCL from the femur using a technique similar to that for the ACL described earlier.

Technique

Visualize the fracture from the anterolateral portal under torniquet control (Fig. 24–4*A*). Through an anteromedial or transpatellar tendon portal, grasp the avulsed fragment and advance it toward the femoral bed, applying an anterior drawer to effect this more easily. Drill holes can be placed directly through a large fragment after reducing it and using a PCL femoral aiming device to drill parallel 2 mm guide wires from the outside in. As in the method described for ACL avulsions, the guide wires are replaced with a pair of suture retrievers, and a loop of No. 5 Tevdek suture is passed around the bony base and tied over a 14 mm plastic button or around a 6.5 mm cancellous screw and smooth washer.

If the bony fragment is small or comminuted, sutures are placed through the base of the PCL itself. Sutures can be placed by using either a curved spinal needle or a commercial suture punch inserted using a cannula (to prevent synovial entrapment) through the anterolateral or a transpatellar tendon portal in lateral to medial direction through the PCL. Three No. 2 or greater-diameter sutures are placed at right angles and brought back through the portal of insertion for safekeeping.

Insert a PCL femoral aiming guide to the center of the femoral bed (usually 8–10 mm posterior to the articular margin near the roof and wall junction) with the external exit site midway between the medial femoral epicondyle and the medial patellar border (Fig. 24–4*B*). Drill a 2 mm guide pin from the outside in. Countersink the ligament and any attached bony fragments into a fresh bony bed, restoring tension if plastic deformation has occurred. Over-ream the femoral guide pin to 6 mm and pass a suture retriever from the outside in. Apply an anterior drawer in 90 degrees of flexion, advance the PCL into the tunnel, and tie the sutures individually over a 14 mm button or around a post and washer (Fig. 24–4*C*). Close the medial skin incision. Apply a compression dressing incor-

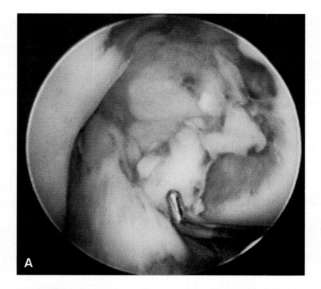

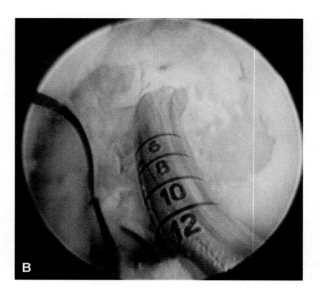

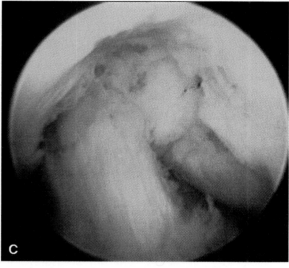

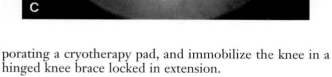

Figure 24–4 • *A,* Avulsion of posterior cruciate ligament from femur with minimal bone. *B,* Aiming guide to select femoral placement site (8 mm posterior to articular margin near roof and wall junction). *C,* Posterior cruciate ligament advanced into bony tunnel with anterior drawer applied and sutures tied over the exterior of the medial femoral condyle.

porating a cryotherapy pad, and immobilize the knee in a hinged knee brace locked in extension.

Postoperative Management

Femoral reattachment of the PCL is treated by immobilization of the knee in extension for 6 weeks. Passive flexion to 60 degrees is started at 4 weeks. Partial weight-bearing is allowed, along with quadriceps isometrics in extension and straight leg raises. Thereafter, unrestricted range-of-motion and quadriceps resistive exercises are started. Hamstring resistive exercises are deferred until 4 months after surgery. Return to activity is allowed when motion is normal and quadriceps strength is at least 90% that of the opposite extremity.

TIBIAL PLATEAU FRACTURES

General Considerations

These fractures typically occur when the knee is subjected to a combination of axial and lateral bending forces. These forces produce articular depression and metaphyseal shearing, most often on the lateral side of the knee. Continuation of valgus loading can rupture the medial collateral ligament. The lateral meniscus, especially, can be torn or entrapped in the fracture. Fracture propagation can involve the tibial insertions of the cruciate ligaments. Potential postfracture problems can include joint stiffness, instability, malalignment, and arthrosis. Appropriate treatment may avoid these potential complications and begins with accurate assessment of the type of fracture.

Assessment of Classification

Clinical examination is important in diagnosing vascular and neurologic injury as well as possible compartment syndrome. Although examination of the knee may be limited due to pain, tenderness over the collateral ligaments may suggest rupture, and mediolateral instability often can be determined.

Routine radiographs with the anteroposterior view angled 10 degrees caudally as well as oblique views may reveal the fracture adequately.[25] However, conventional tomography or computed tomography scanning may be necessary to delineate the degree of articular depression and additional fracture lines.

Although a number of classification schemes have been devised, the AO system remains practical for and applicable to most fractures.[26] There are four general categories of injury: wedge fractures, articular depression fractures, combined wedge and articular depression fractures, and complex Y and T comminuted fractures of both plateaus.

Indications

A diversity of opinion exists as to the merits of arthroscopy in the treatment of tibial plateau fractures. Schatzker[27] maintained that there is no role for arthroscopy other than to rule out entrapment of the lateral meniscus within the fragments of a wedge fracture of the lateral tibial plateau that would otherwise be treated conservatively due to minimal fracture displacement. Others, however, have reported satisfactory results using arthroscopic techniques in selected fractures.[1-4]

Arthroscopy can be useful in removing debris, extracting and repairing meniscal tears, and verifying anatomic reduction of articular fragments. In our experience, arthroscopic-assisted reduction of lateral wedge fractures and subchondral elevation of central depression fractures of the lateral tibial plateau have produced excellent results.

Combined wedge and depression fractures are more tedious to treat by arthroscopic means. Involvement of the eminence and fractures that are categorized as bicondylar or complex or that extend into the diaphysis are best treated by open reduction and internal fixation with buttress plates.[26, 27]

Nonoperative Treatment

In general, fractures that are nondisplaced, have articular depression less than 2–3 mm, and are stable to mediolateral stress are treated nonoperatively in a hinged knee brace, allowing early motion of the joint but protection from weight-bearing until the fracture is healed, usually 8–12 weeks. Follow-up radiographs should be compared with the original studies to prevent missing subtle changes that might dictate the need for operative intervention.

Operative Treatment

Lateral wedge and certain depressed articular fractures are amenable to arthroscopic fixation. Arthroscopic fixation of tibial plateau fractures requires the surgeon to be experienced in and knowledgeable about both arthroscopy and the principles and techniques of fracture fixation. Nonetheless, the authors routinely monitor the leg for the possible occurrence of arthroscopic-induced compartment syndrome, although occurrence is unlikely.[28]

Techniques

Wedge Fractures. With the patient under tourniquet control, perform routine arthroscopy with visualization from the anterolateral portal. It is usually necessary to use either a pump or a separate large-bore inflow with intermittent suction outflow from the arthroscopic cannula. Before inserting the arthroscope in its cannula, lavage and suction the joint to remove blood clots and debris. Continue this until the effluent is clear. Insert the arthroscope and place a probe or grasper in the anteromedial portal to dislodge clots and small fragments of debris. A 5 mm motorized shaver can be helpful in removing debris and clots. Elevate the lateral meniscus, which can be entrapped in the lateral plateau fracture. The lateral meniscus may be torn, and repair may be necessary. Ascertain the stability of the tibial attachment of the ACL.

For reduction of widened but vertically minimally- or non-displaced wedge fractures of the lateral plateau, apply a large reduction forceps clamp percutaneously anterior to the fibular head to compress the lateral and medial plateaus. While confirming anatomic reduction of the articular surface arthroscopically, insert two cannulated 7 mm cancellous screws placed in a lateral to medial direction immediately below the joint. Smooth washers beneath the screws prevent migration of the screw head in soft bone.

Vertically displaced wedge fractures of the lateral plateau can sometimes be reduced by offsetting the reduction forceps on the cortex of the lateral tibial plateau obliquely, resulting in a superior translation effect with compression of the clamp. If reduction is not satisfactory, open reduction is performed.

Depressed Articular Fragments. Certain lateral plateau fractures with central depression can be reduced by arthroscopic-assisted elevation of the depressed fragments. Perform arthroscopy as indicated earlier. Do not repair the torn lateral meniscus, if present, to improve visualization of the articular surface (Fig. 24–5*A*). Elevation of depressed articular fragments can be achieved by a short 1–2 cm incision over the anterior lateral metaphysis of the tibia placed approximately 3 cm distal to the level of the depressed fragments. Making a hinged cortical window, insert a bone tamp and gently elevate the fragments, verifying correct restoration of the articular surface.

Radiographic check of the final elevation is performed before cancellous or synthetic bone grafting and fixation with percutaneously inserted 7 mm cannulated lag screws immediately beneath the elevated fragments and bone graft. Anteroposterior and lateral radiographs are taken in the operating room after fracture fixation. The lateral meniscus is now repaired (Fig. 24–5*B*).

An alternate method developed by one of the authors (Ertl) utilizes an accessory lateral approach just anterior to the fibular head. A short 1–2 cm incision is made, and under fluoroscopic control a 4.5 mm drill is used to penetrate the lateral cortex, inferior to the depressed fragments. Manipulation and definitive lag screw fixation are performed through this lateral opening. Elevation of fragments is performed with arthroscopic and fluoroscopic control, using a custom 4.5 mm reduction instrument (Special Devices Inc., Grass Valley, Calif.) (Fig. 24–6*A*). Iliac crest cancellous graft or a synthetic bone substitute is

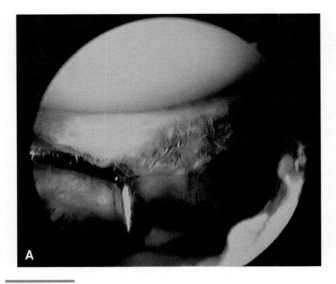

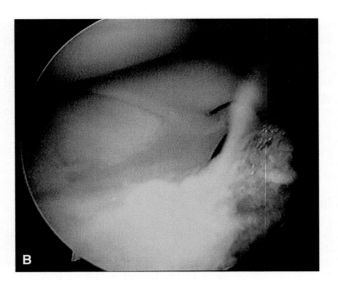

Figure 24–5 • *A*, Improved visualization of tibial plateau fracture by allowing lateral meniscus to remain displaced. *B*, Repair of lateral meniscus tear with restoration of articular congruity of the plateau fracture.

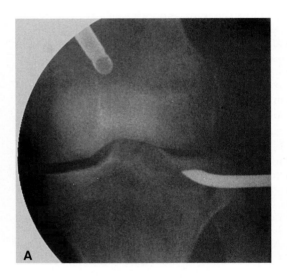

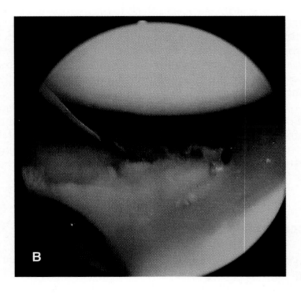

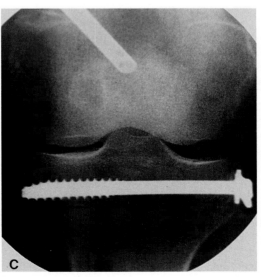

Figure 24–6 • *A*, Elevation of depressed articular fragments with custom instrument. *B*, Arthroscopic confirmation of fracture reduction. *C*, Radiograph confirms completed fixation of plateau fracture.

used to support the elevated fragments; reduction is confirmed by arthroscopy (Fig. 24–6B). The guide wire from a large-fragment cannulated system is introduced through the lateral cortical window and directed to the medial tibial cortex. Determine the length of the engaged guide wire and insert the cannulated drill. A 7 mm cannulated lag screw and smooth washer are now inserted, engaging the medial cortex. Fixation is completed by the parallel placement of a second screw and washer (Fig. 24–6C).

Postoperative Management

Apply a compression dressing that allows use of continuous passive motion during the hospital period. No weight-bearing is allowed for a minimum of 8 weeks; partial weight-bearing is allowed thereafter in wedge fractures only. Full weight-bearing is not allowed until 12 weeks. Active range-of-motion and isometric quadriceps exercises are started initially.

Range of motion is adjusted for collateral ligament injuries. Formal physical therapy using modalities to control swelling and pain (e.g., electrical stimulation, cryocompression) may be beneficial. Return to activity may require 6 months.

Complications

Complications are common to both open and arthroscopic methods of treatment of tibial plateau fractures. Failure to achieve reduction or subsequent loss of fracture reduction (Fig. 24–7) can be minimized by reserving arthroscopic

techniques for indicated fracture patterns, correct use of adequate fixation, and addition of bone grafting when necessary.

SUMMARY

Arthroscopy has a valuable role in the treatment of cruciate ligament avulsions and tibial plateau fractures of the knee. Although arthroscopic techniques are demanding and require cross-training in principles and techniques of fracture surgery, they can minimize soft-tissue dissection. The vascular supply to comminuted fragments is thereby preserved, frequently decreasing the morbidity of the postoperative period and enhancing the functional recovery of the patient.

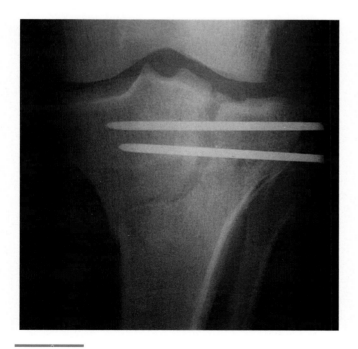

Figure 24–7 • Inadequate fixation of plateau fracture with arthroscopic-assisted reduction and smooth pin insertion demonstrates subsequent varus deformity and fracture displacement.

References

1. Holzach P, Matter P, and Minter J: Arthroscopically assisted treatment of lateral tibial plateau fractures in skiers: use of a cannulated reduction system. J Orthop Trauma 8:273–281, 1994.
2. Jennings JE: Arthroscopic management of tibial plateau fractures. Arthroscopy 1:160–168, 1985.
3. Lemon RA and Bartlett DH: Arthroscopic assisted internal fixation of certain fractures about the knee. J Trauma 25:355–358, 1985.
4. Caspari RB, Hutton PM, Whipple TL, et al.: The role of arthroscopy in the management of tibial plateau fractures. Arthroscopy 1:76–82, 1985.
5. McLennan JG: The role of arthroscopic surgery in the treatment of fractures of the intercondylar eminence of the tibia. J Bone Joint Surg Br 64:477–480, 1982.
6. Duwelius PJ and Connolly JF: Closed reduction of tibial plateau fractures: a comparison of functional and radiographic end results. Clin Orthop 230:116–126, 1988.
7. Noyes FR, DeLucas JL, and Torvik PF: Biomechanics of anterior cruciate ligament failure: an analysis of strain-rate sensitivity and mechanisms of failure in primates. J Bone Joint Surg Am 56:236–253, 1974.
8. Kendall NS, Hsu SY, and Chan K-M: Fracture of the tibial spine in adults and children. J Bone Joint Surg Br 74:848–852, 1992.
9. Clanton TO, DeLee JC, Sanders B, et al.: Knee ligament injuries in children. J Bone Joint Surg Am 61:1195–1201, 1979.
10. Wiley JJ and Baxter MP: Tibial spine fractures in children. Clin Orthop 255:54–60, 1990.
11. Meyers MH and McKeever FM: Fractures of the intercondylar eminence of the tibia. J Bone Joint Surg Am 41:209–222, 1959.
12. Meyers MH and McKeever FM: Fractures of the intercondylar eminence of the tibia: follow-up note. J Bone Joint Surg Am 52:1677–1684, 1970.
13. Berg EE: Comminuted tibial eminence anterior cruciate ligament avulsion injuries: failure of arthroscopic treatment. Arthroscopy 9:446–450, 1993.
14. Fyfe IS and Jackson JP: Tibial intercondylar fractures in children: a review of the classification and the treatment of mal-union. Injury 13:165–169, 1981.
15. Keys GW and Walters J: Nonunion of intercondylar eminence fracture of the tibia. J Trauma 2:870–871, 1988.
16. Zaricznyj B: Avulsion fracture of the tibial eminence: treatment by open reduction and pinning. J Bone Joint Surg Am 59:1111–1114, 1977.
17. Lee HG: Avulsion of the tibial attachments of the crucial ligaments: treatment by operative reduction. J Bone Joint Surg 19:460–468, 1937.
18. Van Loon T and Marti RK: A fracture of the intercondylar eminence of the tibia treated by arthroscopic fixation. Arthroscopy 7:385–388, 1991.
19. Loos WC, Fox JM, Blazina ME, et al.: Acute posterior cruciate ligament injuries. Am J Sports Med 9:86–92, 1981.
20. Moore HA and Larson RL: Posterior cruciate ligament injuries: results of early surgical repair. Am J Sports Med 8:68, 1980.

21. Hughston JC, Bowden JA, Andrews JR, et al.: Acute tears of the posterior cruciate ligament. J Bone Joint Surg Am 62:438–450, 1980.
22. Meyers MH: Isolated avulsion of the tibial attachment of the posterior cruciate ligament of the knee. J Bone Joint Surg Am 54:669–672, 1975.
23. Parolie JM and Bergfeld JA: Long-term results of nonoperative treatment of isolated posterior cruciate ligament injuries in the athlete. Am J Sports Med 14:35–38, 1986.
24. Fowler PJ and Messieh SS: Isolated posterior cruciate ligament injuries in athletes. Am J Sports Med 15:553–557, 1987.
25. Moore TM and Harvey JP: Roentgenographic measurement of tibial plateau depression due to fracture. J Bone Joint Surg Am 56:155–160, 1974.
26. Muller ME, Allgower M, Schneider R, et al.: Manual of Internal Fixation. Techniques Recommended by the AO-Group, 2nd ed. New York, Springer-Verlag, 1979, pp 258–261.
27. Schatzker J: Fractures of the tibial plateau. In Chapman MW (ed.): Operative Orthopaedics, 2nd ed. Philadelphia, J.B. Lippincott Co. 1993, pp 671–684.
28. Peek RD and Hayes DW: Compartment syndrome as a complication of arthroscopy. Am J Sports Med 12:464–468, 1984.

Chapter

25 Patellofemoral Joint

William P. Garth, Jr. • *Kurt T. Stroebel*

Anterior knee pain is one of the most common chief complaints of patients presenting to the physician who takes care of athletes. Although this pain is commonly considered to be patellofemoral in origin, the exact cause or source of the pain can be enigmatic. In the past this pain was often attributed to chondromalacia of the patella. However, experience has shown that the presence or absence of chondromalacia correlates poorly with the degree of pain, and the wise physician is careful to determine a source of the pain with a detailed history and a careful physical examination.[1–7]

Most patients respond to conservative management. In addition to nonsteroidal anti-inflammatory drugs, the cornerstones of conservative management consist of:

1. Rest from high impact activities while substituting low impact training

2. Correction of training errors, such as too rapid an increase in activities

3. Avoidance of climbing activities

4. Correction of structural malalignments associated with pronated feet by the use of orthotics or shoe corrections

5. Correction of strength imbalances with the usual emphasis on the vastus medialis obliques, while restoring flexibility to the muscles crossing the knee joint

Only after all of these conservative measures have been exhausted over a well-supervised period of at least 2–3 months should any consideration be given to surgical management.

PATIENT PRESENTATION

History

The age and activity of the patient presenting to the physician with the complaint of anterior knee pain should trigger an immediate differential diagnosis. For example, the sport of basketball usually results in different disorders in different age groups. The 12 year old basketball player presenting with no history of injury but with one of excessive play likely has pain associated with Osgood-Schlatter disease, Sinding-Larsen-Johansson disease, or patellofemoral malalignment. In contrast, the midadolescent to young adult basketball player commonly has jumper's knee, the common term for infrapatellar tendinitis, or pain associated with patellofemoral malalignment with or without chondromalacia. Athletes presenting in their late twenties and early thirties more commonly have retropatellar pain associated with activities such as quick stops and jumps in sports such as basketball. Pain associated with patellofemoral fissures commonly leads these young adults to adapt and participate in less stressful sports than basketball. As the athlete approaches middle age, osteoarthritic changes may be apparent involving the patellofemoral joint and commonly result in even more restriction of activities.

Once the physician is familiar with the age and activity level of the patient, a history of the event initiating the patient's symptoms should be obtained. Specifically, the physician must note whether the patient is aware of an injury immediately preceding the onset of symptoms or whether the symptoms were associated with an insidious onset with prolonged activity, consistent with overuse. A fall with landing on the knee or the history of an automobile accident in which the patient was sitting in the front seat immediately leads the physician to explore the possibility of a direct blow to the front of the knee leading to painful traumatic chondromalacia or tearing of the posterior cruciate ligament, which may be associated with patellofemoral pain. A blow to the medial knee may result in transient dislocation of the patella or in soft-tissue contusion symptoms of painful clicking caused by a fibrotic plica as the acute injury resolves.[8] A valgus, external rotation twisting injury in the immature patient should elicit concerns of transient patellofemoral instability, whereas in the mature young adult a tear of the anterior cruciate ligament (ACL) and less commonly an episode of patello-

313

femoral instability is likely. Insidious onset of symptoms associated with repetitive activity but without trauma elicits concerns of overuse failure of any structures about the anterior knee. Overuse symptoms may result from repetitive tension on the tendons or bony attachments of the extensor mechanism or excessive compression loads in the patellofemoral joint. Overuse traction injuries or patellofemoral compression syndromes are commonly associated with impact loading activities such as jumping or climbing.

If the patient is not seen after an acute injury, then the history should distinguish whether swelling occurred immediately after the injury, suggestive of hemarthrosis, or whether swelling occurred after 24 hours or more, which is consistent with an effusion. It should be determined whether the swelling was diffuse, which is more consistent with an intra-articular effusion, or localized and more suggestive of extra-articular injury, such as swelling of the inferior pole of the patella associated with acute infrapatellar tendinitis.

Next the physician should elicit a history of the knee giving way prior to the episode leading to the consultation, which may be suggestive of a chronic disorder, or whether the giving way began after a recent activity or event. By careful questioning, the physician should be able to distinguish the difference between the quadriceps release type of giving way and the pivot shift associated with ACL tears. However, transient patellar subluxation can be difficult to differentiate historically from the pivot shift.

The present illness should next include a history of activities that have subsequently provoked pain. Commonly, patellofemoral pain is provoked by repetitive knee flexion or extension activities (e.g., climbing stairs, squatting, or jumping). Often less pain is noted during the activity than is noted after the activity. The so-called "movie sign" (i.e., the onset of pain associated with prolonged sitting with the knee flexed position) is a classic symptom for pathology of the extensor mechanism, such as patellofemoral compression syndrome or infrapatellar tendinitis.

Finally, a family history should be taken. It is common that anterior knee pain or patellofemoral instability has been present in other family members with whom the patient may share patellofemoral malalignment.

Physical Examination

An initial observation of the patient who has anterior knee pain will frequently give some clues that malalignment of the lower extremity may play some role in the etiology of pain or instability. The standing patient is often noted to have squinting patellas, the term used to describe patellas that are facing inward as the feet face straight ahead. Squinting patellas are often associated with varus and external rotation alignment of the tibia with lateral insertion of the infrapatellar tendon, resulting in a high Q-angle.[9] It has been commonly stated that squinting patellas are secondary to femoral anteversion. However, examination of the prone patient for rotation of the hips frequently indicates no significant increase in internal rotation of the femur, indicating no increased femoral anteversion. While the patient is standing, squinting patel-

las can frequently be improved by correcting pronation deformities of the feet, thus indicating that orthotics to correct foot pronation may have some benefit. The high Q-angle persists, however, even if the inward-looking patellas are redirected by orthotics. Observation may also indicate vastus medialis obliquus (VMO) dysplasia or underdevelopment of the medial quadriceps compared with the lateral quadriceps. Less commonly, genu valgus may be present and associated with a high Q-angle.

Range of motion of the knee is inspected and may be restricted following an acute injury associated with hemarthrosis, such as in cases of transient patellar dislocation. Chronic restrictions of range of motion may be the result of arthrofibrosis, which is commonly associated with patella baja and anterior knee pain. J-tracking of the patella (i.e., lateral displacement of the patella as it tracks proximal to the femoral sulcus in terminal knee extension) may be observed during range of motion. The J-tracking is indicative of a tendency for lateral patellar instability.

Much information can be gained from palpation of the knee. During range of motion, palpation may be positive for patellofemoral crepitus, suggesting the presence of chondromalacia of the patella or femoral sulcus. Tenderness is a valuable aid when eliciting the cause of anterior knee pain. Tenderness is present at the tibial tubercle or inferior pole of the patella in the early adolescent who is experiencing traction injury to the immature proximal tibial epiphysis or inferior pole of the patella. Tenderness of the inferior pole of the patella in the midline of the mature adolescent or young adult is typical of infrapatellar tendinitis. Tenderness of the medial patellofemoral ligament (MPFL) may be noted as it originates at the adductor tubercle of the femur or as it inserts deep to the distal edge of the VMO and on the proximal medial pole of the patella. Tenderness of the medial patellomeniscal ligament (MPML) can be noted on the inferior medial pole of the patella extending to the anterior medial joint line. Tenderness confined to the MPFL and MPML, the two most functionally significant portions of the medial retinaculum, is suggestive of patellar instability. This is particularly true if pain is provoked by lateral displacement of the patella, such as in apprehension testing. There are no significant medial retinacular fibers in the triangular area of the medial knee bordered proximally by the MPFL, distally by the MPML, posteriorly by the medial collateral ligament (MCL), and anteriorly by the midpatella. Tenderness in this triangular area may be more indicative of focal synovitis or a symptomatic synovial plica than of sprain of the medial patellar retinaculum. A palpable snapping and tender bandlike structure in this triangle area near the margin of the patella is highly suggestive of a symptomatic plica.[10] Except in cases of displaced bucket handle tears of the medial meniscus with a locked knee, anterior tenderness of the medial joint line is suggestive of a sprain of the MPML, whereas tenderness of the posterior medial joint line is more suggestive of a tear of the medial meniscus. Tenderness of the semimembranous tendon is commonly present in knees that have sustained a valgus injury with an MCL sprain and may be mistaken for joint line tenderness. Tenderness overlying the lateral patellofemoral joint is commonly present in lateral patellofemoral compression syndrome. Through palpation of a fluid wave and patellar ballottement, the examiner should be able to determine the presence of intra-articular effusion or hemarthrosis. The fluid wave may also be present in prepatellar bursitis. However, in that case, palpation should determine the fluid wave to be superficial to the patella and not deep to the patella, which will ballot when the swelling is intra-articular.

Stress examination of the knee, when considered to be positive for significant laxity, should always be compared with the opposite knee as a control for what is normal in the patient being examined. Before an examination provokes pain and causes guarding by the patient, the knee should be checked first for anterior laxity by a Lachman test. Testing for posterior laxity, particularly utilizing the posterior drawer test, is important for patients with anterior knee pain who have experienced trauma directly over the anterior aspect of the knee (e.g., in a dashboard injury). Varus or valgus laxity should be checked. The presence of valgus laxity should not in any way rule out the possibility that patellofemoral dislocation has occurred because a valgus, external rotation injury may result in an MCL sprain but also produce a lateral patellar dislocation. Testing for pivot shift instability should be included, but muscle guarding following an acute injury may result in a false-negative reproduction of the shift. The final stress examination of the knee should be for patellofemoral instability. If a patellofemoral dislocation has occurred, usually the patient will be very apprehensive with lateral manipulation of the patella. If the patient can relax and allow lateral manipulation of the patella to the extent that the degree of hypermobility can be determined, then the degree of hypermobility should be compared with the opposite normal knee for a control.

Generally passive mobility of the patella with manipulation, to the extent that the medial femoral condylar surface of the femoral sulcus can be palpated, should be considered abnormal laxity. By manipulating the patella slightly distally with laterally directed manipulation of the patella, the MPML is relaxed and allows isolated testing of the competence of the MPFL. The patient should be examined throughout the upper and lower extremities as well as the opposite knee for other signs of generalized hypermobility. This can consist of sulcus signs at the shoulder, hyperextension of the elbows, the ability to hyperextend the metacarpophalangeal joints of the fingers to 90 degrees or to touch the thumb to the volar surface of the forearm. In addition, significant recurvatum of the knee, hypermobility of bilateral patellas, and supple pes planus should alert the physician to generalized joint laxity and the possibility of patellofemoral instability with significant congenital predisposition.

Radiographic Examination

A routine radiographic examination of the knee should include the anteroposterior, lateral, merchant, and tunnel views.

The anterior-posterior view of the knee may reveal a bipartite patella, which usually involves the superolateral pole. This can be a source of pain but is frequently asymptomatic.

The lateral examination will indicate patella alta (Insall-Salvetti ratio <0.80) present in approximately 50% of cases of patellofemoral instability.[11] Patella baja, which is suggestive of infrapatellar contraction, may be noted. DeJour has described the intersection sign and the trochlea bump as seen on the lateral radiograph to be commonly associated with both patellofemoral pain and patellofemoral instability. The intersection sign is said to be present when the bottom trochlea line crosses the lateral and medial femoral condyles on the lateral x-ray indicative of a flat trochlea at the level of intersecting lines. A trochlea bump is defined by the distance between the bottom trochlea line and a line extended distally from the anterior cortex of the femoral shaft. The trochlea bump, extending anterior to the shaft of the distal femur, is reportedly indicative of maximal dysplasia of the trochlea (Fig. 25–1). This relative prominence of the femoral trochlea is reported to be associated with increased patellofemoral compression, leading to anterior knee pain and a higher femoral sulcus angle commonly present in knees with patellofemoral instability.[12] Osteochondritis dissecans seen on lateral x-ray of the patella is relatively rare compared with the common location at the medial femoral condyle, which is typically seen in the tunnel view. Care must be taken to distinguish a true osteochondritis dissecans lesion from an osteochondral fracture, which may have occurred with patellofemoral dislocation. In the older patient, the lateral view is helpful in demonstrating a significant thinning of the patellofemoral joint with degenerative spurs associated with osteoarthritis.

The merchant view is, in the authors' opinion, the most helpful of the tangential radiographic views of the patellofemoral articulation. The femoral sulcus angle of more than 144 degrees exceeds one standard deviation of normality and is seen in approximately 70% of patients who have episodic patellofemoral instability. Lateral subluxation of the patella can be measured on the merchant view and is said to be present if the patellofemoral congruence angle is greater than 16 degrees[13] (Fig. 25–2). The lateral patellofemoral angle demonstrates lateral tilting of the patella and is diagnostic of a tight lateral retinaculum[14] (Fig. 25–3). Lateral subluxation of the patella without significant lateral tilt is more indicative of laxity of the MPFL near the margin of the patella and is unlikely to be corrected by release of the lateral retinaculum.[15, 16] The absence of demonstration of lateral subluxation does not rule out significant episodic patellar instability.[15]

The tunnel view is rarely helpful in defining pathology of the patellofemoral joint but is most helpful in demonstrating femoral osteochondritis dissecans of the medial femoral condyle. In addition, the tunnel view allows for inspection of the size of the femoral intercondylar notch, which has significance in ACL injuries.

Computed tomography and kinematic magnetic resonance imaging have been reported to be helpful in demonstrating patellar subluxation.[17, 18] In the authors' opinion, however, with a thorough history and physical examination done on several occasions and routine radiographic studies, these costly modalities are unnecessary in most cases.

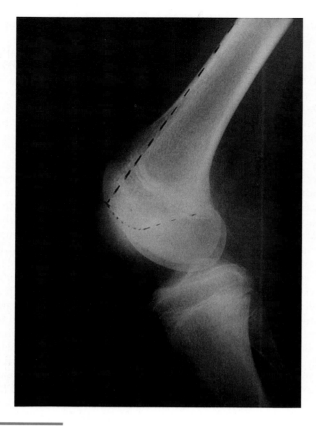

Figure 25–1 • The radiographically demonstrated bottom trochlea line, which is seen on the lateral radiograph, is an anterior extension of the Blumensaat line (roof of the intercondylar notch). The trochlea line is normally parallel to the medial and lateral femoral condyles of the femoral trochlea, extending from the anterior intercondylar notch to the anterior femoral metaphysis without intersecting the two radiographic margins of these condyles. The intersection on the lateral radiograph of the trochlea line with the anterior margins of the femoral condyles is indicative of a flat femoral sulcus, a dysplastic condition leading to patellofemoral instability. A near-perfect lateral radiograph in which the posterior margins of the femoral condyles are interposed is necessary for a completely accurate interpretation of the intersection sign. Fluoroscopy may be required in order to obtain an accurate lateral radiograph. The trochlea bump is a protrusion of the femoral sulcus anterior to a line extended from the anterior surface of the distal shaft of the femur, which has been reported to be associated with anterior knee pain or patellofemoral instability.[12]

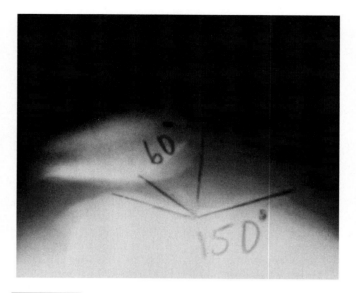

Figure 25–2 • Merchant view. The femoral sulcus angle (150 degrees) is measured by lines drawn parallel to the medial and lateral condyles of the femoral trochlea. The patellofemoral congruence angle (60 degrees) is subtended by a line equally dividing the sulcus angle and a line drawn from the central sulcus to the most posterior point of the patella (i.e., the point on the patella that normally articulates at the center of the sulcus). A femoral sulcus angle greater than 144 degrees and a patellofemoral congruence angle greater than 16 degrees are considered abnormal.

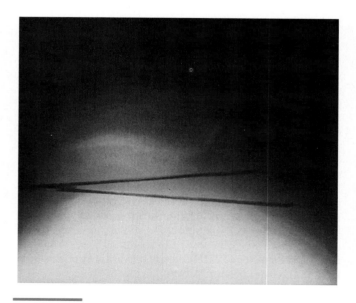

Figure 25–3 • The lateral patellofemoral angle is formed by a line connecting the most anterior points on the femoral condyles of the trochlea (which is abnormally flat in this case) and a second line extending from the vertex of the posterior patella to the posterolateral margin of the patella. The lateral patellofemoral angle so drawn is normally open to the lateral side. An angle that is closed laterally (as shown here) or even parallel is suggestive of lateral subluxation and a taut lateral retinaculum.

Functional Testing

By this time the examiner should have noted the presence or absence of atrophy and atonia of the quadriceps. These two physical findings are indirect evidence of quadriceps weakness. However, significant functional weakness due to pain may exist during some activities in the absence of atrophy or atonia. The authors prefer to test functional strength and compare it with the normal control knee. Initially, the patient is evaluated for the quality of quadriceps setting and straight leg raising. If the patient is unable to perform adequate quadriceps setting or straight leg raising, there is no need to test further for functional strength. If quadriceps setting and straight leg raising are good, the authors then evaluate the strength of leg extension, leg press, and leg curl compared with the opposite extremity. Isolated weakness of leg extension and leg press is usually indicative of symptoms arising from the extensor mechanism. Weakness of the hamstring curl is commonly seen following valgus injuries with an MCL sprain and is commonly associated with tenderness of the semimembranous direct insertion inferior to the medial joint line. In the presence of full leg extension strength but weakness of leg press and leg curl, a valgus knee injury has most likely spared injury to the extensor mechanism and patella.

REHABILITATION

Rehabilitation of the injured knee is begun immediately without antecedent immobilization. There is virtually no advantage to immobilization of the injured knee unless gross dislocation of the tibiofemoral joint has occurred. Immobilization has been shown to be detrimental to joint cartilage,[19] leads to significant muscle atrophy, and, when combined with non–weight-bearing, is associated with disuse osteoporosis of the bone. In addition, ligament healing is slowed. In contrast, controlled mobilization has been shown to facilitate nourishment of the joint cartilage and the healing of extra-articular ligaments about the knee.[19] A proliferation of fibroblasts and the production and strength of new collagen laid down are facilitated by mobilization.[20–22]

Therefore, even after acute patellar dislocation, it is the authors' policy to begin the immediate range of active and passive range of motion of the knee.[23] If significant hemarthrosis is present, it is aspirated to facilitate motion and to reduce tension on the acutely torn medial patellofemoral ligament and patellomeniscal ligament with the hope of allowing these ligaments to heal in a shortened position. Immediate attention is directed toward gaining good quadriceps setting and straight leg raising. This may be facilitated by electrical stimulation of the quadriceps. The goal is to establish immediate restored function of active knee extension, which will allow weight-bearing and reduce the inevitable atrophy that accompanies these injuries. In addition to gaining full active knee extension, an exercise bicycle with attached moveable handle bars allows the injured patient to facilitate active, assistive range of motion, restoring confidence in the knee and in the patient's ability to actively control the knee for ambulation. Nonsteroidal anti-inflammatory drugs are prescribed immediately to facilitate reduction of tenderness and swelling. The knee is fitted with a lateral padded knee sleeve, which is comforting to the patient and probably results in some stabilization effect by virtue of the lateral buttress. The immediate goal is to restore the patient to ambulatory capability without crutches upon leaving the office, even if dislocation of the patella occurred only hours earlier. By this means, it is hoped to take advantage of the beneficial effects of mobilization and speed recovery by reducing the deleterious effects of disuse atrophy and osteoporosis.

SURGICAL MANAGEMENT

Surgical management is considered when a reasonable period of conservative efforts has failed to result in an acceptable resolution of pain or mechanical symptoms. The patient considered for surgery may fit into one of five categories:

1. Persistent pain with evidence of malalignment or functionally significant episodic instability

2. Functionally significant episodic instability without significant pain prevalent between episodes

3. Persistent effusion

4. Internal derangement manifested by internal mechanical locking or catching that typically results in at least intermittent effusions; or clicking and popping associated with pain

5. Idiopathic anterior knee pain without mechanical symptoms may cautiously be considered for diagnostic arthroscopy, if the patient understands the relative unpredictability of arthroscopy in reducing these symptoms

Patellofemoral Pain Syndromes

Contributing to the difficulties in the surgical management of patellofemoral pain is the fact that the exact source of the pain is open for debate. Darracott and Vernon-Roberts recognized that articular cartilage has no nerve endings.[24] These authors hypothesized that patellofemoral pain is frequently caused by the alteration of blood supply in the patella associated with osteoporosis of the subchondral bone. Leslie and Bentley discounted that theory because there was no radiographic evidence of osteoporosis of the subchondral bone, and instead they hypothesized that pain is caused by stimulation of nerve endings in the subchondral bone by cathepsin released from damaged chondrocytes in the deep layers of the articular cartilage.[25] It is difficult to explain by this theory patients who seem to have significant patellofemoral pain and yet no objective evidence of articular cartilage damage.

The poor correlation between chondromalacia and the degree of patellofemoral pain has led to recognition of the importance of malalignment of the patellofemoral joint in association with patellofemoral pain syndromes. Lateral patellar tilt was first described by Ficat, Ficat, and Bailleux and is described as being associated with excessive lateral pressure syndrome.[26] Tenderness of the lateral retinaculum in these cases has been described as a source of lateral patellofemoral pain. The observation of neuromatous degeneration in the taut lateral retinaculum by Fulkerson and colleagues leads credence to that hypothesis.[27] In addition, tenderness of the MPFL and the MPML may be commonly seen in cases of patellofemoral instability and is believed to be the result of traction phenomenon on these medial restraints when the patella subluxates laterally.[28]

Patellofemoral pain does not have to be associated exclusively with malalignment or tilt. During excessive activity resulting in accumulative patellofemoral compressive forces, even subtle grade I chondromalacia of the patella, with damaged deeper layers of articular cartilage, may result in pain when stimulated by patellofemoral compression in the presence of normal alignment. However, less activity may result in pain in the presence of patellofemoral malalignment or lateral tilt. When the patella is malaligned, forces concentrate over a smaller area and increase the stress on local areas of the patellofemoral joint, which may result in chondromalacia. In these cases of lateral patellofemoral tilt, the pain could easily be both retinacular and patellofemoral in origin.

Chondromalacia of the patella cannot be diagnosed definitively on the basis of patellofemoral pain alone. However, the presence of palpable patellofemoral crepitus and grinding with flexion or extension of the knee and intermittent effusions associated with activities loading the patellofemoral joint are highly suggestive of chondromalacia of the patella and lead to the clinical suspicion that chondromalacia may be least in part be responsible for anterior knee pain.

Choice of Surgical Procedure

Lateral release has been shown to be of no predictable benefit in patients with anterior knee pain when there is no evidence that a lateral patellar tilt[17] or a tight lateral retinaculum is present.[29]

In the absence of patellofemoral malalignment or tilt, a tight lateral patellar retinaculum, or hypermobility with positive apprehension testing, arthroscopic débridement of chondral flaps and chondromalacia is probably as likely as any procedure to have the desired result of resolution of mechanical locking, popping, and effusion associated with anterior knee pain. The procedure of choice under these conditions is simply mechanical débridement of articular cartilage to resect flaps that cause catching and mechanical symptoms. Irrigation and débridement also serve to rid the knee of effusion by removing shedding flaps of articular cartilage that stimulate synovitis and a secondary effusion. There is no proven advantage of débriding or drilling through subchondral bone in the hope of stimulating repair or regrowth of mechanically sound articular cartilage. Good results have been noted with limited chondroplasty in approximately half the cases, and some improvement is noted in more than 90% of cases.[30]

Commonly, however, malalignment exists in the symptomatic knee, and débridement alone is unlikely to totally resolve symptoms. Three patterns of malalignment of the patellofemoral joint as imaged on computed tomography from 0 to 30 degrees have been described.[16, 31] These malalignment patterns are:

1. Subluxation without tilt
2. Subluxation with tilt
3. Tilt without subluxation

Subluxation is considered by Schutzer and colleagues on the computed tomography examinations to be a congruence angle more than 0 degrees at 10 degrees knee flexion. Excessive lateral patellar tilt can be relieved substantially by lateral patellar retinacular release. Patellar subluxation, however, is not predictably corrected by either lateral release alone or when combined with distal realignment.[16]

Gecha and Torg defined "mal-loose" signs, which tended to be associated with unsuccessful lateral release. These malalignment and hypermobility factors consist of an increased Q-angle, generalized joint laxity, patellar hypermobility, excessive genu varum or valgum, recurvatum, increased femoral anteversion, increased external tibial torsion, and abnormal foot pronation. A positive Sage sign (inability to displace the patella medially by a distance of one-quarter the width of the patella) is a good prognostic factor for lateral release, whereas positive mal-loose signs cause concern of failure with lateral release. The Gecha and Torg[29] study is consistent with Fulkerson and associates'[16] observation of the inability of lateral release to fully correct lateral subluxation of the patella.

We believe that in the presence of significant medial laxity resulting in persistent symptomatic lateral subluxation of the patella, particularly if episodic dislocations have occurred, lateral release alone is contraindicated. Furthermore, in that scenario, lateral release and medialization of the tibial tubercle are contraindicated because the result has been incomplete correction of subluxation if incompetent medial soft-tissue restraints are not reconstructed. In patients with true instability, the ability to displace the patella laterally at 30 degrees of knee flexion to the extent that more than 1 cm of the medial condyle of the femoral sulcus can be palpated is an indication for delayed repair or reconstruction of the medial patellofemoral ligament and plication of the medial patellomeniscal ligament. In the presence of a high Q-angle, medialization of the tibial tubercle and distal lateral patellar release have been combined with restoration of the medial soft-tissue restraints. We have also identified a subset of patients who have no resting lateral subluxation but exhibit marked dynamic subluxation with active terminal knee extension. These patients experience recurrent dislocations and typically have incompetence of the MPFL posterior to the VMO and generalized MPML laxity. These patients also require open restoration of the medial soft-tissue restraints and reduction of the high Q-angle.[15]

Summary of Indications for Surgical Procedures

1. The ideal candidate for arthroscopic débridement alone is the individual who has failed to respond to conservative measures and has minimal patellar malalignment and hypermobility but has mechanical symptoms suggestive of disruption of the articular surface of the patellar or femoral sulcus.

2. The ideal candidate for limited lateral release without further realignment has significant lateral patellar tilt in the presence of a positive Sage sign without lateral subluxation and no mal-loose signs.

3. The patient who has had a lateral release or has a negative Sage sign but has persistent symptoms and signs of lateral patellofemoral compression and a high

Q-angle may be a candidate for anteromedial medialization of the tibial tubercle, particularly if chondromalacia is documented laterally and distally in the patellofemoral joint.

4. The knee with significant medial laxity and persistent lateral subluxation or recurrent dislocations should have repair or reconstruction of the medial patellofemoral ligament and plication of the medial patellomeniscal ligament. The extent of lateral release and anteromedialization of the tibial tubercle to be included with medial reconstruction depends on the degree of tautness of the lateral retinaculum, the Q-angle, and the presence and location of chondromalacia patella.

Arthroscopic Technique

Arthroscopy for the patellofemoral joint can be performed with or without a thigh holder. However, when patellofemoral pathology is believed to be relatively isolated, the author prefers not to use the thigh holder in order to facilitate the use of proximal portals if desired. The tourniquet is placed about the upper thigh but is inflated only if bleeding is so profuse following lateral release that adequate visualization for cauterization of bleeders is impossible.

Following routine preparation and draping, standard anterolateral and anteromedial portals are utilized. In most cases, adequate visualization of the patellofemoral joint, including evaluation for patellar tilt and subluxation, can be performed through these standard portals without resorting to transpatellar tendon, transquadriceps tendon, or superolateral or superomedial portals. The arthroscope is introduced through the anterolateral portal with initial probing performed through the anteromedial portal. Inspection of the suprapatellar pouch for significant adhesions, synovitis, or potentially symptomatic plicas and loose bodies is performed. If present, these pathologic suprapatellar structures are removed. The arthroscope is then passed through the patellofemoral joint for careful inspection first of the posterior surface of the patella. A thorough probing of the articular cartilage is performed for softness and fissures followed by a thorough evaluation of the entire patellofemoral sulcus. Careful probing of the patella and patellofemoral sulcus is performed to ensure that the edges of the craters are not detached and undermined. Undermined edges inevitably progress to symptomatic flaps. Flaps of articular cartilage are débrided until a stable crater exists. No attempt is made to breech the subchondral bone with drills, burs, or microfracture.

Careful assessment of lateral patellar tilt or subluxation by direct visualization through the arthroscope is performed. Although some authors have recommended the routine use of auxiliary portals,[32, 33] the authors have found standard anterolateral and anteromedial portals to be sufficient in most cases. By utilizing the 25 degree or 30 degree arthroscope, which is inserted through the anterolateral and anteromedial portals at an approximately 25–30 degree angle, a relatively direct view of the patellofemoral joint from the fat pad region is possible.

Arthroscopic Confirmation of Malalignment

Normal and abnormal patellofemoral tracking has been observed during arthroscopy in normal control and malaligned groups of knees.[34] In the normal knee, the lateral facet was seen to align with the femur at a median flexion angle of 20 degrees; the midpatellar ridge aligned with the central patellofemoral sulcus at 35 degrees; and the medial facet of the patella was demonstrated to gain contact with the medial sulcus at 50 degrees of knee flexion. In a comparable group of knees believed to be symptomatic from patellar subluxation, the lateral facet gained contact at 30 degrees, the midpatellar ridge at 55 degrees, and the medial facet at 85 degrees. Statistical analysis indicated significant differences between the control group and the subluxation group with regard to the angle of knee flexion for centralization of the midpatellar ridge and for medial facet contact. Other authors have considered malalignment to be a failure of the midpatellar ridge to align with the femoral groove during the first 45 degrees of knee flexion.[35–37]

Sojbjerg and colleagues[34] defined a stable patella as one centered with lateral and medial articular contact with the femur. Ninety-five percent of normal patients had a centered patella at a knee flexion angle of 55 degrees. Although it is important for the arthroscopist to know these figures, the presence or absence of patellofemoral instability should be discovered before introducing the arthroscope. Arthroscopy is a confirmatory procedure regarding maltracking of the patella. The arthroscope actually adds little further information about the stability of the patellofemoral joint but does document the presence or absence of chondromalacia with or without malalignment. The arthroscope is valuable, however, following lateral release to document improvement of lateral patellar tilt at a knee flexion angle of 55 degrees (Fig. 25–4). Failure of the patella to center following lateral release could mean that inadequate lateral release has been performed or reconstruction of the medial soft-tissue restraints is indicated. Once again, the surgeon should have a good idea of whether or not lateral release alone or medial reconstruction is necessary before entering the operating room.

Lateral Release

Some controversy exists with regard to what is considered to be an adequate lateral patellar retinacular release. Metcalf[37] originally described an adequate lateral release as extended proximally enough to allow a 90 degree tilt of the patella. Henry and colleagues[38] reported good results in cases of patellar subluxation following lateral release extending proximally to allow 90 degree tilt medially (turnup sign).[38] Shea and Fulkerson[17] have also reported that lateral release should be extended to release the oblique fibers of the vastus lateralis, and the release is not adequate unless the patella can be tilted medially 90 degrees.

However, Hughston and Deese reported cases of 50% medial subluxation of the patella in patients with

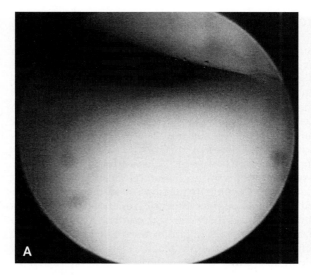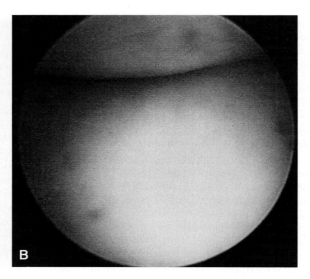

Figure 25–4 • *A,* A taut lateral patellar retinaculum is diagnosed clinically by the inability to displace the patella medially one-fourth of the width of the patella while the knee rests at 20 degrees of flexion and is supported by the lateral patellar tilt demonstrated by x-ray. The arthroscope is used to confirm pathologic lateral tilting as the knee is flexed beyond 55 degrees. The lateral tilting in this figure was visualized through the anteromedial portal with the tip of the scope placed directly infrapatellar. The approximate 30 degree insertion angle of the scope together with the 30 degree angulation of the optics of the arthroscope allows a relatively direct observation of the patellofemoral joint for lateral tilting. *B,* Following arthroscopic visualization of lateral release, correction of the lateral patellar tilt can be confirmed by flexing the knee to 55 degrees and observing congruent articulation of the patella with the femoral trochlea. Congruent reduction was obtained here with a limited lateral release that did not include any of the vastus lateralis oblique insertion and allowed passive medial tilt of the patella to no more than 45 degrees. In our experience, more extensive lateral release is rarely indicated.

symptoms following lateral retinacular release.[39] Shellock and colleagues noted medial subluxation by kinematic magnetic resonance imaging of the patellofemoral joint in 17 of 40 patients with persistent symptoms following lateral patellar retinacular release.[17] These reports have caused concern regarding the use of extensive lateral retinacular release, including a portion of the vastus lateralis in attempting to correct lateral subluxation of the patella.

Subsequently, Metcalf retracted the statement that 90 degrees of turnup is necessary and reported that less extensive lateral release, permitting only a 45 degree tilt of the patella, satisfactorily relieved lateral patellar tilt and avoided complications associated with excessive release. Limited lateral release resulting in only 45 degrees of turnup of the patella is preferred by us in most cases. This limited release relieves excessive tension of the lateral patellar retinaculum and reduces compression forces between the lateral facet and the lateral femoral condyle but avoids excessive lateral laxity resulting in potential medial subluxation of the patella.

Following assessment of the patellofemoral joint for tilt, subluxation, fissuring and softness of the articular cartilage, and necessary débridement of the patella, the remaining knee is inspected for pathology that, when necessary, is treated by débridement or repair. If preoperative assessment revealed a positive Sage sign and indicated that lateral release was desirable, and intraoperative inspection is confirmatory of lateral tilt (particularly if some resistance is encountered at full extension in driving the scope between the lateral facet of the patella and lateral femoral condyle), then the arthroscope is removed from the anterolateral portal and placed in the anteromedial portal for observation of lateral release. Patellofemoral alignment and tilt are again inspected. Lateral patellar retinacular release is performed through the lateral portal.

The technique preferred by the authors consists of severing the lateral patellar retinaculum with Metzenbaum scissors and controlling hemorrhage by electrical cauterization of the edges. Metzenbaum scissors are first inserted deep to the subcutaneous tissue along the superficial surface of the lateral retinaculum. Spreading of the scissor blades separates the subcutaneous tissue from the superficial retinaculum. One edge of the Metzenbaum scissors is then inserted intra-articularly into the knee under arthroscopic guide, while the opposite edge remains in subcutaneous tissue. The scissors are advanced approximately 1 cm posterior to the lateral border of the patella. As the scissors are extended toward the proximal pole of the patella, the author ensures that the convex side of the Metzenbaum scissors is directed anteriorly so that the tips of the scissors are curved slightly posteriorly at the proximal pole of the patella. This helps to prevent severing of any portion of the vastus lateralis tendon. The authors' preference is to extend the lateral release only so far proximally as to permit 45 degree tilting of the patella away from the lateral patellofemoral condyle and to create the capability of the patella to be displaced medially one-quarter of its width. Generally, this extends only to the proximal pole of the patella and just posterior to the distal edge of the vastus lateralis tendon. If full reduction of lateral patellar tilt and subluxation does not occur by 55 degrees of knee flexion, a decision must be made as to whether more extensive lateral release or medial reconstruction is indicated. Under direct arthroscopic visualization, all bleeding is cauterized without inflating the tourniquet. This allows visualization for cauterization of bleeders as they are cut, and we believe that this method reduces the chances of hemarthrosis. Alternatively, with the pneumatic tourniquet inflated for lateral release, the cautery can be run along the edges of the lateral release. Generally as the tourniquet is deflated, further bleeding is noted, and this bleeding can be cauterized prior to discontinuation of the procedure.

Postoperative Complications

Poor results may be caused by inadequate correction of lateral subluxation, a fact that is consistent with Fulkerson and colleagues' observation that patellar subluxation is not reliably corrected by lateral release, resulting in a 90 degree turnup even when combined with distal realignment. Restoration of tension on the medial side of the knee may be indicated in cases of lateral subluxation as opposed to cases with lateral tilt without subluxation, which can be adequately corrected by lateral release alone (Fig. 25–5).

Although an arthroscopic lateral release would appear to be a relatively safe procedure, reports of complications are extensive in the literature. Small reported from a multicenter study that the overall complication rate of lateral retinacular release was 7.2%, and this was the highest complication rate found for all arthroscopic procedures.[40]

Hemarthrosis is the most commonly reported complication that may have a lasting detrimental effect on the result of arthroscopic lateral release.[41, 42] In Small's study, the use of an electrocautery did not influence the rate of hemarthrosis, which is the most common complication in that study. Although we had significant hemarthrosis early in our experience, by utilizing the aforementioned technique, including the electrocautery, significant hemarthrosis has not been a problem in recent years. Another complication recorded to be associated with lateral retinacular release is that of skin burns during the use of the electrocautery. A third-degree skin burn occurred in one of our patients when we first began to use the electrocautery blade to do the actual cutting of the lateral retinaculum. No skin burns have occurred since the technique was modified to utilize the Metzenbaum scissor for cutting, followed by a controlled cauterization of the edges of the retinaculum.

The patient who undergoes a lateral release is at increased risk for a septic knee compared with arthroscopic procedures about the knee that do not involve lat-

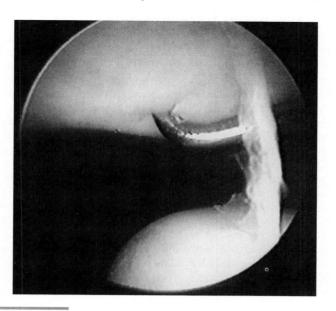

Figure 25–5 • A preoperative physical examination of this patient's knee demonstrated significant laxity of the medial patellofemoral ligament. Arthroscopic observation through the anterolateral portal confirmed significant lateral subluxation of the patella. The central ridge of the patella, softened and fissured as demonstrated by the probe, is noted to articulate with the convex ridge of the lateral femoral condyle. The arthroscopic findings are consistent with the patient's history of recurrent dislocation and chronic pain with activity. Lateral release, although effective in correcting lateral tilt when present, does not correct the lateral displacement of the patella. Open patellar realignment effectively centralized the patella. Pain and instability resolved.

eral release. This increased risk results from the loss of the barrier of the lateral retinaculum between the skin and the joint cavity. A superficial infection of a portal will communicate directly with the knee joint. Our early experience with the septic knee following lateral release led us to utilize intraoperative intravenous antibiotics and postoperative oral antibiotics for 5 days. In addition, if a single suture is placed in the portal, it is either buried beneath the skin or, if penetrating the skin, is removed prior to discontinuation of the oral antibiotics.

Other complications that have been reported peculiar to lateral patellar retinacular release are rupture of the quadriceps tendon and medial subluxation of the patella.[18, 43–46] Complications seen following lateral release (but not necessarily specifically related to lateral release) include deep vein thrombosis, pulmonary embolus, reflex sympathetic dystrophy, and adhesions.[47–55]

The rate of satisfactory results has been reported in the literature to range from 14 to 99%. This large range of results is probably due to differing criteria for selection for the procedure. Provided that none of the aforementioned complications occurs, good to excellent results can be expected following lateral release if proper preoperative indications and planning are utilized.

POSTOPERATIVE REHABILITATION

Postoperative rehabilitation is just as important as preoperative planning, proper selection of candidates for the procedure, and good surgical technique with adequate hemostasis. Immediately following surgery, the patient should be placed in a compressive dressing. Upon awakening from anesthesia, the patient is encouraged to establish good quadriceps setting and straight leg raising. Electrical stimulation of the quadriceps is utilized if the patient is unable to initiate adequate quadriceps setting and straight leg raising. If good quadriceps setting and straight leg raising are demonstrated, full weight-bearing should be encouraged. The patient should be seen in follow-up within 2 days after surgery, at which time the bandage is changed. Care is taken to maintain clean, dry portals, and antibiotics are not discontinued until all drainage has ceased. Drainage usually ceases within 5 days. An exercise bicycle is instituted to facilitate active range of motion. A return to sport is not considered until full quadriceps strength is demonstrated compared with the asymptomatic knee. Generally the patient is not able to return to full-speed running and vigorous physical activity for approximately 8 weeks.

LONG-TERM RESULTS

The literature is mixed with regard to any deterioration of results with time. Some studies fail to show deterioration,[1, 29, 54] whereas other studies indicate some deterioration.[56–60] Factors associated with deterioration of results have been found in patients who were treated by lateral release for recurrent subluxation,[44, 56, 57] and it is likely that these patients were better candidates for a more extensive patellar realignment, including reconstruction of the medial soft-tissue restraints and reduction of the Q-angle. Patients with chondromalacia have been noted to have deterioration of results following lateral release.[60]

CONCLUSION

Once conservative management has failed, the surgeon is faced with the dilemma of whether surgical management offers the realistic possibility of relief of pain or instability or whether to advise the patient to accept some restriction and modification of activities on a permanent basis. The surgeon must assess whether surgical débridement alone is indicated or correction of malalignment associated with anterior knee pain should be performed. Furthermore, if malalignment is judged to be a source of pain, the surgeon must predict whether the patient would be likely to respond to a lateral retinacular release or whether anteromedial displacement osteotomy of the tibial tubercle combined with lateral release would be likely to result in greater relief of pain. A decision must also be made with regard to whether proximal realignment with restoration of medial tensioning to the patellar retinaculum together with restoring mechanical efficiency to the vastus medialis obliquus is indicated.

References

1. Dzioba R: Diagnostic arthroscopy and longitudinal open lateral release: a four year follow-up study to determine predictors of surgical outcome. Am J Sports Med 18:343, 1990.
2. Insall J: Patellar pain. J Bone Joint Surg Am 64:147, 1982.
3. Insall J, Aglietti P, and Tria A: Patellar pain and incongruence. II: Clinical application. Clin Orthop 176:225, 1983.
4. Ficat PR and Hungerford DS: Disorders of the Patello-femoral Joint, 2nd ed. Baltimore, Waverley Press, 1977.
5. Ficat P, Philippe J, Cuzaco PJ, et al.: Le syndrome d'hyperpression externe de la rotule (S.H.P.E.). J Radiol Electrol 53:845, 1972.
6. Insall J, Bullogh PJ, and Burstein AH: Proximal tube realignment of the patella for chondromalacia patella. Clin Orthop 144:63–69, 1979.
7. Radin EL: A rational approach to the treatment of the patello-femoral pain. Clin Orthop 144:107–109, 1979.
8. Patel D: Plica as a cause of anterior knee pain. Orthop Clin North Am 17:273–277, 1986.
9. Cooke TDV, Chir B, Price N, Fisher B, et al.: The inwardly pointing knee: an unrecognized problem of external rotational malalignment. Clin Orthop 260:56–60, 1990.
10. Pipkin G: Knee injuries: the role of the suprapatellar plica and suprapatellar bursa in simulating internal derangement. Clin Orthop 74:161–176, 1971.
11. Insall J and Salvati E: Patella position in the normal knee joint. Radiology 101:101, 1971.
12. DeJour D: Patellofemoral pain evaluation. Presented at 20th Annual Meeting of AOSSM. Palm Desert, California, June 27, 1994.
13. Merchant A, Mercer R, Jacobsen R, et al.: Roentgenographic analysis of patellofemoral congruence. J Bone Joint Surg Am 56:1391, 1974.
14. Laurin C, Dussault R, and Levesque H: The tangential x-ray investigation of the patellofemoral joint: x-ray technique, diagnostic criteria and their interpretation. Clin Orthop 144:16, 1979.
15. DiChristina DG, Garth WP, and Holt G: Chronic patellofemoral instability treated by proximal anatomical repair and distal realignment. J Bone Joint Surg (in press).
16. Fulkerson JP, Schutzer SF, Ramsby GR, et al.: Computerized tomography of the patellofemoral joint before and after lateral release or realignment. Arthroscopy 3:19–24, 1987.
17. Shea KP and Fulkerson JP: Preoperative computed tomography scanning and arthroscopy in predicting outcome after lateral retinacular release. Arthroscopy 8:327–334, 1992.
18. Shellock FG, Mink JH, Deutsch A, et al.: Evaluation of patients with persistent symptoms after lateral retinacular release by kinematic magnetic resonance imaging of the patellofemoral joint. Arthroscopy 6:226–234, 1990.
19. Salter RB: Motion versus rest: why immobilize joints. J Bone Joint Surg Br 64:251, 1982.
20. Caubaud HE, Chatty A, Gildengorin V, et al.: Exercise effects on the strength of the rat anterior cruciate ligament. Am J Sports Med 8:79–86, 1980.
21. Noyes FR, Tavik PJ, Hyde WB, et al.: Biomechanics of ligament failure. II: an analysis of immobilization, exercise and reconditioning effects in primates. J Bone Joint Surg Am 56:1406–1418, 1974.
22. Tipton CM, James SL, Mergner W, et al.: Influence of exercise on strength of medial collateral knee ligaments of dogs. Am J Physiol 218:894–902, 1970.
23. Garth WP, Pomphrey M, and Merrill K: Functional treatment of patellar dislocation in an athletic population. Presented at AOSSM Specialty Day Meeting, February 19, 1995 (in press).
24. Darracott J and Vernon-Roberts B: The bony changes in chondromalacia patellae. Rheumatol Phys Med 11:175–179, 1971.
25. Leslie IJ and Bentley G: Arthroscopy in the diagnosis of chondromalacia patellae. Ann Rheum Dis 37:540–547, 1978.
26. Ficat P, Ficat C, and Bailleux A: Syndrome d'hyperpression externe de la toule (S.H.P.E.). Rev Chir Orthop 61:39, 1975.
27. Fulkerson J, Tennant R, Jaivin J, et al.: Histologic evidence of retinacular nerve injury associated with patellofemoral malalignment. Clin Orthop 197:196, 1985.
28. Conlan T, Garth WP, and Lemons J: Evaluation of the medial

soft-tissue restraints of the extensor mechanism of the knee. J Bone Joint Surg Am 75:682–693, 1993.

29. Gecha S and Torg J: Clinical prognosticators for the efficacy of retinacular release surgery to treat patellofemoral pain. Clin Orthop 253:203, 1990.
30. Schonholtz G, Zahn M, and Magee C: Lateral retinacular release of the patella. Arthroscopy 3:269, 1987.
31. Schutzer S, Ramsby G, and Fulkerson J: Computed tomographic classification of patellofemoral pain patients. Orthop Clin North Am 17:235, 1986.
32. Lindberg U, Hamberg P, Lysholm J, et al.: Arthroscopic examination of the patellofemoral joint using a central, one-portal technique. Orthop Clin North Am 17:263–268, 1986.
33. Johnson L: Comprehensive arthroscopic examination and surgery of the knee. St. Louis, CV Mosby, 1977, p 47.
34. Sojbjerg JO, Lauritzen J, Hvid I, et al.: Arthroscopic determination of patellofemoral malalignment. Clin Orthop 215:243–247, 1987.
35. Casscells SW: The arthroscope in the diagnosis of disorders of the patellofemoral joint. Clin Orthop 144:45, 1979.
36. Grana WA, Hinkley B, and Hollingsworth S: Arthroscopic evaluation and treatment of patellar malalignment. Clin Orthop 1986:122, 1984.
37. Metcalf RW: An arthroscopic method for lateral release of the subluxating or dislocating patella. Clin Orthop 167:9, 1982.
38. Henry JH, Goletz TH, and Williamson B: Lateral retinacular release in patellofemoral subluxation: Indications, results and comparison to open patellofemoral reconstruction. Am J Sports Med 14:121–129, 1986.
39. Hughston JC and Deese M: Medial subluxation of the patella as a complication of lateral release. Am J Sports Med 16:383–388, 1988.
40. Small N: An analysis of complications in lateral retinacular release procedures. Arthroscopy 5:282, 1989.
41. Grana W, Hinkley B, and Hollingsworth S: Arthroscopic evaluation and treatment of patellar malalignment. Clin Orthop 186:122, 1984.
42. Simpson L and Barrett J: Factors associated with poor results following arthroscopic subcutaneous lateral retinacular release. Clin Orthop 186:165, 1984.
43. Blasier R and Ciullo J: Case report: Rupture of the quadriceps tendon after arthroscopic lateral release. Arthroscopy 2:262, 1986.
44. Betz R, Lonergan R, Patterson R, et al.: The percutaneous lateral retinacular release. Orthopedics 5:57, 1982.
45. Hughston J and Deese M: Medial subluxation of the patella as a complication of lateral retinacular release. Am J Sports Med 16:383, 1988.
46. Kolowich P, Paulos L, Rosenbert T, et al.: Lateral release of the patella: indications and contraindications. Am J Sports Med 18:359, 1990.
47. Bray R, Roth J, and Jacobsen R: Arthroscopic lateral release for anterior knee pain: a study comparing patients who are claiming worker's compensation with those who are not. Arthroscopy 3:237, 1987.
48. Busch M and DeHaven K: Pitfalls of the lateral retinacular release. Clin Sports Med 8:279, 1989.
49. Ceder L and Larson R: Z-plasty lateral retinacular release for the treatment of patellar compression syndrome. Clin Orthop 144:110, 1979.
50. Malek M: Arthroscopic lateral retinacular release: functional results in series of 67 knees. Orthop Rev 14:55, 1985.
51. McGinty J and McCarthy J: Endoscopic lateral retinacular release: a preliminary report. Clin Orthop 158:120, 1981.
52. Fox J, Ferkel R, Del Pizzo W, et al.: Electrosurgery in orthopaedics. II: Applications to arthroscopy. Contemp Orthop 8:37, 1984.
53. Henry J, Goletz T, and Williamson B: Lateral retinacular release in patellofemoral subluxation: indications, results, and comparison to open patellofemoral reconstruction. Am J Sports Med 14:121, 1986.
54. Sherman O, Fox J, Sperling H, et al.: Patellar instability: treatment by arthroscopic electrosurgical lateral release. Arthroscopy 3:152, 1987.
55. Betz R, Magill J, and Lonergan R: The percutaneous lateral retinacular release. Am J Sports Med 15:57, 1982.
56. Christensen F, Soballe K, and Snerum L: Treatment of chondromalacia patellae by lateral retinacular release of the patella. Clin Orthop 234:145, 1988.
57. Jackson R, Kunkel S, and Taylor G: Lateral retinacular release for patellofemoral pain in the older patient. Arthroscopy 7:283, 1991.
58. Metcalf R: An arthroscopic method for lateral release of subluxating or dislocating patella. Clin Orthop 167:9, 1982.
59. Kaufer H: Patellar biomechanics. Clin Orthop 144:51, 1979.
60. Osborne A and Fulford P: Lateral release for chondromalacia patellae. J Bone Joint Surg Br 64:202, 1982.

26 Degenerative Arthritis of the Knee

Mary Lloyd Ireland • *Richard I. Williams*

An increased life expectancy and heightened awareness of the importance of maintaining physical fitness throughout adulthood equal more miles on knees.[1-5] There are variations in the patient population with articular surface changes: age, physical demands, goals, and expectations. In the active individual, how do we keep these knees natural, painless, and moving? The wand of the arthroscope does not magically remove the pain from an arthritic, malaligned knee.

The decision to intervene arthroscopically should be based on symptoms of mechanical locking, effusion, and localized painful popping. The light for the future of arthroscopy burns brightly; however, make sure the choice of procedure and equipment is indicated for the patient's problem. Multiple clinical examinations and histories to document symptoms are necessary. Biomechanical assessment of gait, radiographs of the weight-bearing patient, and technetium-99m bone scan are performed.[6-8] In this era of "outcomes review" and close scrutiny of health-care expenditures, the arthroscopist should proceed with caution.[9] Many patients with arthritic knees may not benefit dramatically from arthroscopic intervention.[10] Complications from arthroscopy do occur.[11-13] The superiority of arthroscopy to plain radiography of chondral changes is well recognized.[13-16] The focus of this chapter is degenerative arthritis: its nature and pathophysiology, analysis of the published literature regarding arthroscopic treatment, and areas that warrant further investigation.

RANGE OF CAUSES

There are many causes of arthrosis, not all of which are truly "degenerative."[17] The categories are primary, secondary, and nontraumatic; they are listed in Table 26-1. The order of importance of contributing factors should be ranked. Factors contributing to abnormal joint loading include obesity, congenital or developmental, pathologic, and varus and valgus alignment.[18-20]

The causes of primary osteoarthritis are well recognized. There seems to be a familial component.[21, 22] DNA analysis may predict a predisposition to degenerative joint disease (DJD). Enzymes are released into joint fluid after knee injury.[23] A single-base mutation in the gene coding for type II collagen was identified in a family with chondrodysplasia and osteoarthritis.[24, 25] This enzyme environment from injury or inheritance creates a milieu for destruction of cartilage.

Look for the primary causative factor in the degenerative knee. Is it vascular? Is it ligament instability? Beware of avascular necrosis of the femoral condyles[26] (Table 26-2). Early ligament reconstruction to correct instability and osteotomy to correct malalignment are preventive measures.[27] Longitudinal retrospective studies have illustrated an unfavorable natural history for the anterior cruciate ligament (ACL)–deficient knee.[28-32] Other studies do not support ACL reconstruction to prevent DJD.[33] With mild to moderate DJD with malalignment, ACL reconstruction can be successful.[34] Chronic posterior cruciate ligament instability increases wear and contact forces in the patellofemoral and medial compartments.[35, 36]

Patellar instability with osteochondral fractures and abnormal, excessive patellar loading contribute to localized patellofemoral DJD. The role of patellar instability in the development of patellofemoral arthritis is more debatable.[37] Open patellar realignment procedures must unload the abnormal cartilage to be successful.[38]

The meniscus protects the chondral surfaces of the knee by evening the load distribution, improving joint stability, and assisting in cartilage nutrition.[39] Elegant studies in meniscal biology have been coupled with a clinical understanding of the deleterious results of meniscectomy[26, 40, 41] to create a campaign for meniscal preservation. Allograft meniscal transplantation remains in the investigative stages owing to mixed clinical results.[42-47] Noyes and Barber-Westin[47] reported a 58% failure rate; only 10% of transplants were believed to be "fully healed and functional" after 2–3 years. Experimental synthetic

Table 26-1	**Various Forms of Arthrosis**

I. Primary degenerative arthritis
   A. Osteoarthritis: compartments involved
      1. Angular deformity
         a. Varus: medial compartment
         b. Valgus: lateral compartment
      2. "Isolated" patellofemoral
      3. Tricompartmental
II. Secondary degeneration
   A. Post-traumatic arthritis
      1. Osteochondral fracture (localized lesion)
         a. Loose body
         b. Surface disruption or defect
      2. Osteochondritis dissecans
      3. Intra-articular fracture
         a. Joint surface incongruity
      4. Alteration of force distribution across joint
         a. Femur fracture
         b. Tibia fracture
         c. Leg length inequality
      5. Previous meniscectomy
         a. Medial
         b. Lateral
      6. Post-ligament reconstruction
         a. Posterior cruciate ligament
         b. Anterior cruciate ligament
         c. Medial cruciate ligament
         d. Combined
         e. Patellofemoral
   B. Arthritis associated with instability
      1. Anterior cruciate ligament
      2. Posterior cruciate ligament
      3. Patellofemoral
      4. Combined instabilities
      5. Reconstruction or realignment procedure
III. "Non-traumatic" conditions causing chondral injury and degeneration
   A. Postinfectious
      1. Septic
      2. Tuberculosis, syphilis
      3. Lyme arthritis
   B. Vascular
      1. Avascular necrosis
      2. Osteochondritis dissecans
   C. Inflammatory, crystalline, metabolic
      1. Cartilage matrix deposition
         a. Gout, hemochromatosis, ochronosis, Wilson's disease
      2. Pseudogout (calcium-pyrophosphate deposition)
         a. Calcium-hydroxyapatite crystal deposits
      3. Rheumatoid arthritis
      4. Nonrheumatoid systemic inflammatory conditions
         a. e.g., psoriasis, lupus, ankylosing spondylitis
      5. Other synovial processes
         a. Pigmented villonodular synovitis
         b. Hemophilic arthropathy
   D. Obesity
   E. Genetic

Table 26-2	**Factors Leading to the Development of Joint Degeneration**

I. Direct destruction of cartilage
   A. Infection
   B. Pannus
II. Joint incongruity
   A. "Macroscopic": intra-articular fracture, osteochondritis
   B. "Microscopic": early joint wear, particulate debris
III. Abnormal joint loading
   A. Obesity
   B. Alignment abnormalities
   C. Length discrepancy
   D. Gait abnormalities
IV. Instability
V. Iatrogenic
   A. Meniscectomy
   B. "Over-constraint"
VI. Genetic factors
VII. Activity level

meniscal scaffolds and substitutes are also being developed.[48, 49] Cartilage transplantation is being performed.[50] For localized femoral condyle lesions in a small population, results are encouraging.[50] However, for the truly degenerative knee this highly publicized procedure is not indicated.

Research is being done on the basic science models of chondrocyte transplantation with protective transduced chondrocytes from interleukin-1–induced extracellular matrix degradation.[51] When modified chondrocytes were transplanted into the articular surface of osteoarthritic mice, integration to the articular cartilage occurred. Research is under way in the work-up of deficiencies in cartilage collagens and models for gene therapy.[52]

However—promise of the future notwithstanding—the result remains much the same as in the words of Hunter.[53] In 1743 Hunter wrote "ulcerated cartilage is a troublesome thing . . . once destroyed it is not repaired."[54]

BASIC SCIENCE OF CARTILAGE INJURY

Hyaline cartilage is avascular and aneural. Isolated chondral injury or wear does not generate pain or a significant healing response.[55] The structure of cartilage is predominantly that of an extracellular matrix containing 70–80% water in terms of total weight. Scattered cells in the matrix synthesize the structural macromolecules that comprise this unique composite. The fibrillar components of cartilage are 50% collagen (predominantly type II), 35% proteoglycans, and 15% noncollagenous proteins and glycoproteins. With their low metabolic level, chondrocytes can obtain sufficient nutrition by a process of diffusion through the matrix.[56, 57] The cartilage-bone interface occurs deep to the tidemark with the formation of calcified cartilage, eventually giving way to subchondral bone.[58–60]

Nerve endings and specialized neurosensory organs in the subchondral bone sense pressure changes and, hence, pain. Intraosseous pressure measurements greater than 40 mm Hg and elevation on the femoral side were found in patients with a painful osteoarthritic knee.[61]

The viscoelastic properties from the composite fluid/macromolecular structure and lubrication allow the hyaline cartilage to resist the types of forces seen in joints: shear, tension, and compression. Weeping lubrication occurs on the cartilage surface as water molecules are forced from the extracellular matrix owing to compressive and shearing forces.[62, 63] The coefficient of friction of a Teflon-polyethylene interface is an order of magnitude higher than that of opposing surfaces of hyaline cartilage lubricated by synovial fluid.

Wear occurs from fatigue, impact loading, and interfacial surfaces. Fatigue wear causes intrinsic damage to the molecular structure of collagen. Impact-loading wear results when axial forces do not allow time for stress relaxation of the matrix, again resulting in loss of structural integrity. Interfacial wear, caused by direct contact of irregular surfaces, includes the processes of abrasion and adhesion.[55] Histologic and biochemical evaluation of cartilage in osteoarthritis shows striking changes.[64] Damaged cartilage becomes hyperhydrated,[65] and hydraulic permeability increases, altering the mechanical properties of the tissue.[66, 67]

The three traditional phases of injury response (necrosis, inflammation, and repair) are not always seen following chondral injury.[68–72] In partial-thickness injury, early fibrillation and fissuring occur and are associated with mild hypercellularity and loss of mucopolysaccharides in the superficial and transitional zones.[73] This increase in cellularity appears to result in increased proteoglycan and collagen synthesis.[74, 75] These new cells do not migrate through the matrix toward the site of injury and lack the ability to organize the matrix, resulting in a tissue with inferior mechanical properties.[76, 77] The degradative enzymes produce increased chondral surface damage.[78] As arthritic changes progress, structural clefts extend into the deeper layers, and the hypercellular areas disappear, leaving a hypocellular matrix with marked diminution of proteoglycans. Microfractures in the subchondral bone lead to increased stiffness,[79] and a resulting increase in the peak stresses and impulse loads to articular cartilage accelerates the degenerative process.

After débridement of partial cartilage injuries, ultrastructural studies using electron microscopy show an increase in local fibrillation, degradation, and cell death.[80] After a full-thickness chondral injury, a fibrin clot forms in the defect and develops into granulation tissue with eventual metaplasia on the ingrowth of vascular tufts. The foundation of "abrasion chondroplasty" is based on stimulating the reparative healing of larger chondral defects by creating perforations into the subchondral bone and allowing fibrin clot formation.

Joint motion stimulates increased differentiation of pluripotential cells into chondroblasts.[81] Unfortunately, the fibrocartilaginous repair tissue is inferior to native hyaline cartilage.[82] This repair tissue is higher in concentration of type I collagen and has "inferior" proteoglycan composites. The long-term fate of repair cartilage seems to be fibrillation, degeneration, and deterioration.[83, 84]

NONOPERATIVE TREATMENT

The course of osteoarthritis is insidiously progressive, but the rate of deterioration varies.[85] Some patients improve, others remain unchanged, but most gradually worsen.[86]

It is clear that long-term studies are necessary to evaluate patients undergoing treatment for knee arthritis.[87–91]

In the presence of degenerative wear, the treatment regimen—both nonoperative and operative—must be discussed in detail with the patient.[92] In patients with degenerative wear, postoperative arthroscopy complications and patient dissatisfaction are common. Continued pain, limited motion, popping, and vascular complications can occur. The duration of nonoperative treatment should be long enough that the patient has continued symptoms and localized mechanical signs and is truly convinced an arthroscopy will help. Know your patient. Operate for mechanical signs, not pain.

SURGICAL TREATMENT AND LITERATURE REVIEW OF CARTILAGE LESIONS

Degenerative joint disease of the knee has been treated with arthroscopic lavage during the last 65 years.[93–97] Open débridement has been touted as causing significant improvement in patient comfort level.[98–104]

Washout Procedures

Several investigations have focused on more invasive office procedures for the treatment of degenerative knee conditions, including an office "washout"—closed, flow-through irrigation—with promising and surprising early follow-up. The impetus for this procedure comes from a belief that the benefits of minimal arthroscopic evaluation of a degenerative joint stem from the fluid irrigation of the procedure.[95, 105–107] Eriksson and Haggmark[107] performed needle lavage periodically in follow-up to arthroscopy in a series of avid joggers and found significant, sustained relief. Experimental evidence of joint irritation due to the byproducts of cartilage wear and particulate debris[108] may substantiate the reason for these successes in washing out the "evil humors" of the knee—proteases, hydrolases, and proteoglycans. In a controlled study, Livesley and colleagues[109] found better relief from lavage and physical therapy than from physical therapy alone. Whereas inflammation recurred within 3 months, some relief persisted up to 1 year. Ike et al.[110] prospectively evaluated the results of "tidal irrigation" versus those of medical management, and Edelson, Burks, and Bloebaum[111] reported striking results of irrigation at 2-year follow-up (17/21 good to excellent knees). No additional benefit was gained from the injection of hyaluronate, a substance known to be decreased in osteoarthritic knees.[112] However, not all studies have confirmed this benefit. Dawes, Kirlew, and

Haslock[113] found no evidence that a saline washout provided any more relief than a simple injection of 10 mL of sterile saline in a group of 20 patients studied in a single-blind, random fashion.[111]

Cartilage Débridement Without Abrasion

Aichroth, Patel, and Moyes[114] prospectively studied 254 patients undergoing arthroscopic débridement for pain due to degenerative disease. The average patient age was 49 years, with follow-up being nearly 4 years. Nearly half of the patients had only mild to moderate (Outerbridge grades I and II) changes. Localized abrasion procedures on eburnated tibial bone were utilized in 28% of patients. Reoperation rate was only 14%, and patient satisfaction rate (85%) was high. Younger patients fared significantly better than older patients, and results correlated with the degree of preoperative radiographic degeneration. These authors stated that drilling or abrading small (1–1.5 cm) areas of bone produced satisfactory results with no evidence of harm.

Bonamo, Kessler, and Noah[115] undertook débridement and partial meniscectomy alone in 118 patients older than 40 years of age, all with Outerbridge grades III and IV changes. No abrasion or drilling was performed. After mean follow-up of 3.3 years, this group was compared with a group of 63 patients who had no advanced articular surface changes but who underwent similar meniscal procedures. Whereas the group with degenerative changes fared worse overall, results were gratifying, with an 83% patient satisfaction rate and 75% resumption of recreational athletic activities. In contrast to previous findings by McBride and colleagues,[116] these authors did not find a significant difference in the clinical results between patients with tears classified as degenerative (complex, horizontal, cleavage tears) and those with more nondegenerative (flap, radial, oblique, and bucket-handle) patterns.

Baumgaertner et al.[117] evaluated 49 degenerative knees of 44 patients who underwent arthroscopic cartilage débridement without abrasion chondroplasty or meniscal work. About 67% had "severe" radiographic changes. The procedure involved osteophyte removal and limited débridement. At 33-month average follow-up, 52% of the patients had good or excellent results, and two-thirds of the patients had no visible deterioration. Thirty-nine percent had no improvement, and 9% had only temporary relief. Postoperatively, symptoms of swelling and giving way and walking endurance were markedly improved. Long duration of symptoms, malalignment, and advanced radiographic changes were associated with poorer results. Eight patients with chondrocalcinosis did better as a group. Despite the high percentage (39%) of early failures, the few good results were worth the failures as "no bridges were burned."

Similarly, Timoney et al.[118] reviewed the results of débridement without abrasion in 125 patients, obtaining mean follow-up of 50 months in 92% of the involved knees. Nearly two-thirds of the patients obtained measurable relief for a significant length of time and three-fourths of the patients believed the procedure was beneficial.

However, a 27% failure rate at 6 months was found with most of these patients undergoing total knee replacement during the course of the study. Long duration of symptoms, malalignment, radiographic narrowing down to 1–3 mm joint space, and the presence of eburnated bone at arthroscopy correlated with a poor result. Results deteriorated, averaging nearly 2 years until worsening. Overall, 45% of the knees were rated as good at 50 months. Because of the low complication rate and general satisfaction of the patients, arthroscopic débridement was thought to be a reasonable alternative in selected patients.

Débridement Versus Abrasion Chondroplasty

However, there are no control (nonsurgical) groups in these studies,[117, 118] adding to the difficulty in comparing results. Merchan and Galindo[86] randomized 80 patients older than 50 years of age into one of two treatment groups: arthroscopic limited débridement (no abrasion) and nonoperative treatment. Patients were relatively sedentary, had brief (fewer than 6 months') duration of symptoms, and minimal joint space narrowing and osteophyte formation. Significant angular malalignment and patellofemoral degeneration resulted in exclusion from the study. Both groups underwent similar physical therapy regimens. A greater percentage of the operative group improved subjectively at the mean follow-up time of 25 months. The difference in knee scores (37 for the operative group and 32.76 for the nonoperative group) had a p value of .02. Although deterioration occurred, the authors concluded that meniscal and limited chondral débridement was beneficial in this group of patients.

In surveying the literature, Rand[16] and Bert[119] concurred that abrasion offers little benefit versus débridement and management of degenerative menisci, although both procedures remain unpredictable. Rand's study population demonstrated a 67% rate of continued relief from débridement alone at 5-year follow-up. In contrast, nearly 50% of patients undergoing abrasion required conversion to total knee replacement at 3 years. As such, a trend toward minimal perforation of the subchondral bone (so-called microfracture technique using picks or smaller drills and flexible K-wires) is being seen.[120]

Prior to advancements in arthroscopic techniques, patients were relatively satisfied with short-term follow-up after an arthrotomy and open osteophyte removal and drilling of cancellous bone to improve blood supply. In the early 1970s, diagnostic arthroscopy became more popular for débridement.[105, 121, 122] Subchondral drilling and débridement resulted in 80% subjective good results in 22 patients.[123] Other studies showed overall satisfactory results with drilling.[124, 125] Ficat's original open "spongialization" principles were popularized arthroscopically by Johnson in the form of an abrasion arthroplasty.[126] Intracortical vessel bleeding after motorized débridement of the area resulted in fibrin clot, inflammatory response, and promotion of repair of fibrocartilage. In 95 patients, 75% improved subjectively, and only 7 patients required further surgical intervention at 3-year follow-up. Biopsy samples showed no normal type II collagen fibers, but in some samples the tidemark had reformed. Hjertquist and Lemperg[127] suggested that cortical subchondral bone must be preserved. Hence, the débridement should not go into the cancellous bone. This concern has also been an issue in newer chondrocyte transplantation techniques, in which it is believed to be important not to violate the cancellous base so that the cartilage cells have a tidemark off which to work.[50] In rabbits, if the subchondral plate is violated even with curettage at the base, the defect does not heal spontaneously.[128] The abrasion technique attempts not to violate the cortical layer, avoiding exposure of raw red and cancellous trabeculae.[129]

Abrasion Chondroplasty

Abrasion chondroplasty became very popular; later it was scrutinized.[106] Johnson's strict selection and rehabilitation criteria were believed to select for highly motivated patients who would do well after any procedure.[126] Later authors were unable to duplicate the successes reported earlier. Promising results from procedures, including limited chondral débridement, osteophyte removal, and formal abrasion arthroplasty—such as the favorable report by Chandler[130]—often had less than 2-year average follow-up. Singh, Lee, and Tay[131] reported 50% "improvement" using crude pain and range-of-motion scores in 44 patients with only 3–27-month follow-up; nine patients required further operation during this limited period, and 25% were rated "worse" after surgery. Many surgeons reported abrading large areas of the joint (e.g., the majority of the trochlear surface), contradictory to the recommendations made by Johnson.[126]

In an effort to evaluate the abrasion technique more objectively, studies were attempted[132, 133] comparing two similar groups—débridement and abrasion, and débridement alone. A substantial number of patients in both groups worsened symptomatically following surgery. Joint-space widening on postoperative radiographs did not correlate with reduction in symptoms. At 5-year follow-up, 15 of 59 patients with abrasion and débridement had been converted to total knee replacement. The conclusions were that abrasion was unpredictable and offered no long-term benefit for actual joint resurfacing. Friedman et al.[134] had slightly better results using abrasion techniques when compared with débridement alone, although follow-up was short (12 months), and 83% of patients still had pain, with 63% still taking nonsteroidal anti-inflammatory drugs and 24% using ambulatory aids. Nearly 60% of patients were "unchanged" by the results of surgery.

"Limited" abrasion techniques have been investigated as well. Reports by Jackson, Silver, and Marans[135] and Ogilvie-Harris and Fitsialos[136] showed similar improvement following arthroscopic débridement at 3–4-year follow-up. In the later group[136] of 441 procedures (average patient age was 58 years), 68% of patients obtained at least 2 years of pain relief, 53% remained good at 4.1 years. Mild to moderate (Outerbridge grades I and II) disease was treated with local chondral débridement; limited abrasions were performed when full-thickness defects involv-

ing up to one-half of one condyle were present. All knees were thoroughly lavaged; when no significant meniscal disease was present in the presence of extensive chondral destruction, lavage alone was performed. Immediate weight-bearing was allowed, but reduced impact-loading for at least 6 months was prescribed. Patients with unstable meniscal flap tears fared best, whereas those with bicondylar disease showed the worst results. The extent of patellofemoral degeneration did not seem to affect results; rather, patients with a significant patellofemoral component also had more advanced bicondylar disease, which did correlate with inferior results. Patients with isolated lateral arthrosis fared somewhat better than those with medial side degeneration. Lavage alone failed to provide improvement. Only five patients subjectively worsened, four of whom were in the group with severe degeneration. Patients undergoing abrasion fared slightly worse, but this could have been due to selection bias, as they tended to have more significant lesions.

SURGICAL INTERVENTION AND LITERATURE REVIEW OF MENISCAL TEARS

Radiographically and clinically,[40, 41] total meniscectomy has been shown to lead to progressive arthrosis. Emphasis on leaving stable meniscal rims is based on sound biomechanical principles. When more meniscus is removed, the articular surface is under significantly greater and asymmetric force distribution.[39, 137] Patients with normal preoperative radiographs undergoing medial meniscectomy had a 90% chance of having a good or excellent result, whereas patients with radiographic changes had a 20% chance of a good or excellent result.[26] Careful assessment of standing radiographs and changes for osteonecrosis should be done. Other studies showed joint degeneration in 60% of patients following partial meniscectomy.[138, 139]

In the degenerative knee, medial meniscus tears outnumber lateral meniscus tears by 9:1, and posterior third location occurred in 84% of knees.[140] There are numerous tear patterns in the degenerative knee.[115, 141] It has been suggested to leave stable meniscal tissue alone[9, 142] because such tissue provides a space and scaffold. The most important indicator of successful arthroscopic meniscectomy is preoperative status of severity of degenerative joint disease.[26, 115, 116, 141, 143–145] Lateral meniscus tears in the degenerative knee appeared to do better than medial meniscal tears associated with chondral wear.[42, 136, 139] Many series have evaluated the results of arthroscopic partial and subtotal excisions.[116, 143–146] Patients who cite a specific traumatic event as the cause of symptoms, especially if they are short-term, fare remarkably well, even if the patients have had previous surgery and have suffered reinjury.[146] Chronic symptoms, when associated with significant radiographic changes, tend to lessen overall results. Even in the presence of joint degeneration, though, the results of arthroscopic meniscal resection are promising.[109, 140] In one series, 72% of patients maintained good results at 4.7-year follow-up from partial menisectomy in the presence of advanced degenerative changes.[136]

Patellofemoral Changes

Limited success in patients with significant patellofemoral degenerative changes has been reported.[147, 148] If these changes are localized arthritic defects, procedures to relieve the pressure and transfer it to normal articular surface should be done. Open distal realignments include the Maquet procedure[149–151] and Fulkerson anteromedial tubercle elevation.[38] In patients with patellofemoral arthritis, tibial tubercle advance resulted in 65% excellent or good results at 3-year follow-up.

Spongialization of the patella to the cancellous bone resulted in 79% good or excellent results.[152] The patellofemoral articulation undergoes different forces than do the weight-bearing medial and lateral compartments. In patellar degeneration, resection arthroplasty resulted in 60% of patients being pain-free.[153] Partial cartilage débridement and drilling resulted in 22 of 25 good or excellent results, with patients younger than 30 years of age faring better.

Association with High Tibial Osteotomy

Although MacIntosh[154] routinely performed open joint débridement before high tibial osteotomy with good results, there is controversy whether to do arthroscopy before either high tibial[28, 155–158] or distal femoral osteotomy. With significant angular deformity, the results of valgus tibial osteotomy correlate with the degree of angular correction, not with the involvement of the lateral compartment or patellofemoral joint.[155] There is no clinical evidence to support arthroscopy as a preoperative adjunct to decision-making with respect to unicompartmental versus tricompartmental arthroplasty.[159]

Surgical Indications

However, simple "diagnostic" arthroscopy should not routinely be performed. In-office diagnostic arthroscopy with the patient under local anesthesia is not appropriate for patients undergoing high tibial osteotomies. Failure of conservative treatment constitutes a reasonable indication for arthroscopy in these patients. Clinical signs of a meniscal tear with localized symptoms is the number one indication for arthroscopy.

Radiographic Work-Up

Radiographic work-up includes a standing posteroanterior 30 degree flexed radiograph. Other studies are technetium-99m bone scan and magnetic resonance imaging (MRI).[7] Can MRI effectively replace arthroscopy? The authors think not.[160, 161]

Numerous studies have shown an abnormal MRI signal in menisci that are causing patients no symptoms.[160–162] MRI is gradually evolving in the assessment of articular cartilage injuries; however, at this time, it is not as sensitive and specific as for documentation of meniscal disorders and tear patterns.[162–165] Articles written on correlation of MRI with arthroscopy provide ground for questions as radiologists and orthopaedists protect their diagnostic tools.[160, 161, 163–166]

If the MRI scan is normal, a treatment regimen of time and exercise and no arthroscopy should be suggested.[166] However, the question occurs for a not-too-symptomatic knee patient with mild mechanical signs: should an arthroscopy be done if there is a grade II signal documented by MRI? Often, MRI forces one to proceed with surgery, and questions of trephination and what to do about the grades I and II signals remain. Therapeutic arthroscopy should be done in the degenerative knee for specific mechanical signs and symptoms.

Mechanical limits of extension due to femoral notch and tibial eminence, impingement, and patellofemoral osteophytes can be improved with aggressive arthroscopic débridement.[130] Excision of meniscal flaps and removal of loose bodies, along with resection of notch and tibial spine osteophytes, can improve range of motion in appropriate patients. Improvement of extension range of motion improves gait, lessens hamstring force, and reduces patellofemoral articular pressure. Severe arthrosis and limited range of motion are rarely helped arthroscopically.

It is the knee with more severe chondral damage that poses the greatest dilemma: Can this patient be helped by arthroscopy? What guidelines are there for the treatment of chondral lesions? In fact, even in the knee with severe degenerative changes, the risk-benefit ratio of arthroscopy is relatively favorable when compared with that of more invasive procedures, and for the properly educated patient, arthroscopic evaluation can be considered as a temporizing procedure. It is this class of patients, however, that exhibits the least predictable response to arthroscopic débridement.

INDICATIONS FOR ARTHROSCOPY IN THE DEGENERATIVE KNEE

A review of the literature is appropriate in order to develop a treatment philosophy. The prospective correlation of pre- and postoperative knee-rating questionnaires and evaluating relative improvement and deterioration using combined subjective and objective parameters would help interpret these results, but few such studies have been attempted.[86]

Predictive factors for the success of arthroscopic intervention remain elusive. Gross et al.[167] found that a higher number of significant findings (meniscal tears, osteophytes, chondral lesions) seemed to best predict a negative outcome, as opposed to any particular single pathologic entity. These authors reported high overall success rates in patients with normal limb alignment in whom débridement without formal abrasion was performed. Indeed, the most important negative predictor seems to be significant malalignment (especially valgus).[136] Salisbury, Nottage, and Gardner[168] specifically evaluated the effects of limb alignment on the results of arthroscopic débridement in a series of 52 patients with minimum 2-year follow-up; the researchers showed correlation of poorer results with malalignment (normal being 1–7 degrees valgus), and even the fair results in some of the patients with relative varus tended to deteriorate with

Table 26–3	**Grading of Chondral Surface Lesions**

I. Outerbridge System
- A. Grade I: Softening and swelling of cartilage
- B. Grade II: Fragmentation and fissuring, less than 0.5 inch diameter
- C. Grade III: Fragmentation and fissuring, greater than 0.5 inch diameter
- D. Grade IV: Erosion of cartilage down to exposed subchondral bone

II. Noyes System
- A. Grade 1: Cartilage surface intact (1A = some remaining resilience; 1B = deformation)
- B. Grade 2A: Cartilage surface damaged (cracks, fibrillation, fissuring or fragmentation); with less than one-half of cartilage thickness involved
- C. Grade 2B: Depth of involvement greater than one-half of cartilage thickness but without exposed bone
- D. Grade 3: Bone exposed (3A = surface intact; 3B = surface cavitation)

III. Additional parameters
- A. Measure diameter of lesion(s) in millimeters
- B. Describe the location of lesion(s): which surface and where (patellar facet or anterior, middle, or posterior portions of condylar or plateau surface)
- C. Describe the degree (range) of knee flexion where the lesion is in weight-bearing contact

GRADING OF CARTILAGE LESIONS

Several classification schemes (Table 26–3) for articular lesions have been proposed.[175–177] Previous classifications were based on radiographic findings and did not take into account localized or partial-thickness lesions.[178] The width, depth, and location of the cartilage injury should be documented during arthroscopy.

The Outerbridge classification is based on the following four grades: grade I is softening and swelling of cartilage; grades II and III are fragmentation and fissuring of cartilage (diameter less than 0.5 inch, grade II; greater than 0.5 inch, grade III); grade IV is erosion of cartilage down to exposed subchondral bone. (Fig. 26–1). The Noyes classification is based on three grades, with letters assigned to classification of cartilage resiliency, with the

time. Other negative predictors include prior meniscectomy, additional arthroscopic surgery, tibial surface eburnation, and bilaterality.[136] Age alone does not appear to be a contributory factor in most series, when groups are corrected for amount of degeneration present.[169] The presence of chondrocalcinosis is of unclear significance.[117, 136] In the series by Ogilvie-Harris,[136] worker compensation patients fared the same as other patients when considered as a group, whereas those with pending litigation fared poorly in the Duke study.[169] Collective review of the literature suggests shorter duration of symptoms, mild to moderate radiographic degeneration, and the presence of mechanical symptoms that are associated with better results.

In light of evidence that hyaline-like repair tissue can be seen following corrective osteotomy alone,[170, 171] strong consideration should be given to such a procedure when indicated. Certainly, arthroscopy with removal of loose bodies and limited débridement can be performed in conjunction with an osteotomy. However, there is no firm evidence to support concomitant high tibial osteotomy and arthroscopic débridement and cartilage "stimulation"—abrasion appears to add only morbidity to the postoperative results.[157] Furthermore, Rand and Ritts[170] showed that abrasion arthroplasty is not an effective salvage for failed high tibial osteotomy.

Documentation of the patterns of wear on the patella is necessary to plan any patellar realignment procedures.[172–174] Successful patellofemoral realignment is predictable when the area of overloaded cartilage can be stress-shielded by a realignment.

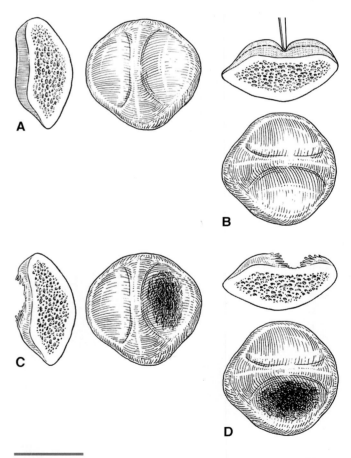

Figure 26–1 • The Outerbridge classification of chondromalacic change is shown diagrammatically. *A*, Normal articular cartilage of the patella is depicted. *B*, Grade I is softening only, without fragmentation or fissuring. *C*, Grades II and III are fissuring and fragmentation, with II being less than 1 inch and III being more than 1 inch. There is no exposed subchondral bone. *D*, Grade IV is down to subchondral bone. Documentation of the grade and size of the arthritic change is helpful, particularly in the patellofemoral articulation, in predicting success and outlining a rehabilitation program.

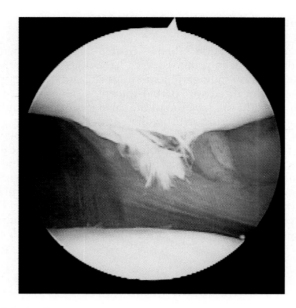

Figure 26–2 • Chondromalacia grade II of the odd patella facet.

surface intact or cavitated. The diameter of the lesion location and degree at which contact of the abnormal cartilage occurs should be documented. Isolated lesions of the patellofemoral articulation are shown of Outerbridge grades II (Fig. 26–2) and III (Fig. 26–3). One should document the grade I degree of flexion when contact occurs to design a rehabilitation program limiting that arc of motion.

Arthroscopic classifications such as that by Bauer and Jackson[179] attempted to describe lesions based on appearance: crack, stellate fracture, flap, crater, and fibrillation. A more comprehensive, specific scheme was developed by Noyes and Stabler[176] that relies on more descriptive data to clarify the size, depth, and relative location of chondral defects. With the addition of minimal descriptive data—measuring the true size of lesions by referencing against the tip of the arthroscopic probe, describing the actual location of the defect with respect to the arc-of-motion angle at which it demonstrates contact with an opposing surface, and differentiating between partial- and full-thickness erosions—more accurate long-term assessment of the results of surgical intervention can be accomplished.

OPERATIVE TECHNIQUES

Principles

The basic principles of arthroscopy for the degenerative knee are to improve biomechanical function. There are many options. The categories are diagnostic, therapeutic, and new technology (Table 26–4). Removal of loose bodies and of free or synovialized osteophytes in the gutters, notch, or tibial eminence; meniscal resection; and addressing chondral lesions are procedures commonly performed in the degenerative knee. A systematic approach must be used. Prioritizing the factors causing the patient's symptoms should be done preoperatively to minimize operating and tourniquet time. Loose bodies should be looked for in the popliteal hiatus and suprapatellar pouch, but when they are located in the Baker cyst they are usually not findable and do not require removal. Synovectomy and plical resection are indicated when there is a true mechanical component or the effusion has created continued loss-of-motion and enzymatic symptoms. Chondrocalcinosis with its punctate calcifications free, imbedded in meniscus and articular cartilage, is commonly seen in the degenerative knee. Radiographic calcifications in the menisci and arthroscopic salt calcifications everywhere are shown in Figure 26–4. Arthroscopic washout and resection of meniscus is usually successful in reducing local symptoms.

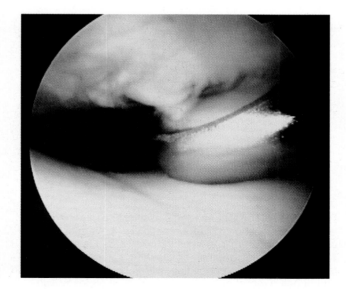

Figure 26–3 • Grade III chondromalacia odd patellar facet without trochlear groove-involvement. Saucerization and débridement with motorized resector is being performed.

Table 26–4	**Arthroscopic Options with Degenerative Joint Disease**

I. Diagnostic
   A. Evaluation
   B. Washout

II. Therapeutic
   A. Débridement
   B. Chondral flap saucerization, débridement
   C. Loose bodies
   D. Meniscectomy, medial or lateral
   E. Abrasion chondroplasty
   F. Removal of osteophytes
   G. Notchplasty

III. New technology: experimental
   A. Laser
   B. Cartilage transplantation

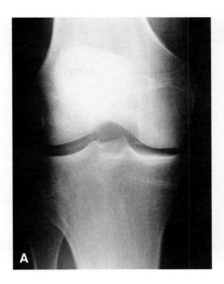 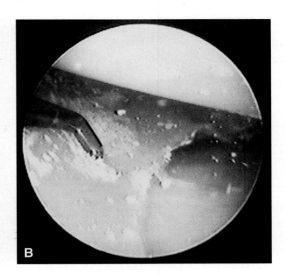

Figure 26–4 • Anteroposterior radiograph of knee showing chondrocalcinosis with calcifications in the meniscus. *A,* Arthroscopic view shows punctate calcification in the articular cartilage, meniscus, and floating free intra-articularly. *B,* Chondrocalcinosis is seen in pseudogout, gout, degenerative joint disease, and following multiple steroid injections.

The methods for changing articular surface defects include removal of loose flaps and saucerization and irrigation to remove cartilaginous loose bodies. Methods for improving blood supply at the base of the grade IV chondromalacic lesion include abrasion chondroplasty, subchondral drilling, and microfracture pick techniques. In the degenerative knee, it is less likely that periosteal grafting, perichondral grafting, and chondrocyte transplantation techniques will be helpful, particularly in femoral and tibial matching lesions. Because of the unique biomechanical aspects of the patellofemoral articulation, débridement of loose cartilage, saucerized, osteophyte removal is done. Abrasion chondroplasty is not suggested as forces are not conducive to better collagen tissue. Reduction of excessive pressure and reduction of cartilaginous free or potentially loose fragment is accomplished by débridement. Use of equipment with which the surgeon is familiar, including graspers, motorized instruments, and curved hand-held instruments, makes this demanding multiple-procedure surgery easier, faster, and more efficient.

Managing Chondral Lesions

In general, the adherence to certain principles will help guide the arthroscopist in the decision-making process. Most significant chondral lesions appear on the surfaces of the femoral condyles and trochlea; patellar defects are also common.

Functional areas of joint cartilage should be preserved at all costs. Occasionally, loose regions of cartilage seem to grow as portions are resected, nearly peeling the entire chondral surface away. Such delamination presents a significant problem, and careful probing of the chondral surface and flap should be performed before beginning removal. The role of transchondral drilling in such circumstances is unclear. Areas of fibrillation and fissuring should not be aggressively débrided; rather, gentle surface resection using a protected ("whisker") shaver should, at most, be performed. Such limited débridement may be beneficial in reducing the total surface area of exposed, damaged cartilage in the joint, thereby reducing the overall inflammatory reaction.

Larger areas of full-thickness cartilage loss and areas of patchy, near–full-thickness erosion where all that remains is a thin layer of fibrillated, degenerative cartilage present the greatest challenge. If the lesions are still well defined (that is, the entire condyle is not involved), then an attempt at cartilage stimulation is reasonable. The first step is to remove loose chondral flaps and create sharp margins of the lesion as outlined previously. This should be followed by débridement or perforation of the subchondral bone to stimulate blood flow into the area. This may be accomplished by abrasion using a bur or perforation using picks or a drill. Abrasion should be performed gently to avoid creating an overly deep crater; edges of the lesion should not be violated. Perforations should be made to an adequate depth to access vascular channels (generally 1–2 mm). Drilling or using a pick to perforate subchondral bone can often be done with precision, avoiding the creation of large, overly deep erosions. Blood flow can often be confirmed by visualization of vascular tufts, not of cancellous trabeculae. Alternatively, stopping arthroscopic inflow can document bleeding. A grade IV multi fragmented flap of medial femoral condyle is shown in Figure 26–5*A*. Débridement of the loose cartilage was performed with a full-radius resector and hand-held duckbill punch (Fig. 26–5*B*), and stimulation of the vascular channel was done by drilling (Fig. 26–5*C*).

Isolated femoral and tibial defects seem best suited to procedures that promote stimulation of fibrocartilage ingrowth. A grade IV isolated femoral lesion, measuring 1.5 × 1 cm, is shown in Figure 26–6*A*. Following abrasion chondroplasty with a motorized bur, the lesion is seen bleeding in Figure 26–6*B*. Follow-up arthroscopy was performed 8 months after the abrasion chondroplasty, with excellent filling-in of the defect (Fig. 26–6*C*). The patient was non–weight-bearing for 8 weeks; immediate motion was started. Although no biopsy was done, the resiliency and appearance of this lesion leads one to question the need for cartilage transplantation.

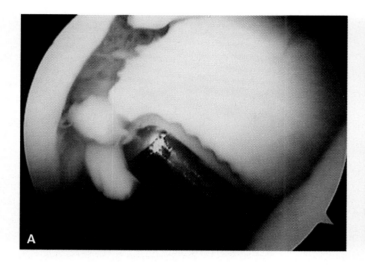

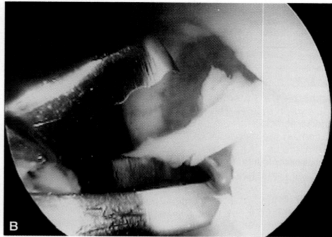

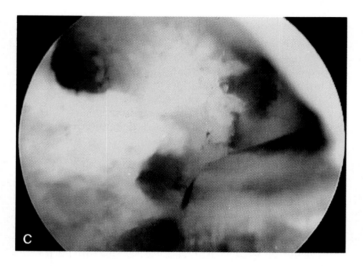

Figure 26–5 • Radiographs were normal in this localized osteochondral flap, which was down to grade II bone. *A,* Cartilage was attached anteriorly only in this medial femoral condyle. *B,* Removal of the loose cartilaginous flap was done with motorized resector and hand held duckbill punch. *C,* Drilling of the defect was performed to allow an improved blood supply and, hence, improved filling in of the collagen and cartilage.

The loss of joint space and the kissing osteophyte lesions from medial gonarthrosis are longitudinal railroad-tie configurations shown diagrammatically in Figure 26–7*A* and *B* and in radiographs in Figure 26–7*D* and *E*. Standing posteroanterior views of both knees show the loss of joint space and varus alignment on the left (Fig. 26–7*C*). A localized tibial lesion was treated with abrasion chondroplasty; this lesion was located just medial to the meniscus, which also had a tear (see Fig. 26–7*B*). Follow-up arthroscopy and x-ray 2 years after tibial abrasion chondroplasty show essentially no change in joint space medially (Fig. 26–7*F*). The abraded area filled in centrally with fibrocartilage at 2-year arthroscopic follow-up (Fig. 26–7*D*). There are reports of actual reconstitution of the joint space following abrasion chondroplasty.[126] If there are matching femoral and tibial grade IV chondromalacic defects, abrasion chondroplasty is not predictably successful. Patients with such advanced surface loss are best treated by minimal débridement, perhaps isolated drilling or picking, and postoperative counseling regarding activity restrictions.

Meniscal Tears

Unstable meniscal tears in the presence of mild or moderate arthrosis without significant malalignment do well with aggressive débridement of the unstable fragments. Using a two-portal technique and gradually allowing access into the difficult posterior medial compartments, partial resection of the meniscus, and saucerization, removal of loose cartilaginous fragments should be performed. Often, once the partial meniscectomy has been started, there is yellowish discoloration of the meniscal fragment and need for further resection, particularly around the tibial side. Most meniscal tears in the degenerative knee are complex. Mechanical symptoms can be relieved by arthroscopic meniscal resection. The lateral meniscal tear in Figure 26–8*A* was causing unpredictable locking and pain localized over the lateral compartment. Subtotal partial lateral meniscectomy was performed. The complex nature of the tear is seen. Arthroscopic resection (Fig. 26–8*B*) shows the exposed popliteal hiatus without lateral meniscus and grade IV tibial articular surface changes. Other meniscal

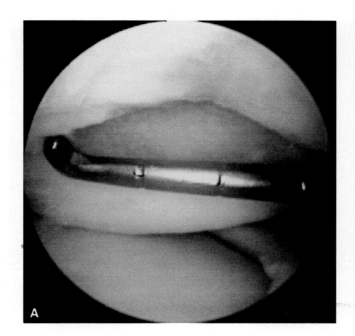

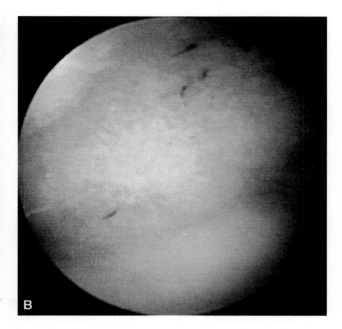

Figure 26–6 • Grade IV chondromalacic localized lesion of the medial femoral condyle measured 1.5 × 1 cm. *A,* Abrasion chondroplasty was performed in this case using a motcrized abrader. Punctate blood supply can be seen. *B,* Follow-up arthroscopy was necessary for another intra-articular problem at 8 months following the abrasion chondroplasty. The excellent filling in of the medial femoral condyle defect is shown. *C,* If abrasion chondroplasty is performed for a localized lesion such as this and it fills in at 8 months, is there a need for cartilage transplantation? No biopsies were performed, but the resiliency by probing of this area was excellent. Postoperatively the patient is doing extremely well without residual pain.

tears show yellowish degeneration, and an adequate resection of the unstable meniscal rim, which is usually the tibial side, should be done. A complex tear of the medial meniscus is shown in Figure 26–9A. Aggressive resection of the unstable tibial surface was performed (Fig. 26–9B and C). Trephination is more successful in the younger patients.[180] Trephination to improve blood supply in the degenerative meniscus is not realistic. Outside-to-inside cyst decompression is done for localized cyst formation from degenerative meniscal tear.

Excision of the meniscus to the periphery essentially eliminates the hoop stress capacity of the meniscus.[181] If the posterior horn cleavage tear of the medial meniscus is removed, there is a two-thirds reduction in energy absorption.[182]

Specific meniscal work should be directed toward the patient's symptoms. Unstable flaps and cartilage fragments should be removed. Horizontal flap meniscal tears require resection on the tibial side. Small superficial stable fissures and chondral lesions should be left alone.

Resection osteophytes and loose bodies, which cause locking, can be treated successfully by removal. Notch osteophytes and the anterior aspect of tibial osteophytes, as well as patellar medial compartment osteophytes, can be removed with osteotome and motorized bur. Limited extension in the knee of this person who had a previous total medial meniscectomy and a symptomatic loose body was treated by arthroscopic notchplasty and removal of the loose body. The standing posteroanterior radiograph (Fig. 26–10A) and notch view (Fig. 26–10B) show no joint space

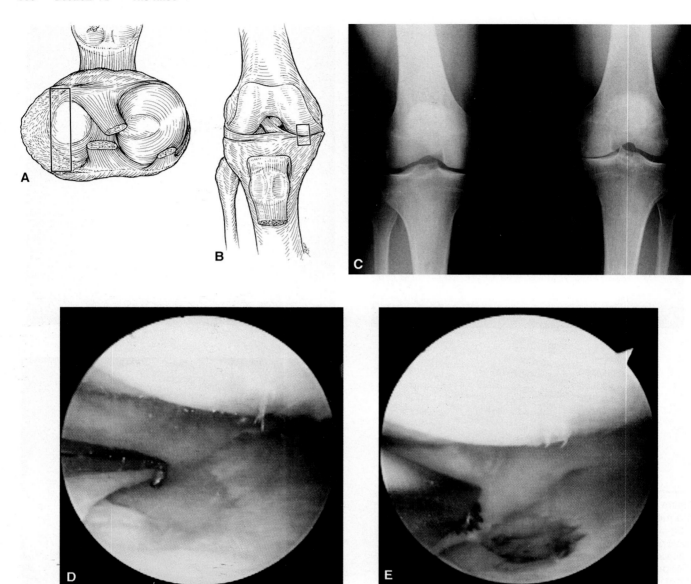

Figure 26–7 • *A,* A varus knee with medial compartment gonarthrosis has a typical rectangular railroad-type longitudinal wear pattern with localized matching lesions on the tibia and femur. *B,* Weight-bearing posteroanterior view is shown diagrammatically, with loss of medial joint space (often after a meniscectomy has been performed). *C,* Patient had left-knee complaints of painful popping and locking for which he underwent arthroscopy. Radiographs showed genu varum loss of joint space. *C,* This film correlates with the diagram. Diagnostic arthroscopy showed localized defect in the medial tibial plateau as shown with probe. *D,* Patient also had medial meniscus tear for which he underwent arthroscopic partial medial meniscectomy. *E,* Localized abrasion chondroplasty of the defect was done.

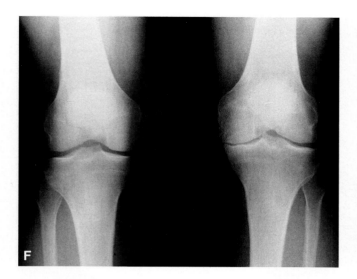

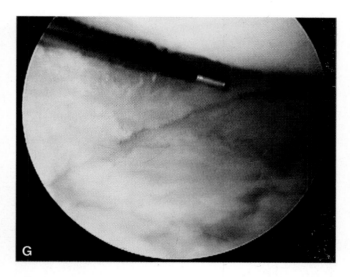

Figure 26–7 • *Continued F,* Two years postoperatively the patient had lateral meniscal complaints. Standing 30 degrees posteroanterior flexed radiographs show no significant progression of the medial gonarthrosis 2 years following his arthroscopic abrasion and chondroplasty of the medial tibial plateau. *G,* Two years postoperatively the central area of the abrasion is well healed. There is some more peripheral articular surface involvement. Partial lateral meniscectomy was performed, and no specific work was done on the articular cartilage in this later arthroscopy. In addition, notch osteophytes and medial osteophytes (not pictured) were removed to reduce pain and improve extension range of motion.

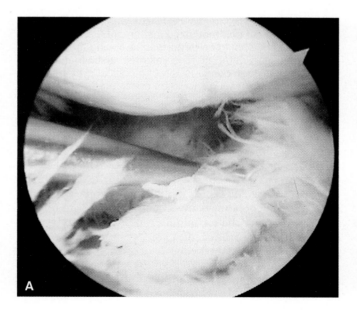

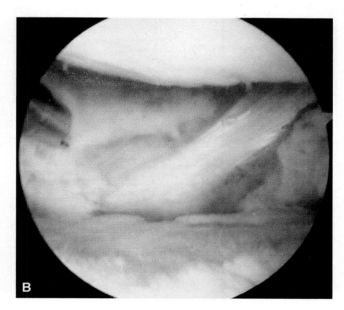

Figure 26–8 • *A,* Complex tear of the lateral meniscus in this left knee was symptomatic in this active farmer. He had localized joint line tenderness. The complex multiple-direction lateral meniscal tear can be seen. *B,* Arthroscopic subtotal lateral meniscectomy was performed, with exposure of grade III chondromalacic changes of the tibial plateau and popliteal hiatus now visible. Postoperatively the patient's symptoms have significantly improved.

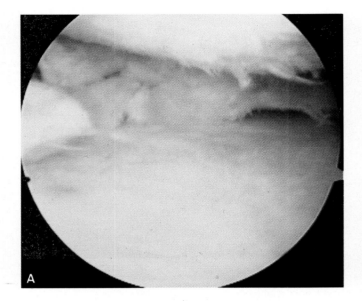

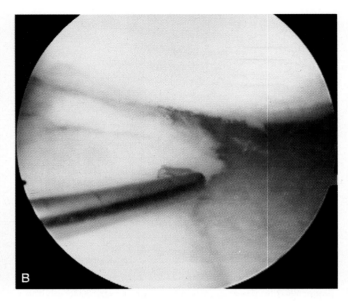

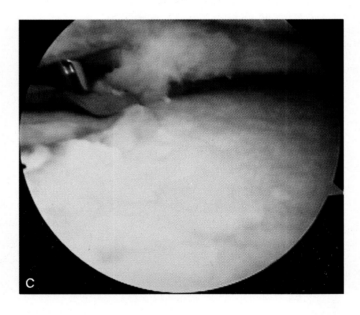

Figure 26–9 • *A,* Complex tear of the medial meniscus is shown and has typical involvement of grade II chondromalacia of the medial femoral condyle and uninvolved medial tibial plateau. *B,* Probe shows a mid third flap tear after the posterior horn of the medial meniscus was removed. *C,* Using hand-held and motorized instruments, an aggressive meniscectomy should be performed removing the unstable meniscal tissue. Often there is yellowish discoloration, and need for outside-in compression of meniscal cyst in the degenerative meniscus should be considered. A good stable rim is the goal.

in this chronic anterior cruciate ligament–insufficient patient who had previous arthrotomy and meniscectomy. The patient had a severe loose body causing locking. Arthroscopic débridement and notchplasty were done (Fig. 26–10*C*). The loose body was removed, and aggressive notchplasty and tibial eminence débridement improved range of motion (Fig. 26–10*D*). Vigorous physical therapy to push range of motion and regain quadriceps strength should be done postoperatively. Counseling and detailed discussion of arthritis severity should be done with a patient like this.

SPECIAL CONSIDERATIONS

Laser Therapy

Laser is an acronym for Light Amplification by the Stimulated Emission of Radiation.[183] One must be cautious in regard to the indication for laser use.[7] The American Academy of Orthopaedic Surgeons (AAOS) position statement is: "Clinical studies reported in orthopaedic literature have not established the benefit provided by lasers when compared to other systems now in use. As further clinical research in laster application becomes available, the Academy encourages investigators to pay attention to these areas where the techniques can be shown to be effective additions to orthopaedic care."[184, 185]

Laser use in arthroscopy is evolving. The ability to deliver focused energy to areas of the knee may prove beneficial as an adjunct to meniscal and chondral healing. Complications of laser use have been cited, including osteonecrosis of the condyle.[186]

Use of lasers for meniscal articular surface problems has been reviewed.[86, 185–187, 190] Use of laser is becoming more widespread with numerous laser tools available in the categories of CO_2, holmium:YAG, neodymium (Nd), and Excimer.[121, 182, 188, 190, 191]

Cases of aseptic necrosis of the femoral condyle following use of a holmium YAG laser have been de-

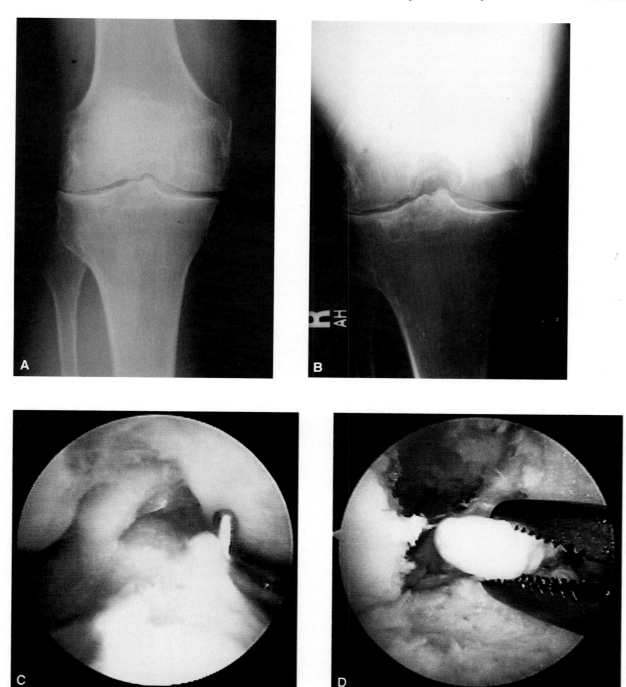

Figure 26–10 • *A,* Previous medial and lateral meniscectomies result in no joint space seen in this radiographic standing posteroanterior 30 degree flexed view. *B,* Patient had an old anterior cruciate ligament injury, and the notch osteophytes are well seen in this notch view. The patient had mechanical symptoms and a palpable loose body. *C,* Arthroscopically shown are the notch osteophytes with kissing lesion of the tibial eminence and medial femoral condyle before notchplasty. There was some tissue in the notch; however, it was not truly that of the anterior cruciate ligament but only scar tissue. *D,* Vigorous notchplasty removal of tibial eminence and notch osteophytes was performed. Loose body removal is shown with Schlissinger clamp. Postoperatively the patient has some improvement of range of motion and no further mechanical signs.

scribed.[188, 191] Inability to regulate depth of thermal energy associated with the CO_2 laser has led to reduced use; the Excimer laser, emitting light energy in the ultraviolet range, is recommended and appears to be superior with fewer thermal complications.[186] The holmium:YAG laser can be used on meniscal tissue with a rate of penetration not dependent on the laser's pulse width.[183] In describing potential risks to patients, one must include thermal energy risks.

In the canine Nd YAG laser, exposure of articular cartilage in low levels stimulates cartilage matrix synthesis, but single exposure may not be sufficient to up-regulate.[192] Similar results have been cited for human cartilage explants exposed to holmium:YAG beams.[193] Limited clinical case reports have shown fibrocartilaginous repair in vivo following laser stimulation.[194–196] However, much of the "praise" for laser technology remains anecdotal, and the AAOS urged caution in an advisory statement: further research is needed before adopting lasers for widespread use. Practice marketing strategies emphasizing such "advances," with implicit suggestions that they are superior to current techniques, should be critically evaluated before lasers are used in the degenerative knee.

Work in chondrocyte transplantation is currently in the early stage. The surgeon needs to beware of patient selection and expectation. Ongoing research into the stimulation of cartilage growth and repair has generated some promising early results with repopulation of damaged surfaces by cultured autogenous chondroblasts, placed back into the defect and covered with a periosteal flap.[51, 197] Work with chondrocyte growth factors,[198–200] direct progenitor cell and matrix composite implantation,[201, 202] artificial scaffolds,[203] periosteal and perichondrial grafts,[204–206] and allograft transplantation[207–209] is now being done.

COMPLICATIONS

In a patient with degenerative joint disease, given the circumstances of multiple procedures, complexity of the arthroscopy, and advanced patient age, complications are more commonly seen. These patients require closer postoperative monitoring if significant pain, calf tightness or calf swelling develops. Historically, the issue of deep venous thrombosis (DVT) prophylaxis has been neglected for arthroscopic procedures. In a series of complications following arthroscopy, Small[12] reported 12 cases of DVT in over 10,000 surgical cases; 8 of the 12 cases involved use of a tourniquet, with an average time of 50 minutes, and 350 mm Hg pressure. Four cases went on to pulmonary embolism, none of which was fatal. This small but significant number of cases may represent the tip of the iceberg in this older population. If there is a history of deep vein thrombosis, there should be preoperative measures of vascular function and avoidance of the use of the tourniquet intraoperatively. Prospective evaluations using Doppler analysis have shown significant levels of DVT following various orthopaedic procedures other than joint replacements, including a 4.4% rate of thrombus formation following arthroscopy in a prospective study of 45 patients screened both pre- and postoperatively with duplex ultrasound.[210] However, at least one study has argued against the need for screening ultrasound following arthroscopy, unless perhaps the patient has a known DVT risk.[211]

A survey done through the Arthroscopy Association of North America and published in 1985[212] revealed the order and frequency of complications. Of all the complications, the order and type are as follows: postoperative hemarthrosis 24%, broken instruments 17%, thrombophlebitis 15%, postoperative infection 10%, neurologic injury 7%, other 6%, anesthesia 5%, reflex sympathetic dystrophy 4.7%, knee ligament injury, 4.4%, and pulmonary embolus 3.4%. As advances in arthroscopy and arthroscopic techniques have occurred, the broken instrument and hemarthrosis complications appear to have been reduced in frequency. Use of a drain, if bony work is done, and compressive devices including the thromboembolic disease hose reduces venostasis. A vigorous postoperative rehabilitation program with early range-of-motion and elevation exercises should be instituted. In the patient with degenerative joint disease of the knee, the age is usually greater, and there is some venous insufficiency. Because of this, venous complications are probably the most common. At the Kentucky Sports Medicine Clinic during the last 7 years, out of 1394 knee arthroscopies, there have been seven deep vein thromboses, for an incidence of .005 (Ireland, unpublished data, 1995). The deep vein thromboses were in older patients who underwent work in the posteromedial compartment. There were no deep vein thromboses associated with anterior cruciate ligament reconstructions.

CONCLUSION

Objective clinical investigations will continue to refine the indications for arthroscopy for the patient with significant degenerative knee problems. Biology and transplantation research in the fields of human genetics, cartilage in animals and humans, and biomedical engineering will result in arthroscopic advancements. The future is bright for treating arthritis arthroscopically.

Patients should be carefully selected for arthroscopy. Decision is based on persistent symptoms despite rehabilitation, unwillingness to undergo a replacement, and a thorough understanding that the arthroscopy is to be a temporizing treatment. The ideal candidate for an arthroscopy has mechanical symptoms, such as locking, catching, or feelings of instability, in the presence of mild to moderate degenerative changes radiographically. If there is significant angular deformity, a corrective osteotomy or a unicompartmental or total knee arthroplasty should be strongly recommended.[213] The following question should be posed to the patient: Is a fair result from a minor operation better than a good result from a major operation?[159]

Above all, however, one must bear in mind that "newer" is not necessarily "better." "Cutting-edge" technological breakthroughs such as laser and cartilage transplantation should be proved successful and cost-effective before use. The orthopaedist should strive to use the tools that work best for the patient in the hands of the individual surgeon.

References

1. Blair SN, Kohl HW III, Paffenbarger RS Jr, et al.: Physical fitness and all-cause mortality: a prospective study of healthy men and women. JAMA 262:2395–2401, 1989.
2. Blair SN, Kohl HW III, Barlow CE, et al.: Changes in physical fitness and all-cause mortality: a prospective study of healthy and unhealthy men. JAMA 273:1093–1098, 1995.
3. Ekelund LG, Haskell WL, Johnson JL, et al.: Physical fitness as a predictor of cardiovascular mortality in asymptomatic North American men: the Lipid Research Clinics mortality follow-up study. N Engl J Med 319:1379–1384, 1988.
4. Lee I-M, Hsieh C-C, and Paffenbarger RS: Exercise intensity and longevity in men: the Harvard Alumni Health Study. JAMA 273: 1179–1184, 1995.
5. Pate RR, Pratt M, Blair SH, et al.: Physical activity and public health: a recommendation from the Centers for Disease Control and Prevention and the American College of Sports Medicine. JAMA 273:402–407, 1995.
6. Rosenberg TD, Paulos LE, Parker RD, et al.: The forty-five degree posteroanterior flexion weight bearing radiograph of the knee. J Bone Joint Surg Am 70:1479–1482, 1988.
7. Dye SF and Chew MH: The use of scintigraphy to detect increased osseous metabolic activity about the knee. J Bone Joint Surg Am 75:1388–1406, 1993.
8. Wang J-W, Kuo KN, Andriacchi TP, et al.: The influence of walking mechanics and time on the results of proximal tibial osteotomy. J Bone Joint Surg Am 72:905–909, 1990.
9. Casscells SW: The torn meniscus, the torn anterior cruciate ligament, and their relationship to degenerative joint disease. Arthroscopy 1:28–32, 1985.
10. Novak PJ and Bach BR: Selection criteria for knee arthroscopy in the osteoarthritic patient. Orthop Rev 22:798–804, 1993.
11. Sherman OH, Fox JM, Snyder SJ, et al.: Arthroscopy—"no problem surgery." J Bone Joint Surg Am 68:256–265, 1986.
12. Small NC: Complications in arthroscopy: the knee and other joints. Arthroscopy 2:253–258, 1986.
13. Small NC: Complications in arthroscopic surgery performed by experienced arthroscopists. Arthroscopy 4:215–221, 1988.
14. Dandy DJ and Jackson RW: The diagnosis of problems after meniscectomy. J Bone Joint Surg Br 57:349–352, 1975.
15. Lysholm J, Hamberg P, and Gillquist J: The correlation between osteoarthrosis as seen on radiographs and on arthroscopy. Arthroscopy 3:161–165, 1987.
16. Rand JA: Role of arthroscopy in osteoarthritis of the knee. Arthroscopy 7:358–363, 1991.
17. Brandt KD and Mankin HJ: Pathogenesis of osteoarthritis. In Kelly WN, Harris ED Jr, Ruddy S, et al. (eds.): Textbook of Rheumatology, 4th ed. Philadelphia, W.B. Saunders Co., 1993, pp 1355–1373.
18. Bartel DL: Unicompartmental arthritis: biomechanics and treatment alternatives. Instr Course Lect 41:73–76, 1992.
19. Felson DT, Andrews JJ, and Naimark A: Obesity and knee osteoarthritis: the Framingham study. Ann Intern Med 109:18–24, 1989.
20. Felson DT, Zhang Y, Anthony JM, et al.: Weight loss reduces the risk of symptomatic knee osteoarthritis in women: the Framingham study. Ann Intern Med 116:535–539, 1992.
21. Mankin HJ: Clinical features of osteoarthritis. In Kelly WN, Harris ED Jr, Ruddy S, et al. (eds.): Textbook of Rheumatology, 4th ed. Philadelphia, W.B. Saunders Co., 1993, pp 1374–1384.
22. Williams CJ and Jimenez SA: Heredity, genes and osteoarthritis. Rheum Dis Clin North Am 19:523–543, 1993.
23. Lohmander LS, Saxne T, and Heinegard DK: Release of cartilage oligomeric matrix protein (COMP) into joint fluid after knee injury and in osteoarthritis. Ann Rheu Dis 53:8–13, 1994.
24. Ala-Kokka L, Baldwin CT, Moskowitz RW, et al.: Single-base mutation in the type II procollagen gene (COL 2A1) as a cause of primary osteoarthritis associated with mild chondrodysplasia. Proc Natl Acad Sci U S A 87:6565–6568, 1990.
25. Knowlton RG, Katzenstein PL, Moskowitz RW, et al.: Genetic linkage of polymorphism in the type II procollagen gene (COL 2A1) to primary osteoarthritis associated with mild chondrodysplasia. N Engl J Med 322:526–530, 1990.
26. Lotke PK, Lekfoe RT, and Ecker ML: Late results following medial meniscectomy in an older population. J Bone Joint Surg Am 63:115–119, 1981.
27. Noyes FR, Barber SD, and Simon R: High tibial osteotomy and ligament reconstruction in varus angulated, anterior cruciate ligament–deficient knees. Am J Sports Med 21:2–12, 1993.
28. Fetto JF and Marshall JL: The natural history and diagnosis of anterior cruciate ligament insufficiency. Clin Orthop 147:29–38, 1980.
29. Hawkins RJ, Misamore GW, and Merritt TR: Follow-up of the acute nonoperated isolated anterior cruciate ligament tear. Am J Sports Med 14:205–210, 1986.
30. Jacobsen K: Osteoarthrosis following insufficiency in the cruciate ligaments in man: a clinical study. Acta Orthop Scand 48:520–526, 1977.
31. McDaniel WJ and Dameron TB: The untreated anterior cruciate ligament rupture. Clin Orthop 172:158–163, 1983.
32. Noyes FR, Mooar PA, Matthews DE, et al.: The symptomatic anterior cruciate–deficient knee. Part I: the long-term functional disability in athletically active individuals. J Bone Joint Surg Am 65:154–162, 1983.
33. Daniel DM, Stone ML, Dobson BE, et al.: Fate of the ACL-injured patient: a prospective outcome study. Am J Sports Med 22:632–644, 1994.
34. Shelbourne KD and Wilckens JH: Intraarticular anterior cruciate ligament reconstruction in the symptomatic arthritic knee. Am J Sports Med 21:685–689, 1993.
35. Keller PM, Shelbourne KD, McCarroll JR, et al.: Nonoperatively treated isolated posterior cruciate ligament injuries. Am J Sports Med 21:132–136, 1993.
36. Skyhar MJ, Warren RF, Ortiz GJ, et al.: The effects of sectioning of the posterior cruciate ligament and the posterolateral complex on the articular contact pressures within the knee. J Bone Joint Surg Am 75:694–699, 1993.
37. Crosby EB and Insall J: Recurrent dislocation of the patella: relation of treatment to osteoarthritis. J Bone Joint Surg Am 58:9–13, 1976.
38. Fulkerson JP: Anteromedialization of the tibial tuberosity for patellofemoral malalignment. Clin Orthop 177:176–181, 1983.
39. Newman AP, Daniels AU, and Burks RT: Principles and decision making in meniscal surgery. Arthroscopy 9:33–51, 1993.
40. Fairbank TJ: Knee joint changes after meniscectomy. J Bone Joint Surg Br 30:664–670, 1948.
41. Tapper EM and Hoover NW: Late results after meniscectomy. J Bone Joint Surg Am 51:517–526, 1969.
42. Arnoczky SP, Warren RF, and McDevitt CA: Meniscal replacement using a cryopreserved allograft: an experiment study in the dog. Clin Orthop 232:121–128, 1990.
43. Garrett JC and Steenson RN: Meniscal transplantation in the human knee: a preliminary report. Arthroscopy 7:57–62, 1991.
44. Jackson DW, McDevitt CA, Simon TM, et al.: Meniscal transplantation using fresh and cryopreserved allografts: an experimental study in goats. Am J Sports Med 20:644–656, 1992.
45. Jackson DW, Whelan J, and Simon TM: Cell survival after transplantation of fresh meniscal allografts. Am J Sports Med 21(4):540–550, 1993.
46. Milachowski KA, Weismeier K, Wirth CJ, et al.: Meniscus transplantation: an experimental study and clinical results (abstract). J Bone Surg Br 71:717, 1989.
47. Noyes FR and Barber-Westin SD: Meniscus allografts in the human knee: a two to five year follow-up study. Presented at the 62nd Annual Meeting of the American Academy of Orthopaedic Surgeons, Orlando, Fla., Feb., 1995.
48. Stone KR, Rodkey WG, Webber RJ, et al.: Collagen-based prosthesis for meniscal regeneration. Clin Orthop 252:129–135, 1990.
49. Stone KR, Rodkey WG, Webber RJ, et al.: Meniscal regeneration and copolymeric collagen scaffolds: in vitro and in vivo studies evaluated clinically, histologically, and biochemically. Am J Sports Med 20:104–111, 1992.
50. Brittberg M, Lindahl A, Nilsson A, et al.: Treatment of deep cartilage defects in the knee with autologous chondrocyte transplantation. N Engl J Med 331:889–895, 1994.
51. Baragi VM, Renkiewicz RR, Jordan H, et al.: Transplantation of transduced chondrocytes protects articular cartilage from interleukin 1-induced extracellular matrix degradation. J Clin Invest 96:2454–2460, 1995.

52. deCrombrugghe B, Katzenstein P, Mukhopadhyay K, et al.: Transgenic mice with deficiencies in cartilage collagens: possible models for gene therapy. J Rheumatol (suppl):43:140–142, 1995.
53. Mankin HJ: Chondrocyte transplantation—one answer to an old question (editorial). N Engl J Med 331:940–941, 1994.
54. Hunter W: On the structure and diseases of articulating cartilage. Philos Trans R Soc Lond (Biol) 9:267, 1743.
55. Mankin HJ, Mow VC, Buckwalter JA, et al.: Form and function of articular cartilage. In Simon SR (ed.): Orthopaedic Basic Science. Rosemont, Ill., American Academy of Orthopaedic Surgeons, 1994, pp 1–44.
56. Buckwalter JA: Articular cartilage. Instr Course Lect 32:349–370, 1983.
57. Buckwalter JA, Rosenberg LC, Cotts R, et al.: Articular cartilage: injury and repair. In Woo SL and Buckwalter JA (eds.): Injury and Repair of the Musculoskeletal Soft Tissues. Park Ridge, Ill., American Academy of Orthopaedic Surgeons, 1988, pp 465–482.
58. Dmitrovsky E, Lane LB, and Bullough PG: The characterization of the tidemark in human articular cartilage. Metab Bone Dis Rel Res 1:115–118, 1978.
59. Muir H, Bullough P, and Maroudas A: The distribution of collagen in human articular cartilage with some of its physiologic implications. J Bone Joint Surg Br 52:554–563, 1970.
60. Poole CA, Flint MH, and Beaumont BW: Morphological and functional interrelationships of articular cartilage matrices. J Anat 138:113–138, 1984.
61. Arnoldi CC, Linderholm H, and Mussibichler H: Venous engorgement and interosseous hypertension in osteoarthritis of the hip. J Bone Joint Surg Br 54:409–421, 1978.
62. Mow VC, Holmes MH, and Lai WM: Fluid transport mechanical properties of articular cartilage. J Biomech 17:377–394, 1984.
63. Mow VC and Rosenwasser MP: Articular cartilage: biomechanics. In Woo SL and Buckwalter JA (eds.): Injury and Repair of the Musculoskeletal Soft Tissues. Park Ridge, Ill., American Academy of Orthopaedic Surgeons. 1988, pp 427–464.
64. Bollet AJ: An essay on the biology of osteoarthritis. Arthritis Rheum 12:152–163, 1969.
65. Maroudas A and Venn M: Chemical composition and swelling of normal and osteoarthritic femoral head cartilage. II: swelling. Ann Rheum Dis 36:399–406, 1977.
66. Armstrong CG and Mow VC: Variations in the intrinsic mechanical properties of human articular cartilage with age, degeneration, and water content. J Bone Joint Surg Am 64:88–94, 1982.
67. Brocklehurst R, Bayliss MT, Maroudas A, et al.: The composition of normal and osteoarthritis articular cartilage from the human knee joints, with special reference to unicompartmental replacement and osteotomy of the knee. J Bone Joint Surg Am 66:95–106, 1984.
68. Calandruccio RA and Gilmer WS: Proliferation, regeneration, and repair of articular cartilage of immature animals. J Bone Joint Surg Am 44:431–455, 1962.
69. DePalma AF, McKeever CD, and Subin DK: Process of repair of articular cartilage demonstrated by histology and autoradiography with tritiated thymidine. Clin Orthop 48:229–242, 1966.
70. Mankin HJ: Reaction of articular cartilage to injury and osteoarthritis: part I. N Engl J Med 291:1285–1292, 1974.
71. Mankin HJ: Reaction of articular cartilage to injury and osteoarthritis: part II. N Engl J Med 291:1335–1340, 1974.
72. Mankin HJ: Response of articular cartilage to mechanical injury. J Bone Joint Surg Am 64:460–466, 1982.
73. Weiss C and Mirow S: An ultrastructural study of osteoarthritic changes in the articular cartilage of human knees. J Bone Joint Surg Am 54:954–972, 1972.
74. Eyre DR, McDevitt CA, Billingham MEJ, et al.: Biosynthesis of collagen and other matrix proteins by articular cartilage in experimental osteoarthritis. Biochem J 188:823–837, 1980.
75. Sandy JD, Adams ME, Billingham MEJ, et al.: In vivo and in vitro stimulation of chondrocyte biosynthetic activity in early experimental osteoarthritis. Arthritis Rheum 27:388–397, 1984.
76. Donohue JN, Buss D, Oegema TR Jr, et al.: The effects of blunt trauma on adult canine articular cartilage. J Bone Joint Surg Am 65:948–957, 1983.
77. Radin EL, Martin RV, Burr DB, et al.: Effects of mechanical loading on the tissue of the rabbit knee. J Orthop Res 2:221–234, 1984.
78. Pelletier J-P, Martel-Pelletier J, Howell DS, et al.: Collagenase and collagenolytic activity in human osteoarthritic cartilage. Arthritis Rheum 26:63–68, 1983.
79. Radin EL and Rose RM: Role of subchondral bone in the initiation and progression of cartilage damage. Clin Orthop 213:34–40, 1986.
80. Schmid A and Schmid F: Results after cartilage shaving study by electron microscopy. Am J Sports Med 14:386–387, 1987.
81. Salter RB, Simmonds DF, Malcolm BW, et al.: The biological effect of continuous passive motion on the healing of full-thickness defects in articular cartilage. J Bone Joint Surg Am 62:1232–1251, 1980.
82. Furukawa T, Eyre DR, Koide S, et al.: Biochemical studies on repair cartilage resurfacing experimental defects in the rabbit knee. J Bone Joint Surg Am 62:79–89, 1980.
83. Shapiro F, Koide S, and Glimcher MJ: Cell origin and differentiation in the repair of full-thickness defects of articular cartilage. J Bone Joint Surg Am 75:532–553, 1993.
84. Mitchell N and Shepard N: Resurfacing of the adult rabbit articular cartilage by multiple perforations of the subchondral bone. J Bone Joint Surg Am 58:230–233, 1976.
85. Hernborg JS and Nilsson BE: The natural course of untreated osteoarthritis of the knee. Clin Orthop 123:130–137, 1977.
86. Merchan EC and Galindo E: Arthroscopic-guided surgery versus nonoperative treatment for limited degenerative osteoarthritis of the femorotibial joint in patients over 50 years of age: a prospective comparative study. Arthroscopy 9:663–667, 1993.
87. McGinty JB, Johnson LL, Jackson RW, et al.: Current concepts review: uses and abuses of arthroscopy: a symposium. J Joint Bone Surg Am 74:1563–1577, 1992.
88. Tegner Y and Lysholm J: Rating systems in the evaluation of knee ligament injuries. Clin Orthop 198:43–49, 1985.
89. Hefti F and Muller W: Current state of evaluation of knee ligament lesions: the new IKDC knee evaluation for. Orthopade 22:351–362, 1993.
90. Ware JE: SF-36 health survey: manual and interpretation guide. Boston, The Health Institute, New England Medical Center, 1993.
91. Lysholm J and Gillquist J: Evaluation of the knee ligament surgery results with a special emphasis on use of a scoring scale. Am J Sports Med 10:150–154, 1982.
92. Bradley J: Nonsurgical options for managing osteoarthritis of the knee. J Musculoskeletal Med 11:14–26, 1994.
93. Finkelstein H and Mayer L: The arthroscope, a new method of examining joints. J Bone Joint Surg 13:583–588, 1931.
94. Burman MS: Arthroscopy for the direct visualization of joints: an experimental cadaver study. J Bone Joint Surg 13:669–695, 1931.
95. Burman MS, Finkelstein H, and Mayer L: Arthroscopy of the knee joint. J Bone Joint Surg 16:255–268, 1934.
96. Bircher E: Die Arthroendoskopie. Zentralbl Chir 48:1460–1461, 1921.
97. Burman MS, Finkelstein H, and Mayer L: Arthroscopy of the knee joint. J Bone Joint Surg 16:255–268, 1934.
98. Haggart GE: Surgical treatment of degenerative arthritis of the knee joint. J Bone Joint Surg Am 22:717–729, 1940.
99. Haggart GE: Surgical treatment of degenerative arthritis of the knee joint. N Engl J Med 236:971–973, 1947.
100. Magnuson PB: Joint débridement: surgical treatment of degenerative osteoarthritis. Surg Gynecol Obstet 73:1–9, 1941.
101. Magnuson PB: Technique of débridement of the knee joint for arthritis. Surg Clin North Am 26:249–266, 1946.
102. Pridie KH: A method of resurfacing osteoarthritic knee joints. J Bone Joint Surg Br 41:618–619, 1959.
103. Insall JN: Intra-articular surgery for degenerative arthritis of the knee: a report of the work of the late KH Pridie. J Bone Joint Surg Br 49:211–228, 1967.
104. Insall JN: The Pridie débridement operation for osteoarthritis of the knee. Clin Orthop 101:61–67, 1974.
105. Jackson RW and Abe I: The role of arthroscopy in the management of disorders of the knee. J Bone Joint Surg Br 54:310–322, 1972.

106. Dandy DJ: Abrasion chondroplasty. Arthroscopy 2:51–53, 1986.
107. Eriksson E and Haggmark T: Knee pain in the middle-aged runner. In Mack RP (ed): Symposium on the Foot and Leg in Running Sports. Park Ridge, Ill., American Academy of Orthopaedic Surgeons, 1980, pp 106–108.
108. Chrisman OD, Ladenbauer-Bellis IM, Panjabi M, et al.: The relationship of mechanical trauma and the early biochemical reactions of osteoarthritic cartilage. Clin Orthop 161:275–284, 1981.
109. Livesley PJ, Doherty M, Needof M, et al.: Arthroscopic lavage of osteoarthritic knees. J Bone Joint Surg Br 73:922–926, 1991.
110. Ike RW, Arnold WJ, Rothschild EW, et al.: Tidal irrigation versus conservative medical management in patients with osteoarthritis of the knee: a prospective randomized study. J Rheumatol 19:772–779, 1992.
111. Edelson R, Burks RT, and Bloebaum RD: Short-term effects of knee washout for osteoarthritis. Am J Sports Med 23:345–349, 1995.
112. Dahl LB, Dahl IMS, Engstrom-Laurent A, et al.: Concentration and molecular weight of sodium hyaluronate in synovial fluid from patients with rheumatoid arthritis and other arthropathies. Ann Rheum Dis 44:817–822, 1985.
113. Dawes PT, Kirlew C, and Haslock I: Saline washout for knee osteoarthritis: results of a controlled study. Clin Rheumatol 6:61–63, 1987.
114. Aichroth PM, Patel DV, and Moyes ST: A prospective review of arthroscopic débridement for degenerative joint disease of the knee. Int Orthop 15:351–355, 1991.
115. Bonamo JJ, Kessler KJ, and Noah J: Arthroscopic meniscectomy in patients over the age of 40. Am J Sports Med 20:422–429, 1992.
116. McBride GG, Constine RM, Hoffman AA, et al.: Arthroscopic partial medial meniscectomy in the older patient. J Bone Joint Surg Am 66:547–551, 1984.
117. Baumgaertner MR, Cannon WD, Vittori JM, et al.: Arthroscopic débridement of the arthritic knee. Clin Orthop 253:197–202, 1990.
118. Timoney JM, Kneisl JS, Barrack RL, et al.: Arthroscopy in the osteoarthritic knee—long-term follow-up. Orthop Rev 19:371–379, 1990.
119. Bert JM: Role of abrasion arthroplasty and débridement in the management of osteoarthritis of the knee. Rheum Dis Clin North Am 19:725–739, 1993.
120. Blevins FT, Rodrigo JJ, Fulstone A, et al.: Treatment of articular cartilage defects in athletes: an analysis of functional outcome and lesion appearance. Presented at the 19th Annual Meeting of the American Orthopaedic Society for Sports Medicine, Sun Valley, Idaho, July, 1993.
121. Jackson RW: The role of arthroscopy in the management of the arthritic knee. Clin Orthop 101:27–35, 1974.
122. Sprague NF: Arthroscopic débridement for degenerative knee joint disease. Clin Orthop 198:118–123, 1981.
123. Richards RN and Lonergan RP: Arthroscopic surgery for relief of pain in the osteoarthritic knee. Orthopedics 7:1705–1707, 1984.
124. Rae PJ and Noble J: Arthroscopic drilling of osteochondral lesions of the knee. J Bone Joint Surg Br 71:534, 1989.
125. Shahriaree H, O'Connor RF, and Nottage W: 7 years follow-up arthroscopic débridement of degenerative knee. Field of View 1:1–7, 1982.
126. Johnson LL: Arthroscopic abrasion arthroplasty: historical and pathological perspective: present status. Arthroscopy 2:54–69, 1986.
127. Hjertquist SO and Lemperg R: Histological, autoradiographic and microchemical studies of spontaneously healing osteochondral articular defects in adult rabbits. Calcif Tissue Res 8:54–72, 1971.
128. Grande DA, Pitman MI, Peterson L, et al.: The repair of experimentally produced defects in rabbit articular cartilage by autologous chondrocyte transplantation. J Orthop Res 7:208–218, 1989.
129. Schonholtz GJ: Arthroscopic débridement of the knee joint. Orthop Clin North Am 20:257–263, 1989.
130. Chandler EJ: Abrasion arthroplasty of the knee. Contemp Orthop 11:21–29, 1985.
131. Singh S, Lee CC, and Tay BK: Results of arthroscopic abrasion arthroplasty in osteoarthritis of the knee joint. Singapore Med J 32:34–37, 1991.

132. Bert JM and Maschka K: The arthroscopic treatment of unicompartmental gonarthrosis: a five-year follow-up study of abrasion arthroplasty plus arthroscopic débridement and arthroscopic débridement alone. Arthroscopy 5:25–32, 1989.
133. Johnson LL: Arthroscopic abrasion arthroplasty. In McGinty JB (ed.): Operative Arthroscopy, 2nd ed. Philadelphia, Lippincott-Raven, 1996, pp 427–446.
134. Friedman MJ, Berasi CC, Fox JM, et al.: Preliminary results with abrasion arthroplasty in the osteoarthritic knee. Clin Orthop 182:200–205, 1984.
135. Jackson RW, Silver R, and Marans R: The arthroscopic treatment of degenerative joint disease. Arthroscopy 2:114, 1986.
136. Ogilvie-Harris DJ and Fitsialos DP: Arthroscopic management of the degenerative knee. Arthroscopy 7:151–157, 1991.
137. Bourne RB, Finlay JB, Papadopoulos P, et al.: The effect of medial meniscectomy on strain distribution in the proximal part of the tibia. J Bone Joint Surg Am 66:1431–1437, 1984.
138. Bolano LE and Grana WA: Isolated arthroscopic partial meniscectomy: functional radiographic evaluation at five years. Am J Sports Med 21:432–437, 1993.
139. Rangger C, Klestil T, Gloetzer W, et al.: Osteoarthritis after arthroscopic partial meniscectomy. Am J Sports Med 23:240–244, 1995.
140. Rand JA: Arthroscopic management of degenerative meniscus tears in patients with degenerative arthritis. Arthroscopy 1:253–258, 1985.
141. Hershman EB and Nisonson B: Arthroscopic meniscectomy: a follow-up report. Am J Sports Med 11:253–257, 1983.
142. Jones RE, Smith EC, and Reisch JS: The effects of medial meniscectomy in patients older than 40 years. J Bone Joint Surg Am 60:783–786, 1978.
143. Boe S and Hansen H: Arthroscopic partial meniscectomy in patients aged over 50. J Bone Joint Surg Br 68:707, 1986.
144. Ferkel RD, Davis JR, Friedman MJ, et al.: Arthroscopic partial medial meniscectomy: an analysis of unsatisfactory results. Arthroscopy 1:44–52, 1985.
145. Jackson RW and Rouse DW: The results of partial meniscectomy in patients older than forty years. J Bone Joint Surg Br 64:481–485, 1982.
146. Friedman MJ, Brna JA, Gallick GS, et al.: Failed arthroscopic meniscectomy: prognostic factors for repeat arthroscopic examination. Arthroscopy 3:99–105, 1987.
147. Jackson AM: Recurrent dislocation of the patella. J Bone Joint Surg Br 74:2–4, 1992.
148. Aglietti P, Pisaneschi A, Buzzi R, et al.: Arthroscopic lateral release for patellar pain or instability. Arthroscopy 5:176–183, 1989.
149. Ferguson AB Jr, Brown TD, Fu FH, et al.: Relief of patellofemoral contact stress by anterior displacement of the tibial tubercle. J Bone Joint Surg Am 61:159–166, 1979.
150. Heatley FW, Allen PR, and Patrick JH: Tibial tubercle advancement for anterior knee pain: a temporary or permanent solution. Clin Orthop 208:215–224, 1986.
151. Siegel M: The Maquet osteotomy: a review of the risks. Orthopedics 10:1073–1078, 1987.
152. Ficat RP, Ficat C, Gedeon P, et al.: Spongialization: a new treatment for diseased patellae. Clin Orthop 144:74–83, 1979.
153. Beltran JE: Resection arthroplasty of the patella. J Bone Joint Surg Br 69:604–607, 1987.
154. MacIntosh DL and Welsh RP: Joint débridement: a complement to high tibial osteotomy in the treatment of degenerative arthritis of the knee. J Bone Joint Surg Am 59:1094–1097, 1977.
155. Keene JS and Dyreby JR: High tibial osteotomy in the treatment of osteoarthritis of the knee. J Bone Joint Surg Am 65:36–42, 1983.
156. Jakob RP and Murphy SB: Tibial osteotomy for varus gonarthrosis: indication, planning, and operative technique. Instr Course Lect 41:87–93, 1992.
157. Fanelli GC and Rogers VP: High tibial valgus osteotomy combined with arthroscopic abrasion arthroplasty. Contemp Orthop 19:547–550, 1989.
158. Morrey BF and Edgerton BC: Distal femoral osteotomy for lateral gonarthrosis. Instr Course Lect 41:77–87, 1992.

159. Burks RT: Arthroscopy and degenerative arthritis of the knee: a review of the literature. Arthroscopy 6:43–47, 1990.
160. Laprade RF, Burnett QM, Veenstra MA, et al.: The prevalence of abnormal magnetic resonance imaging findings in asymptomatic knees. Am J Sports Med 22:739–745, 1994.
161. Spindler KP, Schils JP, Bergfeld JA, et al.: Prospective study of osseous, articular, and meniscal lesions in recent anterior cruciate ligament tears by magnetic resonance imaging and arthroscopy. Am J Sports Med 21:551–557, 1993.
162. Rubin DA and Herzog RJ: Magnetic resonance imaging of articular cartilage injuries of the knee. Oper Tech Sports Med 3:87–95, 1995.
163. Kelly MA, Flock JJ, Kimmel JA, et al.: MR imaging of the knee: clarification of its role. Arthroscopy 7:78–85, 1991.
164. Quinn FF and Brown TF: Meniscal tears diagnosed with MR imaging versus arthroscopy: how reliable a standard is arthroscopy? Radiology 181:843–847, 1991.
165. Quinn SF, Brown TF, and Szumowski J: Menisci of the knee: radial MR imaging correlated with arthroscopy in 259 patients. Radiology 185:577–580, 1992.
166. Ruwe PA, Wright J, Randall RL, et al.: Can MR imaging effectively replace diagnostic arthroscopy? Radiology 183:335–339, 1992.
167. Gross DE, Brenner SL, Estormes I, et al.: The arthroscopic treatment of degenerative joint disease in the knee. Orthopedics 14:1317–1321, 1991.
168. Salisbury RB, Nottage WM, and Gardner V: The effect of alignment on results in arthroscopic débridement of the degenerative knee. Clin Orthop 198:268–272, 1985.
169. Wouters E, Bassett FH, Hardaker WT, et al.: An algorithm for arthroscopy in the over-50 age group. Am J Sports Med 20:141–145, 1992.
170. Rand JA and Ritts GD: Abrasion arthroplasty as a salvage for failed upper tibial osteotomy. J Arthroplasty 4(suppl): 1989, 45–48.
171. Fujisawa Y, Masuhara K, and Shiomi S: The effect of high tibial osteotomy on osteoarthritis of the knee: an arthroscopic study of fifty-four knee joints. Orthop Clin North Am 10:585–608, 1979.
172. Bentley G and Dowd G: Current concepts of etiology and treatment of chondromalacia of the patellae. Clin Orthop 189:209–228, 1984.
173. Ogilvie-Harris D and Jackson RW: The arthroscopic treatment of chondromalacia patellae. J Bone Joint Surg Br 66:660–665, 1984.
174. Fulkerson JP: Patellofemoral pain, disorders, evaluation, and management. J Am Orthop Surg 124–132, 1994.
175. Outerbridge RE: The etiology of chondromalacia patellae. J Bone Joint Surg Br 43:752–757, 1961.
176. Noyes FR and Stabler CL: A system for grading articular cartilage lesions at arthroscopy. Am J Sports Med 17:505–513, 1989.
177. Tippett JW: Articular cartilage drilling and osteotomy in osteoarthritis of the knee. In McGinty JB (ed.): Operative Arthroscopy, 2nd ed. Philadelphia, Lippincott-Raven, 1996, pp 411–426.
178. Ahlback S: Osteoarthritis of the knee: a radiographic investigation. Acta Radiol Diag 277(suppl):7–72, 1968.
179. Bauer M and Jackson RW: Chondral lesions of the femoral condyles: a system of arthroscopic classification. Arthroscopy 4:97–102, 1988.
180. Fitzgibbons RE and Shelbourne KD: "Aggressive" nontreatment of lateral meniscal tears seen during anterior cruciate ligament reconstruction. Am J Sports Med 23:156–159, 1995.
181. Grood ES: Meniscal function. Adv Orthop Surg 7:193–197, 1984.
182. Noble J, Diamond R, Walker G, et al.: The functional capacity of disordered menisci. J R Coll Surg Edinb 27:13–18, 1982.
183. Vangsness CT, Watson T, Saadatmanesh V, et al.: Pulsed Ho:YAG laser meniscectomy: effect of pulsewidth on tissue penetration rate and lateral thermal damage. Lasers Surg Med 16:61–65, 1995.
184. Goble EM, Kane SM, Wilcox TR, et al.: Advanced arthroscopic instrumentation. In McGinty JB (ed.): Operative Arthroscopy, 2nd ed. Philadelphia, Lippincott-Raven, 1996, pp 7–12.
185. Advisory statements: use of lasers in orthopaedic surgery. Bull Am Acad Orthop Surg 41:4, 1993.
186. Prodoehl JA, Rhodes ALB, Cummings RS, et al.: 308 nm excimer laser ablation of cartilage. Lasers Surg Med 15:263–268, 1994.
187. Dillingham MF, Price JM, and Fanton GS: Lasers in orthopedic surgery. Orthopedics 16:563–566, 1993.
188. Garino JP, Lotke PA, Sapega AA, et al.: Osteonecrosis of the knee diagnosed following laser-assisted arthroscopic interventions. Presented at the 62nd Annual Meeting of the American Academy of Orthopaedic Surgeons, Orlando, Fla., Feb. 1995.
189. Sherk HH, Lane GJ, and Black JD: Laser arthroscopy. Orthop Rev 21:1077–1083, 1992.
190. Sisto DJ, Blazina ME, and Hirsh LC: The synovial response after CO_2 laser arthroscopy of the knee. Arthroscopy 9:574–575, 1993.
191. Fink B, Schneider T, Braunstein S, et al.: Holmium:YAG laser–induced aseptic bone necroses of the femoral condyle. Arthroscopy 12:217–223, 1996.
192. Spivak JM, Grande DA, Ben-Yishay A, et al.: The effect of low-level Nd:YAG laser energy on adult articular cartilage in vitro. Arthroscopy 8:36–43, 1992.
193. Smith RL, Montgomery L, Fanton G, et al.: Effects of laser energy on diarthrodial joint tissues: articular cartilage and synovial cell metabolism. In Brillhart AT (ed.): Arthroscopic Laser Surgery: Clinical Applications. New York, Springer-Verlag, 1995, pp 27–31.
194. Brillhart AT: Fibrocartilaginous repair following 2.1 μm holmium:YAG irradiation of human degenerative hyaline cartilage: case report. In Brillhart AT (ed.): Arthroscopic Laser Surgery: Clinical Applications. New York, Springer-Verlag, 1995, pp 33–35.
195. Mooar P: 2.1 μm holmium:YAG arthroscopic laser débridement of degenerative knees: 148 cases. In Brillhart AT (ed.): Arthroscopic Laser Surgery: Clinical Applications. New York, Springer-Verlag, 1995, pp 263–266.
196. Thorpe WP: 2.1 μm holmium:YAG arthroscopic laser chondroplasty: 262 cases. In Brillhart AT (ed.): Arthroscopic Laser Surgery: Clinical Applications. New York, Springer-Verlag, 1995, pp 267–268.
197. Noguchi T, Oka M, Fujino M, et al.: Repair of osteochondral defects with grafts of cultured chondrocytes: comparison of allografts and isografts. Clin Orthop 302:251–258, 1994.
198. Crabb ID, O'Keefe RJ, Puzas JE, et al.: Synergistic effect of transforming growth factor beta and fibroblast growth factor on DNA synthesis in chick growth plate chondrocytes. J Bone Miner Res 5:1105–1112, 1990.
199. Morales TI and Roberts AB: Transforming growth factor-beta regulates the metabolism of proteoglycans in bovine cartilage organ cultures. J Biol Chem 263:12828–12831, 1988.
200. Trippei SB, Wroblewski J, Makower AM, et al.: Regulation of growth-plate chondrocytes by insulin-like growth factor I and basic fibroblast growth factor. J Bone Joint Surg Am 75:177–189, 1993.
201. Goldberg VM and Caplan AI: Biological resurfacing: an alternative to total joint arthroplasty. Orthopedics 17:819–821, 1994.
202. Wakitani S, Goto T, Pineda SJ, et al.: Mesenchymal cell-based repair of large, full-thickness defects of articular cartilage. J Bone Joint Surg Am 76:579–592, 1994.
203. Vacanti CA, Kim WS, Schloo B, et al.: Joint resurfacing with cartilage grown in situ from cell-polymer structures. Am J Sports Med 22:485–488, 1994.
204. Hommga GN, Bulstra SK, Bouwmeester PS, et al.: Perichondrial grafting for cartilage lesions of the knee. J Bone Joint Surg Br 72:1003–1007, 1990.
205. Kreder HJ, Moran M, Keeley FW, et al.: Biologic resurfacing of a major joint defect with cryopreserved allogeneic periosteum under the influence of continuous passive motion in a rabbit model. Clin Orthop 300:288–296, 1994.
206. O'Driscoll SW, Keeley FW, and Salter RB: Durability of regenerated articular cartilage produced by free autogenous periosteal grafts in major full-thickness defects in joint surfaces under the influence of continuous passive motion: a follow-up report at one year. J Bone Joint Surg Am 70:595–606, 1988.
207. Aston JE and Bentley G: Repair of articular surface by allografts of articular and growth-plate cartilage. J Bone Joint Surg Br 68:29–35, 1986.
208. Garrett J: Treatment of osteochondral defects of the distal femur with fresh osteochondral allografts: a preliminary report. Arthroscopy 2:222–226, 1986.

209. Meyers MH, Akeson W, and Convery R: Resurfacing of the knee with fresh osteochondral allograft. J Bone Joint Surg Am 71: 704–713, 1989.

210. Albrigo JL, Branche GC, Tremaine MD, et al.: A prospective study of thrombophlebitis in the knee arthroscopy patient. Presented at the 62nd Annual Meeting of the American Academy of Orthopaedic Surgeons, Orlando, Fla., Feb., 1995.

211. Williams JS Jr, Hulstyn MJ, Lindy P, et al.: Deep vein thrombosis after arthroscopic and anterior cruciate ligament reconstructive surgery: a prospective study. Presented at the 61st Annual Meeting of the American Academy of Orthopaedic Surgeons, New Orleans, Feb., 1994.

212. DeLee JC: Complications of arthroscopy and arthroscopic surgery: results of a national survey. Arthroscopy 1:214–220, 1985.

213. Kozinn SC and Scott RD: Surgical treatment of unicompartmental degenerative arthritis of the knee. Rheum Dis Clin North Am 14:545–565, 1988.

27

Synovial Lesions of the Knee

James R. Andrews • *Kurt C. Schluntz*

RHEUMATOID ARTHRITIS

Of the disease processes involving the synovium of the knee, the most common is rheumatoid arthritis. Rheumatoid arthritis is a pathologic process of unknown cause that creates pain and disability owing to its effects on synovial joints, the synovium being its primary target. The synovium, normally a single cell layer thick, becomes hypertrophied and edematous; inflammatory cells become prominent and active. These cells, triggered by complement components, antibody antigen complexes, and other chemotactic factors, release degradative enzymes that lead to destruction of normal bone, articular cartilage, and other tissues[1-8] (Fig. 27-1).

The hallmark of destruction in rheumatoid arthritis is the pannus, a proliferation of synovial inflammatory cells and fibroblasts. The pannus is an aggressive, locally destructive synovial tissue that directly invades and destroys bone and cartilage along the synovial margins. Treatment of rheumatoid arthritis, therefore, is aimed at controlling the inflammatory process of the synovium as a whole and the more locally aggressive rheumatoid pannus.

Medical treatment, ranging from nonsteroidal antiinflammatory drugs to cytotoxic chemotherapeutic agents, is the first line of defense in rheumatoid arthritis. Controversy exists, however, as to the appropriate treatment of rheumatoid arthritis that is refractory to medical management. Historically, an open synovectomy was the recommended procedure for rheumatoid arthritis that had failed 6 months of medical management. Currently, arthroscopic synovectomy has become more popular owing to its lower morbidity. Other major advantages of arthroscopic synovectomy include cost (it is performed on an outpatient basis), decreased risk of infection, and no loss of motion.[6, 8-11]

Indications and Contraindications

Indications for synovectomy include chronic effusions and a thickened synovium that has failed to improve after 6 months of medical treatment, stage I or stage II disease as defined by the Arthritis Foundation (minimal joint space destruction),[1] and a near-normal range of motion (less than 20 degrees of flexion contracture). Unfortunately, many patients are not considered for synovectomy until their disease has progressed to a point at which joint destruction is too far advanced for synovectomy to have any significant effect. Advanced joint destruction and deformity (stage IV rheumatoid arthritis) should be considered the main contraindications to synovectomy, as many studies have shown no significant benefit in this group of patients.[4, 5, 7, 12-15]

Operative Technique: Arthroscopic Synovectomy

As with open synovectomy, the goal is to remove as much synovium as possible in both the anterior and posterior compartments. Traditionally, the posterior compartment has been the most difficult to treat, requiring a posterior incision, but the advent of arthroscopic synovectomy has made this task easier.[6, 8, 16] Arthroscopic synovectomy generally requires from four to six portals. The procedure should be performed with the patient under tourniquet, and a pressure volume pump providing high flow is beneficial. A combination of synovial resectors is used. Synovial resection should be carried out in a systematic fashion. A useful technique is shown in Figures 27-2, 27-3, and 27-4.[17]

In step 1 the arthroscope is placed in the standard anterolateral portal, with the synovial resector placed in the lateral suprapatellar portal. This allows removal of synovium from the suprapatellar pouch and gutter. In step 2 the arthroscope remains in the anterolateral portal, and the synovial resector is introduced into the anteromedial portal, allowing resection from the intercondylar notch, the medial gutter, and the menisci. In step 3 the arthroscope is placed in the anteromedial portal, with the synovial resector in the anterolateral portal, allowing further work on the intercondylar notch, the menisci, and the lat-

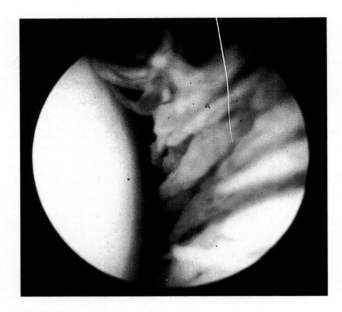

Figure 27–1 • Hypertrophic synovial villi in rheumatoid arthritis of the knee. (From Klein W and Jensen K-U: Arthroscopic synovectomy of the knee joint: indication, technique, and follow-up results. Arthroscopy 4:63–71, 1988.)

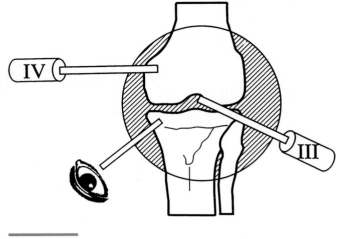

Figure 27–3 • The arthroscope (eye symbol) in the anteromedial portal. In step 3, the synovial resector is introduced through the anterolateral portal (III). In step 4, the synovial resector is introduced through the superomedial portal (IV). (From Ogilvie-Harris DJ and Saleh K: Generalized synovial chondromatosis of the knee: a comparison of removal of the loose bodies alone with arthroscopic synovectomy. Arthroscopy 10:166–170, 1994.)

eral gutter. In step 4 the synovial resector is switched to the superomedial portal, allowing further work on the medial gutter and suprapatellar pouch. Step 5, the most difficult step, involves work in the posterior compartment. With the arthroscope in the anterolateral compartment, and the surgeon visualizing through the intercondylar notch, a posteromedial portal is made at the soft spot along the posteromedial aspect of the medial femoral condyle.

This should be done by first placing the needle at the proposed portal site to ensure appropriate placement. Flexion of the knee to 90 degrees facilitates distention of the posteromedial capsule and also moves the saphenous nerve posteriorly, out of harm's way. This portal allows resection of synovium in the posteromedial compartment. Care should obviously be taken not to violate the posterior capsule while shaving.

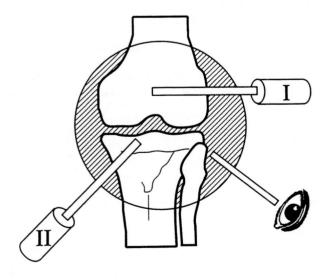

Figure 27–2 • The arthroscope (eye symbol) inserted into the anterolateral portal. In step 1, the synovial resector is introduced through the lateral suprapatellar portal (I). In step 2, the synovial resector is introduced through the anteromedial portal (II). (From Ogilvie-Harris DJ and Saleh K: Generalized synovial chondromatosis of the knee: a comparison of removal of the loose bodies alone with arthroscopic synovectomy. Arthroscopy 10:166–170, 1994.)

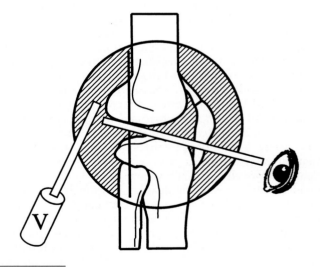

Figure 27–4 • The posterior compartments visualized diagonally across the intracondylar notch (eye symbol). The soft spot at the posterior aspect of the relevant femoral condyle is found to insert the synovial resector (V). The knee must be flexed to 90 degrees. (From Ogilvie-Harris DJ and Saleh K: Generalized synovial chondromatosis of the knee: a comparison of removal of the loose bodies alone with arthroscopic synovectomy. Arthroscopy 10:166–170, 1994.)

The posterolateral compartment is visualized with the arthroscope in the anteromedial portal. Care must be taken in making a posterolateral portal. This portal is established at the joint line posterior to the fibular collateral ligament and anterior to the biceps tendon. This placement prevents damage to the peroneal nerve. Care must also be taken when shaving posteriorly to prevent violation of the posterior capsule and thus damage to the neurovascular structures (Fig. 27–5).

Results

The literature on open synovectomy of the knee is fairly extensive, dating to 1900. Although the results are mixed, in general they have been reported to be about 75–80% good-to-excellent after 2 years, dropping to 60–70% good-to-excellent in 5 years.[4, 5, 14, 18] Several studies looking at arthroscopic synovectomy have been reported, showing similar results with less morbidity.[3, 8, 11, 19]

Recommendations to perform synovectomies only on knees without extensive joint space destruction are based on many studies. In 1966 Vainio[15] reported a series of 201 synovectomies. He had good results in patients with normal articular cartilage, but in those in stage III or later, his good-to-excellent results decreased to one-third. In 1969 Geens et al.[4, 5] also noted that results were directly related to the severity of damage to the joint found at surgery. In 1974 Laurin and colleagues[14] also found better results in patients with less extensive joint destruction, and they noted that flexion deformities of more than 15 degrees portended a poor prognosis. Two-year satisfactory results of 78% dropped to 67% at anywhere from 5 to 17 years after synovectomy. Laurin and colleagues concluded that synovectomy may have a prophylactic effect, not just a palliative effect; their studies showed that the operation appeared to have protected the knee against further damage in the presence of progressive, systemic deterioration. Many others have had similar short-term and medium-term results.

Less enthusiastic findings were reported in controlled studies published by the Arthritis and Rheumatism Council of the British Orthopaedic Association in 1976 and the Arthritis Foundation Committee on Evaluation of Synovectomy in 1977.[1, 2] The British study showed decreased pain, tenderness, and diffusion at 1–3 years but no difference in joint space narrowing. The latter study detected no significant short-term clinical improvement 3–5 years after knee synovectomy. These studies led to a decreased interest in synovectomies.

Studies evaluating the effectiveness of performing synovectomies arthroscopically have been reported. In 1987 Cohen and Jones[3] reported that 1- to 2-year results of arthroscopic synovectomy were similar to those with open procedures but with less morbidity and with an improvement in postoperative range of motion. In 1988 Klein and Jensen[6] reported on 45 knee joints, with an average follow-up period of 2.7 years, again showing results similar to those of open synovectomy but with no postoperative arthrofibrosis or decreased range of motion. In 1990 Smiley and Wasilewski[11] evaluated 25 knees that had undergone arthroscopic synovectomy. At 2 years, 90% of cases had good results, dropping to 57% at 4 years. In 1991, in the largest series to date, Ogilvie-Harris and Basinski[8] reported 2–4 year follow-up on 96 knees treated arthroscopically for rheumatoid arthritis, showing successful control of synovitis and pain. These studies all suggest that if synovectomy is indicated for control of rheumatoid arthritis, similar results with less morbidity and lower cost can be expected if the procedure is performed arthroscopically. Other options include radiation synovectomies, specifically those using short half-life agents such as dysprosium 165, as reported by Sledge et al.[20] Further studies comparing the effectiveness of these two newer techniques need to be done.

PIGMENTED VILLONODULAR SYNOVITIS

Pigmented villonodular synovitis (PVNS) is an uncommon synovial proliferative disorder that has a predilection for the knee. Before the work of Jaffee, Lichtenstein, and Sutro[21] in 1941, PVNS went under many different names and was thought to be a neoplasm. This disorder is characterized by a fibrous stroma, deposition of hemosiderin, a histiocytic infiltrate, and giant cells occurring in the synovial membrane. Most researchers believe that PVNS is an inflammatory process, but no one has been able to determine the cause.

Clinically, PVNS presents 90% of the time in the knee. The onset is insidious and usually occurs in the third or fourth decade of life. Symptoms progress slowly. Recurrent effusions occur and are usually bloody. Owing to the vague symptoms and slow progression, patients often present with a multiple-year history of knee symptoms. The annual incidence is about two cases per million.

Two variants of the disease are found in the knee: diffuse and local. The diffuse form involves multiple areas of the synovial lining; the local form is usually pedunculated but may be sessile. Grossly, specimens are often brown

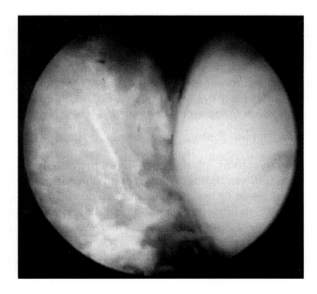

Figure 27–5 • View of subsynovial fibrotic joint capsule after arthroscopic synovectomy. (From Klein W and Jensen K-U: Arthroscopic synovectomy of the knee joint: indication, technique, and follow-up results. Arthroscopy 4:63–71, 1988.)

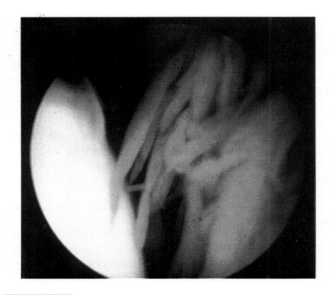

Figure 27–6 • Generalized pigmented villonodular synovitis of the knee. (From Klein W and Jensen K-U: Arthroscopic synovectomy of the knee joint: indication, technique, and follow-up results. Arthroscopy 4:63–71, 1988.)

owing to deposition of iron, but they may also be only mildly pigmented, leading to a yellowish color. The villonodular (or local) form is more often heavily pigmented (Fig. 27–6).

Traditionally, the treatment of choice for PVNS has been open synovectomy, with a total synovectomy for the diffuse form and a local excision for the local form.[22–25] Arthroscopic surgery for this disease has become the treatment of choice.[26, 27] The arthroscopic technique is the same as for rheumatoid arthritis, with local excision recommended for the local form and a total synovectomy for the diffuse form.

Results

Historically, open synovectomy for PVNS has had mixed results. The local, nodular form has responded well to excision, but the diffuse form has had a high recurrence rate, ranging 20–46%. In addition, morbidity has been high, with loss of range of motion common. Johansson and colleagues[25] noted a recurrence rate of approximately one-third (33%) in their study of 18 patients. In addition, manipulations were required postoperatively in an attempt to avoid loss of motion. Rao and Vigorita[28] reported a 21% recurrence rate, and Byers et al.[29] reported a 46% recurrence rate. These high recurrence rates have led some to try radiation synovectomy. Atmore[30] showed no difference in the recurrence rate of open synovectomy versus open synovectomy with radiation therapy. Friedman and Schwartz[10] noted a 20% recurrence rate after treating with radiation therapy alone. However, fear of radiation side effects, especially in younger patients, has decreased interest in this form of treatment.

Since the early 1990s, studies on arthroscopic synovectomy versus open synovectomy have shown improved

results, with much less morbidity. In 1991 Moskovich and Parisien[26] reported on nine patients with localized disease treated by local arthroscopic resection. At mean 48-month follow-up there was no evidence of recurrence. In 1992 Ogilvie-Harris, McLean, and Zarnett[27] reported on 25 patients followed for an average of 4.5 years after arthroscopic treatment. Five patients with localized lesions treated by local resection were improved and without recurrence on follow-up. The remaining 20 had diffuse disease; of these, 11 were treated with total arthroscopic synovectomy and 9 with partial arthroscopic synovectomy. All 11 were improved, with only one recurrence; the 9 treated with partial arthroscopic synovectomy, however, had recurrence of the disease in 5 cases. The researchers concluded, as have others, that total synovectomy remains the treatment of choice for the diffuse form of the disease and that with the advent of arthroscopic surgery a complete synovectomy of the knee joint can be performed with equal or better results and less morbidity than with open synovectomy.

SEQUESTERED SUPRAPATELLAR BURSA

A sequestered suprapatellar bursa can form when the suprapatellar plica persists as a complete septum, preventing communication with the more distal joint space. In 1994 Katz and Levinsohn[31] reported two cases of PVNS in the sequestered suprapatellar bursa. Taps of the knee produced normal results in both cases; only direct taps of the isolated bursa yielded the classic dark brown fluid of PVNS. Both cases were successfully treated by local open resection.

SYNOVIAL CHONDROMATOSIS

Synovial chondromatosis is a rare synovial, proliferative disease that most often affects the knee. Proliferative changes in the synovial membrane cause formation of multiple chondral or osteochondral loose bodies (Figs. 27–7 and 27–8). These loose bodies lead to symptoms of pain, swelling, and locking, and they can lead to joint destruction. The diagnosis is often not made until surgery because radiographs are frequently normal owing to the chondral nature of the disease; in those cases in which osteochondral loose bodies are formed or in which the chondral bodies are calcified, radiographic diagnosis can be made easily (Fig. 27–9).

Controversy exists regarding the treatment of synovial chondromatosis of the knee. Many authors think the removal of loose bodies alone is sufficient, whereas others advocate synovectomy to prevent recurrence. In 1988 Maurice, Crone, and Watt,[32] in their study of 53 cases of synovial chondromatosis, found a recurrence rate of 11.5% was about equal after either synovectomy or removal of loose bodies. Because recurrence may follow either operative technique, they stated that the aim should be to relieve symptoms rather than to be totally curative; they advocated removal of loose bodies if the complaint was of mechanical symptoms and synovectomy if pain and swelling predominated. In 1989 Coolican and Dandy[33]

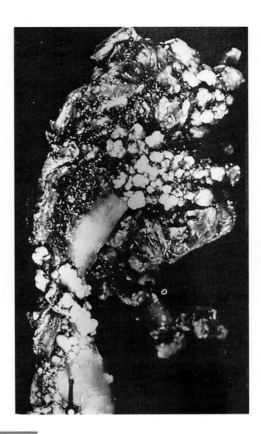

Figure 27–7 • Synovial chondromatosis: proliferating nodules on lateral meniscus and synovium. (From Milgram JW: Synovial osteochondromatosis: a histopathological study of 30 cases. J Bone Joint Surg Am 59:792–801, 1977.)

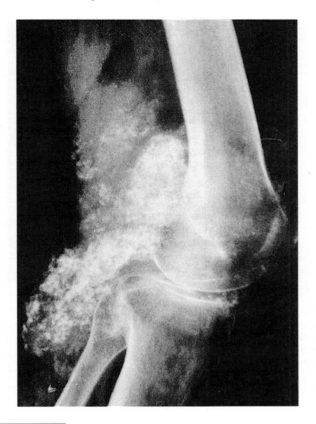

Figure 27–9 • Synovial osteochondromatosis: lateral x-ray of knee, showing large masses of cartilage with stippled calcification. (From Milgram JW: Synovial osteochondromatosis: a histopathological study of 30 cases. J Bone Joint Surg Am 59:792–801, 1977.)

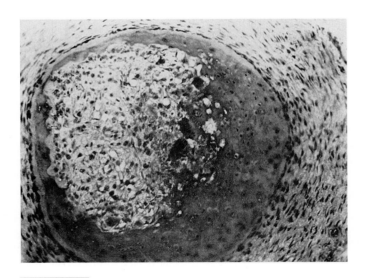

Figure 27–8 • Synovial osteochondromatosis: bone formation in a nodule within a synovial villus. (From Milgram JW: Synovial osteochondromatosis: a histopathological study of 30 cases. J Bone Joint Surg Am 59:792–801, 1977.)

reported on arthroscopic management of synovial chondromatosis of the knee. They advocated removal of any synovium appearing abnormal in addition to removal of loose bodies (Fig. 27–10).

In 1994 Ogilvie-Harris and Saleh[17] reviewed results in 13 patients treated either by removal of loose bodies or by arthroscopic synovectomy. At an average follow-up of 38 months, the authors found no recurrence in the arthroscopic synovectomy group and 60% recurrence in the other group; they therefore recommended arthroscopic synovectomy for patients with generalized synovial chondromatosis. They noted, however, that recurrence can be treated easily by secondary arthroscopic synovectomy, with no expected difference in final outcome.

INTRA-ARTICULAR GANGLIA

Intra-articular ganglia are a rare cause of pain and dysfunction in the knee. They are usually related to the origin of the cruciate ligaments and can manifest with either mechanical symptoms, such as inability to extend fully, or pain and swelling.

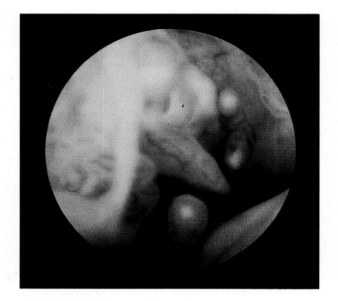

Figure 27–10 • Synovial chondromatosis on a pedicle. (From Dorfmann H, Bierman B, and Soejbergen RM: Arthroscopic treatment of synovial chondromatosis of the knee. Arthroscopy 5:48–51, 1989.)

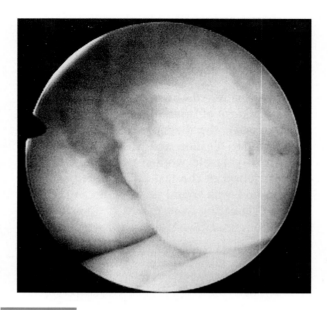

Figure 27–12 • Intra-articular ganglia of the cruciate ligaments shown on arthroscopic view. (From Deutsch A, Veltri DM, Altchek DW, et al.: Symptomatic intra-articular ganglia of the cruciate ligaments of the knee. Arthroscopy 10:219–223, 1994.)

These synovial cysts are thin-walled and are filled with a clear, viscous fluid. The pathogenesis of intra-articular ganglia is unclear, but trauma has been reported as playing a causative role. Cystic degeneration is another theoretical cause. The diagnosis can be made based on the results of magnetic resonance imaging (Figs. 27–11 and 27–12).

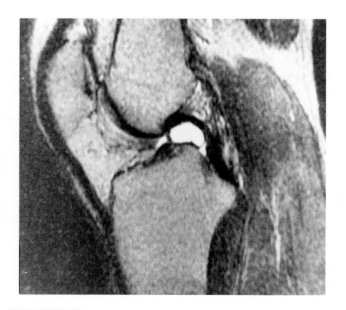

Figure 27–11 • Intra-articular ganglia of the cruciate ligaments shown by magnetic resonance imaging. (From Deutsch A, Veltri DM, Altchek DW, et al.: Symptomatic intra-articular ganglia of the cruciate ligaments of the knee. Arthroscopy 10:219–223, 1994.)

In 1990 Brown and Dandy[34] reported on 38 intra-articular ganglia, 35 of which arose at the insertion of the cruciate ligaments. Of these, 80% involved the anterior cruciate ligament. Nineteen of the ganglia were isolated findings; the remaining knees had degenerative change,[3] meniscal lesions,[29] or partial cruciate ligament tears.[30] Arthroscopic incision produced 100% good-to-excellent results in the isolated group and 89% in the nonisolated group. There were no recurrences.

SYNOVIAL HEMANGIOMA

Synovial hemangioma is a benign vascular lesion arising from synovial tissue. It is rare, and the most frequent site is the knee joint. This lesion becomes symptomatic most often before age 25.

The clinical diagnosis of synovial hemangioma is often difficult to make. Devaney, Vinh, and Sweet,[35] reviewing 20 cases, found that the clinical diagnoses proffered included PVNS (33%), bursitis (22%), hemangioma (22%), and not otherwise specified. Pathologically, this lesion was confused with PVNS 11% of the time. Clinically, most patients have symptoms of pain and swelling, with recurrent bloody effusions.

There are two types of synovial hemangioma: nodular or localized hemangioma and diffuse hemangioma. The localized form, treated by local resection, has a higher cure rate. (Arthroscopy has traditionally been helpful for diagnosis.) The treatment of both is complete resection of the involved synovium. This has traditionally been done open. As this is a benign condition, radiation therapy is not indicated. A pathologic diagnosis is essential for ruling out synovial sarcoma.

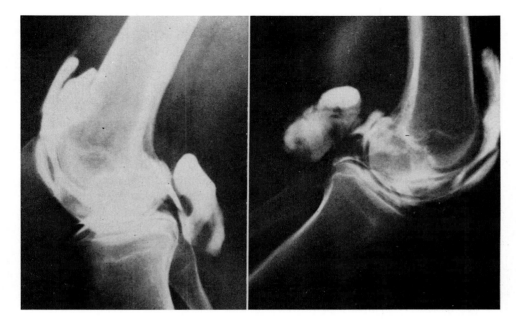

Figure 27–13 • Popliteal cysts shown on lateral arthrograms. (From Bryan RS, DiMichelle JD, and Ford GL: Popliteal cysts. Clin Orthop 50: 203–208, 1967.)

POPLITEAL CYSTS

Popliteal cysts are synovial, fluid-filled cysts usually located between the gastrocnemius semimembranosus muscles in the back of the knee. In adults these cysts most frequently communicate with the knee joint, and it is recognized that the majority are caused by intra-articular lesions, usually a meniscal tear and degenerative joint disease. Frequently the communication between the joint and the popliteal cyst acts as a one-way valve, causing accumulation of fluid in the distended popliteal cyst. This one-way flow has been shown on arthrography; injections of radio-contrast dye into the joint usually communicate with the cyst, whereas injections into the cysts rarely show reverse flow into the joint. Most of these facts were first recognized by Baker in 1877.[36]

The symptoms associated with Baker's cysts often vary, depending on the underlying cause of the cyst; however, they are often painless, with only the swelling being noticed. Some patients note stiffness secondary to the swelling. Others have pain related to underlying meniscal tears or degenerative joint disease. Popliteal cysts may also be confused with deep pain thrombosis, owing to symptoms of pain in the posterior calf.

The diagnosis of a popliteal cyst is usually made clinically. In the past arthrography was often employed to confirm the diagnosis, but magnetic resonance imaging is currently more common because it gives the most useful information on intra-articular lesions causing the secondary popliteal cysts (Fig. 27–13).

Treatment

In the past many treated popliteal cysts with open excision of the cyst. Work by Childress,[37] first reported in the 1950s, showed that meniscal tears were most often the true

lesion and that addressing the intra-articular disease, without surgical resection of the cyst, was curative. Current treatment recommendations are to treat the intra-articular disease only; the popliteal cysts almost always resolve subsequently. Rarely does a popliteal cyst need to be surgically excised.

Popliteal cysts in children differ in their pathogenesis and treatment from those of adults. Most cysts form spontaneously in the semimembranous gastrocnemius bursa. Communication between the joint and the bursa is rare in children, and intra-articular disease is not common. Most of these cysts cause minimal symptoms, and if observed, the majority resolve spontaneously within 1–2 years. Dinham[38] found 73% of untreated cysts resolved, whereas 42% of those treated with excision recurred. As in adults, if an intra-articular lesion is found, it should be addressed, but such a lesion is uncommon in children.

References

1. Arthritis Foundation Committee on Evaluation of Synovectomy: Multicenter evaluation of synovectomy in the treatment of rheumatoid arthritis: report of results at the end of three years. Arthritis Rheum 20:765–771, 1977.
2. Arthritis and Rheumatism Council and British Orthopaedic Association: Control trial of synovectomy of the knee and MCP joints in rheumatoid arthritis. Ann Rheum Dis 35:437–442, 1976.
3. Cohen S and Jones R: An evaluation of the efficacy of arthroscopic synovectomy of the knee in rheumatoid arthritis: 12 to 24 month result. J Rheumatol 14:452, 1987.
4. Geens S: Synovectomy and debridement of the knee in rheumatoid arthritis: historical review. J Bone Joint Surg Am 51:17, 1969.
5. Geens S, Clayton ML, Leidholt JD, et al.: Synovectomy and debridement of the knee in rheumatoid arthritis: clinical and roentgenographic study of 31 cases. J Bone Joint Surg Am 51:626, 1969.
6. Klein W and Jensen K-U: Arthroscopic synovectomy of the knee joint: indication, technique, and follow-up results. Arthroscopy 4:63, 1988.

7. Marmor L: Surgery of the rheumatoid knee: synovectomy and debridement. J Bone Joint Surg Am 55:535, 1973.

8. Ogilvie-Harris DJ and Basinski A: Arthroscopic synovectomy of the knee for rheumatoid arthritis. Arthroscopy 7:91, 1991.

9. Cleland LG, Treganza R, and Dobson P: Arthroscopic synovectomy: a prospective study. J Rheumatol 13:907, 1986.

10. Friedman M and Schwartz EE: A radiation therapy of pigmented villonodular synovitis. Bull Hosp Joint Dis 18:19, 1957.

11. Smiley P and Wasilewski SA: Arthroscopic synovectomy. Arthroscopy 6:18, 1990.

12. Ishikawa H, Ohno O, and Hiiohate K: Long-term results of synovectomy in rheumatoid patients. J Bone Joint Surg Am 68:198, 1986.

13. Jensen CM, Poulson S, Ostergren M, et al.: Early and late synovectomy of the knee in rheumatoid arthritis. Scand J Rheumatol 20:127, 1991.

14. Laurin CA, Desmarchais J, Daziano L, et al.: Long-term results of synovectomy of the knee in rheumatoid patients. J Bone Joint Surg Am 56:521, 1974.

15. Vainio K: Indications and contraindications for surgery in rheumatoid arthritis. Rheumatism 22:10, 1966.

16. Mack RP: Popliteal cysts. In Funk FJ (ed.): American Academy of Orthopaedic Surgeons Symposium of the Athlete's Knee: Surgical Repair and Reconstruction. St. Louis, C.V. Mosby, 1980, p 195.

17. Ogilvie-Harris DJ and Saleh K: Generalized synovial chondromatosis of the knee: a comparison of the removal of the loose bodies alone with arthroscopic synovectomy. Arthroscopy 10:166, 1994.

18. Ranawat CS, Ecker ML, and Straub LR: Synovectomy and debridement of the knee in rheumatoid arthritis (a study of 60 knees). Arthritis Rheum 15:571, 1972.

19. Shibata T, Shiraoka LK, and Takubo N: Comparison between arthroscopic and open synovectomy for the knee in rheumatoid arthritis. Arch Orthop Trauma Surg 105:257, 1986.

20. Sledge CB, Zuckerman JD, Shortkroff S, et al.: Synovectomy of the rheumatoid knee using intra-articular injection of dysprosium-165–ferric hydroxide macroaggregates. J Bone Joint Surg Am 69:970, 1987.

21. Jaffee HL, Lichtenstein L, and Sutro LJ: Pigmented villonodular synovitis. Arch Pathol 31:731, 1941.

22. Bryan RS, DiMichelle JD, and Ford GL: Popliteal cysts. Clin Orthop 50:203, 1967.

23. Flandry F and Hughston JC: Pigmented villonodular synovitis. J Bone Joint Surg Am 69:942, 1987.

24. Granowitz SP, D'Antonio J, and Mankin HL: The pathogenesis and long-term end results of pigmented villonodular synovitis. Clin Orthop 114:335, 1976.

25. Johansson JE, Ajjoub S, Coughlin LP, et al.: Pigmented villonodular synovitis of joints. Clin Orthop 163:159, 1982.

26. Moskovich R and Parisien JS: Localized pigmented villonodular synovitis of the knee: arthroscopic treatment. Clin Orthop 271:218, 1991.

27. Olgivie-Harris DJ, McLean J, and Zarnett ME: Pigmented villonodular synovitis of the knee. J Bone Joint Surg Am 74:119, 1992.

28. Rao AS and Vigorita VJ: Pigmented villonodular synovitis. J Bone Joint Surg Am 66:76, 1984.

29. Byers PD, Cotton RE, Deacon OW, et al.: The diagnosis and treatment of pigmented villonodular synovitis. J Bone Joint Surg Br 50:290–305, 1968.

30. Atmore WG, Dahlin OL, and Ghormley RK: Pigmented villonodular synovitis: a clinical and pathological study. Minn Med 39:196, 1956.

31. Katz DS and Levinsohn EM: Pigmented villonodular synovitis of the sequestered suprapatellar bursa. Clin Orthop 306:204, 1994.

32. Maurice H, Crone M, and Watt I: Synovial chondromatosis. J Bone Joint Surg Br 70:807, 1988.

33. Coolican MR and Dandy DJ: Arthroscopic management of synovial chondromatosis of the knee: findings and results in 18 cases. J Bone Joint Surg Br 71:498, 1989.

34. Brown MF and Dandy DJ: Intra-articular ganglia in the knee. Arthroscopy 6:322, 1990.

35. Devaney K, Vinh TN, and Sweet DE: Synovial hemangioma: a report of 20 cases with differential diagnostic considerations. Hum Pathol 24:737, 1993.

36. Baker WM: On the formation of synovial cysts in the leg in connection with disease of the knee joint. Reprinted Clin Orthop 299:2–10, 1994.

37. Childress HN: Popliteal cysts associated with undiagnosed posterior lesions of the medial meniscus. J Bone Joint Surg Am 52:1487, 1970.

38. Dinham JM: Popliteal cysts in children. J Bone Joint Surg Br 57:69, 1975.

Chapter

28

Anterior Cruciate Ligament Injuries

Barry Phillips

Treatment of anterior cruciate ligament (ACL) injuries requires a careful evaluation of the amount of instability present and of any associated injuries.[1–6] A thorough understanding of the patient's present vocational and recreational activity levels as well as future aspirations is necessary to formulate a rational, individualized treatment plan.[7–10]

ACL injuries are usually caused by deceleration, twisting, cutting, and jumping maneuvers or by hyperextension of the knee.[11, 12] Many patients report hearing or feeling a "pop," after which pain makes it difficult or impossible to continue their activity.[12–14] Swelling of variable severity occurs during the next few hours.[12, 15, 16]

EVALUATION

Physical examination of the injured knee should include an evaluation of the instability caused by the ACL injury, associated ligamentous injuries, and any meniscal or articular cartilage damage.[17–19]

To allow a thorough examination of an acutely injured knee, the patient must be relaxed in the supine position. A pillow should be placed under the thigh to allow the injured knee to be supported and comfortably flexed 25–30 degrees. The uninjured extremity should be examined first to determine normal values for the Lachman and McMurray tests, varus and valgus instability, patellar tracking, and posterior and posterolateral instability.[2, 5, 17, 18, 20, 21] When these parameters have been firmly established, the injured knee is examined, beginning with inspection and palpation of the extremity. Effusion is graded on a scale of 0 to 3, 1 representing slight effusion and 3 representing intense effusion.[22] Areas of tenderness are identified by palpation of the extremity along the joint line, the medial and lateral collateral ligaments, the distal femoral articular cartilage, and the parapatellar soft-tissue structures. The Lachman test is performed with the knee in 25–30 degrees of flexion.[21] To test a right knee, the examiner's left hand is placed on the anterolateral portion

of the distal thigh, and the right hand is placed on the anteromedial portion of the proximal tibia along the medial joint line to evaluate endpoint translation and quality. The Lachman test is graded from 0 to 3 as compared with the grading of the uninjured extremity (Fig. 28–1). The endpoint is graded as soft or firm.[21, 22]

Varus and valgus laxity is checked with the knee in 0 degrees and in 30 degrees of flexion[5, 17, 18]; to evaluate the amount of shift, a gentle flexion rotation drawer test is performed with the hip abducted, the foot slightly rotated externally, and a mild valgus stress applied as the knee is moved from 0 to 50 degrees of flexion.[3, 16, 19, 23–26] Ligamentous instability is graded from 1 to 3, as mild, moderate, and severe as described by the International Knee Documentation Committee[22] (see Fig. 28–1).

A patellar apprehension test is performed to make sure that no extensor mechanism injury or patellar subluxation is associated with the acute knee injury. After patellar tracking and apprehension are evaluated, anterior and posterior drawer tests are performed with the knee in 90 degrees of flexion and the foot in neutral, internal, and external rotation.[5, 13, 19, 27] The quadriceps active test is performed by having the patient place the foot flat on the examining table, then extending the knee against resistance.[28] Anterior displacement of the tibia indicates a posterior sag in the resting position. This is substantiated further by the Godfrey 90 degree sag test.[29] Posterolateral laxity is determined with the knee flexed 30 degrees. The outside of the examiner's hand is placed around the anterolateral portion of the proximal tibia, with the fingers behind the head of the fibula. The degrees and endpoint of external rotation are identified and compared with those of the opposite extremity.[5, 30] A side-to-side 15 degree increase in external rotation indicates a significant posterolateral corner injury.[31] The reverse pivot and external rotation recurvatum tests are also helpful when evaluating posterolateral insufficiency.[31]

Among patients with acute hemarthrosis, over 70% have an acute ACL tear.[15, 16, 32–35] A 3+ hemarthrosis should be aspirated, and 10 mL of 1% lidocaine should be

1993
THE IKDC KNEE LIGAMENT STANDARD EVALUATION FORM

Patient Name _____ Date _____ / _____ / _____ Medical Record # _____

Occupation _____ Sport: 1st Choice _____ 2nd Choice _____

Age _____ Sex _____ Ht _____ Wt _____ Involved Knee: ☐ Right ☐ Left Contralateral Normal: ☐ Yes ☐ No

Cause of Injury: Date of Injury: ___ / ___ / ___   Procedure _____
☐ ADL   ☐ Traffic
☐ Contact   ☐ Noncontact   Date of Index Operation: ___ / ___ / ___   Postop Dx _____

ACTIVITY

	Pre-injury	Pre-Rx	Post-Rx
I. Strenuous Activity jumping, pivoting, hard cutting (football, soccer)			
II. Moderate Activity heavy manual work (skiing, tennis)			
III. Light Activity light manual work (jogging, running)			
IV. Sedentary Activity (housework, ADL)			

Eventual change knee related: ☐ Yes ☐ No

PREVIOUS SURGERY

Arthroscopy: Date (1) _____ (2) _____ (3) _____

Meniscectomy: Dx _____ _____ _____

Stabilization: Procedure _____ _____ _____

MENISCAL STATUS

	N1	1/3	2/3	Total
Med				
Lat				

Morphotype: Lax ——
Normal —— Tight ——
Knee: Varus——
Normal —— Valgus ——

EIGHT GROUPS

1. Patient Subjective Assessment
How does your knee function?
On a scale of 0 to 3, how does your
knee affect your activity level?
2. SYMPTOMS
(Grade at highest activity level
with no significant symptoms.
Exclude 0 to slight symptoms.)
    Pain
    Swelling
    Partial Giving Way
    Full Giving Way
3. Range of Motion Ext/Flex: Index side:
Lack of extension (from 0°)
△ Lack of flexion
4. Ligament Evaluation
(manual, instrumented, x-ray)
△ LACKMAN (25° flex)

  Endpoint: firm/soft
△ Total A.P. Transl. (70° flex)
△ Post. sag(70° flex)
△ Med jt opening(20° flex)(valgus rot)
△ Lat jt opening(20° flex)(varus rot)
△ Pivot shift
△ Reverse pivot shift
5. Compartmental Findings
△ Crepitus patellofemoral
△ Crepitus medial compartment
△ Crepitus lateral compartment
6. Harvest Sight Pathology
7. X-Ray Findings
    Med Joint space
    Lat Joint space
    Patellofemoral
8. Functional Test
One leg hop (% of opposite side)

**FINAL EVALUATION

FOUR GRADES / *GROUP GRADE

	A. Normal	B. Nearly Normal	C. Abnormal	D. Sev. Abnorm.	A	B	C	D
	☐ 0	☐ 1	☐ 2	☐ 3				
	☐ 0	☐ 1	☐ 2	☐ 3	☐	☐	☐	☐
	I. Strenuous Activity	II. Moderate Activity	III. Light Activity	IV. Sedentary Activity				
Pain	☐	☐	☐	☐				
Swelling	☐	☐	☐	☐				
Partial Giving Way	☐	☐	☐	☐				
Full Giving Way	☐	☐	☐	☐	☐	☐	☐	☐
(Ext/Flex)	——/——/	Opposite side:	——/——/					
Lack of extension	☐ < 3°	☐ 3 to 5°	☐ 6 to 10°	☐ <10°	☐	☐	☐	☐
Lack of flexion	☐ 0 to 5°	☐ 6 to 15°	☐ 16 to 15°	☐ >25°				
LACKMAN	☐ −1 to 2mm	☐ 3 to 5mm <-1 to -3 stiff	☐ 6 to 10mm <-3 stiff	☐ >10mm				
Endpoint	☐ firm		☐ soft	☐ >10mm				
Total A.P. Transl.	☐ 0 to 2mm	☐ 3 to 5mm	☐ 6 to 10mm	☐ >10mm				
Post. sag	☐ 0 to 2mm	☐ 3 to 5mm	☐ 6 to 10mm	☐ >10mm				
Med jt opening	☐ 0 to 2mm	☐ 3 to 5mm	☐ 6 to 10mm	☐ >10mm				
Lat jt opening	☐ 0 to 2mm	☐ 3 to 5mm	☐ 6 to 10mm	☐ +++ (gross)				
Pivot shift	☐ equal	☐ + (glide)	☐ ++ (clunk)	☐ gross				
Reverse pivot shift	☐ equal	☐ glide	☐ marked		☐	☐	☐	☐
Crepitus patellofemoral	☐ none	☐ moderate	☐ mild pain (crepitation with)	☐ >mild pain (crepitation with)				
Crepitus medial compartment	☐ none	☐ moderate	☐ mild pain	☐ >mild pain				
Crepitus lateral compartment	☐ none	☐ moderate	☐ mild pain	☐ >mild pain				
Harvest Sight Pathology	☐ none	☐ mild	☐ moderate	☐ severe				
Med Joint space	☐ none	☐ mild	☐ moderate	☐ severe				
Lat Joint space	☐ none	☐ mild	☐ moderate	☐ severe				
Patellofemoral	☐ none	☐ mild	☐ moderate	☐ severe				
One leg hop	☐ ≥90%	☐ 89% to 76%	☐ 79% to 50%	☐ <50%				
FINAL EVALUATION					☐	☐	☐	☐

*Group Grade: The lowest grade within a group determines the group grade. **Final Evaluation: The worst group grade determines the final evaluation for acute and subacute patients. For chronic patients compare preoperative and postoperative evaluations. In a final evaluation, only the first 4 groups are evaluated but all groups must be documented.
△ Difference in involved knee compared to normal or what is assumed to be normal.

IKDC–INTERNATIONAL KNEE DOCUMENTATION COMMITTEE, Members of the Committee:
AOSSM: Anderson, AF, Clancy, WG, Daniel, D, Dehaven, KE, Fowler, PJ, Feagin, J, Grood, ES, Noyes, FR, Terry, GC, Torzilli, P, Warren, RF.
ESKA: Chambat, P, Eriksson, E, Gillquist, J, Hefti, F, Huiskes, R, Jakob, RP, Moyen, B, Mueller, W, Staeubli, H, Vankampen, A.

Figure 28–1 • The Knee Ligament Standard Evaluation Form. (With permission of the International Knee Documentation Committee of the American Orthopaedic Society for Sports Medicine and the European Society for Knee Surgery and Arthroscopy.)

Figure 28–2 • Magnetic resonance imaging may be indicated for acute ACL injuries in some patients.

Indications for MRI

- Inability to determine extent of ligamentous injury

- Meniscal evaluation if conservative treatment is anticipated

- Persistent joint pain or swelling after surgery; evaluate for osteochondral lesion or graft impingement

- Repeat MRI before progressing to impact-loading exercises if occult geographic lesion was present on original MRI and symptoms persist during rehabilitation

- Insurance agreement

injected into the joint to decrease the discomfort and allow better examination of the knee. If an adequate examination still cannot be performed, the knee is re-examined after 5–7 days of conservative therapy for swelling and inflammation.

Magnetic resonance imaging (MRI) is indicated for evaluation of acute knee injuries in some circumstances (Fig. 28–2).[36, 37]

TREATMENT

ACL reconstruction using an autogenous fascia as a graft was first described by Hey Groves[38] in 1917. Reconstruction using the medial portion of the patellar tendon was introduced by Campbell[39, 40] in 1936. Advances in reconstruction techniques were made by Jones,[41–43] who used a patellar bone plug and central third of the patellar tendon, and by Clancy and colleagues,[44–46] who used bone-patellar tendon-bone (BPTB) grafts in eccentrically placed tunnels. The efficacy of ACL reconstructive procedures has steadily increased, and morbidity has decreased. Arthroscopic techniques continue to be modified, concentrating on physiometric and impingement-free placement of the graft.[13, 47–51]

Advances in rehabilitation techniques have resulted in more aggressive conservative and surgical management of ACL-deficient knees.[52–55] With increased knowledge of the natural course of an ACL-deficient knee, treatment decisions can be based on the needs and circumstances of the individual patient (Table 28–1). [4–10, 56–64]

Partial ACL Tears

A partial ACL injury may present as a subclinical, minimally symptomatic partial ACL tear or a tear with significant plastic deformation of the remaining ACL structure.[65–68] Each of these injuries requires a different treatment approach, and the surgical risk factors, outlined by Daniel and Fithian (see Table 28–1),[7] should be considered carefully. For competitive athletes, a KT-1000

arthrometer examination may complement a thorough ligamentous examination.[1, 69, 70] If the patient's history raises suspicion, a partial tear may be evaluated by MRI. Partial tears in highly competitive athletes also should be evaluated by clinical ligamentous examination and arthroscopic examination with the use of general anesthesia.[7, 8, 71, 72]

A 10–12 week rehabilitation program before returning to competitive sports can be effective if KT-1000 testing reveals less than 3 mm of side-to-side difference, Lachman and pivot shift test results are normal on examination with anesthesia, and arthroscopic examination reveals damage to less than 25% of the ligament, with the remainder of the ligaments appearing taut and without visible damage.[7, 8, 73] If instability is present, as indicated by abnormal pivot shift or Lachman test results or by a KT-1000 difference of more than 5 mm, surgical reconstruction should be considered.[7–9, 60, 71, 73, 74]

All patients with ACL-deficient knees should be aggressively treated with either an activity-specific rehabilitation program or an ACL reconstruction, followed by early, progressive, patient-specific rehabilitation.[9, 59–61, 75–77] The most important predictive factor for recurrent knee problems is the total number of hours per year of levels I and II sports participation before injury (see Fig.

Table 28–1 | **Surgical Risk Factor***

KT-1000 Arthrometer Manual Maximum I–N	Sports Hours per Year (Level I or II)		
	<50	*50–199*	*≥200*
<5	Low	Low	Moderate
5–7	Low	Moderate	High
>7	Moderate	High	High

*The risk of meniscal or ligament surgery more than 90 days after index injury in the early KT unstable population. The KT-1000 measurements were performed in the clinic within 14 days of injury. (From Daniel DM, Stone ML, Dobson BE, et al.: Fate of the ACL-injured patient. Am J Sports Med 22:639, 1994.)

28–1).[6–8] Associated injuries, especially reparable meniscal injuries and posterolateral complex injuries, should be treated surgically.[16, 78, 79] The patient should thoroughly understand the rehabilitation process and should have confidence in the rehabilitation team.

Children and Adolescents

Skeletally immature patients with ACL injuries present a perplexing problem, and treatment should be based on social and physiologic maturity.[11, 80] Children tend to have problems with instability because of noncompliance with activity restrictions and progressive stretching of secondary restraints.[11, 14, 81, 82] Treatment decisions are based on evaluation of Tanner sexual characteristics, presence of growth spurt, height relative to siblings and parents, and roentgenographic appearance of the physis.[11, 80–84] In girls, the distal femoral and proximal tibial physes close generally around the age of 14 years or within 2 years of menses, and in boys at 15 years of age or older.[85, 86] In preteen children, bone age should be determined by wrist radiographs (Gruelich and Pyle[85] method) (Fig. 28–3).

Psychological maturity is also important in the long-term treatment of adolescents. Careful preparation before surgery helps adolescents understand the rehabilitation process and allows a period of bonding with and acceptance of the rehabilitation team.

Conservative treatment is emphasized for skeletally immature patients.[3, 11, 80–82, 87, 88] Reduced activity, bracing, exercising, and education may decrease the giving-way episodes and help preserve articular and meniscal functions.[86] If conservative treatment fails, however, intraarticular reconstruction using a soft-tissue graft, preferably an autogenous hamstring graft, placed through a central drill hole in the tibia and over the top of the femur, has been shown to produce good functional results with little or no effect on the physes (Figs. 28–4 and 28–5).[14, 80, 83, 89]

In all patients, meniscal functions should be preserved whenever possible[90–94]; MRI or arthroscopic examination may be necessary to determine the status of the menisci.[16, 36, 37, 94] If conservative treatment is chosen, the child and the parents must understand the importance of compliance with activity restrictions (see Fig. 28–3). A period of bracing may be helpful for protecting associated ligamentous injuries, but long-term functional stability with bracing is questionable.[4, 95–97]

Surgical stabilization is generally indicated for joint instability in patients near skeletal maturity, and the technique is the same as for adult patients.[11, 81, 82, 84, 89] Phy-

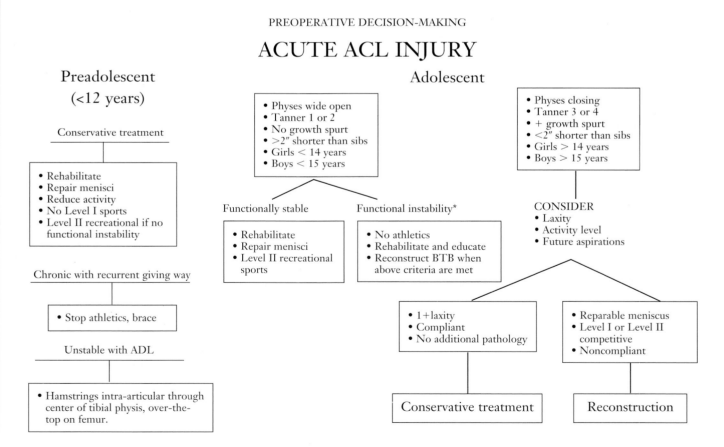

PREOPERATIVE DECISION-MAKING

ACUTE ACL INJURY

Preadolescent (<12 years)

Conservative treatment

- Rehabilitate
- Repair menisci
- Reduce activity
- No Level I sports
- Level II recreational if no functional instability

Chronic with recurrent giving way

- Stop athletics, brace

Unstable with ADL

- Hamstrings intra-articular through center of tibial physis, over-the-top on femur.

Adolescent

- Physes wide open
- Tanner 1 or 2
- No growth spurt
- >2″ shorter than sibs
- Girls < 14 years
- Boys < 15 years

Functionally stable
- Rehabilitate
- Repair menisci
- Level II recreational sports

Functional instability*
- No athletics
- Rehabilitate and educate
- Reconstruct BTB when above criteria are met

- Physes closing
- Tanner 3 or 4
- + growth spurt
- <2″ shorter than sibs
- Girls > 14 years
- Boys > 15 years

CONSIDER
- Laxity
- Activity level
- Future aspirations

- 1+laxity
- Compliant
- No additional pathology

- Reparable meniscus
- Level I or Level II competitive
- Noncompliant

Conservative treatment

Reconstruction

* Functional instability indicates repeat episodes of complete or partial giving way

Figure 28–3 • Treatment algorithm for ACL injuries in children and adolescents.

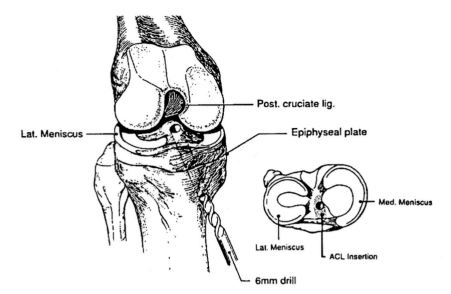

Figure 28–4 • Technique for ACL allograft reconstruction in skeletally immature patients. A 7-mm hole is drilled through the anteromedial aspect of the tibia, passing through the center of the tibial physis in a perpendicular fashion slightly posterior to the anatomic ACL insertion. (From Andrews A, Noyes FR, and Barber-Westin SD: Anterior cruciate ligament allograft reconstruction in the skeletally immature athlete. Am J Sports Med 22:50, 1994.)

seal abnormalities have not been clinically significant after ACL reconstruction in older adolescents.[11, 14, 80, 82, 89]

Adults

In adult patients (16 to 40 years of age) with ACL injuries, surgical risk factors (see Fig. 28–3) should be determined before making treatment recommendations (Fig. 28–6).[6–8, 62] Shelbourne and others[98–101] showed that ACL reconstruction can be performed successfully in patients with chronic instability and mild-to-moderate degenerative joint changes; functional scores are improved despite previous partial medial or lateral meniscectomies. Patients with more severe degenerative changes and primary complaints of pain and swelling should be treated with a non-impact strengthening program.[98]

In an ACL-deficient knee with medial joint space narrowing, varus alignment, and a varus thrust caused by lateral joint opening (double varus knee), successful treatment may depend on correction of gait abnormalities.[102, 103] Noyes et al.[103] stressed the importance of careful gait analysis, combined with analysis of the tibiofemoral alignment, in this patient group. Patients with "double varus" and "triple varus" (double varus plus excessive recurvatum caused by arcuate ligament complex laxity) are treated operatively if conservative therapy fails to decrease symptoms of pain, swelling, and instability that may lead to rapid deterioration of the joint.[102, 103] These patients should have the gait abnormality corrected by therapy that stresses a partially flexed knee gait before surgical intervention.[99, 103] If indicated by symptoms and varus alignment, lateral closing wedge osteotomy may be performed. A staged ACL reconstruction may be performed if symp-

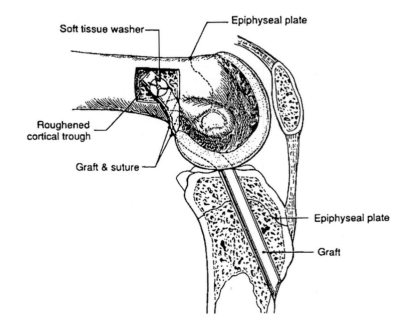

Figure 28–5 • Technique for ACL allograft reconstruction in skeletally immature patients. Over-the-top position in the lateral femoral condyle, with elevation of periosteal "H" flaps and roughening of the femoral cortical trough. (From Andrews A, Noyes FR, and Barber-Westin SD: Anterior cruciate ligament allograft reconstruction in the skeletally immature athlete. Am J Sports Med 22:50, 1994.)

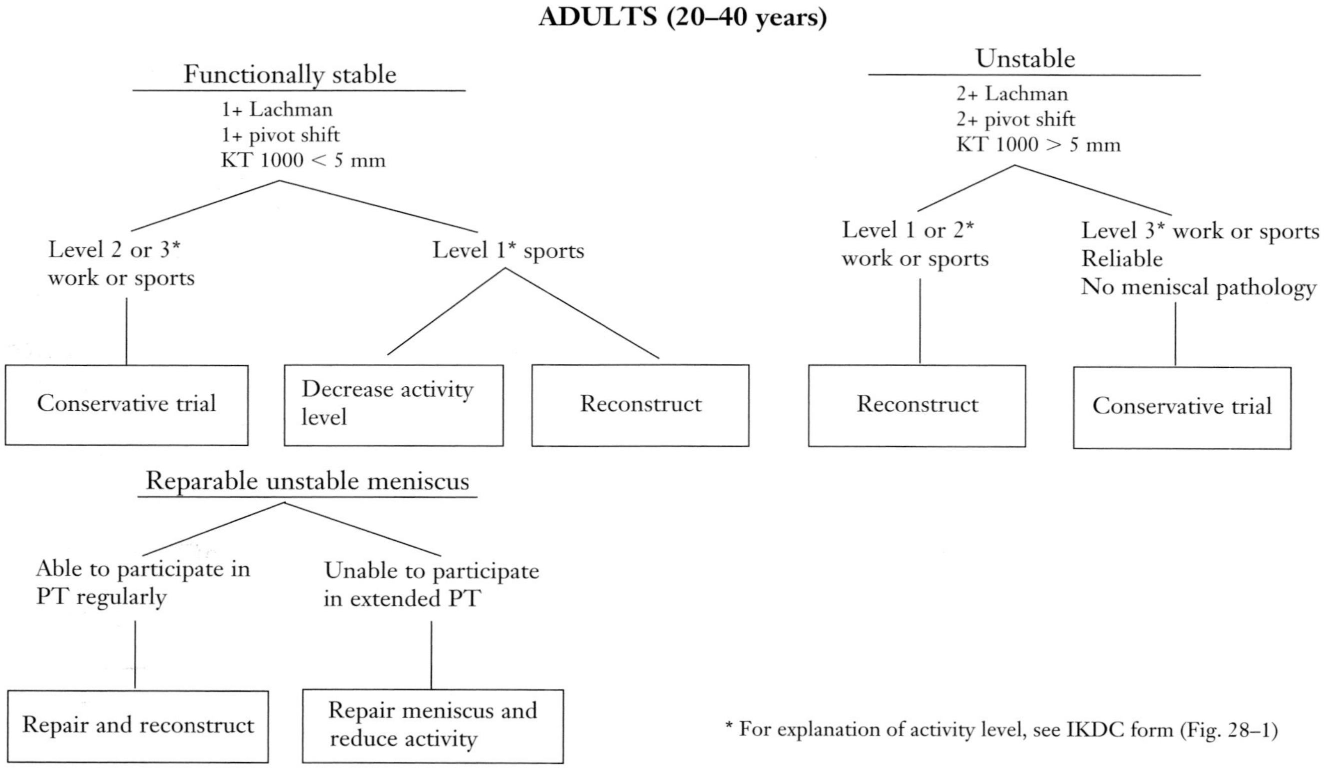

ADULTS (20–40 years)

Functionally stable
1+ Lachman
1+ pivot shift
KT 1000 < 5 mm

Unstable
2+ Lachman
2+ pivot shift
KT 1000 > 5 mm

Level 2 or 3* work or sports

Level 1* sports

Level 1 or 2* work or sports

Level 3* work or sports
Reliable
No meniscal pathology

Conservative trial

Decrease activity level

Reconstruct

Reconstruct

Conservative trial

Reparable unstable meniscus

Able to participate in PT regularly

Unable to participate in extended PT

Repair and reconstruct

Repair meniscus and reduce activity

* For explanation of activity level, see IKDC form (Fig. 28–1)

Figure 28–6 • Treatment algorithm for ACL injuries in patients 20–40 years of age.

toms warrant after correction of alignment and completion of extensive rehabilitation (Fig. 28–7).[56, 102]

Associated Injuries

Meniscus

The importance of preserving meniscal functions cannot be overemphasized.[79, 104] These functions include load transmission, joint stabilization, joint nutrition, and joint lubrication.[90, 105] Disruption of these meniscal functions has been shown to lead to progressive joint deterioration.[64, 90–94, 106–108] Meniscal healing has been reported to be best when ACL reconstruction is performed concurrently with the meniscal repair.[78, 79, 104, 105, 109, 110] Shelbourne and colleagues[101] reported decreased likelihood of arthrofibrosis when a staged meniscal repair-rehabilitation-ACL reconstruction program was followed. This author's approach is to perform the meniscal repair and ligament reconstruction at a single surgical setting, thus avoiding a second anesthesia.

Medial Collateral Ligament

A medial collateral ligament tear in association with an acute ACL tear may be treated conservatively when the knee is stabilized by ACL reconstruction.[57, 111–114] Mild, asymptomatic valgus laxity may persist, but the chance of arthrofibrosis decreases.[111, 114] If the medial opening to valgus stress is more than 1 cm with the knee extended,

significant posterior oblique and posterior capsular injury is present; the injury should be carefully re-evaluated after arthroscopic ACL reconstruction at 7–10 days when the capsule has sealed and inflammatory response has decreased.[19, 30, 57, 111, 114] If more than 1+ laxity in extension persists after ACL reconstruction, open repair of the medial collateral ligament and posteromedial corner is indicated.[57, 111, 112] Some authors recommend that the medial structures be repaired surgically to seal the joint before arthroscopic ACL reconstruction.[115] Whether the medial structures are surgically repaired or not, full range-of-motion exercises are stressed, making sure that full extension is accomplished. A brace to prevent valgus stress to the knee should be used in the early weeks of rehabilitation.[109, 112]

Posterolateral Corner

Early ACL reconstruction is indicated for an associated acute posterolateral corner injury.[31, 116, 117] Best results with posterolateral injuries are obtained with early repair.[118, 119] Failure to stabilize this injury results in a gait abnormality that produces a varus thrust (lateral compartment opening). This produces a high tensile stress on the ACL graft and will likely doom it.[103, 118, 120]

Extra-Articular Procedures

Procedures using the iliotibial band tenodesis alone or in combination with an intra-articular reconstruction have

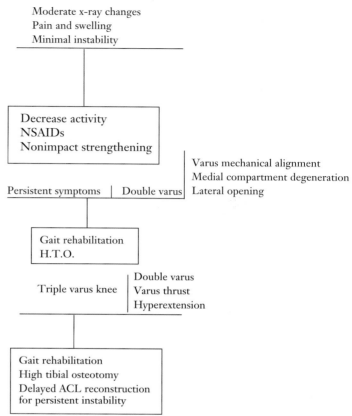

ADULTS (>40 years)

ACUTE ACL INJURY

Mild to moderate x-ray changes
(standing 30°–45° PA view)

Treat according to surgical
risk factors in Table 28–1
• Age
• Activity level
• Instability level
• Aspirations
• Ability to complete physical
  therapy

CHRONIC ACL INJURY

Moderate x-ray changes
Pain and swelling
Minimal instability

Decrease activity
NSAIDs
Nonimpact strengthening

Varus mechanical alignment
Medial compartment degeneration
Lateral opening

Persistent symptoms | Double varus

Gait rehabilitation
H.T.O.

Triple varus knee | Double varus
Varus thrust
Hyperextension

Gait rehabilitation
High tibial osteotomy
Delayed ACL reconstruction
for persistent instability

Figure 28–7 • Treatment algorithm for ACL injuries in patients older than 40 years of age.

been shown to increase morbidity, lateral knee pain, and loss of motion without producing increased long-term functional stability.[121–124]

Timing of Reconstruction

Early ACL reconstruction has been shown to be a contributing factor in the development of arthrofibrosis.[64, 101, 125–127] Surgery should be performed when the acute inflammation has resolved, motion has been regained, and quadriceps function has been restored (no extension lag). Surgery can be scheduled to accommodate school or work routines, and the athlete's schedule of future competitive events should be considered.[11]

CONSERVATIVE TREATMENT

Conservative treatment of an acute ACL injury can be divided into three phases, usually extending throughout a 10- to 14-week period:

• Phase 1: Inflammatory stage; treatment aimed at decreasing inflammation and regaining range of motion and quadriceps tone.

• Phase 2: Strengthening, with emphasis on closed-chain exercises.

• Phase 3: Sport-specific rehabilitation, working on increased balance and reflexes and avoiding subluxation episodes (see ACL rehabilitation protocol, Fig. 28–3). The rehabilitation protocol may be accelerated according to the patient's overall fitness, desired goals, and amount of soft-tissue inflammation.

SURGICAL TREATMENT

Surgical treatment of an ACL-deficient knee allows early progressive, patient-specific rehabilitation, but it is not without risks.[4, 124, 127–133] Early surgical failure may result from loss of fixation, graft impingement, or nonisometric graft position.[4, 44, 47, 51, 106, 127, 128, 131, 133–135] Strong grafts correctly placed and firmly secured help avoid many early complications.[130, 131] Noyes et al.[136] found that the central 14 mm of the patellar tendon has more than adequate strength to replace the normal ACL (Table 28–2). A 10-mm graft is initially stronger (approximately 120%) than the normal ACL and probably regains more than 80% of the ACL's original strength during a 6-month

Table 28–2 **Maximum Loads for the Human Anterior Cruciate Ligament and Its Replacements***

	Maximum Load (N)	Percent of Anterior Cruciate	Maximum Load/ Unit Width (N/mm)	Maximum Stress (MPa)
Measured values				
Anterior cruciate ligament-bone (n = 6)[†]	1725 ± 269	100	[†]	37.8 ± 3.8
Bone-patellar tendon-bone				
Central third (n = 7)	2900 ± 260[‡]	168	208 ± 24	58.3 ± 6.1[‡]
Medial third (n = 7)	2734 ± 298[‡]	159	162 ± 13	56.7 ± 4.4[‡]
Semitendinosus (n = 11)	1216 ± 50	70	[†]	88.5 ± 5.0[¶]
Gracilis (n = 17)	838 ± 30[§]	49	[†]	111.5 ± 4.0[¶]
Distal iliotibial tract (18-mm width) (n = 10)	769 ± 99[§]	44	44 ± 6	19.1 ± 2.9[#]
Fascia lata (16-mm width) (n = 18)	628 ± 35[#]	36	39 ± 2	78.7 ± 4.6[¶]
Quadriceps-patellar retinaculum-patellar tendon				
Medial (n = 7)	371 ± 46[¶]	21	24 ± 4	15.4 ± 3.4[#]
Central (n = 6)	266 ± 74[¶]	15	17 ± 3	16.1 ± 1.8[¶]
Lateral (n = 7)	249 ± 54[¶]	14	19 ± 4	9.7 ± 1.5[¶]
Calculated values**				
Distal iliotibial tract				
25-mm width	1068	62		
Plus adjacent 10 mm of fascia	1468	85		
Plus adjacent 20 mm of fascia	1868	108		
Fascia lata (45-mm width)	1800	104		

*Data are given as mean and standard error of the mean. (From Noyes FR, Butler DL, Grood ES, et al.: Biomechanical analysis of human ligament grafts used in knee-ligament repairs and reconstruction. J Bone Joint Surg Am 66:344, 1984.)
[†]Width measurements were not made.
[‡]Statistically different from the maximum value for the anterior cruciate ligament: p<.05.
[§]p<.01.
[#]p<.005.
[¶]p<.001.
**Calculated by adjusting test values to new specimen widths.

period.[137–139] Laboratory tests have shown the strength-to-failure of a double-gracilis/double-semitendinosus graft to be more than 200% of that of the ACL.[139–142]

Early fixation strength is the weak link in ACL reconstruction. Fixation that can endure over 445 N of stress[136] (that seen in activities of daily living) may best be accomplished by fixation of a soft-tissue graft in a figure-of-eight manner around two bicortical screws and washers.[143] Fixation of soft-tissue grafts may also be adequately secured using a Krackow double whipstitch technique (Fig. 28–8).[144] The most secure fixation of a BPTB graft is obtained with a combination of interference screw and post fixation of both bone plugs. Excellent fixation strength is also obtained by using an appropriately sized interference screw and by using a post technique for one plug with interference screw fixation of the opposite end.[143, 145] Some authors believe that post fixation provides some graft protection with early motion by letting the graft settle in a nonconstrained position and by placing tension on the sutures rather than on the graft.[115, 146] Studies have shown bioabsorbable screws with long resorption times to provide comparable pullout strength to metallic screw fixation.[147, 148]

When early full motion and aggressive rehabilitation are stressed, morbidity with a BPTB graft is comparable to

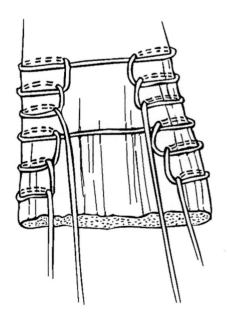

Figure 28–8 • Krackow double whipstitch for fixation of soft-tissue grafts.

morbidity with an autogenous hamstring graft.[81, 149–152] Because of the BPTB graft's strength, rigidity, early fixation stability (early bone-to-bone healing at 6–8 weeks), and history of good results,[44–46, 152–156] the author prefers it. A quadruple hamstring graft provides excellent graft strength, but according to Rodeo and colleagues[157] approximately 12 weeks for substantial healing to the bony tunnel is required. Grana et al.[158] showed healing as early as 3–4 weeks. Thus, the true healing time has not been firmly established. The large cross sectional area of the quadrupled graft may allow for better bony contact and healing than once thought.[139] Due to ease of harvest and low morbidity from harvest, the surgeon should learn the hamstring graft technique and the BPTB graft technique.[159–161] Hamstring graft may be the graft of choice in patients with moderate patellofemoral arthritis or with recurrent patellofemoral instability.[73, 162, 163] This graft is also an alternative when revision surgery is necessary.[73, 164, 165]

Endoscopic ACL reconstruction has the advantage of eliminating postoperative pain and scarring produced by a lateral incision. It also allows thorough examination of the femoral tunnel and allows some correction of the tunnel before final reaming.[166] The disadvantage of this technique is the learning curve that is required to avoid complications and surgical failure.

Before ACL reconstruction, roentgenograms of the knee should be carefully evaluated, including a standing 30–45 degree posteroanterior view, a 45 degree lateral view, and a 45 degree Merchant view.[167, 168] In patients with patella alta or Osgood-Schlatter disease, a longer than normal graft is required, and endoscopic technique may be difficult.[169] A tibial trough to secure the bone plug distally or recession of the graft 5–6 mm up into the femoral tunnel may be successful, but further recession up into the tunnel may cause problems with fixation, graft injury, graft impingement, and changes in isometry.[130, 170] Another alternative is the use of a two-incision technique to provide a longer bone tunnel. When the tibial ossicle is of substantial size and quality, it need not be excised.

BONE-PATELLAR TENDON-BONE GRAFT: ENDOSCOPIC TECHNIQUE

Set-Up

Place the patient supine on the operating table. After general endotracheal anesthesia is administered, examine the uninjured knee to obtain a reference examination for ligamentous laxity. Examine the injured knee and record Lachman and pivot shift instability. Apply a tourniquet around the upper thigh and a well-padded lateral post. Secure a 5-L intravenous saline solution bag to the table to act as a stop to maintain 90 degrees of knee flexion (Fig. 28–9). Prepare and drape the extremity with standard arthroscopy drapes, and use an Esmarch wrap for exsanguination. Inflate the tourniquet to 100 mm Hg above the patient's systolic pressure. If preoperative examination revealed significant laxity, proceed with patellar tendon harvesting. Arthroscopic joint portals may be made through this initial skin incision. If there is any question as

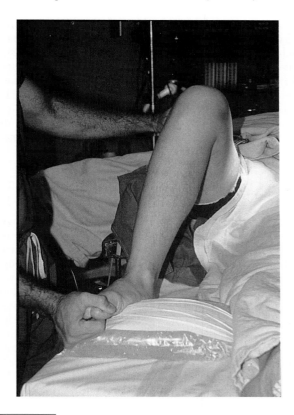

Figure 28–9 • Patient positioning for endoscopic bone-patellar tendon-bone graft reconstruction.

to the status of the ACL, or if more than 90 minutes of tourniquet time is anticipated for completion of the procedure, standard arthroscopy portals should be made for joint evaluation and notch débridement before making the skin incision for harvest of the patellar tendon. Injecting the portals with lidocaine and epinephrine is helpful to control bleeding, as is maintaining hypotensive anesthesia. An arthroscopy pump can be used to maintain proper joint distention and to decrease bone bleeding.

Graft Harvest

With the knee held in 90 degrees of flexion, make a 6-cm midline incision starting over the inferior pole of the patella and extending distally over the tibial tuberosity. The length of this incision depends on the size of the patient. Expose the patella and tendon by subcutaneous dissection. Make a straight midline incision through the peritenon. Dissect the peritenon from the patellar tendon, taking the flaps medially and laterally. With the knee held flexed to maintain some tension on the patellar tendon, measure the width of the tendon.

Harvest a graft 10 mm wide, or one-third of the tendon, whichever is smaller, from the central portion of the tendon, extending distally from the palpable inferior tip of the patella. Maintain straight, single-fiber plane incisions while harvesting the tendon. Use an oscillating saw with a blade 1 cm wide to make the bone cuts. Run the saw parallel to the anterior cortex of the patella, keeping 2 mm of the saw blade visible, to make a cut 8 mm deep. The cut should be about 10 mm wide and 27 mm long, measured from the bony tip of the patella. Make similar cuts distally, and free the tibial graft with a curved osteotome. Place a towel clip through the tendon. An assistant should hold the towel clip at all times to make sure that the graft is not contaminated. Complete the patellar cut, 7–8 mm deep and parallel to the anterior cortex, with an osteotome placed at the inferior pole of the patella.

Graft Preparation

Secure the graft to the top drape on a previously prepared table that holds appropriately sized bone plug trials, rongeurs, a 2 mm drill bit, a Silastic block, a skin marker, and four No. 5 Tevdec sutures on Keith needles. Contour the graft with the rongeurs so that it fits through the 10-mm trial, making sure that the complete graft will pass through the trial. Place a single drill hole in the patellar plug about 3 mm from the end. Round the end of the bone plug to make passage easier. Place three drill holes in the tibial bone plug. Place a No. 5 nonabsorbable suture through each of the bone plug drill holes, and use the sutures to maintain tension on the graft (with the help of a tension board or an assistant) while using a No. 2 absorbable suture to roll the graft edges together with a running suture through only the anterior fibers of the graft. Mark the bone-tendon junction on the cancellous side of the graft at both ends, and measure the total graft length (Fig. 28–10).

Notch Preparation

Use the electrocautery to make an inverted L-shaped flap through the tibial periosteum, starting about 2.5 cm distal to the joint line and then extending distally 1 cm medial to the tibial tuberosity. Reflect the flap medially with a periosteal elevator to expose the proximal tibia for later placement of the tibial tunnel. Make standard anteromedial and anterolateral arthroscopy portals, taking care not to damage the remaining portion of the patellar tendon. If a separate inflow is being used for the arthroscopy pump, make a portal just medial to the inferior pole of the patella so that the cannula can be placed just superior to the notch for an unobstructed flow. Examine the knee systematically, and evaluate and treat any associated intra-articular disease. Perform meniscal suturing before securing the ACL graft. Tie the meniscal sutures after completing the ACL reconstruction.

With the arthroscope in the anterolateral portal and a 5.5 mm full-radius resector in the anteromedial portal, release the ligamentum mucosum, and partially resect the fat pad to allow full exposure of the joint during the procedure. Resect the soft tissue from the intercondylar notch and from the tibial stump by sliding the resector between the remaining stump of the ACL and the posterior cruciate ligament (PCL). The opening of the blade should always be pointed superiorly or laterally to avoid damage to the PCL. Leave the outline of the tibial footprint intact as a reference guide. Avoid damaging the intermeniscal ligament just anterior to the tibial stump. Completely resect the femoral stump posteriorly to allow full exposure of the over-the-top position (Fig. 28–11).

With the knee in 30 degrees of flexion to visualize the opening of the notch, evaluate the available space between the PCL and lateral wall and the architecture of the roof. Use a 5.5 mm bur to enlarge the notch as indicated. The notch should be opened to look like an inverted U. Take care not to extend the notchplasty too far medially or superiorly, which would interfere with the patellofemoral articulation. Often the opening needs to be enlarged 2–3 mm superiorly and laterally. The bur may be placed in reverse to remove the articular fringe and smooth the initial notchplasty. As the notchplasty proceeds posteriorly, flex the knee 45–60 degrees; when the notchplasty is com-

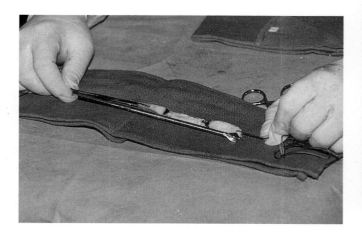

Figure 28–10 • After the bone-tendon junction at each end of the graft is marked, the total graft length is measured.

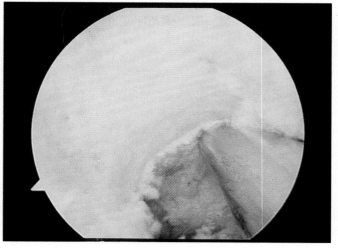

Figure 28–11 • The femoral stump should be completely resected posteriorly to allow full exposure of the over-the-top position.

plete, the knee should be at 90 degrees of flexion. Use controlled strokes with the bur from posterior to anterior. Posteriorly, open the notch enough to accommodate the 10 mm endoscopic reamer. Smooth the edges of the tunnel by placing the bur in reverse or by using an arthroscopic rasp.

With a curved curet, make a femoral starting point about 6 mm anterior to the over-the-top spot at approximately the 11-o'clock position on the right knee or the 1-o'clock position on the left knee.[127, 171, 172] The knee must be flexed at least 80–90 degrees to visualize the over-the-top spot accurately.

Tibial Tunnel Preparation

When placing the tibial guide, be aware of the intended tunnel length and direction so that the graft may be secured in a physiometric, impingement-free position.[173] Proper length and direction of the tunnel require a starting point at least 3 cm distal to the joint line and about 1.5 cm medial to the tuberosity (Fig. 28–12).[174] Intra-articular reference points for the guide include the ACL stump, the inner edge of the anterior horn of the lateral meniscus, the medial tibial spine, and the PCL.

When evaluating pin placement in a two-dimensional picture, in the anteroposterior plane the guide wire should

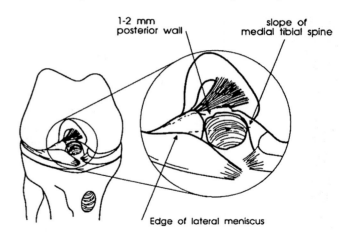

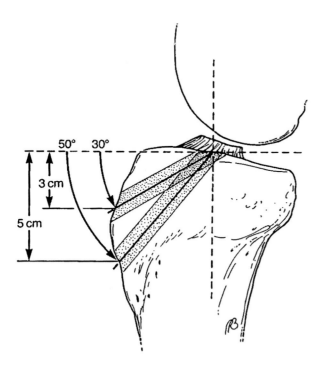

Figure 28–12 • Starting point of the tibial tunnel must be at least 3 cm distal to the joint line and about 1.5 cm medial to the tibial tuberosity to allow sufficient tunnel length and appropriate direction. (From Christian CA and Indelicato PA: Allograft anterior cruciate ligament reconstruction with patellar tendon: an endoscopic technique. Oper Tech Sports Med 1:50, 1993.)

Figure 28–13 • Reference line to be approximated by guide wire in anteroposterior plane extends medially from the inner edge of the lateral meniscus. (From Jackson DW and Gasser SI: Tibial tunnel placement in ACL reconstruction. Arthroscopy 10:124, 1994.)

approximate a reference line extended medially from the inner edge of the lateral meniscus (Fig. 28–13). This point should be approximately 7 mm anterior to the PCL and about 2–3 mm anterior to the peak of the medial spine (Fig. 28–14).[48, 51, 171, 173] In the mediolateral plane, the wire should enter at the base of the medial spine, in the center or just slightly medial to the center of the ACL footprint, and centered in the notch opening (Fig. 28–15).[175]

The unaltered roof of the intercondylar notch normally forms an angle of 35–40 degrees with the long axis of the femur (Fig. 28–16).[173] To prevent impingement, an internal notchplasty as previously described is necessary, as is appropriate tunnel placement.[135, 176] Use the tibial and

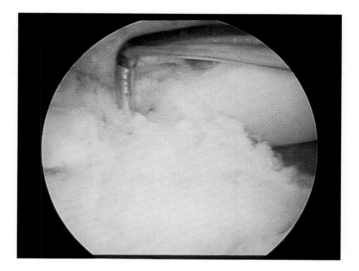

Figure 28–14 • Drill guide should enter approximately 7 mm anterior to the posterior cruciate ligament and about 2–3 mm anterior to the peak of the medial spine.

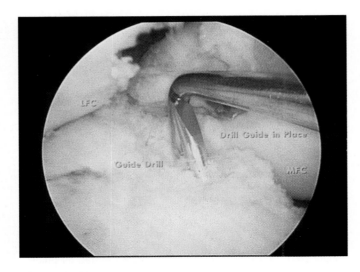

Figure 28–15 • In the medial-lateral plane, the wire enters at the base of the medial spine, in the center or just slightly medial to the center of the ACL footprint, centered in the notch opening.

femoral landmarks described previously, and place the guide at 50–60 degrees to the tibial plateau surface to obtain sufficient tunnel length and an angle that allows the graft angle to approximate that of the altered roof. Determine minimum acceptable tunnel length by measuring the length of the entire graft and subtracting 60 mm (30 mm for femoral tunnel length, allowing for 5 mm of graft recession, and 30 mm for intra-articular distance from the femur to the tibial tunnel). Tibial tunnel length can be measured directly off the guide calibrations. Tunnel length should be sufficient to allow at least 2 cm of bone to be secured in the tibial tunnel for stable fixation.[140, 177]

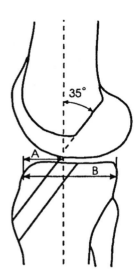

Figure 28–16 • The normal intercondylar notch forms an angle of 35–40 degrees with the long axis of the femur. (From Jackson DW and Gasser SI: Tibial tunnel placement in ACL reconstruction. Arthroscopy 10:128, 1994.)

Using the guide, advance the wire approximately 2 cm into the knee while observing through the arthroscope. Move the knee through a range of motion to make sure that the wire passes within 2 mm of the PCL and does not impinge on the medial or lateral walls or the roof of the intercondylar notch. Make small corrections in position to prevent impingement and to allow the wire to be aimed close to the previously chosen pilot hole on the femoral condyle, with the knee in 70–90 degrees of flexion. Making small corrections at this point can make femoral tunnel reaming and graft passage much easier in the later steps of the procedure.

With the knee flexed 70–90 degrees, advance the tibial guide wire to abut the anticipated site of the femoral tunnel opening. By subtracting the length of the wire remaining outside the tibia from the total wire length, the length of the tibial tunnel and the anticipated intra-articular portion of the graft can be determined. To the number obtained by the guide wire measurement (tibial tunnel plus intra-articular length), add 25 mm (graft length to occupy femoral tunnel). This number is compared with the total graft length. The fact that the graft may be recessed 5 mm is offset by the 5 mm loss in potential tunnel length caused by the obliquity of the tunnel openings. For example, for a total graft length of 95 mm, TT = tibial tunnel, IA = intra-articular length, and FT = femoral tunnel:

$$(TT + IA) + FT = 95$$

$$70 + 25 = 95$$

In this case, the tibial tunnel should be sufficient. If TT and IA were 65, one might wish to increase the tunnel angle to 60 degrees to obtain additional tunnel length.

Place the open end of the full-radius resector over the intra-articular end of the Kirschner wire to prevent advancement. Ream over the wire with an 8 mm reamer. Leave the protruding end of the reamer in the tunnel and examine the tunnel for appropriate impingement-free position as the knee is moved through a full range of motion. Make necessary adjustments with the 8 mm reamer. Bow-stringing of the ACL graft over the PCL is prevented by leaving a 2-mm posterior wall between the tibial tunnel and the PCL. By directing the tunnel just lateral to the PCL, the graft will lie on the PCL without bowing around the ligament. Ream the tunnel with the 10 mm reamer and use the full-radius resector to contour the edges of the tunnel and resect any remaining soft tissue that might block extension. Place a rasp through the tunnel to complete contouring, and make certain that the external portion of the tunnel is free of soft tissue.

Femoral Tunnel Preparation

With the knee flexed approximately 90 degrees, confirm the previously chosen femoral pilot hole with an Arthrex 6 mm offset femoral guide passed through the tibial tunnel. Make sure that 1–2 mm of bone remains as a posterior wall. The starting point is at the 11-o'clock position on the right knee or approximately 8 mm lateral to the

PCL.[171, 178, 179] Maintain correct visual orientation by keeping the tibia vertical and the knee flexed 90 degrees. Advance a long guide wire through the guide to the chosen physiometric point on the posterolateral portion of the femoral condyle. Advance the wire so that it exits the distal anterolateral femoral cortex. Use wire plier handles to stabilize the skin and soft tissues so that the wire advances externally and does not traverse the thigh more proximally. Before placement of the guide wire, an Isotac and isometer centered in the tibial tunnel can be used to evaluate isometry,[179–183] although the functional efficacy of isometry measurements is still being evaluated. Ideally, the graft will tighten 1–2 mm with knee extension from 45 degrees down to full extension. If the isometer tightens more than 1 mm with knee flexion more than 45 degrees, move the pilot hole posteriorly or inferiorly in the notch.[166]

Pass a 10 mm endoscopic reamer over the previously placed wire. With the knee in 80–90 degrees of flexion to avoid posterior wall ream-out, advance the reamer to make a slight print at the entry point in the femoral condyle. If the reamer print cannot be seen, remove any debris with a shaver. If the print is adequately posterior, leaving a 1–2 mm posterior wall, advance the reamer to 35 mm (5-mm increment marks on the reamer can be visualized arthroscopically). Retract the reamer carefully, and remove it from the joint, making sure not to enlarge the tunnel and ream-out the posterior wall of the femur. During the reaming of the femoral tunnel, a bone wax plug placed around the reamer at the external mouth of the tibial tunnel helps maintain joint distention and improves visualization. Smooth the edges of the femoral tunnel with a full-radius resector. Use an AO screwdriver to make a slot at the 12-o'clock position in the femoral tunnel. The slot should be about 3 mm deep and 5 mm long. This derotation slot keeps the interference screw from migrating posteriorly during insertion and allows observation of the graft after recessing it approximately 5 mm into the tunnel (Fig. 28–17).[126]

Graft Passage

Use the eyed guide wire to pass the patellar bone plug guide suture up through the femoral tunnel and then out through the lateral thigh. With the suture, pull the graft up into the knee, and use a probe to help guide the graft up into the femoral tunnel, with the cancellous portion of the graft pointing directly anteriorly (Fig. 28–18). If difficulty is encountered in passing the graft, use an Allis clamp to grab the graft and ease it up into the tunnel. If the graft is still difficult to pass, resize it and make sure that no soft tissue impedes the passage. When the graft is about halfway into the femoral tunnel, either pass a flexible guide wire through the medial portal or make a central fat-pad portal, whichever makes the straightest line with the femoral tunnel. Place the wire anterior to the graft and, with the wire parallel to the graft, advance both up into the tunnel. Make certain at least 2 cm of bone plug remains in the tibial tunnel for later fixation; if necessary, recess the graft in the femoral tunnel up to 5 or 6 mm. If recession does not allow adequate bone in the tibial tunnel, place the

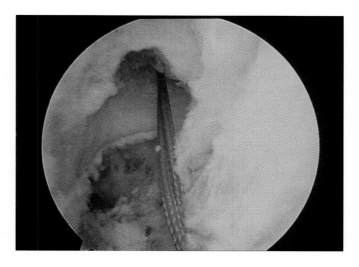

Figure 28–17 • Derotation slot allows observation of the graft after it is recessed approximately 5 mm into the femoral tunnel and prevents posterior migration of the interference screw.

graft even with the mouth of the femoral tunnel, and make a trough in the tibia just distal to the tibial tunnel.

Graft Fixation

Place an 8 mm cannula with a cannulated screw with noncutting threads through the medial portal or central patellar portal. Flex the knee to about 110 degrees. Lever the cannula inferiorly and make a straight line with the femoral tunnel (Fig. 28–19). Close observation is necessary during this step and is made possible by placing the arthroscope above the graft and looking down at the graft during placement of the screw. For secure fixation, the screw

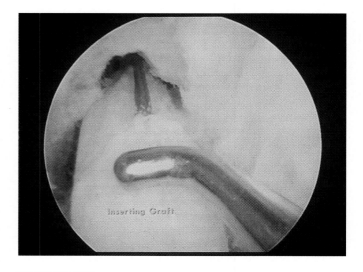

Figure 28–18 • A probe is used to help guide the graft into the femoral tunnel.

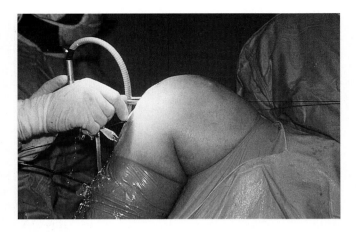

Figure 28–19 • An 8 mm cannula with a cannulated screw is placed through the medial or central patellar portal. With the knee flexed about 110 degrees, the cannula is levered inferiorly to make a straight line with the femoral tunnel.

should not diverge from the line of the tunnel or bone plug by more than 15 degrees.[140] Advance the screw into the tunnel, and place the screw head even with the bone plug, verifying its position by observation and palpation with the screwdriver. Use the distal sutures to tug on the graft to make sure that it is securely fastened in the femoral tunnel. Move the knee through a range of motion while holding tension distally on the graft to make sure that there is no impingement or pistoning of the graft. If the graft tightens more than 2 mm with knee flexion, remove the graft, and using a convex arthroscopic rasp, move the femoral tunnel or both tunnels slightly posteriorly. Slight tightening during knee extension is normal. Rotate the cancellous portion of the tibial bone plug so that it points laterally to reproduce the 90 degree rotation of the ACL.[184] This rotation also helps to move the graft away from the lateral wall and adds some strength through fiber tensioning.[185] If no graft pistoning or impingement is evident, hold the tension on the graft for approximately 3 minutes to allow for collagen fiber stress relaxation.[186] If the graft tends to impinge in one direction, use the screw to push the bone graft in the opposite direction. Tension the graft with about 6–8 lb of pull, depending on the ligamentous laxity of the opposite knee.[183] Overtensioning of the graft may cause failure because of joint capture or graft necrosis.[131, 187–189] Secure the graft with a 7 mm screw if the bone plug-to-tunnel gap is less than 3 mm; use a 9 mm screw if the gap is 3 mm or more. If the gap is more than 5 mm, add a cancellous screw and washer post 1.5 cm distal to the tibial tunnel.[140] While holding tension on the No. 5 sutures, secure them around the post with two square knots, then tighten the screws securely.

If the bone remaining in the tibial tunnel is not long enough (less than 2 cm), tie the three sutures over a cancellous screw and metal washer post.[145] Alternatively, use an osteotome to outline a trough just distal to the tibial tunnel, and punch the trough in with a bone punch. Place the graft into the trough and tie the sutures over a post, or use two Richards staples to secure the plug in the trough.

Move the knee through a full range of motion and make sure that there is no evidence of capture of the knee joint. Observe and probe the graft arthroscopically to make certain that it is taut. The graft should be slightly tighter than a normal ACL. Make certain that there is no impingement and that no bone or screw protrudes into the joint from the tibial or femoral tunnel.

Closure

Loosely approximate the patellar tendon with simple interrupted absorbable sutures through the anterior portion of the fiber of the tendon. Bone-graft the patellar defect and close the peritenon. Remove the sutures from the thigh proximally and from the tibial bone plug distally. Remove any protruding bone, leaving a smooth surface distally. Close the periosteal flap back over the tunnel. Pass 3 in of drain tubing through the medial pump inflow sheath and into the suprapatellar pouch, making sure that the drain does not curl back on itself. Remove the sheath, leaving the drain in the suprapatellar pouch. Make a small stab incision with a No. 11 blade just proximal to the superior portion of the skin incision, and use a hemostat to pull the drain out through the skin. Close the subcutaneous tissues with interrupted 2-0 Vicryl sutures and approximate the skin with a running subcuticular 3-0 Prolene suture. Apply adhesive strips loosely over the closure, and apply a sterile dressing, a cooling sleeve, and an elastic wrap.

When the patient is alert in the recovery room, the limb is placed in a CPM machine. Ketorolac tromethamine (Toradol) (30 mg IV) is given before tourniquet inflation. Antibiotics are given before inflation of the tourniquet, and two additional doses are given postoperatively (see stage I physical therapy protocol).

BONE-PATELLAR TENDON-BONE GRAFT: TWO-INCISION TECHNIQUE

Place the patient supine on the operating table, and apply a tourniquet and a lateral post around the upper thigh. Tape a 5-L saline solution bag to the table to maintain the knee in 90 degrees of flexion (see Fig. 28–9). Use waterproof arthroscopy drapes for standard draping.

Graft Harvest

Graft harvest is performed as described for the endoscopic technique.

Graft Preparation

At a separate table, have an assistant contour the graft until it fits through a 10-mm trial without difficulty. Secure the graft to the top table drape while preparing. Contour the ends of the bone plugs in a bullet-type fashion, and place a No. 5 nonabsorbable suture through each drill hole; the first drill hole should be approximately 3 mm from each end of the graft. Roll the graft with a running 2-0 Vicryl suture while maintaining the graft under tension. Mark the tendon-bone interface with a methylene blue pencil.

Notch Preparation

With the electrocautery, make an inverted L incision, starting 2.5 cm below the joint line and extending distally 2 cm, approximately 1.5 cm medial to the tibial crest. Use a periosteal elevator to raise the periosteal flap. Place an inflow cannula medial to the inferior pole of the patella. Make medial and lateral parapatellar arthroscopic portals for observation and instrumentation.

Examine the knee thoroughly to evaluate all damaged structures. Place meniscal sutures as indicated to be tied at the end of the procedure. Use a 5.5 mm full-radius resector to resect the soft tissue from the intercondylar notch, and resect the tibial stump, leaving a visible footprint. Flex the knee to 90 degrees to see the over-the-top position clearly, and complete the resection of the posterior fringe of the ACL femoral stump.

Extend the knee to 30 degrees, and identify the notch architecture. Use a 5.5 mm bur to open the notch to an inverted U shape if there is evidence of stenosis of the opening.[135, 176] Superiorly and laterally 2–3 mm of bone is usually removed. Place the bur in reverse to smooth the edges of the resected fringe. Increase the flexion of the knee and, working posteriorly, use controlled posterior-to-anterior strokes to widen the roof and lateral wall. Flex the knee to 90 degrees so that the over-the-top position is clearly visible, then complete the notchplasty. For the rear-entry technique, taper the notch posteriorly, making sure not to remove excessive bone in the posterior part of the notch. Use a full-radius resector or an arthroscopic rasp for final smoothing of the roof and wall of the notch.

Visualize the femoral notch architecture thoroughly, and use a curved curet to make a pilot hole about 6 mm anterior to the over-the-top spot at the 1-o'clock position on the right knee (approximately 8 mm lateral to the PCL).[127, 171, 172]

Tibial Tunnel Preparation

With a tibial guide, place a Kirschner wire at least 3 cm distal to the joint line and 1.5 cm medial to the tibial crest. The wire should enter the joint in the center of the ACL footprint approximately 2 mm anterior to the peak of the medial tibial spine, which is approximately 7 mm anterior to the PCL.[51, 171, 173, 175] A third reference point in the anteroposterior plane is that of the inner edge on the anterior horn of the lateral meniscus. A line extended medially from the inner edge of the meniscus should approximate the guide wire (see Fig. 28–13).[51, 171, 173] In the mediolateral plane, the wire should enter at the base of the medial spine (see Fig. 28–14). Advance the guide wire into the

joint, and carefully identify its direction of passage just lateral to the PCL in the general direction of the previously chosen femoral starting portal (see Fig. 28–15). The guide wire should not impinge on the roof or the walls of the notch during knee range of motion.[175]

Lateral Exposure

Make a 4-cm lateral incision, starting 1.5 cm proximal to the flare of the lateral condyle, centered directly over the iliotibial band. Carry the dissection down to the iliotibial band, and expose it with wide subcutaneous dissection. Divide the iliotibial band in its midline, and extend proximally and distally from the skin incision. The lower edge of the distal portion of the vastus lateralis can be felt by sweeping a finger along the intramuscular septum. Slide a periosteal elevator under the edge of the vastus lateralis, and lift the muscle anteriorly over the lateral part of the femur without injuring the muscle belly. Place a Z retractor over the femur to hold the vastus lateralis superiorly. Use the electrocautery to make a longitudinal incision through the periosteum just proximal to the flare of the condyle, and extend it proximally for about 2.5 cm. Use a periosteal elevator to expose the bone and the over-the-top spot where the flare of the condyle and the metaphysis of the femur meet. Coagulate the lateral genicular vessel in this area.

Femoral Tunnel Preparation

With an arthroscope in the anteromedial portal, pass the gaff for the rear-entry guide through the anterolateral portal. Make sure that the gaff does not hook the PCL and that it passes directly over the over-the-top spot, hugging the posterior edge of the condyle. This opening may have to be enlarged with a periosteal elevator to ease the passage of the rear-entry guide. Hook the appropriate side (right or left) of the guide through the eyelet in the graft. While holding slight tension on the rear-entry guide, use the gaff to bring the guide into the knee, and release the gaff from the guide without any twisting motion that might break the tip of the gaff (Fig. 28–20). Place the guide in the previously chosen pilot hole on the femoral condyle, 6 mm anterior to the over-the-top spot in approximately the 11-o'clock position on the right knee or the 1-o'clock position on the left knee. This point should coincide with the junction of the arch of the roof and the lateral wall of the condyle approximately 8 mm lateral to the PCL (Fig. 28–21).[46, 190] The pilot hole should be deep enough to be seen when trying to place the guide but not deep enough to allow more than 2 mm recession of the tip of the guide into the bone. If the guide is recessed too far into the bone, the guide wire will pass the tip of the guide and enter the joint anterior to the desired location. The external landmark for the guide is the midportion of the femur, approximately 3 cm proximal to the over-the-top spot. The angle of the wire should be approximately 45 degrees to the femur and should be as close as possible to the plane of the

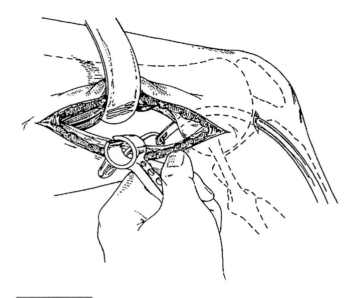

Figure 28–20 • Gaff is used to bring rear-entry guide into the knee. (From Technique for Rear Entry ACL Guide. Acufex Microsurgical, Inc., Norwood, Mass., 1988.)

previously placed tibial guide wire. Make sure that at least 2 cm of lateral cortex remains posterior to the wire to prevent troughing of the condyle (Fig. 28–22).

Verify placement of the wire with the arthroscope in the anterolateral or central patellar portal. Use a curved curet to palpate the placement of the wire, making sure that it is 6 mm anterior to the over-the-top spot. It is important to have the knee flexed 90 degrees to be able to observe the posterior position of the guide wire. When accurate wire placement is confirmed with both observation and palpation, begin the femoral tunnel with an 8 mm reamer, make any necessary corrections with the 8 mm tibial reamer, and complete the tunnel with a 10 mm reamer after checking isometry if desired. Prevent guide wire advancement during reaming with the open end of a full-radius resector or with a Kelly clamp. After reaming and smoothing the edges of the tunnel with a full-radius resector and an arthroscopic rasp, place a plastic plug in the femoral tunnel.

Tibial Tunnel Preparation

Ream over the previously placed tibial wire with the 8 mm reamer. Place the reamer tip in the joint, and leave it there while the knee is moved through a range of motion. Look for potential impingement on the roof or walls. To help evaluate isometry, place a suture through a button, pull the

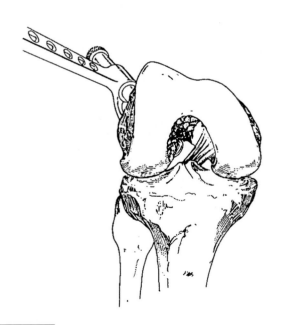

Figure 28–21 • The rear-entry guide is placed in the pilot hole on the femoral condyle, at a point coinciding with the junction of the arch of the condylar roof and the lateral condylar wall, approximately 8 mm lateral to the PCL. (From Technique for Rear Entry ACL Guide. Acufex Microsurgical, Inc., Norwood, Mass., 1988.)

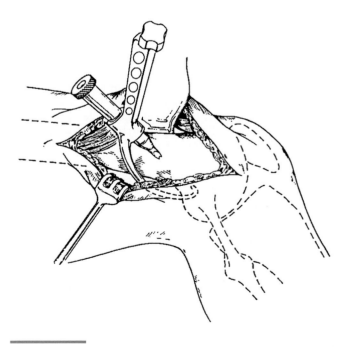

Figure 28–22 • At least 2 cm of lateral cortex should remain posterior to the wire to prevent troughing of the condyle. (From Technique for Rear Entry ACL Guide. Acufex Microsurgical, Inc., Norwood, Mass., 1988.)

suture through the 8 mm femoral tunnel, and place a centered isometer in the tibial tunnel.

With an 8 mm reamer, make necessary corrections to the tunnels before over-reaming with a 10 mm reamer. Most corrections are necessary because the tunnels are too far anterior, resulting in graft tightening during knee flexion. If this is a problem, the femoral tunnel may be widened posteriorly or inferiorly in the notch; likewise, the tibial tunnel may be moved posteriorly if indicated.[166] Contour the edges of the tunnels with a rasp to prevent graft abrasion.

Graft Fixation

Place a slight (15 degree) bend into a suture passer to help the passer slide along the femoral tunnel as it is passed proximally through the tibial tunnel. Pass the graft from the femoral tunnel into the tibial tunnel with the suture passer. As the graft is passed distally from the femoral tunnel out through the tibial tunnel, the cancellous portion of the bone in the femoral tunnel should point anteriorly to maximize posterior placement of the graft; the cancellous portion in the tibial tunnel should point laterally to reproduce the 90 degree fiber rotation of the normal ACL.[184] This rotation has been shown to increase graft strength by fiber recruitment.[185] Secure the graft with an appropriately sized interference screw placed anterior to the graft in the femur, thus pushing the graft posteriorly.

Move the knee through a range of motion to make sure that no pistoning or impingement of the graft is present. If the graft tightens more than 2 mm with knee flexion, remove the graft and enlarge the femoral tunnel posteriorly, or inferiorly in the notch if the tunnel is as far posterior as possible. If the tunnel or tunnels are moved after having been reamed with the 10 mm reamer, a larger interference screw or a bone grafting technique may be necessary. Place the knee in extension, and maintain tension on the graft for approximately 3 minutes before securing the graft to the tibia with an interference screw.[186] This screw is usually placed medial to the graft in the tunnel but may be placed laterally if this centers the graft in the notch better. If less than 2 cm of bone plug is available for secure fixation in the femoral and tibial tunnels, use a bicortical screw and washer post for distal fixation.[143]

Observe the graft arthroscopically, and probe it to make sure that it is adequately tight and that no screw or bone is left protruding. Check the stability of the knee by Lachman and pivot shift maneuvers. The knee should be just slightly tighter than the uninjured knee.

Place a Hemovac drain intra-articularly into the suprapatellar pouch, making sure that it does not curl upon itself. Place a drain laterally before closure of the iliotibial band. Bone-graft the patellar defect, and approximate the patellar tendon loosely with interrupted No. 0 Vicryl sutures, closing just the anterior fibers. Close the paratenon with 2-0 Vicryl sutures, and then close the skin with a running subcuticular 3-0 Prolene suture. Apply adhesive strips and a sterile dressing.

Postoperative routine is as described earlier.

HAMSTRING GRAFT: TWO-INCISION TECHNIQUE

Place the patient supine on the operating table, and apply a padded lateral post and tourniquet around the upper thigh. Tape a 5-L saline solution bag to the table to use as a foot stop to maintain the knee in 90 degrees of flexion during the procedure (see Fig. 28–9). Exposure is easier with the extremity placed in a *figure-of-four* position (Fig. 28–23*A*).[73]

Graft Harvest

Make a 4-cm incision anteromedially on the tibia, starting approximately 4 cm distal to the joint line and 3 cm medial to the tibial tuberosity (Fig. 28–23*B*). Expose the pes anserinus insertion with subcutaneous dissection. Palpate the upper and lower borders of the sartorius tendon, and

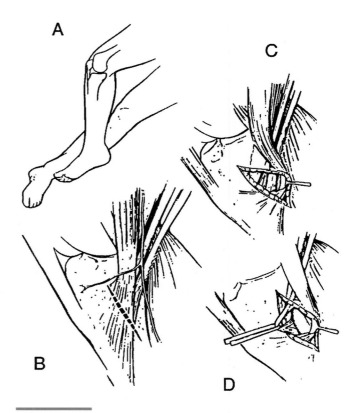

Figure 28–23 • *A*, Figure-of-four position makes exposure and graft harvest easier. *B*, A 4-cm incision is made on the anteromedial tibia, starting approximately 4 cm distal to the joint line and 3 cm medial to the tibial tuberosity. *C*, A short incision is made in line with and through the first layer of the gracilis tendon, being careful not to injure the underlying medial collateral ligament. *D*, A Penrose drain is placed around the gracilis tendon, and its fibrous extension to the gastrocnemius and semimembranosus muscles is released. (From Warner JJP, Warren RF, and Cooper DE: Management of acute anterior cruciate ligament injury. Instr Course Lect 40:225, 1992.)

identify the palpable gracilis and semitendinosus tendons 3–4 cm medial to the tendinous insertion. Make a short incision in line with the upper border of the gracilis tendon, and carry the incision just through the first layer, taking care not to injure the underlying medial collateral ligament (Fig. 28–23C). With Metzenbaum scissors, carry the dissection proximally up the thigh. Stay in the same plane, and maintain adequate exposure by use of properly placed retractors. Careful observation of structures is necessary to avoid injuring the saphenous vein or nerve by straying from the plane of dissection. With a curved hemostat, dissect the gracilis and semitendinosus tendons from the surrounding soft tissues about 3 cm medial to their insertion into the tibia. After carefully identifying each tendon, place a Penrose drain around the gracilis tendon, and release its fibrous extensions to the gastrocnemius and semimembranosus muscles (Fig. 28–23D). These fibrous extensions come off the hamstring tendons at approximately 6–7 cm proximal to their distal attachment. Before releasing the tendon with an open-end tendon stripper, palpate all sides of the tendon to make sure that there are no fibrous extensions. If firm resistance is felt, redissect around the tendon with a periosteal elevator and Metzenbaum scissors. Release the tendon proximally by controlled tension on the tendon while advancing the stripper proximally. The muscle should slide off the tendon as the stripper is advanced proximally. Use the same procedure to release the semitendinosus tendon. Subperiosteally dissect the tendons medially to the insertion, and release them sharply. Take care not to damage or release the sartorius tendon. At another table, separate the muscle from the tendon with a No. 10 blade. Place a Krackow-type whipstitch in both ends of each tendon with No. 2 nonabsorbable sutures[144] (see Fig. 28–8). Fold both tendons in half to form four strands of tendon. Place a No. 5 nonabsorbable suture through the loop end of both tendons.

Notchplasty and Tunnel Placement

Use a 5.5 mm bur to enlarge the opening of the intercondylar notch as necessary to form an inverted U. Within the notch, remove approximately 2 mm of bone superiorly and laterally to make sure that there is no wall or roof impingement. Extend the notchplasty over to the PCL medially. The notchplasty should funnel posteriorly to avoid altering the posterior architecture.[135, 176]

Use the lateral incision described for rear-entry ACL reconstruction with BPTB.

Tunnel placement and reaming are similar to those for the central-third patellar tendon graft technique. Place the doubled gracilis and semitendinosus tendons through the sizer sleeve to determine appropriate tunnel size. Place the tibial and femoral guide wires according to the landmarks described earlier. Place the femoral tunnel approximately 5 mm anterior to the over-the-top spot, leaving 1–2 mm of bone posterior to the tunnel. Ream initially with a reamer 2 mm smaller in diameter than the final tunnel size. Make adjustments in the tunnel as necessary, using the smaller 7 mm or 8 mm reamer. Com-

plete the reaming with a 9 mm or 10 mm reamer, depending on the graft size. Ream the tibial tunnel in a similar manner, making sure to adjust to leave approximately 2 mm of bone between the posterior wall of the tunnel and the PCL and ensuring that there is no roof or wall impingement.[51, 127, 171–175] Contour the edges of the tunnels to prevent graft abrasion.

Graft Fixation

Place three No. 5 Ti-cron anchor sutures through the loop in the doubled graft. Use a methylene blue pencil to make a line 2.5 cm proximal to the loop end. With a suture passer placed through the tibial tunnel and up through the femoral tunnel, pass the graft down from the femur into the tibia. Use an osteotome to fish-scale the area of intended graft fixation on the femur. Recess the graft into the tibial tunnel, making sure that at least 2 cm of graft remains in the tunnel; verify this by checking the previously placed mark on the graft. Place a bicortical screw and metal washer 2 cm distal to the tibial tunnel. The screw should be 5 mm longer than the measured length to allow for sutures and washer. Tie a single square knot in one of the anchor sutures around the post, and tighten the screw to hold the graft in the tibial tunnel. With 8–10 lb of tension on the graft, secure the graft to the femur with two bicortical screws and spiked soft-tissue washers.[187] Pass the graft in a figure-of-eight fashion (Fig. 28–24).[162] The

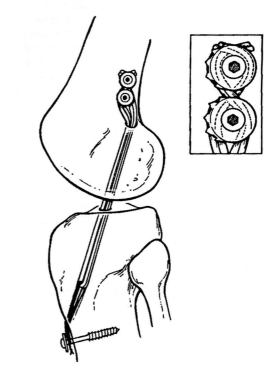

Figure 28–24 • Graft fixation with bicortical screws and spiked soft-tissue washers. (From Brown CH Jr, Steiner ME, and Carson EW: The use of hamstring tendons for anterior cruciate ligament reconstruction. Clin Sports Med 12:745, 1993.)

most distal screw should be just proximal to the femoral tunnel. If sufficient graft is not available for placement of two screws in this manner, secure the graft by wrapping it around a bicortical screw and spiked washer, two strands clockwise and two strands counterclockwise. The whip-stitch sutures can then be tied around a bicortical screw, and a metal washer can be placed more proximally. After securing the graft on the femur, retighten the tibial sutures. With approximately 8–10 lb of tension on the graft and the knee in 0 degrees of extension, pull the graft down taut and hold tension for 3 minutes.[186, 187] Place two square knots in each of the three sutures. Tighten the screw and washer over the knots to secure the fixation. Check the knee again for stability and range of motion to make sure that no impingement of the graft is present. Examine and probe the graft arthroscopically to make sure that it is taut and securely anchored.

Place an intra-articular drain, and close the deep layers with No. 0 absorbable sutures, the subcuticular tissues with No. 2 absorbable sutures, and the skin with running subcuticular sutures.

Rehabilitation after this procedure is the same as that after BPTB graft reconstruction.

HAMSTRING GRAFT: ENDOSCOPIC TECHNIQUE

Set-up, graft harvest, and graft preparation are performed as described for the two-incision hamstring technique.

Place two running, interlocking No. 2 nonabsorbable Krackow-type whipstitches in each end of each hamstring so that the graft can be passed as a single quadruple graft or as two separate doubled grafts.[144, 165, 166] (see Fig. 28–8). Perform notchplasty and tunnel placement as described for the endoscopic BPTB technique. Ream the tibial tunnel at 50 degrees to the tibial articular surface. Ream the femoral tunnel or tunnels to a depth of approximately 30 mm. Determine the size of the femoral tunnel by measuring the graft with the sizer sleeve. Snug fit of the graft is essential for early healing. A single tunnel 9–10 mm can be reamed, or a "double-barrel" tunnel with a small bony bridge between may be formed by reaming two 6- or 7-mm tunnels, the first at the 1-o'clock position and the second just lateral to it.[165, 166] This technique may be beneficial for revisions to place the revision posterior to the original failed graft.

Advance a 2.7 mm, 15-in drill tip passing pin through the tibial and femoral tunnels and out through the antero-lateral femoral cortex. Maintain the knee at approximately 90 degrees of flexion during passage of the pin. Ream the 4.5 mm endobutton drill bit over the passing pin, exiting the anterolateral cortex (Fig. 28–25). Remove this assembly, and use the calibrated depth probe to measure the total femoral tunnel length (Fig. 28–26). Secure polyester tape 4–6 mm wide to the endobutton(s) and the quadrupled or doubled grafts (Fig. 28–27). Subtract the length of graft to be recessed in the tunnel (usually 20 mm) from the total femoral tunnel length (obtained from the calibrated depth probe) to obtain the appropriate length of tape (Fig.

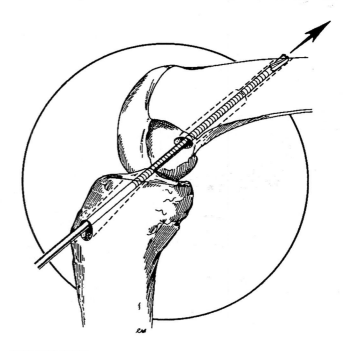

Figure 28–25 • The 4.5 mm endobutton drill bit is reamed over the passing pin to exit the anterolateral cortex. (From Rosenberg TD and Graf B: Techniques for ACL reconstruction with Multi-Trac drill guide. Technique manual, Acufex Microsurgical, Inc., Mansfield, Mass., 1994.)

28–28). Use a marker to make a line 6 mm distal to the intended insertion length on each graft. Place a No. 5 non-absorbable lead suture in one end of the endobutton and a No. 2 nonabsorbable suture in the opposite end (Fig. 28–29). Pass the drill-tip passing pin back through both tunnels and out through the anterolateral thigh. Use the pin to pull both the lead and the trail suture of the endobutton-graft complex out through the skin proximally (Fig. 28–30). Use the No. 5 lead suture to pass the assembly through both tunnels and the button out through the anterolateral femoral cortex. When the mark on the graft enters the mouth of the tunnel, pull the No. 2 suture to rotate the button into place. When this rotation is felt, pull the graft distally to confirm seating of the button.

Pull the graft taut, and move the knee through a range of motion to ensure that no impingement or excessive graft pistoning occurs. Maintain 8–10 lb of tension for 3 minutes before distal fixation over a bicortical screw and washer fixation post (Fig. 28–31).[186, 187] Examine and probe the graft arthroscopically to ensure secure fixation and tautness just slightly more than those of the normal ACL.

Closure and postoperative management are as described earlier.

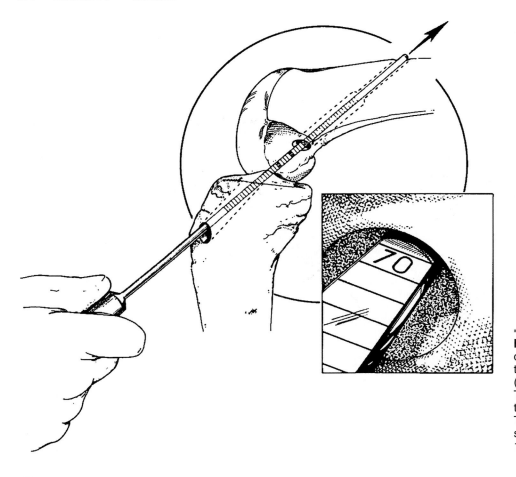

Figure 28–26 • The calibrated depth probe is used to measure total length of the femoral tunnel. (From Rosenberg TD and Graf B: Techniques for ACL reconstruction with Multi-Trac drill guide. Technique manual, Acufex Microsurgical, Inc., Mansfield, Mass., 1994.)

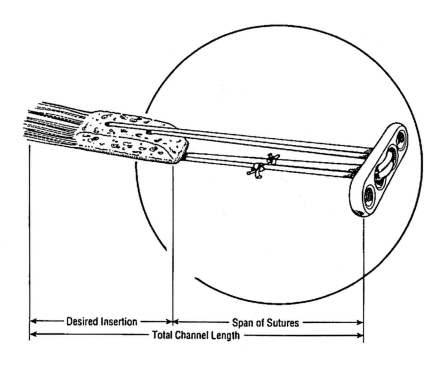

Figure 28–27 • Polyester tape is secured to the endobutton(s) and the quadrupled or doubled grafts. (From Rosenberg TD and Graf B: Techniques for ACL reconstruction with Multi-Trac drill guide. Technique manual, Acufex Microsurgical, Inc., Mansfield, Mass., 1994.)

Desired Insertion — Span of Sutures
Total Channel Length

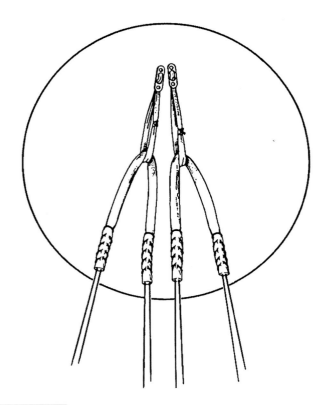

Figure 28–28 • The appropriate length of tape is determined by subtracting the length of the graft to be recessed in the tunnel (usually 20 mm) from the total femoral tunnel length. (From Rosenberg TD and Graf B: Techniques for ACL reconstruction with Multi-Trac drill guide. Technique manual, Acufex Microsurgical, Inc., Mansfield, Mass., 1994.)

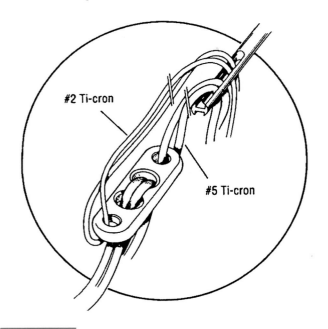

Figure 28–29 • A No. 5 nonabsorbable suture is placed in one end of the endobutton, and a No. 2 nonabsorbable suture in the other end. (From Rosenberg TD and Graf B: Techniques for ACL reconstruction with Multi-Trac drill guide. Technique manual, Acufex Microsurgical, Inc., Mansfield, Mass., 1994.)

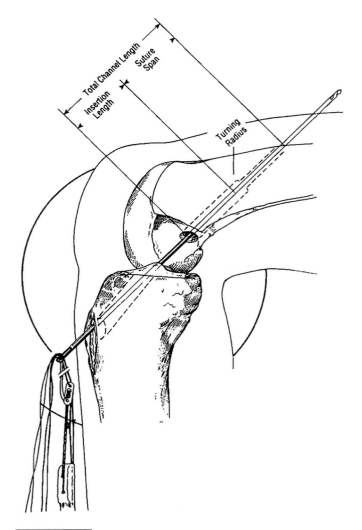

Figure 28–30 • The drill-tip passing pin is used to pull sutures and the endobutton-graft complex out through the skin. (From Rosenberg TD and Graf B: Techniques for ACL reconstruction with Multi-Trac drill guide. Technique manual, Acufex Microsurgical, Inc., Mansfield, Mass., 1994.)

COMPLICATIONS

Complications of ACL injuries can occur preoperatively, intraoperatively, or postoperatively.[124, 130, 164] The surgeon must have a thorough understanding of the potential complications, how to avoid them, and how to treat them to prevent surgical failures.

Preoperative Complications

Skeletally Immature Patients

Preoperative treatment dilemmas may occur in children and adolescents. In a skeletally immature patient, when all attempts at conservative therapy have failed, the physician, the patient, and the parents must weigh the risk of further

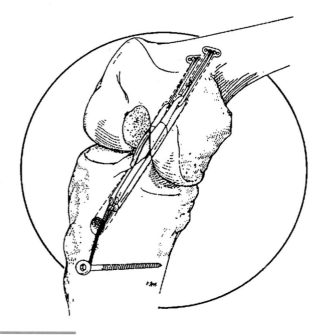

Figure 28–31 • The dual-tunnel graft is fixed distally over a bicortical screw and washer fixation post. (From Rosenberg TD and Graf B: Techniques for ACL reconstruction with Multi-Trac drill guide. Technique manual, Acufex Microsurgical, Inc., Mansfield, Mass., 1994.)

intra-articular damage against the risks of the potential for physeal problems (see Fig. 28–3).[11, 82] This matter should be discussed at length with the parents. Several reports of ACL reconstruction in skeletally immature patients have cited minimal complications.[11, 14, 82, 84, 89] Good results have been reported using a soft-tissue graft placed through a small drill hole centered in the ACL stump or just slightly posterior to the center of the ACL stump.[11, 14, 80–83] Care must be taken to avoid injury to the tibial tuberosity, which may cause a recurvatum deformity.[80] The most severe complication of ACL surgery in skeletally immature patients occurs when the lateral femoral physis is damaged. This can be avoided by taking the soft-tissue graft over the top of the femur and making certain that proximal fixation is in metaphyseal bone away from the physis (see Fig. 28–5).[83] Extra-articular reconstructions in these patients usually result in loosening and instability that require a second procedure.[11, 14, 82] If an extra-articular procedure is performed, the physis should be avoided at all costs.

Osgood-Schlatter Disease

If an ossicle is noted on preoperative roentgenograms, a 3.5 cm tibial plug should be harvested when taking the graft. If the ossicle is good bone and securely attached, it may be saved; otherwise, it should be excised, which will effectively lengthen the BPTB graft. The added length

may be compensated for by a graft recession, a tibial trough, or use of a two-incision technique.[165]

Patellofemoral Abnormalities

The status of the patellofemoral joint, especially in the case of patellar subluxation or degenerative change, should be evaluated on preoperative roentgenograms.[73, 162, 163, 191] A lateral release may be indicated for symptomatic subluxation, but more extensive realignment procedures are not indicated because of difficulty with rehabilitation. Marked patellofemoral changes and a history of patellofemoral pain are relative indications for use of the hamstrings for reconstruction and are contraindications for the use of open-chain exercises postoperatively.[73, 162, 163, 192] Patients with moderate arthritis usually benefit from reconstructive procedures, whereas patients who primarily have pain and swelling from degenerative changes respond better to mechanical realignment (see Fig. 28–7).[2, 99, 100–103]

Synovitis

Preoperative traumatic synovitis should be allowed to subside before surgery. Several studies have shown that waiting until the acute inflammatory reactions have resolved and range of motion and quadriceps tone have been regained is beneficial in the early postoperative period.[101, 125, 126, 169, 193, 194]

Meniscal Problems

Treatment of associated meniscal tears is based on the symptoms. If locking with activity is present, activity should be greatly reduced before reconstruction, and partial weight-bearing on crutches should be stressed while the patient is regaining motion and quadriceps function.[105, 108, 110, 195] For a locked meniscus, early reconstruction and repair of the meniscus are indicated, followed by early patient-specific progressive rehabilitation.[92] Johnson and Shelbourne[195] recommended repairing the meniscus, then performing a second-stage ACL reconstruction. This may be beneficial if extensive meniscal repair is necessary, but in general this author tries to avoid a second operative procedure. Only minimal problems with stiffness have been encountered when an aggressive postoperative rehabilitation program has been followed.[92]

Bone Infractions

Bone infractions (bone bruises) are reported to occur in over 80% of patients with complete ACL injuries.[36, 196, 197] The lateral compartment is involved in 80%. Vellet and colleagues[196] classified these bone infractions according to the architectural appearance, the spatial relationship to cortical bone, and the short-term osteochondral seque-

Table 28–3	MRI Classification of infractions of the Knee Associated with ACL injury

Occult subcortical infractions
  Reticular
  Geographic I and II
  Linear
Osteochondral
  Chondral
  Displaced
  Impaction

From Fowler PJ: Bone injuries associated with anterior ligament disruption. Arthroscopy 10:453, 1994.

lae (Table 28–3). In their study, more than 70% of bone infractions consisted of reticular lesions involving the cancellous bone, all of which had resolved on follow-up MRI. Most of the remaining infractions were occult geographic or impaction fractures involving damage to the subcortical bone. The lateral compartment was involved in 84% of patients with geographic lesions, all of whom also had reticular fractures of the posterior tibial margin owing to the amount of subluxation of the knee joint that resulted in the ACL injury. Follow-up MRI showed chronic defects from geographic lesions in 67% of these patients.

Intraoperative Complications

Set-up

The prevention of intraoperative complications begins with attention to the details of operative set-up. A tourniquet should be applied high enough to avoid problems of sterility. A lateral post should be used, or the end of the table should be dropped to allow full range of motion of the knee during the procedure.[130] A separate table with all the necessary instruments for preparation of the graft should be set up before the procedure. The graft itself should be secured to the table drapes with sutures to prevent it from being dropped.

Graft Harvest

Complications with graft harvest can be avoided by making exact cuts of known depths and by making a single straight incision in the same fiber plane when making the cuts.[130] While harvesting hamstring tendons, clear isolation of the tendons is required, using appropriately placed retractors. Neurovascular injury can be avoided by staying in the same plane and maintaining clear visualization.[73] Adequate length is ensured by releasing all fibrous extensions with a combination of sharp and blunt dissection before using a tendon stripper.[162] The stripper should pass

8–10 cm up the thigh before meeting soft resistance. If inadequate hamstring tissue is available, conversion to a BPTB procedure is indicated.

Graft Contamination

If graft contamination occurs during preparation, an alternate graft (such as the hamstrings) can be used, or the graft can be soaked in 4% chlorhexidine gluconate for 30 minutes, then soaked in a triple antibiotic solution for 30 minutes, and finally washed with saline solution.[198, 199] This has been shown to eliminate virulent organisms present in the operating room suite.[199]

Graft Passage

Problems with passage of the graft can be eliminated by making sure that fat tissue is removed and by making sure that the whole graft passes through the trial. Also, slightly contouring the lead end of the graft and placing the lead guide hole 3 mm from the end of the patellar plug, making sure that both plugs are 25–27 mm in length, and measuring the length of the complete graft can help prevent problems in passage.[130] Marking the bone-tendon edges and rolling the graft make accurate placement easier.

Patellar Fracture

Fractures of the patella are rare and can be prevented by avoiding excessive force during graft harvest. Most patellar fractures can be secured with a cerclage suture. Resisted knee extension should be avoided during the first 4–6 weeks after surgery. Flexion progresses as quickly as possible, depending on the stability of the patellar fracture, which usually is nondisplaced and stable.[200]

Posterior Wall Ream-out

Problems with posterior ream-out of the femoral wall during an endoscopic technique can be minimized by obtaining adequate visualization through careful attention to soft-tissue resection and notchplasty and by requiring at least 80–90 degrees of knee flexion.[130] Use of a femoral offset guide is also helpful, and the reamer footprint should be identified before reaming progresses. If ream-out occurs, a two-incision rear-entry technique may be used for recovery. Significant posterior wall ream-out may require placing the graft through a trough over the top and securing it over a bicortical screw and post.[130, 164, 201] If enough of the posterior wall is intact, the tunnel can be rerouted by using the rear-entry guide to pass a Kirschner wire to enter the mouth of the previously reamed tunnel.[130, 164, 201] The tunnel is then rerouted, beginning with an 8 mm reamer and advancing to a 10 mm reamer. The graft should be secured with an appropriately sized interference screw. If the necessary equipment is available and the surgeon is familiar with the technique, an endobutton can be used for secure graft fixation when the posterior wall is inadequate for interference screw fixation.[165, 166]

Ream-out of the femoral tunnel during the rear-entry technique can be avoided by making sure that the starting portal for the guide wire is at least 1.5 cm anterior to the posterior cortex of the lateral femur.[172] If ream-out occurs, a trough technique should be used, with the graft secured over a post.[166, 172]

Guide Wire Breakage

Guide wire breakage during the two-incision rear-entry technique can be avoided by carefully monitoring reaming over the femoral guide wire to make sure that the reamer is advancing appropriately. Metal filings may indicate crimping and cutting into the guide wire. If no filings are noted, progression of reaming can be attempted. If unsuccessful, the wire should be removed, checked for crimping, and replaced as necessary.

Postoperative Complications

Complications Related to Graft Source

Use of a central-third BPTB autograft may result in activity-related anterior knee pain, which generally is self-limiting.[130] With an accelerated rehabilitation program, persistent weakness of the quadriceps mechanism is rarely functionally significant.[77, 130, 202] After harvest of a hamstring graft, a 15–20% hamstring deficiency may occur, but it is usually functionally insignificant.[130, 151, 203] Because of delayed maturation, it has become more evident that allografts are approximately half as strong as autografts at 6 months after surgery, and elongation of allografts may occur for up to 2 years.[163, 204–206] The addition of ligament augmentation devices and extra-articular

tenodesis procedures has been reported to increase complications without significantly increasing stability with allograft or autograft ligament reconstructions.[119, 122, 206] Resorption around the tunnels is also a concern after allograft reconstructions.[207]

Loss of Motion

Extension block is most often caused by graft impingement or nonisometric placement of the graft.[134, 135, 187, 193] This problem should be corrected during surgery.[134] Postoperatively, extension may also be impeded by notch fibrosis, a "cyclops" lesion (fibrotic soft-tissue remnant), or graft hypertrophy at 4–6 months.[208, 209] If notch fibrosis is suspected, rehabilitation should stress early full-knee extension (prone hangs, pillow under heel), whereas graft hypertrophy is an indication to stop open-chain extension exercises (which reproduce the symptoms) during the maturation phase. A cyclops lesion may require resection of the impeding soft tissue.[203] If extension problems persist, excellent results can be obtained with arthroscopic resection of impinging soft tissue and further notchplasty.[134, 208–213]

Arthrofibrosis

Arthrofibrosis can be minimized by delaying reconstruction until acute inflammatory reaction of the knee has resolved and knee motion and quadriceps tone have been regained.[101, 125] After surgery, motion problems can be prevented by emphasis on early full extension, patellar mobilization, and active range of motion.[54, 77, 212] If stiffness develops, prone hangs and the use of modalities such as heat and ultrasound should be used to regain extension (Fig. 28–32).[54, 212] A drop-out cast or similar device may be necessary. Surgical intervention is indicated in the absence of progress (Fig. 28–33).[211–216]

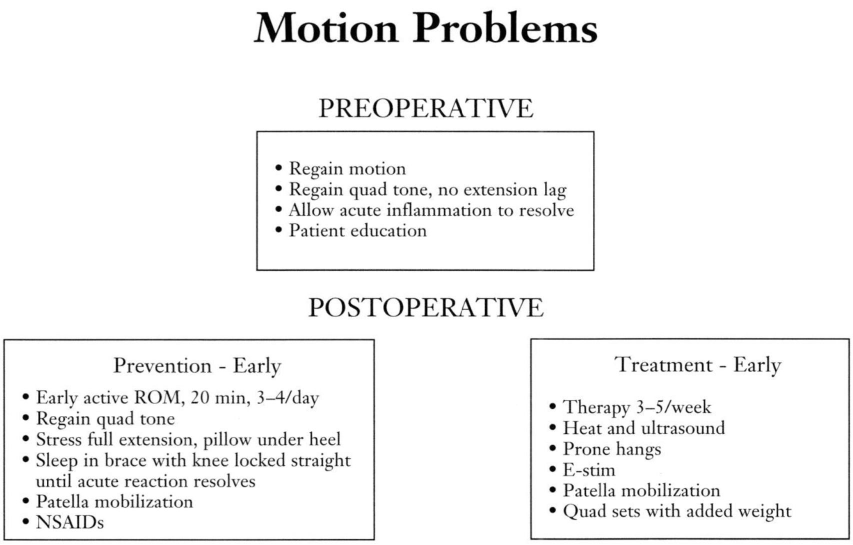

Motion Problems

PREOPERATIVE

- Regain motion
- Regain quad tone, no extension lag
- Allow acute inflammation to resolve
- Patient education

POSTOPERATIVE

Prevention - Early

- Early active ROM, 20 min, 3–4/day
- Regain quad tone
- Stress full extension, pillow under heel
- Sleep in brace with knee locked straight until acute reaction resolves
- Patella mobilization
- NSAIDs

Treatment - Early

- Therapy 3–5/week
- Heat and ultrasound
- Prone hangs
- E-stim
- Patella mobilization
- Quad sets with added weight

Figure 28–32 • Treatment algorithm for motion problems after ACL surgery.

MANIPULATION INDICATED IF

- < 5° gain/week × 2 weeks +
  < 90° after 4 weeks of supervised therapy

  OR

- < 5° gain/week × 2 weeks +
  < 120° after 6 weeks of supervised therapy

ARTHROSCOPIC RELEASE INDICATED IF

- Firm endpoint to manipulation
Consider if:
- > 9° weeks from surgery

LATERAL RELEASE INDICATED IF

- Decreased patellar mobility (<1 quadrant medial passive glide) after arthroscopic débridement

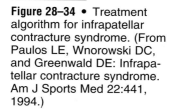

Figure 28–33 • Indications for surgical treatment of motion problems after ACL surgery.

If full-blown infrapatellar contracture syndrome develops (indicated by peripatellar soft-tissue enduration, restricted patellar mobility, and limited knee motion), knee extension should be emphasized, but aggressive therapy should be avoided during the inflammatory stage.[211] Quadriceps and hamstring strengthening exercises are beneficial. Open release is usually necessary at approximately 3 months (Fig. 28–34).[54] If the contracture causes significant patella baja (more than 8 mm), a DeLee-type osteotomy (Fig. 28–35) may be indicated.[211, 212, 217]

Joint Effusion

Joint effusion in the early postoperative period is usually caused by joint overuse in therapy; effusion can be treated with the use of nonsteroidal anti-inflammatory drugs, the use of modalities, and reduction of repetitive joint stress.[77, 127, 218] Effusion may also be caused by graft impingement, graft rupture, or joint capture.[127, 130, 164, 201, 219] An effusion that does not resolve with activity restriction should be aspirated for cultures.[127, 220, 221] Leukocyte counts from a joint aspirate may be in the range of 50,000–70,000 if intra-articular synthetic material has been used.[220, 221] If a 2+–3+ effusion persists despite conservative treatment and culture results are negative, MRI may be helpful to evaluate for graft impingement or partial rupture (see Fig. 28–2).[37, 222–224]

Figure 28–34 • Treatment algorithm for infrapatellar contracture syndrome. (From Paulos LE, Wnorowski DC, and Greenwald DE: Infrapatellar contracture syndrome. Am J Sports Med 22:441, 1994.)

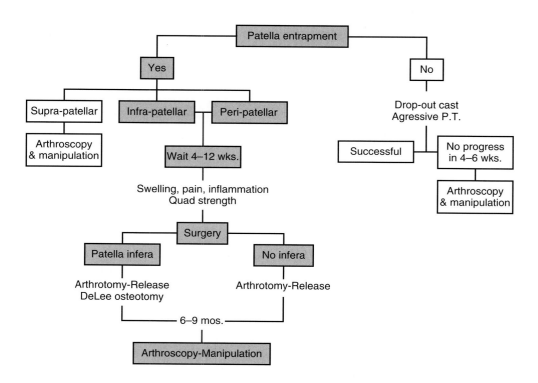

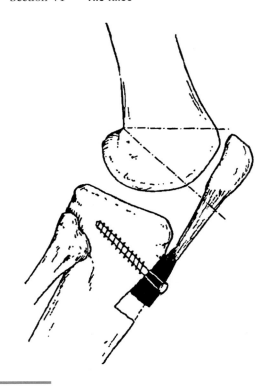

Figure 28–35 • DeLee oblique osteotomy for proximal tubercle slide and patellofemoral joint unloading. (From Paulos LE, Wnorowski DC and Greenwald DE: Infrapatellar contracture syndrome. Am J Sports Med 22:442, 1994.)

Extensor Mechanism Problems

Extensor mechanism problems that may develop during rehabilitation include patellar tendinitis, which is activity-related and usually self-limiting. Therapy should stress closed-chain exercises.[75, 127, 225–227]

Ruptures of both the patellar tendon and the quadriceps have been reported, but they are rare after ACL reconstruction.[228] Ruptures of either should be repaired early and reinforced with a cerclage suture. Range-of-motion exercises progress as tolerated by the security of the repair, but active extension, especially resisted extension, should be avoided during the early healing phase.[228–231]

Loss of Stability

Loss of stability during the early postoperative period (3–4 weeks) may be caused by inadequate graft fixation.[130–133, 140, 141, 145–148, 158, 164, 201] Attention to the details of secure fixation and ensuring that proper rehabilitation protocols are followed (avoidance of open-chain exercises, especially in the flexion range of 0–45 degrees) can eliminate most of these problems.[130, 131] If fixation failure occurs, the screws can be removed, and the graft can be secured with a larger

interference screw or with post fixation.[140, 141, 145, 146, 158, 232] Daniel[233] suggested that interference screw fixation strength is greatest when the outer screw diameter is 4 mm greater than the tunnel-bone gap; for example, if the gap is less than 3 mm, a 7 mm screw should be used; for a gap of 5 mm or less, a 9 mm screw should be used. A gap of 6 mm or more requires fixation over a post, which can be supplemented with a 9 mm interference screw. If screw replacement is necessary, it is imperative that the tunnels be placed appropriately and that there be no impingement or capture of the joint.[131, 133, 164, 201] The replacement screw is placed parallel to the graft for more secure fixation.[140, 145, 233]

Late loss of stability may be caused by traumatic disruption of the graft or failure of incorporation of the graft.[130, 131, 133, 164, 201] Jackson and colleagues[138] showed that the critical factors affecting graft maturation strength were appropriate graft tension and orientation. Before any revision procedure, anteroposterior and lateral roentgenograms should be obtained to determine the placement of previous tunnels and fixation devices and to evaluate for tunnel enlargement. If the fixation screws can be removed without excessive difficulty or excessive removal of bone from the femoral condyle, they should be removed. If screw removal appears difficult, the lateral roentgenogram should be carefully evaluated to determine if a rear-entry technique, which changes the orientation of the tunnel to a more horizontal position, would allow the new graft to be secured without removing the previously placed femoral screw.[131, 133] Another alternative is to secure the graft in a trough in the over-the-top position.[127, 131, 133] An excellent graft source for revision is a BPTB graft from the opposite extremity, which allows larger bone plugs to be taken and results in a graft as strong as the original graft. Other techniques include the ipsilateral hamstring quadruple graft and doubled grafts taken through dual 6- to 7-mm tunnels with endoscopic fixation.[149, 165, 166, 234] The smaller-diameter tunnels may allow the revision graft to be placed in good bone posterior to the original tunnel (see Fig. 28–31).[165, 166] An allograft may be used if the patient understands the possible complications of the use of allograft material.[163, 201, 235] When revision ACL surgery is considered, the patient should be informed that a two-stage procedure may be necessary. If a cavernous enlargement of the tunnels is noted on radiographs or at surgery, the defect should be grafted with autogenous bone. A second-stage revision may be performed when the graft has healed solidly at approximately 2 months.[127]

REHABILITATION

Successful ACL reconstruction depends on appropriate rehabilitation based on the concepts of tissue maturation and biomechanical effects of stress to tissues during the maturation process.[137, 236–238] A rehabilitation program should take into consideration stability of fixation, strength and maturation rate of the graft, anticipated loads to be applied to grafts, and patient reliability (Fig. 28–36).[225, 236, 237]

CONCEPTS AFFECTING EARLY REHABILITATION

- 0–4 weeks - weak point at fixation
- 4–6 weeks - graft synovialization
- 3–12 weeks - ligament to tunnel healing
- 6–8 weeks - bone plug to tunnel healing
- 6–12 weeks - graft at weakest point
- 6 months - graft strength comparable to ACL

- Graft at 3 weeks - viable and vascular

Stage of repopulation	2 months
Stage of rapid remodeling	2–12 months
Maturation	1–3 years
Quiescence	3 years

- Stability of fixation

- Strength of graft

- Maturation rate of graft

- Anticipated loads to be applied to graft

- Reliability of patient

PATIENT INDIVIDUALIZATION

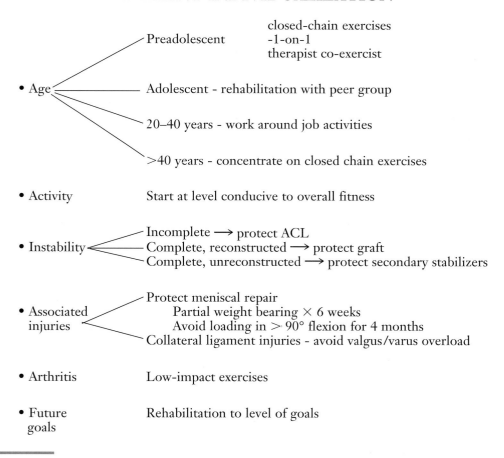

- Age
  - Preadolescent — closed-chain exercises -1-on-1 therapist co-exercist
  - Adolescent - rehabilitation with peer group
  - 20–40 years - work around job activities
  - >40 years - concentrate on closed chain exercises

- Activity — Start at level conducive to overall fitness

- Instability
  - Incomplete → protect ACL
  - Complete, reconstructed → protect graft
  - Complete, unreconstructed → protect secondary stabilizers

- Associated injuries
  - Protect meniscal repair
    - Partial weight bearing × 6 weeks
    - Avoid loading in > 90° flexion for 4 months
  - Collateral ligament injuries - avoid valgus/varus overload

- Arthritis — Low-impact exercises

- Future goals — Rehabilitation to level of goals

Figure 28–36 • Rehabilitation should consider stability of fixation, strength and maturation rate of the graft, anticipated loads, and patient reliability.

When a BPTB or quadrupled gracilis semitendinosus graft is used, the initial strength of the graft is more than adequate, compared with that of the normal ACL.[137, 239, 240] According to Rougraff and colleagues,[241] Shino et al.,[242] and Abe and coworkers,[243] grafts probably do not go through an extensive necrotic stage as was once believed. Rougraff and colleagues[241] described four stages of ligamentization after reconstruction (see Fig. 28–36).

Earlier studies showed the grafts to be at their weakest 6–9 weeks after surgery and approximately equal in strength to the normal ACL at 6 months.[137, 138] The grafts continue to gain strength until 12–18 months and then remain the same during the maturation process.

Based on biological and biomechanical concepts, rehabilitation is divided into six stages (Table 28–4).[77, 230, 241, 242] In the immediate postoperative period, cold therapy by one of the commercially available units has been shown to be beneficial in decreasing pain and swelling.[218] Use of a continuous passive motion machine immediately after surgery has been shown to decrease pain and assist in pumping fluid from the soft tissues, but prolonged use has not been shown to be beneficial or cost-effective.[244, 245] In fact, aggressive use of a continuous passive motion machine for flexion in the initial postoperative period may be detrimental to the graft, depending on isometry of the graft, stability of fixation, and impingement wear on the tunnel edges.[170, 246] Electrical stimulation of the thigh muscles has been reported to be effective during the early postoperative course,[247] but Sisk et al.[248] found little benefit with the routine use of electrical stimulation. This modality probably should be used on an individualized basis as an adjuvant to muscle re-education when the return of quadriceps function is progressing slowly.[249]

The progression of the ACL rehabilitation protocol and the patient's return to contact or cutting sports vary. The concept of accelerated rehabilitation and earlier stress was advanced by Shelbourne and Nitz,[77] who emphasized that the rehabilitation process should be monitored with periodic KT-1000 evaluations of the graft. Other studies reported no difference in long-term results in patients who returned to sports earlier as compared with those who returned later.[24, 250] In a long-term study of autogenous grafts, Harter et al.[251] found no propensity for grafts to elongate with activity throughout a long time. Barber-Westin and Noyes,[236] on the other hand, found that, in allografts, one-third of the abnormal displacement seen on follow-up KT-1000 developed more than 2 years after surgery. These findings and others show that allografts take longer to incorporate than autografts and may be subject to progressive stretching.[163, 206, 252–254] Earlier return to activity (6 months) of patients with autografts is acceptable.[77, 138, 241] Clinical studies and laboratory evaluation, including electron microscopy, have shown rapid tissue remodeling more than 1 year after surgery.[242–244] Possible variations in the maturation process among individuals must be considered, and return to activity before 6 months may put some patients at risk.[242, 253]

Table 28–4	**Staging of Rehabilitation**
Stage I Goals	Immediate postoperative • Decrease pain • Control swelling • Crutch ambulation • Extremity control • Muscle tone • Active and passive range of motion • Patient education
Protocol	• Quad sets 10–15 (15–20 s) hourly • Straight leg raises 15–20 hourly (assist as necessary) • Ankle pumps 15–20 hourly • Sitting slides (active and active-assisted) 15–20 min 3/daily • Brace locked straight except for range-of-motion exercises • Emphasize full extension 　Pillow under heel while resting 　Sleep in brace with knee straight
Stage II	• Regain motion • Regain muscle tone • Decrease inflammation (modalities) • Achieve normal gait • Protect graft • Continue patient education
Stage III	• Protected strengthening 　Quads: antagonistic to ACL 0–45 degrees of flexion • Proprioceptive feedback • Allow continued graft maturation
Stage IV	• Advanced strengthening • Full range of motion • Plyometrics • Jogging, running
Stage V	• Sport-specific exercises • Agility training • Mental preparation
Stage VI	• Return to sport • Maintenance exercises 2–3/wk

The six stages of rehabilitation, which are detailed in Table 28-5, allow the patient to return to sports activity at approximately 6 months after surgery. Use of an ACL protective brace is not encouraged but may be used by some individuals. During the rehabilitation process, the patient should be observed closely, every 1–2 weeks initially and every 4–6 weeks later in the protocol, for evaluation of swelling, patellofemoral problems, and motion or stability problems. Appropriate adjustments—decreasing joint stress, emphasizing closed-chain exercises, and changing the frequency and duration of exercises—may be necessary.

Table 28–5	**ACL Rehabilitation Protocol**

Stage I
0–2 weeks
- Patellar mobilizations (emphasize superior/inferior glides)
- Motion control brace 0–90
- Quad sets/straight-leg raises all planes (emphasize straight-leg raise without extension lag)
- Prone/standing hamstring curls
- Passive extension (emphasize full extension)
    - Prone hangs
    - Pillow under heel
- Passive, active, and active-assisted range-of-motion knee flexion
    - Wall slides
    - Sitting slides
    - Prone towel pulls
- Edema control—compression pump
- Electrical stimulation for muscle re-education if poor quadriceps set
- Cryotherapy
- Partial weight-bearing 50–75% with crutches or weight-bearing to tolerance without crutches if motion control brace locked in full extension
- Sleep in brace locked in extension

GOALS:
- Full knee-extension range of motion
- 90° knee-flexion range of motion
- Good quad set
- Emphasize normal gait pattern

Stage II
2–4 weeks
- Motion control brace full range of motion
- Progress range of motion to 120 by 4 weeks
- Progress straight-leg raises and prone/standing hamstring curls with weights
- Bike for range of motion, begin low-resistance program when range of motion adequate
- Stool scoots
- Full weight-bearing with crutches, discontinue crutches when ambulating without limp
- Begin double-leg biomechanical ankle platform system, progress to single-leg
- Begin double-leg press with light weight/high repetitions
- Wall sits at 45-degree angle with tibia vertical; progress time
- Lateral step-ups (4 in) when able to perform single-leg quarter squat
- Hip machine and hamstring machine when able to perform straight-leg raises with 10 lb
- Treadmill (forward and backward) with emphasis on normal gait
- Knee extension 90–60 degrees (submaximal) with manual resistance by therapist

GOALS:
- Range of motion 0–120 degrees
- Full weight-bearing without crutches, no limp

4–6 weeks
- Progress to full range of motion by 6 weeks
- Begin Kin-Com hamstring progression (isotonic/isokinetic)
- Begin Kin-Com quad work 90–40 isotonics with antishear pad
- Stairmaster (forward and backward)
- Progress closed-chain exercises
- At 6 weeks, begin Kin-Com quad work 90–40 isokinetics
    (start with higher speed and work endurance)
- Aquatic exercises

8–10 weeks
- Progress above exercises
- Slow-form running with sport-cord (forward and backward)
- Isokinetic quad work at different speeds (60, 90, 120)
- Begin lunges
- At 10 weeks, begin Fitter, slide board

Table continued on following page

Table 28-5 **ACL Rehabilitation Protocol (*Continued*)**

Stage III
12–16 weeks
- Full-range isotonics on Kin-Com (begin moving antishear pad down)
- Knee extension machine with low weight/high repetition
- Lateral sport-cord drills (slow, controlled)
- Kin-Com test hamstrings, discontinue isokinetic hamstrings if 90% of well-leg strength
- Progress isokinetic quads to full extension by 16 weeks
- Plyometric exercises start at 14 weeks

Stage IV
16–18 weeks
- Kin-Com test quads, retest hamstrings if necessary
- Progress plyometric program with shuttle, minitramp, jump rope if quad strength 65%, no effusion, full range of motion, stable knee
- Begin jogging program if quad strength (same criteria as above)

Stage V
5–6 months
- Agility training
- Sport-specific drills (carioca, cutting at a 45 degree angle, figure 8, etc.)
- Retest quads if necessary

Stage VI
6 months
- Return to sport if:
  Motion > 130 degrees
  Hamstrings > 90% of strength of well leg
  Quads > 85%
  Sport-specific agility training completed
- Maintenance exercises 2–3/wk

References

1. Bach BR, Warren RF, Flynn WM, et al.: Arthrometric evaluation of knees that have a torn anterior cruciate ligament. J Bone Joint Surg Am 72:1299, 1990.
2. Girgis FG, Marshall JL, and Al Monajem ARS: The cruciate ligaments of the knee joint: anatomical, functional and experimental analysis. Clin Orthop 106:216, 1975.
3. Grood ES, Noyes FR, Butler DL, et al.: Ligamentous and capsular restraints preventing straight medial and lateral laxity in intact human cadaver knees. J Bone Joint Surg Am 63:1257, 1981.
4. Johnson RF, Beynnon BD, Nichols CE, et al.: Current concepts review: the treatment of injuries of the anterior cruciate ligament. J Bone Joint Surg Am 74:140, 1992.
5. Noyes FR and Grood ES: Classification of ligament injuries: why an anterolateral laxity or anteromedial laxity is not a diagnostic entity. Instr Course Lect 36:185, 1987.
6. Odensten M and Gillquist J: Functional anatomy of the anterior cruciate ligament and a rationale for reconstruction. J Bone Joint Surg Am 67:257, 1985.
7. Daniel DM and Fithian DC: Current concepts: indications for ACL surgery. Arthroscopy 10:434, 1994.
8. Daniel DM, Stone ML, Dobson BE, et al.: Fate of the ACL-injured patient: a prospective outcome study. Am J Sports Med 22:632, 1994.
9. Noyes FR, Mooar PA, Matthews DS, et al.: The symptomatic anterior cruciate–deficient knee: part I: the long-term functional disability in athletically active individuals. J Bone Joint Surg Am 65:154, 1983.
10. Ray JM: A proposed natural history of symptomatic anterior cruciate ligament injuries of the knee. Clin Sports Med 7:697, 1988.
11. McCarroll JR, Shelbourne KD, Porter DA, et al.: Patellar tendon graft reconstruction for midsubstance anterior cruciate ligament rupture in junior high school athletes: an algorithm for management. Am J Sports Med 22:478, 1994.
12. Torg JS, Conrad W, and Kalen V: Clinical diagnosis of anterior cruciate ligament instability in the athlete. Am J Sports Med 4:84, 1976.
13. Kennedy JC, Weinberg HW, and Wilson AS: The anatomy and function of the anterior cruciate ligament, as determined by clinical and morphological studies. J Bone Joint Surg Am 56:223, 1974.
14. Lipscomb AB and Anderson AF: Tears of the anterior cruciate ligament in adolescents. J Bone Joint Surg Am 68:19, 1986.
15. DeHaven KE: Arthroscopy in acute trauma. Presented at the American Academy of Orthopaedic Surgeons Continuing Education Course on the Athlete's Knee: Surgical Repair and Reconstruction—Diagnostic Arthroscopy and Arthrography. Hilton Head Island, S.C., June, 1978.
16. Noyes FR, Bassett RW, Grood ES, et al.: Arthroscopy in acute traumatic hemarthrosis of the knee: incidence of anterior cruciate tears and other injuries. J Bone Joint Surg Am 62:687, 1980.
17. Hughston JC, Andrews JR, Cross MJ, et al.: Classification of knee ligament instabilities: part I: the medial compartment and cruciate ligaments. J Bone Joint Surg Am 58:159, 1976.
18. Hughston JC, Andrews JR, Cross MJ, et al.: Classification of knee ligament instabilities: part I: the lateral compartment. J Bone Joint Surg Am 58:173, 1976.
19. Kennedy JC and Fowler PJ: Medial and anterior instability of the knee. J Bone Joint Surg Am 53:1257, 1971.
20. Butler DL, Noyes FR, and Grood ES: Ligamentous restraints to anterior-posterior drawer in the human knee: a biomechanical study. J Bone Joint Surg Am 62:259, 1980.
21. Rosenberg TD and Rasmussen GL: The function of the anterior cruciate ligament during anterior drawer and Lachman's testing: an in vivo analysis in normal knees. Am J Sports Med 12:318, 1984.
22. International Knee Documentation Committee of the American Orthopaedic Society for Sports Medicine and the European Society for Knee Surgery and Arthroscopy: Knee ligament standard evaluation form, 1993.
23. Fetto JF and Marshall JL: Injury to the anterior cruciate ligament producing the pivot-shift sign: an experimental study on cadaver specimens. J Bone Joint Surg Am 61:710, 1979.
24. Galway HR and MacIntosh DL: The lateral pivot shift: a symptom and sign of anterior cruciate ligament insufficiency. Clin Orthop 147:45, 1980.

25. Warren LF, Marshall JL, and Girgis F: The prime static stabilizer of the medial side of the knee. J Bone Joint Surg Am 56:665, 1974.
26. Warren LF and Marshall JL: The supporting structures and layers on the medial side of the knee: an anatomical analysis. J Bone Joint Surg Am 61:56, 1979.
27. Marshall JL, Wang JB, Furman W, et al.: The anterior drawer sign: what is it? J Sports Med 3:152, 1975.
28. Daniel DM, Stone ML, Barnett P, et al.: Use of the quadriceps active test to diagnose posterior cruciate ligament disruption and measure posterior laxity of the knee. J Bone Joint Surg Am 70:386–1988.
29. Godfrey JD: Ligamentous injuries of the knee. Curr Pract Orthop Surg 5:56, 1973.
30. Warren RF and Marshall JL: Injuries of the anterior cruciate and medial collateral ligaments of the knee: a long-term follow-up of 86 cases: part II. Clin Orthop 136:198, 1978.
31. Veltri DM and Warren RF: Posterolateral instability of the knee. Instr Course Lect 44:441, 1995.
32. Butler JC and Andrews JR: The role of arthroscopic surgery in the evaluation of acute traumatic hemarthrosis of the knee. Clin Orthop 228:150, 1988.
33. DeHaven KE: Diagnosis of acute knee injuries with hemarthrosis. Am J Sports Med 8:9, 1980.
34. DeHaven KE: Arthroscopy in the diagnosis and management of the anterior cruciate ligament deficient knee. Clin Orthop 172:52, 1983.
35. Hardacker WT, Garrett WE Jr, and Bassett FH III: Evaluation of acute traumatic hemarthrosis of the knee joint. South Med J 83:640, 1990.
36. Rose MS, Jackson DW, and Burger PE: Occult osseous lesions associated with ACL ruptures documented by magnetic resonance imaging. Arthroscopy 7:45, 1991.
37. Schwartz ML: Magnetic resonance imaging of knee ligaments and tendons. Oper Tech Sports Med 3:27, 1995.
38. Hey Groves EW: Operation for the repair of the crucial ligaments. Lancet 1:674, 1917.
39. Campbell WC: Reconstruction of the ligaments of the knee. Am J Surg 43:473, 1939.
40. Campbell WC: Repair of the ligaments of the knee: report of a new operation for repair of the anterior crucial ligament. Surg Gynecol Obstet 62:964, 1936.
41. Jones KG: Reconstruction of the anterior cruciate ligament: a technique using the central one-third of the patellar ligament. J Bone Joint Surg Am 45:925, 1963.
42. Jones KG: Reconstruction of the anterior cruciate ligament: a technique using the central one-third of the patellar ligament: a follow-up report. J Bone Joint Surg Am 52:1302, 1970.
43. Jones KG: Results of use of the central one-third of the patellar ligament to compensate for anterior cruciate ligament deficiency. Clin Orthop 147:39, 1980.
44. Clancy WG Jr, Nelson DA, Reider B, et al.: Anterior cruciate ligament reconstruction using one-third of the patellar ligament, augmented by extra-articular tendon transfers. J Bone Joint Surg Am 64:352, 1982.
45. Clancy WG Jr: Anterior cruciate ligament functional instability: a static intra-articular and dynamic extra-articular procedure. Clin Orthop 172:102, 1983.
46. Clancy WG Jr: Arthroscopic anterior cruciate ligament reconstruction with patellar tendon. Tech Orthop 2:13, 1988.
47. Howell SM and Clark JA: Tibial tunnel placement in anterior cruciate ligament reconstruction and graft impingement. Clin Orthop 283:187, 1992.
48. Morgan CD and Galinat BJ: The tibial attachment of the ACL: where is it? Exhibit, American Academy of Orthopaedic Surgeons Meeting, San Francisco, Calif., Feb., 1993.
49. O'Donoghue DH, Frank GR, Jeter GL, et al.: Repair and reconstruction of the anterior cruciate ligament in dogs: factors influencing long-term results. J Bone Joint Surg Am 53:710, 1971.
50. O'Donoghue DH, Rockwood CA Jr, Frank GR, et al.: Repair of the anterior cruciate ligament in dogs. J Bone Joint Surg Am 48:503, 1966.
51. Yaru NC, Daniel DM, and Penner D: The effect of tibial attachment site on graft impingement in an anterior cruciate ligament reconstruction. Am J Sports Med 20:217, 1992.
52. Cabaud HE, Rodkey WG, and Feagin JA: Experimental studies of acute anterior cruciate ligament injury and repair. Am J Sports Med 7:18, 1979.
53. Noyes FR, Butler DL, Paulos LE, et al.: Intra-articular cruciate reconstruction: I: perspectives on graft strength, vascularization, and immediate motion after replacement. Clin Orthop 172:71, 1983.
54. Noyes FR, Mangine RE, and Barber-Westin SD: The early treatment of motion complications after reconstruction of the anterior cruciate ligament. Clin Orthop 277:217, 1992.
55. Shelbourne KD and Nitz P: Accelerated rehabilitation after anterior cruciate ligament reconstruction. Am J Sports Med 18:292, 1990.
56. Feagin JA Jr, Cabaud HE, and Curl WW: The anterior cruciate ligament: radiographic and clinical signs of successful and unsuccessful repairs. Clin Orthop 164:54, 1982.
57. Indelicato PA: Non-operative treatment of complete tears of the medial collateral ligament of the knee. J Bone Joint Surg Am 65:323, 1983.
58. Shelbourne KD and Porter DA: Anterior cruciate ligament–medial collateral ligament injury: nonoperative management of medial collateral ligament tears with anterior cruciate ligament reconstruction: a preliminary report. Am J Sports Med 20:283, 1992.
59. Noyes FR, McGinniss GH, and Grood ES: The variable functional disability of the anterior cruciate ligament–deficient knee. Orthop Clin North Am 16:47, 1985.
60. Noyes FR and McGinniss GH: Controversy about treatment of the knee with anterior cruciate laxity. Clin Orthop 198:81, 1985.
61. Pattee GA, Fox JM, Del Pizzo W, et al.: Four-to ten-year followup of unreconstructed anterior cruciate ligament tears. Am J Sports Med 17:430, 1989.
62. Sherman MF, Warren RF, Marshall JL, et al.: A clinical and radiographical analysis of 127 anterior cruciate ligament–insufficient knees. Clin Orthop 227:229, 1988.
63. Tegner Y and Lysholm J: Rating systems in the evaluation of knee ligament injuries. Clin Orthop 198:43, 1985.
64. Wasilewski SA, Covall DJ, and Cohen S: Effect of surgical timing on recovery and associated injuries after anterior cruciate ligament reconstruction. Am J Sports Med 21:338, 1993.
65. Kennedy JC, Hawkins RJ, Willis RB, et al.: Tension studies of human knee ligaments: yield point, ultimate failure, and disruption of the cruciate and tibial collateral ligaments. J Bone Joint Surg Am 58:350, 1976.
66. Lintner DM, Kamaric E, Moseley JB, et al.: Partial tears of the anterior cruciate ligament: are they clinically detectable? Am J Sports Med 23:111, 1995.
67. Noyes FR, DeLucase JL, and Torvik PJ: Biomechanics of anterior cruciate ligament failure: an analysis of strain-rate sensitivity and mechanisms of failure in primates. J Bone Joint Surg Am 56:236, 1974.
68. Rijke AM, Perrin DH, Goitz HT, et al.: Instrumented arthrometry for diagnosing partial versus complete anterior cruciate ligament tears. Am J Sports Med 22:294, 1994.
69. Fleming BC, Beynnon BD, and Johnson RJ: The use of knee laxity testers for the determination of anterior-posterior stability of the knee. In Jackson DW (ed.): The Anterior Cruciate Ligament: Current and Future Concepts. New York, Raven Press Ltd., 1993, pp 239–250.
70. Harter RA, Osternig LR, and Singer KM: Instrumented Lachman tests for the evaluation of anterior laxity after reconstruction of the anterior cruciate ligament. J Bone Joint Surg Am 71:975, 1989.
71. Buckely SL, Barrack RL, and Alexander AH: The natural history of conservatively treated partial anterior cruciate ligament tears. Am J Sports Med 17:221, 1989.
72. Sandberg R and Balkfors B: Partial rupture of the anterior cruciate ligament: natural course. Clin Orthop 220:176, 1987.
73. Warner JJP, Warren RF, and Cooper DE: Management of acute anterior cruciate ligament injury. Instr Course Lect 40:219, 1991.
74. Noyes FR, Mooar LA, Moorman CT III, et al.: Partial tears of the anterior cruciate ligament: progression to complete ligament deficiency. J Bone Joint Surg Br 71:825, 1989.
75. Anderson AF and Lipscomb AB: Analysis of rehabilitation techniques after anterior cruciate reconstruction. Am J Sports Med 17:154, 1989.
76. Odensten M, Hamberg P, Nordin M, et al.: Surgical or conservative treatment of the acutely torn anterior cruciate ligament: a ran-

domized study with short-term follow-up observations. Clin Orthop 198:87, 1985.

77. Shelbourne KD and Nitz P: Accelerated rehabilitation after anterior cruciate ligament reconstruction. Am J Sports Med 18:292, 1990.

78. Buseck MS and Noyes FR: Arthroscopic evaluation of meniscal repairs after anterior cruciate ligament reconstruction and immediate motion. Am J Sports Med 19:489, 1991.

79. DeHaven KE, Black KP, and Griffiths JH: Open meniscus repair: technique and two- to nine-year results. Am J Sports Med 17:788, 1989.

80. Nottage WM and Matsuura PA: Management of complete traumatic anterior cruciate ligament tears in the skeletally immature patient: current concepts and review of the literature. Arthroscopy 10:569, 1994.

81. Brief LP: Anterior cruciate ligament reconstruction without drill holes. Arthroscopy 7:350, 1991.

82. McCarroll JR, Rettig AC, and Shelbourne KD: Anterior cruciate ligament injuries in the young athlete with open physes. Am J Sports Med 16:44, 1988.

83. Andrews M, Noyes FR, and Barber-Westin SD: Anterior cruciate ligament allograft reconstruction in the skeletally immature athlete. Am J Sports Med 22:48, 1994.

84. Sullivan JA: Ligamentous injuries of the knee in children. Clin Orthop 255:44, 1990.

85. Gruelich W and Pyle S: Radiographic Atlas of Skeletal Development of the Hand and Wrist, 2nd ed. Stanford, Stanford University Press, 1959.

86. Hensinger RN: Standards in Pediatric Orthopaedics. New York, Raven Press, 1986.

87. Kannus P and Jarvinen M: Knee ligament injuries in adolescents. J Bone Joint Surg Br 70:772, 1988.

88. Parker AW, Drez D Jr, and Cooper JL: Anterior cruciate ligament injuries in patients with open physes. Am J Sports Med 22:44, 1994.

89. Angel KR and Hall DJ: Anterior cruciate ligament injury in children and adolescents. Arthroscopy 5:197, 1989.

90. Bolano LE and Grana WA: Isolated arthroscopic partial meniscectomy. Am J Sports Med 21:432, 1993.

91. Caldwell GL Jr, Allen AA, and Fu FH: Functional anatomy and biomechanics of the meniscus. Oper Tech Sports Med 2:152, 1994.

92. Cannon WD Jr: Techniques, indications, results of meniscal repair. Presented at the Arthroscopy Association of North America Specialty Day, Orlando, Fla., Feb. 19, 1995.

93. Jaureguito JW, Elliot JS, Lietner T, et al.: The effects of arthroscopic partial lateral meniscectomy in an otherwise normal knee: a retrospective review of functional, clinical, and radiographic results. Presented at the Arthroscopy Association of North America Specialty Day, Orlando, Fla., Feb. 19, 1995.

94. Roos H, Lindberg H, Gärdsell P, et al.: The prevalence of gonarthrosis and its relation to meniscectomy in former soccer players. Am J Sports Med 22:219, 1994.

95. Zarins B: Knee arthroscopy: basic technique. Contemp Orthop 6:63, 1983.

96. Beynnon B, Wertheimer C, Fleming B, et al.: An in-vivo study of the anterior cruciate ligament strain biomechanics during functional knee bracing. Trans Orthop Res Soc 15:223, 1990.

97. Cawley PW, France EP, and Paulos LE: The current state of functional knee bracing research: a review of the literature. Am J Sports Med 19:226, 1988.

98. O'Brien SJ, Warren RF, Pavlov H, et al.: Reconstruction of the chronically insufficient anterior cruciate ligament with the central third of the patellar ligament. J Bone Joint Surg Am 73:278, 1991.

99. Shelbourne KD: Symposium: ACL insufficiency and osteoarthritis: ACL reconstruction. Presented at the American Orthopaedic Society for Sports Medicine Specialty Day, Orlando, Fla., Feb. 19, 1995.

100. Shelbourne KD and Wilckens JH: Intraarticular anterior cruciate ligament reconstruction in the symptomatic arthritic knee. Am J Sports Med 21:685, 1993.

101. Shelbourne KD, Wilckens JH, Mollabashy A, et al.: Arthrofibrosis in acute anterior cruciate ligament reconstruction: the effect of timing of reconstruction and rehabilitation. Am J Sports Med 19:332, 1991.

102. Noyes FR, Barber-Westin SD, and Simon R: High tibial osteotomy and ligament reconstruction in varus-angulated, anterior cruciate ligament–deficient knees: a two- to seven-year follow-up study. Am J Sports Med 21:2, 1993.

103. Noyes FR, Schipplein OD, Andriacchi TP, et al.: The anterior cruciate ligament–deficient knee with varus alignment: an analysis of gait adaptations and dynamic joint loadings. Am J Sports Med 20:707, 1992.

104. Henning CE, Lynch MA, and Clark JR: Vascularity for healing of meniscus repairs. Arthroscopy 3:13, 1987.

105. McConville OR, Kipnis JM, Richmond JC, et al.: The effect of meniscal status on knee stability and function after anterior cruciate ligament reconstruction. Arthroscopy 9:431, 1993.

106. DeLee JC: Complications of arthroscopy and arthroscopic surgery: results of a national survey. Arthroscopy 1:214, 1985.

107. Fairbanks TJ: Knee joint changes after meniscectomy. J Bone Joint Surg Br 30:664, 1948.

108. Weiss CB, Lundberg M, Hamberg P, et al.: Non-operative treatment of meniscal tears. J Bone Joint Surg Am 71:811, 1989.

109. Henning CE, Clark JR, Lynch MA, et al.: Arthroscopic meniscus repair with a posterior incision. Instr Course Lect 37:209, 1988.

110. Rokito AS, Kvitne RS, Lee MR, et al.: Long-term results following meniscal repair. Presented at the American Orthopaedic Society for Sports Medicine Specialty Day, Orlando, Fla., Feb. 19, 1995.

111. Indelicato PA: Isolated medial collateral ligament injuries in the knee. JAAOS 3:9, 1995.

112. Indelicato PA, Hermansdorfer J, and Huegel M: Nonoperative management of complete tears of the medial collateral ligament of the knee in intercollegiate football players. Clin Orthop 256:174, 1990.

113. Jones RE, Henley MB, and Francis P: Nonoperative management of isolated grade III collateral ligament injury in high school football players. Clin Orthop 213:137, 1986.

114. Shelbourne KD and Porter DA: Anterior cruciate ligament–medial collateral ligament injury: nonoperative management of medial collateral ligament tears with anterior cruciate ligament reconstruction: a preliminary report. Am J Sports Med 20:283, 1992.

115. Andrews JR: Personal communication, 1994.

116. Martin SD and Clancy WG Jr: Posterolateral instabilty of the knee: treatment using the Clancy biceps tenodesis. Presented at the 62nd Annual Meeting of the American Academy of Orthopaedic Surgeons, Orlando, Fla., Feb. 18, 1995.

117. Noyes FR and Barber-Westin SD: Surgical reconstruction of severe chronic posterolateral complex injuries of the knee using allograft tissues. Am J Sports Med 23:2, 1995.

118. Albright JP, Tearse DS, and Dodds JA: Chronic posterolateral instability of the knee: evaluation of the posterolateral corner sling procedure. Presented at the 62nd Annual Meeting of the American Academy of Orthopaedic Surgeons, Orlando, Fla., Feb. 18, 1995.

119. Terry GC and LaPrade RF: Injury patterns and their correlation to clinical instability in posterolateral knee injuries. Presented at the 62nd Annual Meeting of the American Academy of Orthopaedic Surgeons, Orlando, Fla., Feb. 18, 1995.

120. Markolf KL, Wascher DC, and Finerman GA: Direct in vitro measurements of forces in the cruciate ligaments: part II: the effect of section of the posterolateral structures. J Bone Joint Surg Am 75:387, 1993.

121. Aglietti P, Buzzi R, D'Andria S, et al.: Long-term study of anterior cruciate ligament reconstruction for chronic instability using the central one-third patellar tendon and a lateral extraarticular tenodesis. Am J Sports Med 20:38, 1992.

122. Noyes FR and Barber-Westin SD: The effect of an extra-articular procedure on allograft reconstructions for chronic ruptures of the anterior cruciate ligament. J Bone Joint Surg Am 73:882, 1991.

123. O'Brien SJ, Warren RF, Wickiewicz TL, et al.: The iliotibial band lateral sling procedure and its effect on the results of anterior cruciate ligament reconstruction. Am J Sports Med 19:21, 1991.

124. Strum GM, Fox JM, Ferkel RD, et al.: Intraarticular versus intraarticular and extraarticular reconstruction for chronic anterior cruciate ligament instability. Clin Orthop 245:188, 1989.

125. Cosgarea AJ, Sebastianelli WJ, and DeHaven KE: Prevention of arthrofibrosis after anterior cruciate ligament reconstruction using

the central third patellar tendon autograft. Am J Sports Med 23:87, 1995.

126. Harner CD, Irrgang JJ, Paul J, et al.: Loss of motion after anterior cruciate ligament reconstruction. Am J Sports Med 20:499, 1992.

127. Rubinstein RA Jr and Shelbourne KD: Preventing complications and minimizing morbidity after autogenous bone-patellar tendon-bone anterior cruciate ligament reconstruction. Oper Tech Sports Med 1:72, 1993.

128. Strum GM, Friedman MJ, Fox JM, et al.: Acute anterior cruciate ligament reconstruction: analysis of complications. Clin Orthop 253:184, 1990.

129. Aglietti P, Buzzi R, D'Andria S, et al.: Arthroscopic anterior cruciate ligament reconstruction with patellar tendon. Arthroscopy 8:510, 1992.

130. Gillogly SD, Andrews JR, and Soffer SR: Pitfalls and complications of anterior cruciate ligament reconstruction. AOSSM Instr Course Lect, Palm Desert, Calif., June 26, 1994.

131. Johnson DL and Fu FH: Anterior cruciate ligament reconstructions: why do failures occur? Instr Course Lect 44:391, 1995.

132. Raab DJ, Fischer DA, Smith JP, et al.: Comparison of arthroscopic and open reconstruction of the anterior cruciate ligament: early results. Am J Sports Med 21:680, 1993.

133. Uribe JW and Zvijac JE: Surgical management of failed intra-articular anterior cruciate ligament reconstructions. J South Orthop Assoc 3:181, 1994.

134. Howell SM: Arthroscopic roofplasty: a method for correcting an extension deficit caused by roof impingement of an anterior cruciate ligament graft. Arthroscopy 8:375, 1992.

135. Howell SM and Taylor MA: Failure of reconstruction of the anterior cruciate ligament due to impingement by the intercondylar roof. J Bone Joint Surg Am 75:1044, 1993.

136. Noyes FR, Butler DL, Grood ES, et al.: Biomechanical analysis of human ligament grafts used in knee-ligament repairs and reconstructions. J Bone Joint Surg Am 66:344, 1984.

137. Clancy WG, Narechania RG, Rosenberg TD, et al.: Anterior and posterior cruciate ligament reconstruction in Rhesus monkeys: a histological, microangiographic and biomechanical analysis. J Bone Joint Surg Am 63:1270, 1981.

138. Jackson DW, Grood ES, Goldstein JD, et al.: A comparison of patellar tendon autograft and allograft used for anterior cruciate ligament reconstruction in the goat model. Am J Sports Med 21:176, 1993.

139. Larson RV: The use of the hamstring tendons in anterior cruciate ligament surgery. Presented at the Arthroscopy Association of North America Specialty Day, Orlando, Fla., Feb. 19, 1995.

140. Butler JC, Branch TP, and Hutton WC: Optimal graft fixation: the effect of gap size and screw size on bone plug fixation in anterior cruciate ligament reconstruction. Presented at the 62nd Annual Meeting of the American Academy of Orthopaedic Surgeons, Orlando, Fla., Feb. 16, 1995.

141. Hulstyn M, Fadale PD, Abate J, et al.: Biomechanical evaluation of interference screw fixation in a bovine patellar bone-tendon-bone autograft complex for anterior cruciate ligament reconstruction. Arthroscopy 9:417, 1993.

142. Shapiro JD, Cohn BT, Jackson DW, et al.: The biomechanical effects of geometric configuration of bone-tendon-bone autografts in anterior cruciate ligament reconstruction. Arthroscopy 8:453, 1992.

143. Steiner ME, Hecker AT, Brown CH Jr, et al.: Anterior cruciate ligament graft fixation: comparison of hamstring and patellar tendon grafts. Am J Sports Med 22:240, 1994.

144. LeGeyt MT and Fulkerson JP: Comparison of Kurosaka screw versus Krackow whipstitch/screw fixation for anterior cruciate ligament graft fixation. Presented at the 62nd Annual Meeting of the American Academy of Orthopaedic Surgeons, Orlando, Fla., Feb. 16, 1995.

145. Alicea JA, Scuderi GR, Scott WN, et al.: Endoscopic anterior cruciate ligament reconstruction: is there a clinical difference in tibial fixation techniques? Presented at the 62nd Annual Meeting of the American Academy of Orthopaedic Surgeons, Orlando, Fla., Feb. 16, 1995.

146. Paschal SO, Seemann MD, Ashman RB, et al.: Interference fixation versus postfixation of bone-patellar tendon-bone grafts for anterior cruciate ligament reconstruction: a biomechanical comparative study in porcine knees. Clin Orthop 300:281, 1994.

147. McGuire DA, Barber FA, Elrod BF, et al.: Use of bioabsorbable interference screws in anterior cruciate ligament reconstruction: mid-term results. Presented at the 62nd Annual Meeting of the American Academy of Orthopaedic Surgeons, Orlando, Fla., Feb. 16, 1995.

148. Stahelin AC, Feinstein R, and Friederich NF: Clinical experience using a bioabsorbable interference screw for anterior cruciate ligament reconstruction. Presented at the 62nd Annual Meeting of the American Academy of Orthopaedic Surgeons, Orlando, Fla., Feb. 16, 1995.

149. Aglietti P, Buzzi R, Zaccherotti G, et al.: Patellar tendon versus doubled semitendinosus and gracilis tendons for anterior cruciate ligament reconstruction. Am J Sports Med 22:211, 1994.

150. Karlson JA, Steiner ME, Brown CH, et al.: Anterior cruciate ligament reconstruction using gracilis and semitendinosus tendons: comparison of through-the-condyle and over-the-top graft placements. Am J Sports Med 22:659, 1994.

151. Marder RA, Raskind JR, and Carroll M: Prospective evaluation of arthroscopically assisted anterior cruciate ligament reconstruction: patellar tendon versus semitendinosus and gracilis tendons. Am J Sports Med 19:478, 1991.

152. Shaffer BS and Tibone JE: Patellar tendon length change after anterior cruciate ligament reconstruction using the mid-third patellar tendon. Am J Sports Med 21:449, 1993.

153. Arnoczky SP: Comparison of bone and soft tissue fixation strength in ACL surgery. Presented at the Arthroscopy Association of North America Specialty Day, Orlando, Fla., Feb. 19, 1995.

154. Jackson DW, Heinrich JT, and Simon TM: Biologic and synthetic implants to replace the anterior cruciate ligament. Arthroscopy 10:442, 1994.

155. Shelbourne KD, Rettig AC, Hardin G, et al.: Miniarthrotomy versus arthroscopic-assisted anterior cruciate ligament reconstruction with autogenous patellar tendon graft. Arthroscopy 9:72, 1993.

156. Shelbourne KD, Whitaker HJ, McCarroll JR, et al.: Anterior cruciate ligament injury: evaluation of intraarticular reconstruction of acute tears without repair. Am J Sports Med 18:484, 1990.

157. Rodeo SA, Arnoczky SP, Torzilli PA, et al.: Tendon-healing in a bone tunnel: a biomechanical and histological study in the dog. J Bone Joint Surg Am 75:1795, 1993.

158. Grana WA, Egle DM, Mahnken R, et al.: An analysis of autograft fixation after anterior cruciate ligament reconstruction in a rabbit model. Am J Sports Med 22:344, 1994.

159. Holmes PF, James SL, Larson RL, et al.: Retrospective direct comparison of three intraarticular anterior cruciate ligament reconstructions. Am J Sports Med 19:596, 1991.

160. Sgaglione NA, Del Pizzo W, Fox JM, et al.: Arthroscopic-assisted anterior cruciate ligament reconstruction with the semitendinosus tendon: comparison of results with and without braided polypropylene augmentation. Arthroscopy 8:65, 1992.

161. Sgaglione NA, Del Pizzo W, Fox JM, et al.: Arthroscopically assisted anterior cruciate ligament reconstruction with the pes anserine tendons: comparison of results in acute and chronic ligament deficiency. Am J Sports Med 21:249, 1993.

162. Brown CH Jr, Steiner ME, and Carson EW: The use of hamstring tendons for anterior cruciate ligament reconstruction. Clin Sports Med 12:723, 1993.

163. Noyes FR and Barber-Westin SD: Allograft reconstruction of the anterior and posterior cruciate ligaments: report of ten-year experience and results. Instr Course Lect 42:381, 1993.

164. Greis PE, Johnson DL, and Fu FH: Revision anterior cruciate ligament surgery: causes of graft failure and technical considerations of revision surgery. Clin Sports Med 12:839, 1993.

165. Rosenberg TD: Revision of failed ACL reconstruction with semitendinosus autograft. Presented at the Arthroscopy Association of North America Specialty Day, Orlando, Fla., Feb. 19, 1995.

166. Rosenberg TD and Graf B: Techniques for ACL reconstruction with Multi-Trac drill guide. Technique manual, Acufex Microsurgical, Inc., Mansfield, Mass., 1994.

167. Franklin JL, Rosenberg TD, Paulos LE, et al.: Radiographic assessment of instability of the knee due to rupture of the anterior cruciate ligament. J Bone Joint Surg Am 73:365, 1992.

168. Harner CD, Paulos LE, Greenwald AE, et al.: Detailed analysis of patients with bilateral anterior cruciate ligament injuries. Am J Sports Med 22:37, 1994.

169. Cosgarea AJ, Weng MS, and Andrews M: Case report: Osgood-

Schlatter's disease complicating anterior cruciate ligament reconstruction. Arthroscopy 9:700, 1993.

170. Graf BK, Henry J, Rothenberg M, et al.: Anterior cruciate ligament reconstruction with patellar tendon: an ex vivo study of wear-related damage and failure at the femoral tunnel. Am J Sports Med 22:131, 1994.

171. Dodds JA and Arnoczky SP: Anatomy of the anterior cruciate ligament: a blueprint for repair and reconstruction. Arthroscopy 10:132, 1994.

172. Rosenberg TD: Technique for rear entry ACL guide. Technique manual, Acufex Microsurgical, Inc., Mansfield, Mass., 1988.

173. Jackson DW and Gasser SI: Tibial tunnel placement in ACL reconstruction. Arthroscopy 10:124, 1994.

174. Christian CA and Indelicato PA: Allograft anterior cruciate ligament reconstruction with patellar tendon: an endoscopic technique. Oper Tech Sports Med 1:50, 1993.

175. Romano VM, Graf BK, Keene JS, et al.: Anterior cruciate ligament reconstruction: the effect of tibial tunnel placement on range of motion. Am J Sports Med 21:415, 1993.

176. Berns GS and Howell SM: Roofplasty requirements in vitro for different tibial hole placements in anterior cruciate ligament reconstruction. Am J Sports Med 21:292, 1993.

177. Shaffer B, Gow W, and Tibone JE: Graft-tunnel mismatch in endoscopic anterior cruciate ligament reconstruction: a new technique of intraarticular measurement and modified graft harvesting. Arthroscopy 9:633, 1993.

178. Bylski-Austrow DE, Grood ES, Hefzy MS, et al.: Anterior cruciate ligament replacements: a mechanical study of femoral attachment location, flexion angle at tensioning, and initial tension. J Orthop Res 8:522, 1990.

179. Colville MR and Bowman RR: The significance of isometer measurements and graft position during anterior cruciate ligament reconstruction. Am J Sports Med 21:832, 1993.

180. Flandry F, Terry GC, Montgomery RD, et al.: Accuracy of clinical isometry and preload testing during anterior cruciate ligament reconstruction. Clin Orthop 279:214, 1992.

181. Fleming B, Beynnon BD, Johnson RJ, et al.: Isometric versus tension measurements: a comparison for the reconstruction of the anterior cruciate ligament. Am J Sports Med 21:82, 1993.

182. Good L and Gillquist J: The value of intraoperative isometry measurements in anterior cruciate ligament reconstruction: an in vivo correlation between substitute tension and length change. Arthroscopy 9:525, 1993.

183. Sapega AA, Moyer RA, Schneck C, et al.: Testing for isometry during reconstruction of the anterior cruciate ligament: anatomical and biomechanical considerations. J Bone Joint Surg Am 72:259, 1990.

184. Clark JM and Sidles JA: The interrelation of fiber bundles in the anterior cruciate ligament. J Orthop Res 8:180, 1990.

185. Cooper DE, Burstein AL, and Warren R: The strength of the central third patellar tendon graft: a biomechanical study (abstract). Orthop Trans 16:639, 1992.

186. Losse GM, Howard ME, and Cawley PW: Bone-patellar tendon-bone grafts for anterior cruciate ligament reconstruction: the effects of pretensioning. Presented at the 62nd Annual Meeting of the American Academy of Orthopaedic Surgeons, Orlando, Fla., Feb. 16, 1995.

187. Burks RT and Leland R: Determination of graft tension before fixation in anterior cruciate ligament reconstruction. Arthroscopy 4:260, 1988.

188. Rubinstein RA and Shelbourne KD: Graft selection, placement, fixation and tensioning for anterior cruciate ligament reconstruction. Oper Tech Sports Med 1:10, 1993.

189. Yoshiya S, Andrish JT, Manley MT, et al.: Graft tension in anterior cruciate ligament reconstruction: an in vivo study in dogs. Am J Sports Med 15:464, 1987.

190. VanMeter CD, Sallay P, and McCarroll JR: Reconstruction through the patellar tendon defect. Oper Tech Sports Med 1:40, 1993.

191. Shino K, Nakagawa S, Inoue M, et al.: Deterioration of patellofemoral articular surfaces after anterior cruciate ligament reconstruction. Am J Sports Med 21:206, 1993.

192. Sachs RA, Daniel DM, Stone ML, et al.: Patellofemoral problems after anterior cruciate ligament reconstruction. Am J Sports Med 17:760, 1989.

193. Mohtadi NG, Webster-Bogaert S, and Fowler PJ: Limitation of motion following anterior cruciate ligament reconstruction: a case-control study. Am J Sports Med 19:620, 1991.

194. Noyes FR, Mangine RE, and Barber-Westin SD: The early treatment of motion complications after reconstruction of the anterior cruciate ligament. Clin Orthop 277:217, 1992.

195. Johnson GE and Shelbourne KD: Patient selection for anterior cruciate ligament reconstruction. Oper Tech Sports Med 1:16, 1993.

196. Vellet AA, Marks PH, Fowler PJ, et al.: Occult post-traumatic osteochondral lesions of the knee: prevalence, classification, and short-term sequelae evaluated with MR imaging. Radiology 178:271, 1991.

197. Fowler PJ: Bone injuries associated with anterior cruciate ligament disruption. Arthroscopy 10:453, 1994.

198. Cooper DE, Arnoczky SP, and Warren RF: Contaminated patellar tendon grafts: incidence of positive cultures and efficacy of an antibiotic solution soak: an in vitro study. Arthroscopy 7:272, 1991.

199. Goebel ME, Drez D Jr, Heck SB, et al.: Contaminated rabbit patellar tendon grafts: in vivo analysis of disinfecting methods. Am J Sports Med 22:387, 1994.

200. Rubenstein RA Jr, Shelbourne KD, VanMeter DC, et al.: Isolated autogenous bone-patellar tendon-bone graft site morbidity. Am J Sports Med 22:324, 1994.

201. Harner CD: Revision anterior cruciate ligament reconstruction using fresh-frozen allograft tissue. American Academy of Orthopaedic Surgeons Instr Course Lect, Orlando, Fla., Feb. 16, 1995.

202. Lephart SM, Kocher MS, Harner CD, et al.: Quadriceps strength and functional capacity after anterior cruciate ligament reconstruction: patellar tendon autograft versus allograft. Am J Sports Med 21:738, 1993.

203. Jackson DW and Schaefer RK: Cyclops syndrome: loss of extension following intra-articular anterior cruciate ligament reconstruction. Arthroscopy 6:171, 1990.

204. Kramer J, Nusca D, Fowler P, et al.: Knee flexor and extensor strength during concentric and eccentric muscle actions after anterior cruciate ligament reconstruction using the semitendinosus tendon and ligament augmentation device. Am J Sports Med 21:285, 1993.

205. Drez DJ, DeLee J, Holden JP, et al.: Anterior cruciate ligament reconstruction using bone-patellar tendon-bone allografts: a biological and biomechanical evaluation in goats. Am J Sports Med 19:256, 1991.

206. Indelicato PA, Bittar ES, Prevot TJ, et al.: Clinical comparison of freeze-dried and fresh-frozen patellar tendon allografts for anterior cruciate ligament reconstruction of the knee. Am J Sports Med 18:335, 1990.

207. Noyes FR and Barber-Westin SD: The effect of a ligament-augmentation device on allograft reconstructions for chronic ruptures of the anterior cruciate ligament. J Bone Joint Surg Am 74:960, 1992.

208. Lane JG, Daniel DM, and Stone ML: Graft impingement after anterior cruciate ligament reconstruction: presentation as an active extension "thunk." Am J Sports Med 22:415, 1994.

209. Marzo JM, Bowen MK, Warren RF, et al.: Intraarticular fibrous nodule as a cause of loss of extension following anterior cruciate ligament reconstruction. Arthroscopy 8:10, 1992.

210. Fisher SE and Shelbourne KD: Arthroscopic treatment of symptomatic extension block complicating anterior cruciate ligament reconstruction. Am J Sports Med 21:558, 1993.

211. Paulos LE, Rosenberg TD, Drawbert J, et al.: Infrapatellar contracture syndrome: an unrecognized cause of knee stiffness with patella entrapment and patella infera. Am J Sports Med 15:331, 1987.

212. Paulos LE, Wnorowski DC, and Greenwald AE: Infrapatellar contracture syndrome: diagnosis, treatment, and long-term followup. Am J Sports Med 22:440, 1994.

213. Shelbourne KD, Porter DA, and Rozzi W: Use of a modified Elmslie-Trillat procedure to improve abnormal patellar congruence angle. Am J Sports Med 22:318, 1994.

214. Shelbourne KD and Johnson GE: Outpatient surgical management of arthrofibrosis after anterior cruciate ligament surgery. Am J Sports Med 22:192, 1994.

215. Cosgarea AJ, DeHaven KE, and Lovelock JE: The surgical treatment of arthrofibrosis of the knee. Am J Sports Med 22:184, 1994.

216. Klein W, Shah N, and Gassen A: Arthroscopic management of postoperative arthrofibrosis of the knee joint: indications, technique, and results. Arthroscopy 10:591, 1994.

217. Tria AJ Jr, Alicea JA, and Cody RP: Patella baja in anterior cruciate ligament reconstruction of the knee. Clin Orthop 299:229, 1994.

218. Cohn BT, Draeger RI, and Jackson DW: The effects of cold therapy in the postoperative management of pain in patients undergoing anterior cruciate ligament reconstruction. Am J Sports Med 17:344, 1989.

219. Steadman JR, Seemann MD, and Hutton KS: Revision ligament reconstruction of failed prosthetic anterior cruciate ligaments. Instr Course Lect 44:417, 1995.

220. Grewe SR and Paulos LE: Prosthetic replacement of the anterior cruciate ligament with expanded polytetrafluoroethylene. Instr Course Lect 40: 213, 1991.

221. Gillquist J and Odensten M: Reconstruction of old anterior cruciate ligament tears with a Dacron prosthesis: a prospective study. Am J Sports Med 21:358, 1993.

222. Howell SM, Berns GS, and Farley TE: Unimpinged and impinged anterior cruciate ligament grafts: MR signal intensity measurements. Radiology 179:639, 1991.

223. Maywood RM, Murphy BJ, Uribe JW, et al.: Evaluation of arthroscopic anterior cruciate ligament reconstruction using magnetic resonance imaging. Am J Sports Med 21:523, 1993.

224. Rak KM, Gillogly SD, Schaefer RA, et al.: Anterior cruciate ligament reconstruction: evaluation with MR imaging. Radiology 178:553, 1991.

225. Aglietti P, Buzzi R, D'Andria S, et al.: Patellofemoral problems after intraarticular anterior cruciate ligament reconstruction. Clin Orthop 288:195, 1993.

226. Berg EE: Intrinsic healing of a patellar tendon donor site defect after anterior cruciate ligament reconstruction. Clin Orthop 278:160, 1992.

227. Meisterling RC, Wadsworth T, Ardill R, et al.: Morphologic changes in the human patellar tendon after bone-tendon-bone anterior cruciate ligament reconstruction. Clin Orthop 289:208, 1993.

228. DeLee J and Craviotto DF: Rupture of the quadriceps tendon after a central third patellar tendon anterior cruciate ligament reconstruction. Am J Sports Med 19:415, 1991.

229. Furman W, Marshall JL, and Girgis FG: The anterior cruciate ligament: a functional analysis based on postmortem studies. J Bone Joint Studies 58:179, 1976.

230. Grood ES, Suntay WJ, Noyes FR, et al.: Biomechanics of the knee-extension exercise: effect of cutting the anterior cruciate ligament. J Bone Joint Surg Am 66:725, 1984.

231. Takeda Y, Xerogeanes JW, Livesay GA, et al.: Biomechanical function of the human anterior cruciate ligament. Arthroscopy 10:140, 1994.

232. Robertson DB, Danile DM, and Biden E: Soft tissue fixation to bone. Am J Sports Med 14:398, 1986.

233. Daniel DM: Principles of knee ligament surgery. In Daniel DM, Akeson WH, and O'Connor JJ (eds.): Knee Ligaments: Structure, Function, Injury, and Repair. New York, Raven Press, 1990.

234. Linn RM, Fischer DA, Smith JP, et al.: Achilles tendon allograft reconstruction of the anterior cruciate ligament–deficient knee. Am J Sports Med 21:825, 1993.

235. Meyers JF, Caspari RB, Cash JD, et al.: Arthroscopic evaluation of allograft anterior cruciate ligament reconstruction. Arthroscopy 8:157, 1992.

236. Barber-Westin SD and Noyes FR: The effect of rehabilitation and return to activity on anterior-posterior knee displacements after anterior cruciate ligament reconstruction. Am J Sports Med 21:264, 1993.

237. Beynnon BD, Fleming BC, Johnson RJ, et al.: Anterior cruciate ligament strain behavior during rehabilitation exercises in vivo. Am J Sports Med 23:24, 1995.

238. Good L, Odensten M, and Gillquist J: Sagittal knee stability after anterior cruciate ligament reconstruction with a patellar tendon strip: a two-year follow-up study. Am J Sports Med 22:518, 1994.

239. Butler DL, Grood ES, Noyes FR, et al.: On the interpretation of our anterior cruciate ligament data. Clin Orthop 196:26, 1985.

240. Noyes FR and Grood ES: The strength of the anterior cruciate ligament in humans and Rhesus monkeys: age-related and species-related changes. J Bone Joint Surg Am 58:1074, 1976.

241. Rougraff B, Shelbourne KD, Gerth PK, et al.: Arthroscopic and histologic analysis of human patellar tendon autografts used for anterior cruciate ligament reconstruction. Am J Sports Med 21:277, 1993.

242. Shino K, Inoue M, Horibe S, et al.: Maturation of allograft tendons transplanted into the knee: an arthroscopic and histological study. J Bone Joint Surg Br 70:556, 1988.

243. Abe S, Kurosaka M, Iguchi T, et al.: Light and electron microscopic study of remodeling and maturation process in autogenous graft for anterior cruciate ligament reconstruction. Arthroscopy 9:394, 1993.

244. Richmond JC, Gladstone J, and MacGillivray J: Continuous passive motion after arthroscopically assisted anterior cruciate ligament reconstruction: comparison of short- versus long-term use. Arthroscopy 7:39, 1991.

245. Rosen MA, Jackson DW, Atwell EA: The efficacy of continuous passive motion in the rehabilitation of anterior cruciate ligament reconstructions. Am J Sports Med 20:122, 1992.

246. O'Meara PM, O'Brien WR, and Henning CE: Anterior cruciate ligament reconstruction stability with continuous passive motion: the role of isometric graft placement. Clin Orthop 277:201, 1992.

247. Snyder-Mackler L, Ladin Z, Schepsis AA, et al.: Electrical stimulation of the thigh muscles after reconstruction of the anterior cruciate ligament: effects of electrically elicited contraction of the quadriceps femoris and hamstring muscles on gait and on strength of the thigh muscles. J Bone Joint Surg Am 73:1025, 1991.

248. Sisk TD, Stralka SW, Deering MB, et al.: Effect of electrical stimulation on quadriceps strength after reconstructive surgery of the anterior cruciate ligament. Am J Sports Med 15:215, 1987.

249. Wojtys EM, Carpenter JE, and Ott GA: Electrical stimulation of soft tissues. Instr Course Lect 42:443, 1993.

250. Glasgow SG, Gabriel JP, Sapega AA, et al.: The effect of early versus late return to vigorous activities on the outcome of anterior cruciate ligament reconstruction. Am J Sports Med 21:243, 1993.

251. Harter RA, Ostering LR, Singer KM, et al.: Long-term evaluation of knee stability and function after surgical reconstruction for anterior cruciate insufficiency. Am J Sports Med 16:434, 1988.

252. Noyes FR, Barber-Westin SD, and Mangine RE: Bone-patellar ligament-bone and fascia lata allografts for reconstruction of the anterior cruciate ligament. J Bone Joint Surg Am 72:1125, 1990.

253. Shino K, Inoue M, Horibe S, et al.: Reconstruction of the anterior cruciate ligament using allogenic tendon: long-term follow-up. Am J Sports Med 18:457, 1990.

254. Howell SM, Knox KE, Farley TE, et al.: Revascularization of a human anterior cruciate ligament graft during the first two years of implantation. Am J Sports Med 23:42, 1995.

29 | Posterior Cruciate Ligament

Scott D. Kuiper • *William G. Clancy, Jr*

Both cruciate ligaments play an important role in normal knee kinematics. During the past several years a resurgence of interest has developed in studying the treatment of posterior cruciate ligament (PCL) anatomy, function, biomechanics, and injury. Although controversy still exists regarding the natural history of the PCL-deficient knee and treatment recommendations, a better general understanding of this structure and its importance is developing.

Basic scientific research has provided new insight into the complex anatomy and functional biomechanics of the PCL. This information, along with a better understanding of the natural history of the PCL-deficient knee, will hopefully help to provide the clinician with better, more reliable, and more successful treatment programs.

ANATOMY AND BIOMECHANICS

The PCL derives its name from its insertion site on the posterior aspect of the proximal tibia. The ligament fibers are enveloped by a fold of synovium, essentially providing it with an extrasynovial milieu. Early studies by Girgis, Marshall, and Al Monajem reported that the average length of the PCL is 38 mm, and the average midportion width is 13 mm.[1] The cross-sectional area of the PCL decreases from its proximal origin to its distal insertion and has been reported to be 50% and 51% larger than the anterior cruciate ligament (ACL) at the midsubstance and proximal sections respectively at 30 degrees of knee flexion.[2]

The femoral and tibial PCL insertion site anatomy is complex and has not been previously well described. An understanding of these insertion sites is critical if one is to perform surgical reconstruction. In our laboratory ten fresh-frozen cadavers were dissected for anatomic and radiographic studies. Barium sulfate cream was injected into the PCL fibers, and radiographs were obtained at 0, 45, and 90 degrees of flexion to establish radiographic landmarks that can be utilized by the clinician. Our studies indicate that the PCL femoral insertion originates high

on the notch roof and low on the medial femoral condyle (Fig. 29–1). The PCL insertion width was an average of 9 mm anteriorly (AB) but gradually broadened to its greatest width of 14 mm (EF) and then narrowed as the insertion became more posterior compared with the notch roof. The PCL insertion length was an average of 29 mm proximally (AK) and 35 mm distally (BK). The distal fibers inserted within 1 mm of the anterior and inferior articular cartilage and tapered away posteriorly. From the posteroanterior (PA) projection (Fig. 29–2), the insertion covered two-thirds of the notch roof. The tibial insertion of the PCL is a tilted rectangle on a recessed shelf below the joint line in a fossa between the tibial plateaus (Fig. 29–3). The proximal and distal width was an average of 11 mm and 13 mm, respectively. The average medial and lateral insertion lengths were 14 mm and 16 mm, respectively. The root of the medial meniscus overlaps the PCL insertion an average of 6 mm. The proximal insertion fibers of the insertion start at an average of 1.6 mm distal to the root of the medial meniscus. The distal fibers, which blend with the posterior capsule attachment, are bound by the popliteus muscle, which overlaps the distal insertion fibers an average of 1.5 mm.

Barium injection radiographic findings confirm the importance of the Blumensaat line and a line drawn as a continuation of the trochlear groove line as landmarks for the femoral insertion on a lateral radiograph of the knee (Fig. 29–4). For the tibial insertion, the distal fibers were noted to intersect with the tibial physeal scar and the proximal tip of the fibula. The most important landmark, however, was identification of the posterior tibial ridge on which the PCL inserts (Fig. 29–5).

The PCL has been described as consisting of two to four bundles or bands. Traditionally, authors have described an anterior or anterolateral bundle and a posterior or posteromedial bundle. O'Brien and colleagues described two fiber bundles, the first being an anterior bundle, representing 95% of the ligament, and the second being a posterior oblique bundle, consisting of approximately 5% of the ligament.[3] Kurosawa and colleagues and

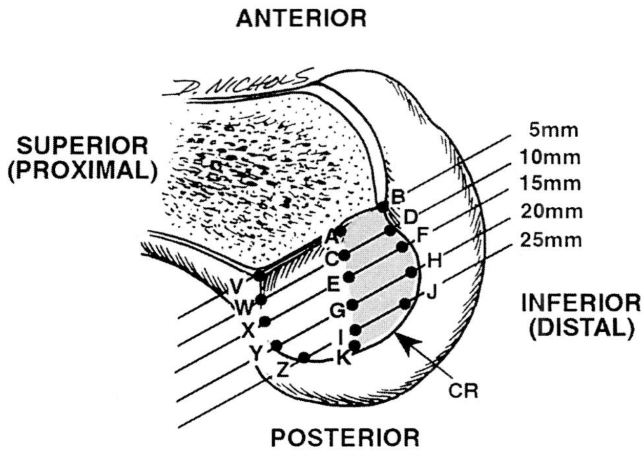

ANTERIOR

SUPERIOR
(PROXIMAL)

5mm
10mm
15mm
20mm
25mm

INFERIOR
(DISTAL)

POSTERIOR

Figure 29–1 • Lateral view of the posterior cruciate ligament (PCL) femoral insertion site. Insertion site width measurements at 5 mm intervals are depicted. The anterior PCL insertion width (AB) averaged 9 mm. Its greatest average width was 14 mm (EF). The insertion narrowed posteriorly. PCL insertion length (AK) averaged 29 mm proximally and 35 mm distally (BK).

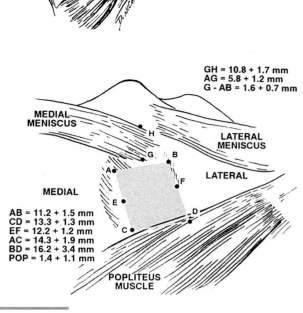

GH = 10.8 + 1.7 mm
AG = 5.8 + 1.2 mm
G - AB = 1.6 + 0.7 mm

MEDIAL
MENISCUS

LATERAL
MENISCUS

LATERAL

MEDIAL

AB = 11.2 + 1.5 mm
CD = 13.3 + 1.3 mm
EF = 12.2 + 1.2 mm
AC = 14.3 + 1.9 mm
BD = 16.2 + 3.4 mm
POP = 1.4 + 1.1 mm

POPLITEUS
MUSCLE

Figure 29–3 • Posterior cruciate ligament (PCL) tibial insertion site measurements. The average proximal width (AB) was 11 mm. The average distal width (CD) was 13 mm. The average medial PCL insertion length (AC) was 14 mm. The average lateral insertion length (BD) was 16 mm. The PCL insertion site is crossed proximally by the root of the medial meniscus and distally by the popliteus muscle. Both landmarks are borders of the PCL insertion.

Trent, Walker, and Wolf described anterior, middle and posterior fiber bundles.[4, 5] Recent anatomic studies are now characterizing the PCL as a continuum of fibers that provide stability to the knee through a full range of motion. Covey and associates have subdivided these fibers into so-called fiber regions on the basis of functional and morphologic criteria.[6] The four fiber regions are called the anterior, central, posterior longitudinal, and posterior oblique. The anterior and central fiber regions make up

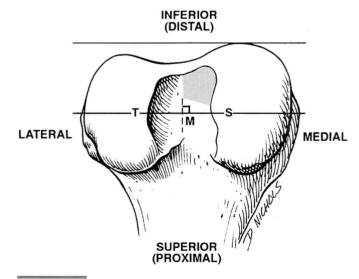

INFERIOR
(DISTAL)

LATERAL

MEDIAL

SUPERIOR
(PROXIMAL)

Figure 29–2 • Posteroanterior projection of the distal femur illustrating the posterior cruciate ligament (PCL) insertion site on the notch roof. MS divided by TS times 100 was used to calculate the percent notch roof crossed by the PCL insertion, and this average was 66%.

85–90% of the ligament bulk, whereas the posterior longitudinal and posterior oblique fibers account for only 10–15% of the mass. These fiber regions are based on their osseous attachment sites and spacial orientation of fibers and differences in mechanical fiber behavior during joint motion.[6]

Two additional structures that are variably present are the ligament of Humphry and the ligament of Wrisberg. They have been reported to be present between 70 and 100% of the time.[7–9] Each of these ligaments has a femoral attachment that is discrete and distinguishable from that of the PCL fibers. The mean total cross-sectional area of the meniscofemoral was determined to be approximately 20% of the cross-sectional area of the PCL.[2] Heller and Langman found the anterior portion (ligament of Humphry) in 36% of the knees that they dissected, and the ligament was never larger than one-third that of the diameter of the PCL.[8] The more posterior band (ligament of Wrisberg), when present, courses from the posterior aspect of the PCL insertion on the medial femoral condyle to insert onto the posterolateral aspect of the lateral meniscus. This was found in 35% of knees and could be up to one half of the diameter of the PCL.[8] Girgis, Marshall, and Al Monajem never observed both meniscofemoral ligaments together and found that they

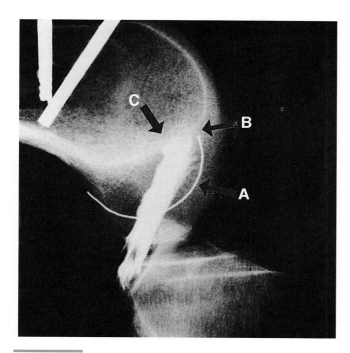

Figure 29–4 • A lateral radiograph of a knee with a barium-injected posterior cruciate ligament (PCL). A wire has been placed along the articular cartilage margin (*arrow A*). Note the PCL fibers insert within 1–2 mm of the articular cartilage margin (*arrow B*). They originate at the intersection of the Blumensaat line and the femoral trochlear groove line (*arrow C*).

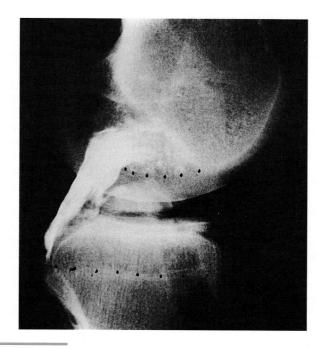

Figure 29–5 • A lateral radiograph of a knee with a barium-injected posterior cruciate ligament (PCL). Note the distal insertional fibers on the tibia intersect with the tibial physeal scar line, which is outlined with black dots. The superior aspect of the fibular head is 4 mm distal to the distal insertional fibers. The posterior tibial ridge on which the PCL inserts can be clearly visualized.

were absent in 30% of their specimens.[1] In contrast, Kaplan found one or the other in all knees dissected.[9]

FUNCTIONAL BIOMECHANICS

To better understand how injury to the PCL affects knee functioning, one must have a clear understanding of the kinematic behavior of the PCL. Arms, Johnson, and Pope studied PCL fiber strain in various regions of the ligament.[10] They noted that when the knee was flexed from 10 to 120 degrees, the strain in the anterior fibers increased significantly.[10] Hefzy, Grood, and Lindenfeld also noted that the linear distance between the femoral and tibial attachment sites of most PCL fibers increased with knee flexion, although there were regional variations in the amount of lengthening noted.[11] This change in distance between the insertion sites appears to be more sensitive to femoral insertion site variations than to changes in the fiber insertions on the tibial attachment.[12-17] Grood, Hefzy, and Lindenfeld studied the changes in distance between tibial and femoral attachment sites and found no isometric point within the femoral attachment zone.[18] However, Friederich, Müller, and O'Brien noted that sites located at the posterior superior margin of the femoral origin and at the posterolateral margin of the tibial insertion exhibit isometric behavior.[19, 20] This was later confirmed by Covey and associates with an in vitro study under various load conditions and knee motions.[6, 21] They concluded the posterior oblique fibers, which make up approximately 5% of the entire PCL substance, were the only isometric fibers within the PCL. The posterior longitudinal fiber group previously described also exhibited variable but near isometric behavior.

The results of these studies would indicate the fibers in the anterior central or anterolateral portion of the PCL are nonisometric in that only a very small group of posterior fibers approximate isometric behavior. Indeed, if there is a reciprocal behavior between the two major bundles of the PCL, the reciprocating fiber regions are certainly not balanced with regard to region size or mass. The greatest bulk of the ligament appears to tighten as the knee is brought into flexion. It appears that the PCL as a whole does act as a continuum through the knee range of motion with various fiber groups providing stability, dependent on knee flexion and loading conditions.

While isometric graft placement has been recommended,[20] other investigators have reported improved biomechanical results when nonisometric graft placement is utilized. Bomberg and colleagues performed a biomechanical study on fresh cadaveric knees.[22] Their results were superior when the PCL femoral tunnel was located slightly anterior to the center of the femoral PCL attachment site. This allowed the graft to progressively tighten with knee flexion. This appeared to more effectively eliminate the tibial sag that is produced with increased knee flexion. Graft attachment sites, which demonstrated an increase in linear separation distance of 4.5 mm between 0 and 90 degrees of flexion, produced a more successful normalization of the anteroposterior tibial laxity profile and fiber strain in the surrounding ligaments. Knees that were reconstructed with a more isometric graft placement had a less satisfactory result biomechanically.[22] Galloway and associates reported that centering the graft at the PCL femoral origin resulted in a more physiologic pattern of knee kinematics and stability than when an isometric reconstruction was undertaken.[23]

Recent biomechanical studies of the kinematic behavior of the PCL and posterolateral complex have led to an improved understanding of the PCL's role in providing stability to the knee. It has been long accepted that the PCL is the primary restraint to straight posterior translation of the tibia at almost all positions of knee flexion.[24–27] The absolute amount of translation increases progressively from 0 to 90 degrees of flexion. No significant increase in varus-valgus rotation or tibial internal or external rotation occurred with isolated PCL injury without concomitant injury to the secondary extra-articular restraints.[25, 27, 28] When both the PCL and posterolateral complex are torn, significantly increased varus angulation and tibial external rotation are observed when the knee is flexed 90 degrees. When the posterolateral complex is torn and a varus moment or external tibial rotation torque is applied to the knee, an increase in the force within the PCL is noted between 45 and 90 degrees of knee flexion.[29] These results indicate that a PCL or posterolateral complex injury can be best detected by examining for posterior translation, varus rotation, and external rotation of the tibia. The isolated PCL injury should cause maximum posterior translation between 75 and 90 degrees of knee flexion and less posterior translation between 0 and 30 degrees of flexion. External tibial rotation and varus-valgus angulation would not be expected to change. An isolated posterolateral corner disruption would be expected to demonstrate increased varus rotation, posterior translation, and tibial external rotation at 30 degrees of knee flexion. If increased tibial external rotation is noted at both 30 degrees and 90 degrees of flexion, this should alert the examiner to the possibility of a complete tear of the PCL. When both the posterolateral corner and the PCL are ruptured, an increase in posterior translation, tibial external rotation, and varus angulation would be expected at all angles of knee flexion.

Skyhar and associates studied the effect of sectioning the PCL and posterolateral structures on the articular contact pressures of the medial, lateral, and patellofemoral compartments of the knee.[30] Medial compartment pressures were significantly increased after isolated sectioning of the PCL and combined sectioning of the PCL and posterolateral structures. Patellofemoral compartment pressures increased with isolated PCL sectioning and combined PCL and posterolateral sectioning with peak pressures at 90 degrees of knee flexion. They postulated that a medial shift in the joint center of rotation and alteration of the tibiofemoral contact areas during joint motion resulted in increased medial compartment pressures recorded after ligament sectioning. It is hypothesized that these increased contact pressures in the medial and patellofemoral compartments of the knee may lead to the high incidence of patellofemoral and medial compartment articular degenerative changes described by Clancy and colleagues on arthroscopic inspection of chronic PCL injuries.[31]

INCIDENCE OF INJURY

Although injury to the PCL is less common than injury to the ACL, the PCL is probably injured more frequently than is generally recognized. Numerous studies have been performed, all reporting different injury rates relative to the PCL. O'Donoghue reported that the PCL was injured in about 9% of patients in his 1950 series.[32] However, in 1955, he only reported a 3.4% injury rate.[33] The PCL was found to be injured in 16% of cases in Kennedy and Grainger's series[34] and 20% in Clendenin, DeLee, and Heckman's series.[35] Clancy and colleagues reviewed a series of acute and chronic severe knee ligament injuries and found that the PCL was injured 10% of the time.[31] The different percentages reported in these studies may be a reflection of differences in patient population. Because injuries to the PCL do not always cause a large, tense effusion and painful knee, many patients do not seek medical care and can easily be misdiagnosed. In addition, because physical findings can be subtle in the isolated PCL-deficient knee, the diagnosis can be missed even by an experienced examiner. A high index of suspicion and also a careful history and physical examination are very important. A recent study was performed to determine the accuracy of the clinical examination in the setting of isolated chronic PCL tears.[36] The overall accuracy of the clinical examination for all orthopaedists was 96%. The accuracy for detecting a PCL tear was 96% with a 90% sensitivity and a 99% specificity. However, the sensitivity for grade I injuries was only 70%.

MECHANISM OF INJURY

Isolated injuries to the PCL generally occur by one of three mechanisms. The first and most common mechanism is a blow to the flexed knee, either via a dashboard injury or after a fall onto the flexed knee with the foot plantar flexed.[37, 38] With the dashboard type of mechanism, the knee is generally flexed approximately 90 degrees, and a posteriorly directed force is applied to the proximal tibia by the dashboard during impact. With this knee position the posterior capsule is lax, while the anterolateral bundle of the PCL is taut. The result is an isolated PCL rupture, which in some cases includes an avulsion fracture of the tibial attachment site. When the patient falls on the flexed knee with the foot plantar flexed, the tibial tubercle is driven posteriorly relative to the femur, which can lead to a complex interstitial PCL tear or sometimes to a failure in continuity. If the foot remains in a dorsiflexed position during impact, the forces are generally directed at the patellofemoral joint and up the shaft of the femur, thus avoiding injury to the PCL.

The second mechanism for isolated PCL injury is forced knee hyperflexion with the foot plantar flexed or dorsiflexed (Fig. 29–6A–D). It is believed that forced hyperflexion may place excessive strain on the anterolateral bundle of the PCL as it tightens with flexion. Fowler and Messieh reported that this mechanism commonly led to interstitial failure of the PCL and was actually the most common mechanism of injury in their series.[39]

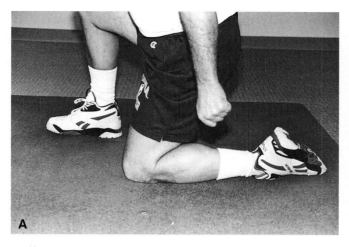
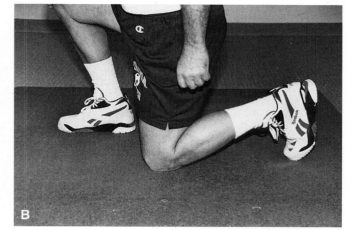
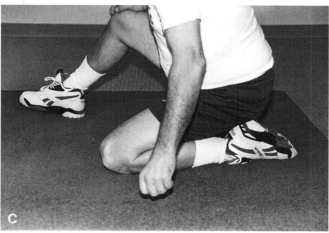
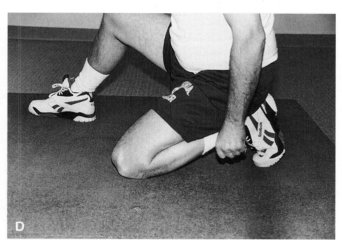

Figure 29–6 • *A–D* illustrate the mechanisms of injury to the posterior cruciate ligament (PCL) in sports when one falls on his or her knee. *A,* A fall on the flexed knee with the foot in plantar flexion. The blow is delivered to the tibial tubercle driving the tibia posteriorly. If the foot is in dorsiflexion (*B*), the blow is delivered to the patellofemoral joint. *C* and *D,* A fall on the hyperflexed knee with the foot plantar or dorsiflexed, which may produce a failure in situ of the PCL. (From Andrews JR, Edwards JC, and Satterwhite YE: Isolated posterior cruciate ligament injuries: history, mechanism of injury, physical findings, and ancillary tests. Clin Sports Med 13:519–530, 1994.)

PCL injury has also been reported when an athlete attempts to change direction rapidly while shifting weight from one foot to the other.[40] The foot becoming unloaded is planted with the knee minimally flexed. The femur internally rotates and translates anteriorly as the player's body quickly rotates, which creates a relative external rotation and posterior force to the tibia with subsequent PCL failure.

Other mechanisms of injury tend to injure the PCL along with other ligamentous structures, causing a combined ligament disruption. These mechanisms include forced hyperextension of the knee, which commonly tears the ACL, PCL, and posterior capsule. Severe varus or valgus stress injuries to the knee can disrupt both primary and secondary restraints. This generally leads to a combination injury to either the medial or lateral collateral structures and the PCL.

NATURAL HISTORY OF THE PCL-DEFICIENT KNEE

Controversy persists regarding the best treatment for acute and chronic PCL injuries, mainly because of the continued debate over what the natural history of the PCL-deficient knee is. Most authors agree that combined injuries do not fare well with conservative treatment. However, they continue to recommend nonoperative treatment for the isolated PCL injured knee, citing the lack of functional instability that accompanies the acute

PCL injury.[39, 41–44] A critical review of these studies, however, shows that many patients were not entirely satisfied with their knees after nonoperative or conservative treatment protocols.

Dandy and Pusey reported on 20 patients with chronic, isolated PCL deficiency.[44] Forty-five percent of these patients had complaints of the leg giving way when they walked on uneven ground. Fifty-five percent of patients had pain while walking down steps, and 70% had pain when walking long distances. These symptoms prompted 10 of the 20 patients to undergo diagnostic arthroscopy.

Cross and Powell reported on 116 cases of PCL injury in which 67 patients were treated nonoperatively with a quadriceps strengthening program.[43] Thirty-six percent of these patients had retropatellar pain that started between 3 months and 5 years after the injury. Of the 67 patients treated nonoperatively, 49 (42%) had enough symptoms to undergo either repair, reconstructive surgery, or palliative surgery. The authors concluded that eventual degenerative changes were probably inevitable despite maintenance of good quadriceps tone.

Parolie and Bergfeld reported on 25 patients with chronic isolated PCL insufficiency at a 6-year average follow-up.[41] Eleven patients were seen acutely, and 85% were considered to be satisfied with their knees. On further review, however, only 68% were able to return to their previous sport without disability. Fifty-two percent of the patients had knee pain, and 48% had stiffness after prolonged sitting. Intermittent clicking was noted in 28% of patients, and 20% of patients had episodes of instability. Results were better in patients who had quadriceps strength equal to or greater than that of the opposite leg.

Keller and associates reviewed nonoperatively treated isolated PCL injuries in 40 patients with an average 6 year follow-up from injury.[45] Sixty-five percent of these patients reported a limited activity level after the injury, and 49% indicated that full recovery was not achieved despite a rehabilitation program that returned their quadriceps:hamstring ratio equal to their opposite knee. Ninety percent of these patients had pain in their knee with activities, and 43% complained of problems while walking. Diminished function of the knee was reported as the time interval from injury increased.

Dejour and colleagues reported an 89% incidence of knee pain in patients with isolated PCL injuries at an average of 15 years after the injury.[46] They described three post-injury phases based on their findings: (1) functional adaptation (3–18 months); (2) functional tolerance (1–20 years); and (3) osteoarthritic deterioration (approximately 25 years).[47]

To help better understand what abnormalities are seen in the acute versus chronic setting after PCL injury, Geissler and Whipple studied intra-articular abnormalities in 88 arthroscopically proven PCL tears in symptomatic patients.[48] In the 33 patients studied acutely, four patients (12%) had chondral defects involving the lateral femoral condyle and patella. Nine patients (27%) had meniscal tears (six lateral and three medial). In the 55 patients with chronic PCL tears, 27 (49%) had chondral defects and 20 patients (36%) had meniscal tears (7 lateral and 17 medial). In this group, chondral defects of the medial femoral condyle were more common. This study reported an increased incidence of articular defects and meniscal tears in patients with chronic PCL injury, both lesions primarily involving the medial compartment.

Clancy and colleagues noted no articular damage in 15 acute PCL injuries, although they reported medial compartment changes in chronically PCL-deficient knees.[31] Nine of ten patients who underwent PCL reconstruction more than 4 years after their original injury had moderate to severe articular damage to the medial compartment. Clancy also reviewed 191 patients with either acute or symptomatic chronic PCL insufficiency. Articular cartilage defects were mapped and recorded, along with the interval between the time of injury and the time of surgery.[49] Articular lesions were noted to mainly involve the medial femoral condyle, the patella, and eventually the lateral compartment. It was noted that as the interval increased between the time of injury and the time of surgery, the percentage of patients with grade III or grade IV chondromalacic lesions increased significantly. The clinical findings in this study seem to correlate well with the in vitro biomechanical findings reported by Skyhar and colleagues, indicating increased forces on the patellofemoral joint and medial femoral condyle in the PCL-deficient knee.[30]

While functional instability may not be a prominent problem in the isolated PCL-deficient knee, it appears that the abnormal biomechanics produced lead to poor long-term sequela in a significant percentage of knees.

DIAGNOSIS

A diagnostic work-up begins with a careful, thorough and detailed history, including the time and mechanism of injury. When a specific mechanism of injury is known, the clinician can have a high index of suspicion for PCL and associated ligamentous injuries. Whether the injury is acute, subacute, or chronic is, of course, very important in guiding one's physical examination and eventual treatment recommendations. It is important to know whether the patient is having complaints of instability, giving way, or pain relative to the functional disability.

The physical examination begins with inspection of the knee. Ecchymosis and abrasions over the anterior proximal tibial region should alert the clinician to a possible PCL injury. Although there may be an effusion, it may not be as large as one might expect after an ACL injury. A thorough examination of the neurovascular status of the injured limb is very important, especially when there is evidence of a combined ligamentous injury of the knee, which may represent a spontaneously reduced, low-velocity knee dislocation. If a recent knee dislocation is suspected, whether it is low or high velocity, arteriography should be considered to rule out vascular injury. Peroneal nerve function should also be closely examined, especially in knees that have sustained a varus mechanism of injury. Injury to the peroneal nerve has been reported to occur from 10 to 30% of the time in association with lateral and posterolateral ligament disruptions.[50–52]

After the neurovascular examination is completed, an examination of the knee for ligamentous stability can be initiated. In the acute setting, swelling and guarding can make an evaluation difficult. All ligamentous structures must be tested to ascertain whether an isolated or combined injury has occurred. In Clancy and colleagues' earlier series,[31] 40% of 191 PCL injuries reviewed were isolated, and the remainder were combined injuries.

Patients with an acute isolated PCL injury generally can fully extend the knee with minimal discomfort and can flex at least to 90 degrees. Several physical examination techniques have been described to determine the integrity of the PCL. Biomechanical studies have demonstrated that isolated PCL injuries should allow maximum posterior tibial translation with a posterior-directed force performed at 90 degrees of flexion.[25, 28, 53] This is the basis for using the 90 degree knee flexion angle when performing the posterior drawer test or observing the posterior sag sign. Both tests are performed with the patient in the supine position, with the knee flexed to 90 degrees and the foot stabilized. The posterior sag sign, described by Insall and Hood is the gravity-assisted posterior tibial sag, which results from an absence of the restraining function of the PCL in this knee position after injury.[54] Occasionally quadriceps muscle spasm, a knee effusion, or pretibial swelling may decrease or hide the posterior sag that is present. This effectively decreases the sensitivity of this test.

It is important to palpate the normal anteromedial and anterolateral tibial plateau step-off in the normal knee at 90 degrees of flexion and compare this with the injured knee (Fig. 29–7). A posterior drawer test can then be performed by placing both thumbs on the proximal tibia and applying a posteriorly directed force with the knee in 90 degrees of flexion.[25, 28, 53] Normally the anterior tibial plateau lies approximately 1 cm anterior to the femoral

condyles. If the step-off is less than 10 mm, but is still palpable, this is graded as a 1+ posterior drawer. If the anterior tibial crest lies flush with the femoral condyles, which represents approximately a 10 mm posterior subluxation, this is graded as a 2+ posterior drawer. When the tibial crest can be translated or subluxed posterior to the femoral condyles with the posterior drawer test, this is graded as a 3+ posterior drawer and indicates significant injury to the posterior capsule or posterolateral structures in addition to the PCL. Palpation should occur at both the anteromedial and anterolateral crest, because significant injury can occasionally obliterate either the anterolateral or anteromedial step-off.

A concomitant posterolateral complex injury may increase the posterior translation of the lateral tibial plateau in a posterior drawer test. Internal rotation of the tibia will reduce the external rotation component of the posterior drawer found in this combined injury. Internal rotation of the tibia, however, may decrease the posterior drawer in an isolated PCL injury, depending on the integrity of the meniscofemoral ligaments of Humphry and Wrisberg. It has been proposed that internal tibial rotation tightens the meniscofemoral ligaments, allowing them to act as secondary restraints to posterior tibial translation[49]; however, data suggest that the superficial MCL may be responsible for this clinical observation.[55] The meniscofemoral ligaments, if present, are generally intact after an isolated PCL injury.[31]

A modification of the posterior drawer test has been described by Whipple and Ellis.[56] To improve patient relaxation and thigh stability, the patient is placed prone, and a posteriorly directed force is applied to the tibia with the knee flexed at 45 and 90 degrees of flexion. By observ-

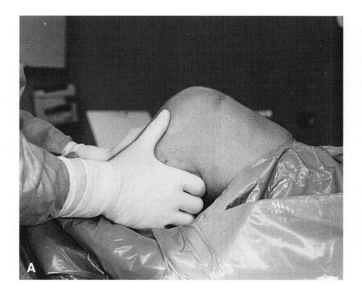
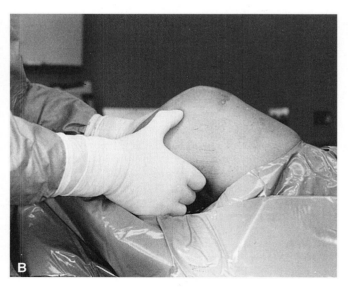

Figure 29–7 • *A*, With the knee flexed to 90 degrees, gravity drops the tibia posteriorly in a posterior cruciate ligament (PCL)-deficient knee. Palpation of the anterior tibial step-off shows it to be flush with the femoral condyles. *B*, With an anterior drawer the posteriorly displaced tibia is reduced, thus re-establishing the normal anterior tibial stepoff. (From Clancy WG Jr and Timmerman LA: Arthroscopically assisted PCL reconstruction using an autologous patella tendon graft. Op Tech Sports Med 1:129–135, 1993.)

ing the rotation of the foot, injury to the posteromedial or posterolateral structures may also be assessed. Shelbourne and associates described an adjuvant test called the dynamic posterior shift test.[57] The patient is positioned supine with the hip and knee flexed to 90 degrees. With a PCL disruption the tibia will sag posteriorly in this position, aided by hamstring tension. The examiner slowly extends the knee towards full extension. In the PCL-deficient knee, the posteriorly subluxed tibia will reduce with a palpable or visible shift. This may also reproduce the patient's symptoms. A dynamic shift may also occur if posterolateral instability is present. However, in that situation, the lateral tibial plateau will sublux further posteriorly than the medial tibial plateau (external tibial rotation).

Daniel and colleagues described the quadriceps active test, which is a useful test used to demonstrate the posterior tibial subluxation after a PCL rupture.[58] In the normal knee there is a shear component of patellar tendon vector forces, which at a certain angle (quadriceps neutral angle) is eliminated during quadriceps contraction. The quadriceps neutral angle range is from 60 to 90 degrees with a mean of 71 degrees. At angles less than the quadriceps neutral angle, the quadriceps contraction produces an anterior tibial subluxation. If the knee is flexed greater than the quadriceps neutral angle, a quadriceps produces a posterior tibial subluxation. A PCL rupture is diagnosed by using the quadriceps active test to demonstrate posterior tibial subluxation. At 90 degrees of flexion (in the normal knee), a quadriceps contraction should generally produce no movement or a slight posterior shift. If the PCL is ruptured, the tibia is already sagging posteriorly, and the patella tendon vector is subsequently directed anteriorly. Contraction of the quadriceps in the PCL-deficient knee then causes an anterior shift of the tibia, which should be visible whether the injury is chronic or acute. The test is performed by placing the patient supine and flexing the knee to 90 degrees with the foot resting on the table in a stabilized position. The patient is asked to gently push or slide the foot down the table with a quadriceps contraction.

ANCILLARY TESTS

As an aid to physical examination, the KT-1000 (Med Metric Corporation, San Diego, Calif.) testing device may be used to demonstrate and quantitate anterior-posterior displacement of the tibia relative to the femur. The test begins with an evaluation for any potential posterior tibial sag at 90 degrees of flexion. If there is a positive sag and PCL disruption is suspected, measurements with the KT-1000 are performed at the quadriceps neutral angle described earlier. Once the quadriceps neutral angle is identified in the normal knee, anterior-posterior measurements are utilized or obtained at 15 lb, 20 lb, and 30 lb in manual maximum loading. Finally, a quadriceps contraction to lift the weight of the leg and testing device is performed. The forward displacement of the tibia can be measured. The distance measured can then be added to the posterior tibial displacement measured in the injured knee and subtracted from the anterior tibial displacement measured with the testing device. This effectively negates

the initial posterior sag, which can potentially give a falsely elevated anterior displacement reading. To obtain sensitive and accurate results with good testing reproducibility, the patient must be relaxed, the instrument should be properly positioned, and the position or technician performing the test must be familiar with the testing device. Rubinstein and colleagues reported only a 33% sensitivity for diagnosing grade I PCL tears and an 86% sensitivity for grade II and III tears by a single qualified KT-1000 examiner.[36]

A series of plain x-rays should be used to evaluate for signs of PCL disruption or associated ligamentous injury. Avulsion fractures can sometimes be demonstrated, especially off the proximal posterior tibia, which may influence the form of treatment provided. If a posterolateral disruption is associated with a PCL injury, occasionally fibular head avulsion or avulsion of Gerdy's tubercle can be diagnosed as well. Lateral radiographs of the knee taken with the hip and knee flexed to 90 degrees with an applied anterior and posterior drawer can be used to demonstrate posterior tibial translation. A line is drawn parallel to the tibial plateau. A second line is drawn parallel to the first on a tangent to the lowest point on the femoral condyle. A perpendicular line is drawn to that line at the lowest point. A perpendicular line is then drawn through the center of the tibial spine. Comparison of these two perpendicular lines after anterior and posterior stress testing can be compared in the normal and injured knees to diagnose PCL disruption.

Magnetic resonance imaging (MRI) is another useful diagnostic modality and has been confirmed by arthroscopic findings to be as accurate as 99%.[59] A normal PCL appears as a dark homogeneous band on MRI. Its orientation is near vertical; thus, the PCL can often be visualized in its entirety on a single sagittal projection. Changes in signal intensity noted within the ligament or loss of continuity can be visualized.

TREATMENT GUIDELINES FOR ACUTE BONY AVULSIONS OF THE PCL

Surgical repair of PCL bony avulsion has been recommended by almost all authors, and good to excellent objective results have been reported by Trickey,[60] Meyers,[61] Lee,[62] and Torisu.[63] A combined arthroscopic and open approach is generally utilized. The procedure begins with an examination under anesthesia to evaluate for all ligamentous instabilities. A diagnostic arthroscopy can then be performed to evaluate the menisci and articular cartilage for injury. A direct posterior approach has been described by Trickey,[60] which allows visualization of the avulsion fracture and direct internal fixation with a screw. A combined anteromedial arthrotomy and posteromedial arthrotomy through a medial parapatellar "hockey stick" skin incision has been described by Hughston and colleagues.[64]

It is imperative to test the provisionally fixed avulsion fracture fragment once it has been reduced into its bony bed to determine if plastic deformation has occurred within the ligament, resulting in a permanently lengthened structure. If this is the case, despite anatomic fixation of the avulsion fraction, instability will continue to persist.

If this is noted intraoperatively, the bony avulsion fragment can be countersunk into the proximal tibia to restore the proper functional length of the PCL and improve the biomechanical stability of the repair. If the fracture fragment is large enough to accept a cancellous screw, this is generally the recommended fixation technique.[60, 65] However, if the bony fragment is small, sutures should be placed through the ligamentous structure as well as the bony fragment and delivered through drill holes, which are drilled from the anterior tibia into the posterior bony bed and tied anteriorly while applying an anterior drawer to the knee flexed at 90 degrees.[66, 67]

TREATMENT OF ISOLATED INTERSTITIAL PCL RUPTURES

To date, the greatest controversy in treatment of PCL injury exists in the group of patients with an isolated PCL interstitial tear. The authors believe that with any PCL injury, the kinematic function and biomechanical stability of the knee are compromised, which leads to accelerated articular cartilage wear. Although more is being learned about surgical reconstruction of the PCL, there continues to be considerable controversy regarding femoral and tibial tunnel position, type of fixation, knee positioning at the time of graft tensioning, and graft source. No procedure has been shown to completely restore objective biomechanical stability to the knee. Therefore, an operative procedure is indicated only if it can consistently produce a zero or trace posterior drawer, thus improving the stability of the injured knee.

It has been our experience that interstitial failures in continuity of the PCL can occur and can be diagnosed with MRI. This injury represents a plastic deformation of the PCL with an intact synovial sheath. If a proper rehabilitation program is utilized, in many cases the PCL appears to contract and possibly heal, thus reducing a 1 or 2+ posterior drawer to a 1+ or trace posterior drawer over several months (Fig. 29–8).

A clear dialogue must be maintained between the surgeon and the patient. The uncertainty of the natural history must be explained, and the patient must understand that it is difficult to consistently obtain excellent biomechanical stability after PCL reconstruction. It has been the author's experience that isolated PCL injury will lead to medial femoral condyle and patellofemoral degenerative changes over time.[31] The variability occurs in the degree of degenerative changes that will ultimately occur and over what period of time. Muscular development, activity level, and genetic predisposition all play a role in determining if a patient will sustain this irreversible damage over a relatively short period of time or over a period of decades.

The authors have found that bone scanning is a useful screening measure in patients who have a chronic isolated PCL injury. A positive result on a bone scan indicates that there has been a breakdown in the tangential layer of the articular surface or of the articular cartilage with increased subchondral bone activity, indicating that considerable degenerative changes are taking place. Because we believe that these patients will continue to undergo further progressive arthritic changes with the instability present, a stabilization procedure is warranted. While it may be argued that the time to operate would be before the result of the bone scan is positive to obviate the otherwise inevitable arthritic process, no long-term studies have demonstrated that PCL reconstruction prevents potential degenerative arthritic changes. When clinical studies can

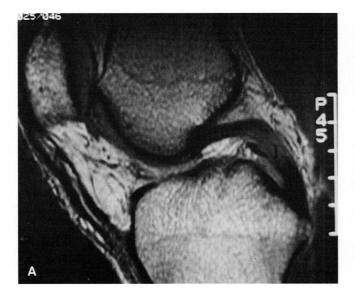 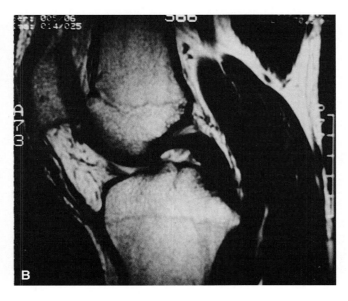

Figure 29–8 • *A,* Magnetic resonance imaging (MRI) at 3 days post injury depicts an in situ tear of the posterior cruciate ligament (PCL). *B,* MRI at 8 weeks depicts healing of the in situ rupture of the PCL after conservative management. (From Kaplan MJ and Clancy WG Jr: Alabama sports medicine experience with isolated and combined posterior cruciate ligament injuries. Clin Sports Med 13:545–552, 1994.)

show that PCL reconstruction is predictively successful and offer the patients biomechanical stability, not just functional stability, then patients can then be offered a PCL reconstruction, even in the acute setting.

ISOLATED, CHRONIC PCL-DEFICIENT KNEE—ASYMPTOMATIC

Many patients remain pain free and have little or no functional instability after PCL injury. We believe that periodic bone scanning or MRI to evaluate the articular surface and underlying subchondral bone is indicated. If no degenerative changes are seen, the authors would not recommend an operative stabilization procedure. Patients should be followed over a period of time, and if functional instability becomes a significant clinical factor or if pain develops, a PCL reconstruction may then be indicated.

ISOLATED, CHRONIC PCL-DEFICIENT KNEE—SYMPTOMATIC

If a patient presents with pain or functional instability, he or she must then be considered for appropriate ligamentous reconstruction. Patients should be categorized by physiologic age and activity level. In patients who are younger than 40 years of age and who are active and have functional instability or pain, a reconstructive procedure is then recommended. In patients who are middle-aged (40–60 years of age), treatment depends on both knee alignment and the patient's symptoms. In the patient with severe genu varum, it is appropriate to correct the varus deformity first with a valgus osteotomy. If the patient does poorly with regard to pain, he or she may be a candidate for a total joint procedure rather than a secondary PCL reconstruction. If after the valgus osteotomy the patient goes on to have frank instability without pain, a PCL reconstruction may be indicated if the patient is physiologically young. If the patient is older than 60 years of age, he or she is generally not a candidate for PCL reconstruction but would do better with a PCL stabilized total knee arthroplasty if pain is the primary complaint.

OPERATIVE TECHNIQUE

As with any surgical procedure, careful preoperative planning will better enable the surgeon to perform a successful reconstruction. The surgeon must first decide on a graft source. The authors generally use a patellar tendon autograft from the ipsilateral knee. If associated ligamentous instabilities require additional graft sources or if revision surgery is being performed, a contralateral patellar tendon graft is occasionally utilized. If this is not available or is not in the patient's best interest, an allograft can be utilized. Some special equipment should be planned in order to be available. We utilize a 0 degree arthroscope for use during the procedure. In addition, a 30 and 70 degree arthroscope should be available for use in special circumstances. Additionally, a drill guide system for PCL reconstruction

should also be available, along with a graft passer (DePuy, Warsaw, Ind.), and special right-angled curettes (Acufex, Norwood, Mass.). Intraoperative radiographs are also useful to confirm tibial tunnel pin placement prior to drilling the tunnel. It has been our experience that radiographs are more accurate than is fluoroscopy.

The procedure begins with a careful examination under anesthesia to confirm the diagnosis of PCL instability and to determine any other associated ligamentous injuries. The leg is prepared and draped free without the use of a leg holder. A tourniquet is placed on the thigh; however, it is generally not utilized unless visualization is a problem. With the surgeon in a seated position, the leg is placed over the side of the table with the foot slightly externally rotated on the outside of the surgeon's thigh (Fig. 29–9). One percent lidocaine with epinephrine is injected at the portal site positions to aid in hemostasis. A medial parapatellar portal and anteromedial collateral portal are made, and a routine diagnostic arthroscopy is performed. The condition of the articular surfaces and menisci is carefully evaluated. Associated lesions are addressed at this time. The condition of both cruciate ligaments is carefully assessed. Specifically, the condition of the ligaments of Humphry and Wrisberg, if present, is evaluated, because these may still be intact even with complete rupture of the main portion of the PCL.

Once the diagnosis is confirmed, a straight longitudinal incision is made to the distal tip of the tibial tubercle, incorporating the medial parapatellar portal. A middle-third patellar tendon graft 10 mm wide is harvested with bone plugs from the patella and the tibial tubercle, which measure 25 mm in length and 4 mm in depth. Three small drill holes are placed in each bone block with a 0.062 K-wire. No. 5 nonabsorbable sutures are then passed through the holes in each bone block with Keith needles (Fig. 29–10).

A central fat pad portal is then established through the patellar tendon defect. The arthroscope is placed in the medial parapatellar portal with a shaver in the central fat pad portal to perform débridement of the residual PCL fibers and stump. While débriding the femoral insertion fibers, the footprint of the PCL on the medial femoral condyle and in the intercondylar notch is noted. To allow for better visualization of the medial femoral condyle, the arthroscope can be placed in a lateral parapatellar portal.

Attention is then directed to the tibial insertion of the PCL. Residual stump fibers are débrided, and the posterior capsule is then elevated and punctured with a small right-angle curette at the distal insertion site of the PCL on the posterior tibial ridge (Fig. 29–11). Below the posterior tibial ridge rests the popliteus muscle fibers, which can be viewed with the arthroscope. Occasionally an angled arthroscope (30 or 70 degrees) can be utilized to improve visualization over the posterior aspect of the tibia. An Arthrex PCL tibial drill guide (Arthrex, Naples, Fla.) is then introduced through the central fat pad portal and is tipped positioned centrally on the distal aspect of the posterior tibial ridge. Anteriorly, the drill guide is placed in the center of the tibia just distal to the bone defect from the graft harvest site in cortical bone (Fig. 29–12). The graft harvest site is not used because the cancellous bone is soft, and the drill may not remain correctly centered. In

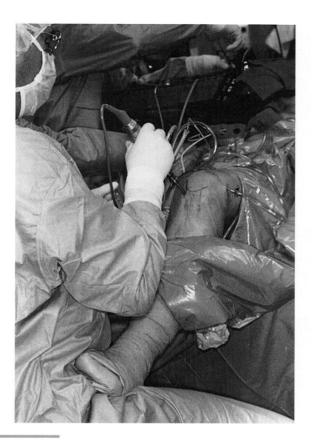

Figure 29–9 • The involved knee is placed over the side of the table, and the heel is positioned into the surgeon's groin. The arthroscope is placed initially in the medial parapatellar portal. (From Clancy WG Jr and Timmerman LA: Arthroscopically assisted PCL reconstruction using an autologous patella tendon graft. Op Tech Sports Med 1:129–135, 1993.)

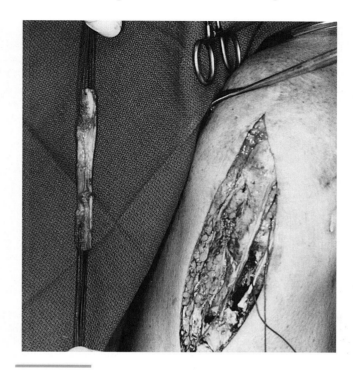

Figure 29–10 • The central portion of the patellar tendon measuring 10 mm in width is taken along with its patellar and tibial bony attachments measuring 10 mm in width, 4 mm in depth, and 25 mm in length. Three No. 5 nonabsorbable sutures are placed in the bone blocks. (From Clancy WG Jr and Timmerman LA: Arthroscopically assisted PCL reconstruction using an autologous patella tendon graft. Op Tech Sports Med 1:129–135, 1993.)

the cortical bone distal to the cancellous bone, the pin remains centered. A guide pin is then drilled from anterior to posterior. It is critical to feel the penetration of the posterior cortex. An arthroscope can be used through the center of the notch to visualize the pin as it exits, or a medial parapatellar portal can be utilized to place a curette posteriorly to help protect the neurovascular structures. In addition, the knee is kept in a flexed position to allow the neurovascular structures to fall away from the posterior capsule.

A lateral roentgenogram is then obtained to confirm K-wire placement (Fig. 29–13). The pin should exit at the distal portion of the posterior tibial ridge, which can be viewed. Other associate landmarks on a lateral knee radiograph include the superior aspect of the fibular head and also the tibial physeal scar proximally. Once the correct placement of the guide pin is confirmed, a 10 mm reamer is used to overdrill the pin. Once again, extreme caution is utilized when the drill penetrates the posterior cortex to prevent injury to neurovascular structures. Once the tunnel is complete, the periosteum and soft tissues should be completely débrided from the tunnel in order to aid in the eventual graft passage.

Attention is then directed to the femoral condyle for femoral tunnel placement. As noted previously, the femoral PCL insertion is broad and expansive. PCL fibers insert high on the intercondylar notch roof and actually cross the midline of the roof and also extend down low and posterior on the medial femoral condyle. Fibers insert within 1 mm of the articular cartilage distally. The femoral tunnel is critical because this determines which portion of the PCL is to be reconstructed with a single graft source. If it is placed high and anterior, it will better represent the anterolateral bundle of the PCL. If an attempt is made to place the graft low and posterior, it will better represent the more isometric fibers of the PCL insertion. We, however, believe that clinical results are improved if one reconstructs the larger anterolateral portion of the PCL. To date, we have generally used a single patellar tendon graft. However, we have explored utilizing a split patellar tendon graft to help reconstruct both the anterolateral and posteromedial bundles. While this technique seems promising, our clinical experience has been limited and cannot be generally recommended at this time.

A small curette is used to mark the proposed guide pin exit site on the medial femoral condyle. As stated earlier, the femoral tunnel is placed anterior and distal. The guide pin should exit approximately 5 mm proximal to the distal edge of the articular surface of the medial femoral condyle at approximately 1:30 for a right knee and 10:30 for a left

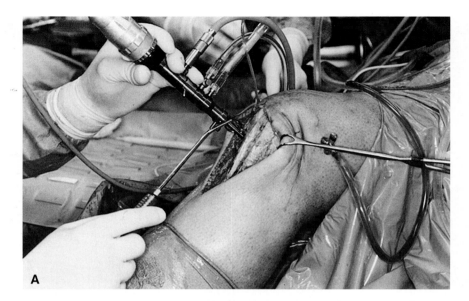

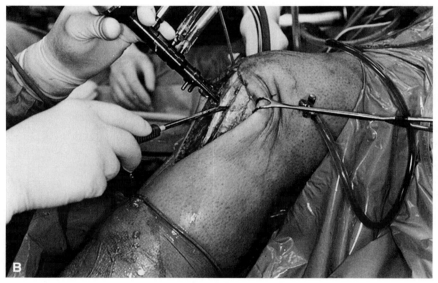

A

B

Figure 29–11 • *A,* The arthroscope is placed in the medial parapatellar portal, and a right-angle curette is placed through the central fat pad portal where the patellar tendon graft has been taken. *B,* The curette is used to free the posterior capsule from tibial insertion just inferior to the posterior cruciate ligament insertion area. (From Clancy WG Jr and Timmerman LA: Arthroscopically assisted PCL reconstruction using an autologous patella tendon graft. Op Tech Sports Med 1:129–135, 1993.)

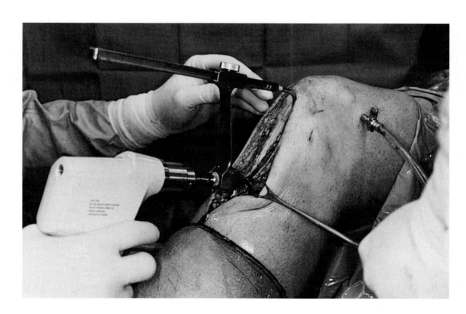

Figure 29–12 • The drill guide has been passed through the central fat pad portal and placed just below the posterior tibial ridge. The anterior portion of the drill guide is placed in the midline of the tibia just below the tibial tubercle where the patellar tendon graft has been harvested. (From Clancy WG Jr and Timmerman LA: Arthroscopically assisted PCL reconstruction using an autologous patella tendon graft. Op Tech Sports Med 1:129–135, 1993.)

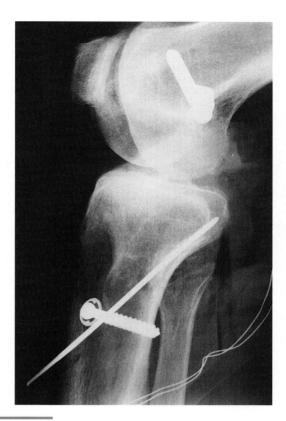

Figure 29–13 • The roentgenogram shows that the K-wire has exited the posterior aspect of the tibia just at the posterior tibial ridge. (From Clancy WG Jr and Timmerman LA: Arthroscopically assisted PCL reconstruction using an autologous patella tendon graft. Op Tech Sports Med 1:129–135, 1993.)

knee (Fig. 29–14). By placing the guide pin 5 mm posterior or proximal to the articular surface edge, the 10 mm reamer will exit right at the articular margin.

A small skin incision is made medially overlying the vastus medialis obliquus (VMO) insertion into the medial intermuscular septum. The VMO is identified and retracted laterally with a Slocum retractor after dissecting

it off the intermuscular septum. The Arthrex PCL femoral drill guide is then introduced through the medial parapatellar portal with the intra-articular side placed in the selected site on the medial femoral condyle. The opposite end is placed just above the medial femoral epicondyle such that the guide pin can be drilled from proximal to distal at a slight angle so that the articular cartilage is not undermined on the medial femoral condyle. Once the guide pin is placed in a satisfactory position, a 10 mm reamer is then used to overdrill the tunnel.

A Hewson suture passer (Richards, Memphis, Tenn.) is fashioned by curbing the distal tip of the passer so that it can be passed through the tibial tunnel from anterior to posterior and visualized with the arthroscope in the medial parapatellar portal. A grasper is used to pull the suture passer out the central fat pad portal. A No. 5 nonabsorbable suture is then passed so that one end exits the central fat pad portal and the other end leaves the tibial tunnel anteriorly. A second suture is passed through the femoral tunnel to exit the same central fat pad portal. The latter suture is then tied to the three sutures on one end of the graft, and the graft is passed through the femoral tunnel from outside to inside and then out through the central fat pad portal. The sutures that are exiting the medial femoral tunnel are then tied over a button (Fig. 29–15). The bone block is oriented in the femoral tunnel such that the cancellous bone faces posteriorly and the cortical bone anteriorly so that the patellar tendon will effectively insert closer to the articular surface and not ride over the posterior edge of the tunnel. The sutures from the bone block exiting the central fat pad portal are then passed through a DePuy (Warsaw, Ind.) graft passer, which has been cut to the appropriate size. These sutures are then tied to the suture previously passed through the tibial tunnel. The knee is flexed to 90 degrees, and an anterior drawer is applied to the proximal tibia. The sutures are pulled back through the central fat pad portal into the joint and then into the tibial tunnel with the graft following (Fig. 29–16).

The arthroscope is then placed into the tibial tunnel to visualize the presence of the bone block to confirm that it has been delivered into the tibial tunnel properly. The anterolateral muscle is then elevated off the proximal tibia just lateral to the tibial tubercle and distal to the tibial tunnel. A 25 mm long 6.5 mm AO cancellous screw (Synthes,

Figure 29–14 • The medial femoral tunnel placements are depicted in a right knee and a left knee. The desired site on the right knee is approximately at 1:30 and for the left knee it is approximately at 10:30. (From Clancy WG Jr and Timmerman LA: Arthroscopically assisted PCL reconstruction using an autologous patella tendon graft. Op Tech Sports Med 1:129–135, 1993.)

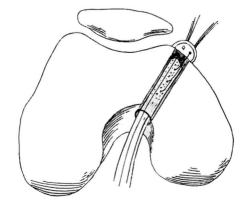
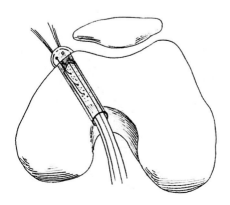

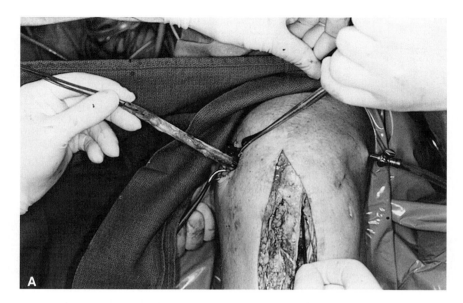

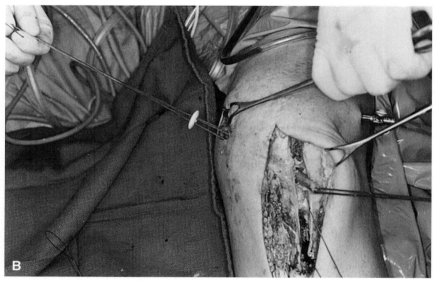

Figure 29–15 • *A*, The patellar tendon graft is pulled through the medial femoral condyle and out through the central fat pad portal. *B*, The sutures attached to the bone block within the medial femoral tunnel are then tied over a button. (From Clancy WG Jr and Timmerman LA: Arthroscopically assisted PCL reconstruction using an autologous patella tendon graft. Op Tech Sports Med 1:129–135, 1993.)

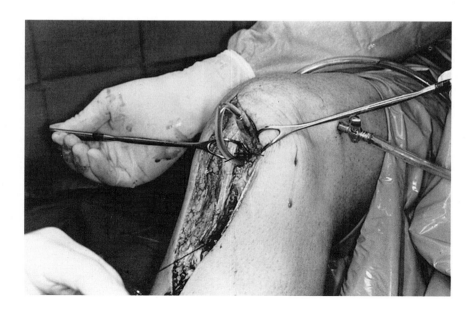

Figure 29–16 • The graft passer, along with the inferior portion of the patellar tendon graft, is pulled back through the central fat pad portal, into the knee joint and then into the posterior tibial tunnel while at the same time performing the anterior drawer. (From Clancy WG Jr and Timmerman LA: Arthroscopically assisted PCL reconstruction using an autologous patella tendon graft. Op Tech Sports Med 1:129–135, 1993.)

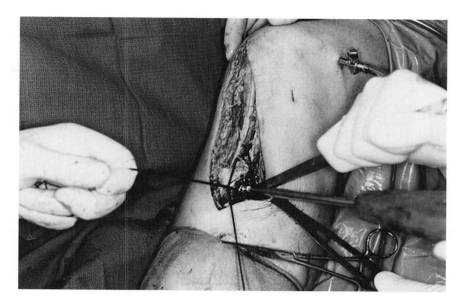

Figure 29–17 • The anterior lateral muscle insertions have been retracted to place a 25 mm cancellous screw and washer into the tibia just below the tibial tunnel entrance. (From Clancy WG Jr and Timmerman LA: Arthroscopically assisted PCL reconstruction using an autologous patella tendon graft. Op Tech Sports Med 1:129–135, 1993.)

U.S.A., Paoli, Pa.) and a washer are placed in the lateral tibia. Sutures are placed around this to be ultimately tied over this post (Fig. 29–17). An anterior drawer is placed on the externally rotated tibia with the knee first flexed to 90 degrees and then to 30 degrees. The sutures are then tied under tension. The knee is examined to ensure that the normal tibial step-off has been restored. No posterior drawer should be detected. To compensate for graft tension relaxation, the suture ends from the button on the medial femoral condyle are tied around the staple, which is placed approximately 5 mm proximal to the button.

The wounds are closed over suction drains, and the knee is then placed in a brace locked in extension. Postoperatively an aggressive specific rehabilitation program is utilized. On the first postoperative day, range of motion from 0 to 60 degrees is allowed, and this is continued for the first 6 weeks. Range of motion is then advanced to 90 degrees at 6 weeks. Full weight-bearing with crutches is allowed immediately postoperatively, and crutches can be discarded at 2 weeks. Minisquats from 0 to 40 degrees, swimming, bicycle exercising, and quadriceps progressive-resistant exercises are utilized, starting at week 6. Hamstring strengthening is begun at 4 months, and a running program is allowed at that time as well. Noncontact sports are allowed at 6 months, and contact sports are allowed at 9 months.

COMBINED PCL INSTABILITY

PCL disruption, combined with disruption of one or more of the other major ligamentous structures, can be a devastating injury as well as produce significant functional instability. When presented with such a case, an accurate diagnosis must be made and stabilization of torn structures performed to help provide a satisfactory result. This approach has been well documented in literature.[68–71]

ACUTE PCL AND MCL COMBINED INJURY

A combined injury of the PCL and MCL is more rarely encountered than combined injuries involving the ACL/PCL and PCL and posterolateral corner. The clinician must first determine the degree of MCL injury, because this dictates the type of treatment to be performed. The knee should be examined for stability to valgus stress in full extension and at 30 degrees of flexion. Grade III tibial collateral ligament rupture without a posterior oblique ligament tear will give greater than 10 mm of laxity at 30 degrees of knee flexion, but only 1 or 2 mm laxity at 0 degrees flexion with valgus stress. If indeed the posterior oblique portion of the MCL or the tibial collateral ligament is intact, the authors' approach is to reconstruct the PCL and treat the MCL injury conservatively with postoperative range of motion brace, utilizing a standard PCL postoperative protocol.

If gross laxity is encountered at 0 degrees of extension and 30 degrees of knee flexion, both the posterior oblique ligament and the superficial tibial collateral ligament have been disrupted. In this scenario the clinician must also be very suspicious of a concomitant ACL injury. Treatment for this injury is to reconstruct the PCL arthroscopically and to explore the MCL and posterior oblique ligament for direct repair as indicated. This combined repair can be performed at one operative setting.

COMBINED PCL AND ACL INJURY

A combined injury to the PCL and ACL suggests the possibility of an acute dislocated knee with spontaneous reduction and is often associated with concomitant medial collateral or lateral collateral ligament/posterolateral corner injury. A high index of suspicion must be maintained for neurovascular injury. Appropriate work-up for clinical or occult arterial injury should be performed, including femoral arteriography. A detailed ligamentous examination must also be performed to plan any potential reconstruction. This includes tests for external rotation at 90 degrees of knee flexion and 30 degrees of knee flexion and also varus and valgus stress testing at 0 and 30 degrees.

Past recommendations have been for repair or reconstruction of all torn ligament structures.[33, 72, 73] Sisto and Warren reviewed 13 patients with knee dislocations who underwent complete ligament repair.[74] Although clinical instability did not seem to be a problem postoperatively, 46% of these patients had a reported loss of range of motion, chronic pain, and disability. Meyers and Harvey reported good results after ligamentous repair (returned to normal occupation or daily living).[73] However, 25% of their patients had significant pain and instability.

With the improved results reported after reconstruction versus repair of the ACL and PCL injuries, reconstruction has become the method of choice in combined injuries as well. Shelbourne has recommended a stabilizing procedure centered on the PCL with an aggressive rehabilitation program, because he feels that this procedure will give acceptable stability and a more functional range of motion and outcome.[75] However, based on our own experiences, we have not found a loss of range of motion with combined reconstruction of the ACL and PCL to be a significant problem.[76]

With an acute combined ACL and PCL injury, the authors recommend a delay in surgical intervention of approximately 7–10 days if possible. Controlled motion is initiated during this period. At the time of surgery both cruciate injuries are addressed simultaneously to re-establish the neutral position of the tibia on the femur. Whenever possible, a patellar tendon autogenous graft is utilized for reconstruction of the PCL, and a similar graft is harvested from the contralateral knee for the ACL reconstruction. If this is not feasible, hamstring tendons may be utilized for the ACL reconstruction.

SURGICAL TECHNIQUE

After careful evaluation of the knee under anesthesia, both legs are prepared and draped free without the use of a leg holder. One percent lidocaine with epinephrine is injected into the portal sites, and a routine diagnostic arthroscopy is performed. After a complete evaluation of the knee, patellar tendon grafts are harvested from both legs. On the injured leg, the medial parapatellar portal is extended below the tibial tubercle to allow for patellar tendon harvest. A 10 mm wide graft is obtained with 10 mm wide by 4 mm deep by 25 mm long patellar and tibial bone plugs. A similar graft is taken from the contralateral knee for ACL reconstruction. Bone blocks are drilled with a 0.062 K-wire, and No. 5 nonabsorbable sutures are placed into each bone block. The knee is then prepared, and tunnels are made for PCL reconstruction as described for isolated PCL reconstruction. When this is complete, attention is turned toward ACL reconstruction. An incision is made on the lateral thigh just proximal to the metaphyseal flare of the lateral femoral condyle. The fascia lata is divided, and the vastus lateralis is elevated. A gaff is passed through

the knee and out the lateral incision to allow a rear-entry guide to be placed into the knee joint. A K-wire is drilled, followed by a 10 mm reamer for placement of the femoral ACL tunnel. The tibial drill guide is introduced through the medial parapatellar portal with the tip of the guide slightly anterior and medial to the center of the ACL insertion. The K-wire is drilled, followed by a 10 mm reamer, after proper position has been confirmed.

The previously prepared grafts are then passed. The PCL graft is passed first, followed by the ACL graft. Once the PCL graft has been passed as described previously, the ACL graft is then passed through the femoral tunnel and out the tibial tunnel with the use of a Hewson suture passer (Richards, Memphis, Tenn.). The femoral bone block is secured around a button similar to the PCL proximal bone block. Both grafts are then fixed distally using unicortical 25 mm, 6.5 mm cancellous screws with washers. A cortical bone bridge of approximately 1 cm is left between the two tibial tunnels. The anterolateral musculature is elevated just distal to the tibial PCL tunnel, and the screw and washer are placed into the lateral tibia. With the knee at 30 degrees of flexion, both grafts are simultaneously tensioned and tied around the respective screws. This centers the tibia in its normal neutral position on the femur. Knee motion is then assessed; the Lachman test is performed; and the tibial stepoff is examined. To compensate for graft tension relaxation, the suture ends from the button fixing each proximal graft are tied around a staple, which is placed approximately 5–10 mm proximal to the button. Aggressive rehabilitation is begun on the first postoperative day, but range of motion is limited from 0 to 60 degrees during the first 6 weeks.

The results of combined arthroscopic reconstruction of the ACLs and PCLs have been studied.[76] We reviewed 17 patients who underwent a combined procedure and were evaluated at a minimum 2-year follow-up. Group A consisted of nine patients who were reconstructed within 2 weeks of a knee dislocation. Group B consisted of eight patients with chronic combined insufficiency of both cruciates. In final follow-up seven of nine patients in group A were graded as nearly normal and two patients as abnormal by the IKDC Evaluation Scale. All patients in group A returned to their preinjury activity level. In the chronic reconstruction group (group B), four patients were almost normal; two patients were abnormal; and two patients were severely abnormal. Only three patients were able to return to their preinjury activity level. Based on these results, we believe that an acute reconstruction of combined ACL and PCL injuries is an effective procedure for achieving static and functional stability of the dislocated knee. It was also noted that acute reconstructions fared better than did chronic reconstructions using this technique.

COMBINED PCL/POSTEROLATERAL INSTABILITY

PCL disruption, combined with posterolateral instability, produces a significant functional instability. Posterolateral instability results in excess of external rotation of the tibia, which is most pronounced at 30 degrees of knee flexion.

This rotational instability moves the tibial insertion of the PCL medially and anteriorly, effectively shortening the distance to the PCL femoral insertion, producing a functionally lax ligament. Therefore, reconstruction of the PCL without achieving adequate posterolateral instability will yield a poor result. After a PCL reconstruction is performed, the knee should be carefully examined for evidence of posterolateral instability so that this does not go untreated.

Treatment of this injury begins with reconstruction of the PCL as described previously in this chapter. After the graft has been passed and fixed proximally and distally, the posterolateral structures are thoroughly evaluated. If significant posterolateral instability is present, operative repair or reconstruction is indicated. In the acute situation, direct repair can be performed with good results. The posterolateral capsule is repaired, and the popliteus and fibular collateral ligament are repaired or reattached to bone as indicated. If in the acute setting repair is not possible, then the second choice would be to proceed with a biceps tenodesis. A biceps tenodesis should only be performed, however, if the biceps tendon is adequately attached to the fibular head. If this is not possible, a third alternative is to use an allograft Achilles tendon to create a "posterolateral cruciate." Once the posterolateral structures have been addressed, the posterior cruciate graft is again tightened over a staple proximally to remove any potential slack in the graft.

If the PCL posterolateral insufficiency is chronic, limb alignment must be closely evaluated and considered. If significant varus angulation exists, either secondary to medial compartment degenerative disease or congenital varus alignment, consideration must be made for performing a valgus high tibial osteotomy in conjunction with a posterolateral reconstruction. In these situations, primary repair is rarely possible. In our experience, posterolateral reconstruction by anterior and superior advancement of the lateral gastrocnemius tendon, superior posterolateral capsule, fibular collateral ligament, and the popliteus tendon, as advocated by Hughston and Jacobsen,[77] has not provided consistently good results. Popliteus tendon resection on the femur as recommended by Jakob, Hassler, and Staeubli has also produced inconsistent results in the authors' hands.[78] Our procedure of choice has become a posterolateral stabilization performed by rerouting the biceps tendon to the lateral femoral epicondyle, while leaving the distal tendon attached to the fibula. This creates a new fibular collateral ligament and effectively tightens the deep inferior posterolateral arcuate complex, which is firmly attached to the biceps tendon complex.[79, 80]

SURGICAL TECHNIQUE: POSTEROLATERAL RECONSTRUCTION WITH BICEPS FEMORIS

The skin incision starts laterally at Gerdy's tubercle and is carried superiorly in a curvilinear fashion approximately 15 cm proximal. The iliotibial band is incised longitudinally over the lateral femoral epicondyle. The biceps tendon is dissected free from its surrounding soft tissue. The biceps muscle and tendon are freed from their attachments to the lateral gastrocnemius muscle. Dissection of the per-

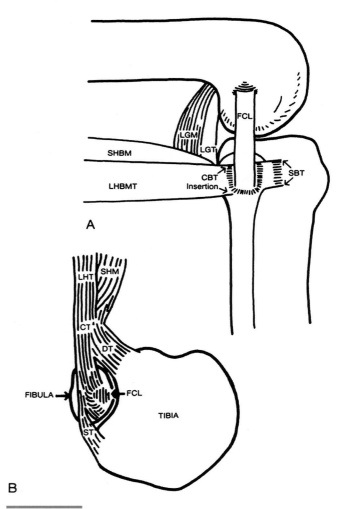

Figure 29–18 • *A,* The superior insertion of the fibular collateral ligament on the inferior two-thirds of the lateral epicondyle. The common biceps tendon inserts on the fibula, completely surrounding the inferior insertion of the fibular collateral ligament. *B,* This cross-sectional drawing of the proximal fibula and tibia demonstrates the insertions of the common biceps tendon into the arcuate complex posteriorly and its horseshoe insertion around the fibular collateral ligament. Superior advancement of the common biceps tendon will tighten the arcuate complex and enable isometric reconstruction of the fibular collateral ligament. (From Clancy WG Jr: Repair and reconstruction of the posterior cruciate ligament. In Chapman MW [ed.]: Operative Orthopaedics, 2nd ed, vol 3. Philadelphia, J.B. Lippincott Co., 1993.)

oneal nerve is performed carefully at the inferior portion of the biceps tendon. Once dissected free, the nerve is protected throughout the procedure. The biceps muscle is retracted laterally, exposing the peroneal nerve as it courses in a vertical proximal direction. The biceps tendon and muscle can then be brought underneath the inferior portion of the iliotibial band so that the tendon can be fixed to the lateral femoral epicondyle. Soft tissues are freed and dissected off the lateral femoral epicondyle, allowing visualization of the superior insertional fibers of the fibular collateral ligament (Fig. 29–18). A trough is

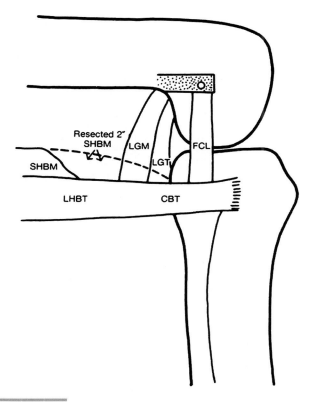

Figure 29–19 • A trough 10 mm wide and 2.5 cm long is made into the upper third of the lateral femoral epicondyle where there are no fibers of the fibular collateral ligament insertion. The distal 5 cm of the biceps muscle is removed from the common tendon to allow the tendon to be fixed to the lateral femoral epicondyle. (From Clancy WG Jr: Repair and reconstruction of the posterior cruciate ligament. In Chapman MW [ed.]: Operative Orthopaedics, 2nd ed, vol 3. Philadelphia, J.B. Lippincott Co., 1993.)

created approximately 1 cm wide and 2 cm long in the upper portion of the lateral femoral epicondyle, just proximal to the flare of the lateral femoral epicondyle (Fig. 29–19). A 3.2 mm hole is drilled in the trough just superior to the lateral femoral epicondyle. The hole should be aimed slightly cephalad to avoid the PCL tunnel in the femur. The distal 3–4 cm of biceps muscle is dissected away from the tendon to improve fixation of the tendon to the lateral femoral epicondylar trough. A 6.5 mm partially threaded cancellous screw with spiked washer is then placed. The tendon is brought up over the anterior aspect of the screw, effectively tightening the arcuate ligament complex through its attachments to the biceps tendon. The screw is then seated firmly, bringing the tendon into the trough (Fig. 29–20). The knee is placed through a full range of motion and again varus laxity, valgus laxity, external rotation, and anteroposterior translation are all closely checked for static stability. Postoperatively, the knee is held in full extension for 6 weeks, followed by a rehabilitation program designed for posterior cruciate reconstruction, emphasizing quadriceps strength.

SURGICAL TECHNIQUE: POSTEROLATERAL CRUCIATE

A curvilinear incision is made as described earlier for the biceps tendon transfer. The iliotibial band is incised over the lateral femoral epicondyle. The biceps tendon and lateral gastrocnemius muscle are retracted to allow visualization of the posteromedial aspect of the fibula and tibia.

A K-wire is placed below Gerdy's tubercle and drilled posteriorly to exit just medial to the fibular head. This is overdrilled with a 10 mm drill. A No. 5 nonabsorbable suture is placed from anterior to posterior through this tunnel using a Hewson suture passer (Richards, Memphis, Tenn.). The suture is brought out anteriorly and superiorly under the inferior portion of the iliotibial band and attached to an Isotac (Acufex, Mansfield, Mass.), which has

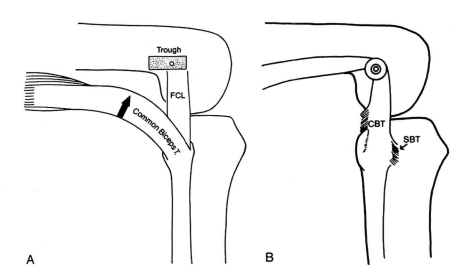

Figure 29–20 • A, Once the appropriate amount of short head biceps muscle has been resected, with care taken not to injure the common tendon, the common biceps tendon is brought anteriorly to be fixed in the previously developed trough. B, An AO cancellous screw and plastic washer is placed inferior to the tendon and tightened to hold the tendon in place. The entire tendon lies on top of the screw. (From Clancy WG Jr: Repair and reconstruction of the posterior cruciate ligament. In Chapman MW [ed.]: Operative Orthopaedics, 2nd ed, vol 3. Philadelphia, J.B. Lippincott Co., 1993.)

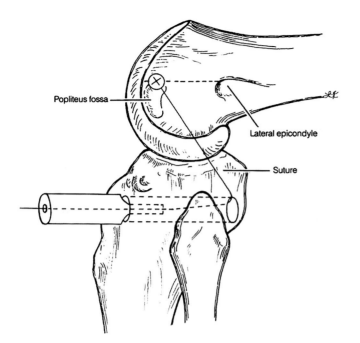

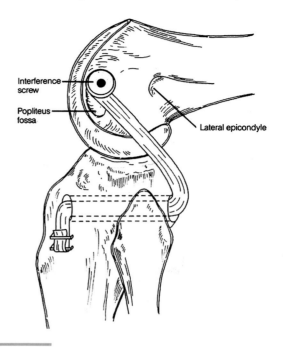

Figure 29–21 • Method for finding the most physiometric area for placement of the Achilles tendon allograft for the creation of a "posterolateral cruciate ligament." The suture is fixed to the lateral femoral condyle and then run posteriorly into the tibial tunnel and anteriorly attached to a strain gauge. The knee is placed through a full range of motion, and measurements are recorded. (Andrews JR, Baker CL, Curl WW, et al.: Surgical repair of acute and chronic lesions of the lateral capsular ligamentous complex of the knee. In Feagin JA Jr [ed.]: The Crucial Ligaments, 2nd ed. Churchill Livingstone, New York, 1994.)

Figure 29–22 • When the desired area of physiometry is located, a 10 mm tunnel is created and the Achilles tendon bone block is fixed in this site. The remaining tendon is pulled posteriorly and placed into the tibial tunnel. The graft is then fixed anteriorly over two staples. (Andrews JR, Baker CL, Curl WW, et al.: Surgical repair of acute and chronic lesions of the lateral capsular ligamentous complex of the knee. In Feagin JA Jr [ed.]: The Crucial Ligaments, 2nd ed. Churchill Livingstone, New York, 1994.)

been placed in the anteriormost part of the popliteus hiatus and lateral aspect of the lateral femoral condyle. The knee is placed through a full range of motion and the Isotac (Acufex, Mansfield, Mass.) is moved until the strain gauge isolates an isometric or physiometric area for attachment of the Achilles tendon graft (Fig. 29–21).

A 10 mm hole is made in this spot to a depth of 25 mm. An Achilles tendon allograft is fashioned, and a bone block is made to fit into the tunnel. Once the graft has been placed in the tunnel, it is held in place with an interference screw. The tendon is then passed medially to the iliotibial tract and under the fibular collateral ligament and brought posterior to anterior in the previously drilled tibial tunnel. The graft is secured with two staples (Fig. 29–22).

Accompanying lateral laxity must also be corrected if it exists after reconstruction of the posterolateral corner. This can be performed with either a biceps tendon transfer or by using a patellar tendon autograft or allograft. Postoperatively, the knee is placed in a full extension splint for 6 weeks. A range of motion from 0 to 90 degrees is allowed, as is full weight-bearing. At 6 weeks, full range of motion is begun. This protocol can be modified if an ACL or PCL reconstruction is performed.

References

1. Girgis FG, Marshall JL, and Al Monajem ARS: The cruciate ligaments of the knee joint: anatomical, functional and experimental analysis. Clin Orthop 106:216–231, 1975.
2. Harner CD, Livesay GA, Choi NY, et al.: Evaluation of the sizes and shapes of the human anterior and posterior cruciate ligaments: a comparative study. Trans Orthop Res Soc 17:123, 1992.
3. O'Brien WR, Friederich NF, Muller W, et al.: Functional anatomy of the cruciate ligaments and their substitutes. Presented as a Scientific Exhibit at the Annual Meeting of the American Academy of Orthopaedic Surgeons, Las Vegas, Nevada, February 9–14, 1989.
4. Kurosawa H, Yamakoshi KL, Yasuda K, et al.: Simultaneous measurement of changes in length of the cruciate ligaments during knee motion. Clin Orthop 265:223–240, 1991.
5. Trent PS, Walker PS, and Wolf B: Ligament length patterns, strength and rotational axes of the knee joint. Clin Orthop 117:263–270, 1976.
6. Covey DC, Sapega AA, Sherman GM, et al.: Testing for "isometry" during posterior cruciate ligament reconstruction. Trans Orthop Res Soc 17:665, 1992.
7. Brantigan OC and Voshell AF: The mechanics of the ligaments and menisci of the knee joint. J Bone Joint Surg 23:44–66, 1941.
8. Heller L and Langman J: The menisco-femoral ligaments of the human knee. J Bone Joint Surg Br 46:307–313, 1964.
9. Kaplan EB: Some aspects of functional anatomy of the human knee joint. Clin Orthop 23:18–29, 1962.
10. Arms SW, Johnson RJ, and Pope MH: Strain measurement of the

human posterior cruciate ligament. Trans Orthop Res Soc 9:355, 1984.

11. Hefzy MS, Grood ES, and Lindenfeld TL: The posterior cruciate ligament: a new look at length patterns. Trans Orthop Res Soc 11:128, 1986.

12. Bach BR, Daluga DJ, Mikosz R, et al.: Force displacement characteristics of the posterior cruciate ligament. Am J Sports Med 20:67–72, 1992.

13. Bradley J, FitzPatrick D, Daniel D, et al.: Orientation of the cruciate ligament in the sagittal plane: a method of predicting its length-change with flexion. J Bone Joint Surg Br 70:94–99, 1988.

14. Ogata K and McCarthy JA: Measurements of length and tension patterns during reconstruction of the posterior cruciate ligament. Am J Sports Med 20:351–355, 1992.

15. Ogata K, McCarthy JA, Dunlap J, and Manske PR: An experimental study of posterior sag of the tibia in posterior cruciate deficient knee. Trans Orthop Res Soc 13:279, 1988.

16. Sidles JA, Larson RV, Garbini JL, et al.: Ligament length relationships in the moving knee. J Orthop Res 6:593–610, 1988.

17. Trus P, Gotzen L, and Petermann J: Wiederherstellende Eingriffe am hinteren Kreuzband—Experimentelle Untersuchungen zur Isometrie. Teil I: Untersuchungen am Fadenmodell. Unfallchirurgie 95:349–353, 1992.

18. Grood ES, Hefzy MS, and Lindenfeld TN: Factors affecting the region of most isometric femoral attachments. I: The posterior cruciate ligament. Am J Sports Med 17:197–207, 1989.

19. Friederich NF, Müller W, and O'Brien WR: Klinische Anwendung biomechanischer und funktionell anatomischer Daten am Kniegelenk. Orthopade 21:41–50, 1992.

20. Presented as a Scientific Exhibit at the Annual Meeting of the American Academy of Orthopaedic Surgeons, New Orleans, Louisiana. February 8–13, 1990.

21. Covey DC, Sapega AA, Sherman GM, et al.: Anatomical and biomechanical factors governing the choice of bone tunnel location during posterior cruciate ligament reconstruction. Presented as a Scientific Exhibit at the Annual Meeting of the American Academy of Orthopaedic Surgeons, San Francisco, California, February 18–23, 1993.

22. Bomberg BC, Acker JH, Boyle J, et al.: The effect of posterior cruciate ligament loss and reconstruction on the knee. Am J Knee Surg 3:85–96, 1990.

23. Galloway M, Mehalik J, Grood E, et al.: Tibial displacement following reconstruction of the posterior cruciate ligament: the effect of knee position during graft fixation. Orthop Trans 17:225, 1993.

24. Butler DL, Noyes FR, and Grood ES: Ligamentous restraints to anterior-posterior drawer in the human knee: a biomechanical study. J Bone Joint Surg Am 62:259–270, 1980.

25. Gollenhon DL, Torzilli PA, and Warren RF: The role of the posterolateral and cruciate ligaments in the stability of the human knee: a biomechanical study. J Bone Joint Surg Am 69:233–242, 1987.

26. Nielsen S and Helmig P: Posterior instability of the knee joint: an experimental study. Arch Orthop Trauma Surg 105:121–125, 1986.

27. Nielsen S, Ovesen J, and Rasmussen O: The posterior cruciate ligament and rotatory knee instability: an experimental study. Arch Orthop Trauma Surg 104:53–56, 1985.

28. Grood ES, Stowers SF, and Noyes FR: Limits of movement in the human knee. Effect of sectioning the posterior cruciate ligament and posterolateral structures. J Bone Joint Surg Am 70:88–97, 1988.

29. Markolf KL, Wascher DC, and Finerman GAM: Direct in vitro measurement of forces in the cruciate ligaments. II: The effect of section of the posterolateral structures. J Bone Joint Surg Am 75:387–394, 1993.

30. Skyhar MJ, Warren RF, Ortiz GJ, et al.: The effects of sectioning of the posterior cruciate ligament and the posterolateral complex on the articular contact pressure within the knee. J Bone Joint Surg Am 75:694–699, 1993.

31. Clancy WG Jr, Shelbourne KD, Zoellner GB, et al.: Treatment of knee joint instability secondary to rupture of the posterior cruciate ligament: report of a new procedure. J Bone Joint Surg Am 65:310–322, 1983.

32. O'Donoghue DH: Surgical treatment of fresh injuries to the major ligaments of the knee. J Bone Joint Surg Am 32:721, 1950.

33. O'Donoghue DH: Analysis of end results of surgical treatment of major injuries to ligaments of the knee. J Bone Joint Surg 37:1, 1955.

34. Kennedy JC and Grainger RW: The posterior cruciate ligament. J Trauma 7:367–377, 1967.

35. Clendenin MB, DeLee JC, and Heckman JD: Interstitial tears of the posterior cruciate ligament of the knee. Orthopedics 3:764–772, 1980.

36. Rubenstein RA, Shelbourne KA, and McCarroll JR, et al.: The accuracy of the clinical examination in the setting of posterior cruciate ligament injuries. Am J Sports Med 4:550–557, 1994.

37. Abbot LC, Saunders JB, and Bost FC, et al.: Injuries to the ligaments of the knee joint. J Bone Joint Surg 26:503–521, 1944.

38. Lee HG: Avulsion fracture of the tibial attachment of the posterior cruciate ligament of the knee. J Bone Joint Surg 57:669–672, 1975.

39. Fowler PJ and Messieh SS: Isolated posterior cruciate ligament injuries in athletes. Am J Sports Med 15:553–557, 1987.

40. Shelbourne KD: Posterior cruciate ligament injuries. In Reider B (ed.): Sports Medicine: The School-Aged Athlete. Philadelphia, W.B. Saunders Co., 1991.

41. Parolie JM and Bergfeld JA: Long-term results of nonoperative treatment of isolated posterior cruciate ligament injuries in the athlete. Am J Sports Med 14:35–38, 1986.

42. Torg JS, Barton TM, Pavlov H, et al.: Natural history of the posterior cruciate ligament-deficient knee. Clin Orthop 246:208–216, 1989.

43. Cross MJ and Powell JF: Long-term followup of posterior cruciate ligament rupture: a study of 116 cases. Am J Sports Med 12:292, 1984.

44. Dandy DJ and Pusey RJ: The long-term results of unrepaired tears of the posterior cruciate ligament. J Bone Joint Surg Br 64:92, 1982.

45. Keller PM, Shelbourne KD, McCarroll JR, et al.: Nonoperatively treated isolated posterior cruciate ligament injuries. Am J Sports Med 21:132–136, 1993.

46. Dejour H, Walch G, Peyrot J, et al.: The natural history of rupture of the posterior cruciate ligament. Orthop Trans 11:146, 1987.

47. Dejour H, Walch G, Peyrot J, et al.: Histoire naturelle de la rupture du ligament croisé postérieur. Rev Chir Orthop 74:35–43, 1988.

48. Geissler WB and Whipple TL: Intra-articular abnormalities in association with posterior cruciate ligament injuries. Am J Sports Med 21:846, 1993.

49. Clancy WG: Repair and reconstruction of the posterior cruciate ligament. In Chapman MW (ed.): Operative Orthopedics, 2nd ed. Philadelphia, J.B. Lippincott Co., 1993, pp 2093–2107.

50. Hughston JC and Jacobson KE: Chronic posterolateral rotatory instability of the knee. J Bone Joint Surg Am 67:351–359, 1985.

51. DeLee JC, Riley MB, and Rockwood CA, Jr.: Acute posterolateral rotatory instability of the knee. Am J Sports Med 11:199–207, 1983.

52. Baker CL Jr, Norwood LA, and Hughston JC: Acute posterolateral rotatory instability of the knee. J Bone Joint Surg Am 65:614–618, 1983.

53. Wascher DC, Markolf KL, Shapiro MS, et al.: Direct in vitro measurement of forces in the cruciate ligaments. I: The effect of multiplane loading in the intact knee. J Bone Joint Surg Am 75:377–386, 1993.

54. Insall JN and Hood RW: Bone-block transfer of the medial head of the gastrocnemius for posterior cruciate insufficiency. J Bone Joint Surg 64:691–699, 1982.

55. Katchis SD, Bergfeld JA, Edelson R, et al.: Isolated sectioning of the posterior cruciate ligament, meniscofemoral ligaments, the superficial MCL and the posteromedial ligament complex: The influence on posterior tibial translation with neutral and internal tibial rotation. Presented at the AASM 21st Annual Meeting, Toronto Ontario, Canada, July 16–19, 1995.

56. Whipple TL and Ellis FD: Posterior cruciate ligament injuries. Clin Sports Med 10:515–527, 1991.

57. Shelbourne KD, Benedict F, McCarroll JR, et al.: Dynamic posterior shift test: an adjuvant in elevation of posterior tibial subluxation. Am J Sports Med 17:275–277, 1989.

58. Daniel DM, Stone ML, Barnett P, et al.: Use of the quadriceps active test to diagnose posterior cruciate-ligament disruption and measure posterior laxity of the knee. J Bone Joint Surg Am 70:386–391, 1988.

59. Fischer SP, Fox JM, Del Pizzo W, et al.: Accuracy of diagnoses from magnetic resonancy imaging of the knee. J Bone Joint Surg Am 73:2, 1991.
60. Trickey EL: Injuries to the posterior cruciate ligament: diagnosis and treatment of early injuries and reconstruction of late instability. Clin Orthop 147:76–81, 1980.
61. Meyers MH: Isolated avulsion of the tibial attachment of the posterior cruciate ligament of the knee. J Bone Joint Surg Am 57:669, 1975.
62. Lee HG: Avulsion fracture of the tibial attachments of the cruciate ligaments: treatment by operative reduction. J Bone Joint Surg 29:460, 1937.
63. Torisu T: Avulsion fracture of the tibial attachment of the posterior cruciate ligament: indications and results of delayed repair. Clin Orthop 143:107, 1979.
64. Hughston JC, Bowden JA, Andrews JR, et al.: Acute tears of the posterior cruciate ligament: results of operative treatment. J Bone Joint Surg Am 62:438–450, 1980.
65. Burks RT and Schaffer JJ: A simplified approach to the tibial attachment of the posterior cruciate ligament. Clin Orthop 254:216–219, 1990.
66. Loos WC, Fox JM, Blazina ME, et al.: Acute posterior cruciate ligament injuries. Am J Sports Med 9:86–92, 1981.
67. Suprock MD and Rogers VP: Posterior cruciate avulsion. Orthopedics 13:659–662, 1990.
68. Barrett GR and Savoie FH: Operative management of acute PCL injuries with associated pathology: long-term results. Orthopedics 14:687–692, 1991.
69. Clancy WG, Jr. and Smith L: Arthroscopic anterior and posterior cruciate ligament reconstruction technique. Ann Chir Gynaecol 80:141–148, 1991.
70. Cooper DE, Warren RF, and Warner JJP: The posterior cruciate ligament and posterolateral structures of the knee: anatomy, function, and patterns of injury. In Instructional Course Lectures, The American Academy of Orthopaedic Surgeons, Vol. 40, pp 249–270. Park Ridge, IL, The American Academy of Orthopaedic Surgeons, 1991.
71. Kannus P, Bergfeld J, and Jarrinen M, et al.: Injuries of the posterior cruciate ligament of the knee. Sports Med 12:110, 1991.
72. Kennedy JC: Complete dislocation of the knee joint. J Bone Joint Surg 45:989, 1963.
73. Meyers M and Harvey JP: Traumatic dislocation of the knee joint: a study of 18 cases. J Bone Joint Surg Am 53:16, 1971.
74. Sisto DJ and Warren RF: Complete knee dislocation. Clin Orthop 198:94–101, 1985.
75. Shelbourne KD, Porter DA, and Clingman JA, et al.: Low-velocity knee dislocation. Orthop Rev 20:995–1004, 1991.
76. Sclafani MA, Clancy WG, and Wilk K: Combined arthroscopic reconstruction of the anterior and posterior cruciate ligaments. Presented at the AASM 21st Annual Meeting, Toronto, Ontario, Canada, July 16–19, 1995.
77. Hughston JC and Jacobsen KE: Chronic posterolateral rotatory instability of the knee. J Bone Joint Surg Am 67:351, 1985.
78. Jakob RP, Hassler H, and Staeubli H-U: Observations on rotary instability of the lateral compartment of the knee. Acta Orthop Scand 191(suppl):1–32, 1981.
79. Marshall JL, Girgis FG, and Zelho R: The biceps femoris tendon and its functional significance. J Bone Joint Surg 54:1444, 1972.
80. Seebacker JR, Angles AE, Marshall JL, et al.: The structure of the posterolateral aspect of the knee. J Bone Joint Surg Am 64:53, 1982.

Complications of Knee Arthroscopy

Neal C. Small • *Mehrdad M. Malek*

OVERVIEW

During the last three decades, knee arthroscopy has become the most commonly performed orthopaedic procedure in the United States. Despite the fact that arthroscopic surgery was brought to the North American continent in 1964, efforts to document and analyze complications in arthroscopy came somewhat later. The Arthroscopy Association of North America (AANA) began tracking complications in knee arthroscopy in 1983.[1] A second retrospective survey of complications found by arthroscopic surgeons was published in 1986.[2] This second survey, in addition to data on knee arthroscopy, compiled data on complications in other joints. This survey compiled the results of 395,566 arthroscopic procedures. Among these were 375,069 knee arthroscopies. The complication rate for knee arthroscopy was found to be less than 1%. In 1988 a more comprehensive, multicenter study was completed.[3] This study was more controlled. Data were collected monthly, from August 1986 through February 1988, from arthroscopic surgeons practicing in the United States and Canada. The study tabulated 8,791 knee procedures (Table 30–1). There were 162 complications among these knee procedures, resulting in a complication rate of 1.85%.

The most common complication in each of these three large studies was hemarthrosis (Table 30–2). It was determined that hemarthrosis requiring aspiration or surgical evacuation occurs in approximately 1% of all arthroscopic procedures. The second most frequent complication was infection. There were 19 knee infections in the multicenter prospective study, resulting in an incidence of .02% (1 per 500 knee arthroscopies). Thromboembolic disease and anesthetic complications were also relatively common following arthroscopic surgery. The incidence was .01% (1 per 1,000 procedures) for both these complications. The 1988 study found that the incidence of instrument failure, neurologic complications, and significant vascular complications was reduced from that of the previous two studies.

The procedure with the highest complication rate was lateral retinacular release. The complication rate for this procedure was 7.2% (Table 30–3). All the complications occurring with lateral retinacular release were hemarthroses. The complication rate for meniscectomy was, surprisingly, higher than that for meniscal repair. Various types of anterior cruciate ligament (ACL) reconstructions were studied. The highest complication rate was found among the synthetic ACL reconstructions (3.7%). The complication rate for allograft ACL reconstructions (3.3%) was somewhat lower. Autogenous bone-tendon-bone ACL reconstructions had a lower complication rate (1.7%) than that for either synthetic or allograft ACL reconstructions.

COMPLICATIONS OF ARTHROSCOPIC MENISCAL SURGERY

The initial retrospective surveys, performed by the AANA in 1983 and 1986, showed complication rates for arthroscopic partial meniscectomy to be under 1%. The multicenter controlled study completed in 1988 indicated that the complication rate for arthroscopic partial meniscectomy was higher. The complication rate for partial medial meniscectomy was 1.8%; the complication rate for partial lateral meniscectomy was 1.5%; and the complication rate for arthroscopic medial meniscal repair was 1.5%. There were no complications reported in 60 lateral meniscal repairs. Overall, the complication rate for meniscectomy was found to be 1.7% as compared with 1.3% for meniscal repair.

The infection rate in meniscal repair was found to be consistent with the infection rate for arthroscopic procedures of all types. There has been a substantial decrease in the infection rate for meniscal repair since the technique that required sutures to be tied externally over buttons or bolsters was abandoned. Currently, most techniques advo-

Table 30–1 **Multicenter Registry of Complications in Arthroscopic Surgery, 1988**

Total Number of Procedures and Complications Reported Overall Rate 1.68% or 168 per 1,000

	Procedures	%	*Complications*	%
Knee	8,791	85.5	162	93.64
Shoulder	1,184	11.51	9	5.2
Ankle	146	1.42	1	0.58
Elbow	79	0.77	0	0
Wrist	68	0.66	0	0
Hip	14	0.14	1	0.58
Total	10,282	100	173	100

Table 30–2 **Types of Complications**

	173 Complications	
	Number of All Complications	*Percentage of All Complications*
Hemarthrosis/Hematoma	104	60.1
Infection	21	12.1
Thromboembolic disease	12	6.9
Anesthetic	11	6.4
Instrument failure	5	2.9
Reflex sympathetic dystrophy	4	2.3
Ligament injury	2	1.2
Fracture	1	0.6
Neurologic injury	1	0.6
Miscellaneous	12	6.9
Vascular injury	0	0
Total	173	100

Table 30–3 **Complication Rate for Specific Procedures***

	Percentage
Lateral retinacular release	7.17
ACL synthetic reconstruction	3.70
ACL allograft reconstruction	3.30
Shoulder staple capsulorrhaphy	3.30
Arthroscopic synovectomy	3.12
Abrasion arthroplasty	1.89
Outside-in meniscal repairs	1.89
Medial meniscectomy	1.78
Plica excision	1.71
ACL autogenous reconstruction	1.71
Shaving chondroplasty	1.60
Medial meniscal repair	1.52
Lateral meniscectomy	1.48
Anterior acromioplasty	1.10
Débridement of glenoid labrum tear	.50
Lateral meniscal repair	0.00

*In decreasing order of frequency.

cate sutures tied either intra-articularly or on the capsular surface deep to the subcutaneous tissues. The use of prophylactic antibiotics for meniscal repair may also have played a role in this reduced infection rate. There was found to be no statistically significant difference in the complication rate for inside-out versus outside-in meniscal repair. No complication data have been collected on use of the inside-in (endoscopic) technique of meniscal repair.

There was a reduction in the number of neurovascular complications when comparing the later data (1988) with data from the earlier surveys (1983 and 1986). The use of accessory posteromedial and posterolateral incisions, as advocated by Henning et al.,[4] Barber and Stone,[5] and others, contributed to the decreased incidence of complications in meniscal repair. The proximity of neurovascular structures on the medial and lateral sides allows easy injury if repair needles penetrate soft tissues beyond the capsular layer (Fig. 30–1). Attention to knee positioning is of utmost importance during medial and lateral meniscal repair. For medial meniscal repair, the saphenous nerve and vein are most likely to be injured when posterior horn tears are repaired with the knee in flexion. When the knee is closer to full extension, the saphenous nerve and vein are situated anteriorly to the needle exit sites (Fig. 30–2). For lateral meniscal repair the knee is best flexed 60–90 degrees to allow the popliteal neurovascular structures to displace posteriorly, away from the posterolateral capsule. In extension these structures are in close proximity to the capsule (Fig. 30–3).

Suturing through the ipsilateral portal while viewing through the contralateral portal places the more posteriorly situated neurovascular structures more at risk (Fig. 30–4). Ideally the tear should be viewed through the ipsilateral portal while sutures are inserted throughout the contralateral portal. A deflecting retractor is used to

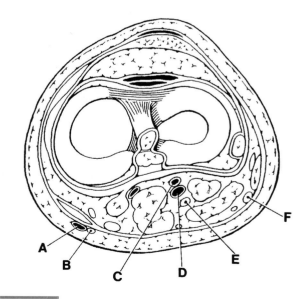

Figure 30–1 • Neurovascular structures at risk during arthroscopic meniscal repair. *A*, Saphenous vein. *B*, Saphenous nerve. *C*, Popliteal artery. *D*, Popliteal vein. *E*, Tibial nerve. *F*, Peroneal nerve.

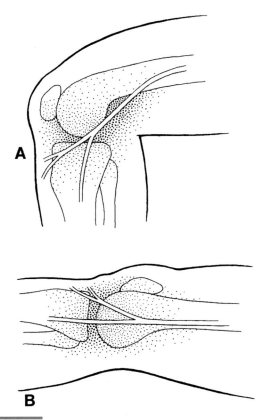

Figure 30–2 • The positioning of the knee for medial meniscal repair at (*A*) 90 degrees of flexion and (*B*) full extension. The saphenous nerve is more likely injured when posterior horn tears of the medial meniscus are repaired with the knee in flexion because of the posterior exit sites of the repair needles. With the repair performed with the knee close to full extension, the needles exit posteriorly to the saphenous nerve and vein.

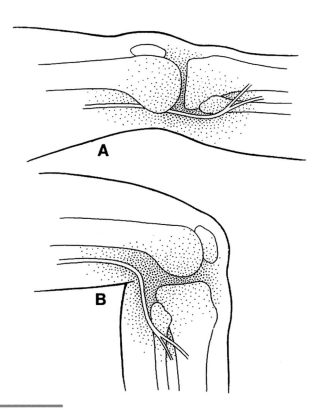

Figure 30–3 • The position of the knee for lateral meniscal repair at (*A*) full extension and (*B*) 90 degrees of flexion. The nerve is more removed from the posterolateral capsule and likely needle exit sites when the knee is flexed 60–90 degrees.

deflect the needle away from the neurovascular structures at risk (Fig. 30–5).

Considering the preceding information, technical considerations useful in avoiding complications during meniscal repair include using prophylactic antibiotics; appropriate knee positioning in flexion or extension for meniscal repair; suturing through the contralateral portal while viewing through the ipsilateral portal, when possible; using accessory posteromedial and posterolateral incisions for posterior horn tears; using deflecting retractors; and tying sutures intra-articularly or extracapsularly.

COMPLICATIONS OF ARTHROSCOPIC ACL PROCEDURES

Several complications that can occur in ACL reconstruction are identical to complications seen in other arthroscopic knee procedures. Complications that are not procedure-specific include hemarthrosis, hematoma, sepsis, skin necrosis, arthrofibrosis, deep venous thrombosis, recurrent effusions, sensory nerve injury, reflex sympathetic dystrophy, tourniquet paralysis, tissue irritation over metallic devices, and compartment syndrome.

The most common complication encountered in ACL reconstructions is arthrofibrosis, resulting in loss of knee flexion, extension, or both.[6] Many studies have focused on complications resulting from graft fixation techniques.[7]

When comparing types of ACL reconstructions, the highest complication rate was in synthetic ligament substitutes (see Table 30–3). The complication rate in 27 synthetic ACL reconstructions was 3.7%. In 151 allograft ACL reconstructions the complication rate was 3.3%. For 469 autogenous ACL reconstructions the complication rate was 1.7%. There were no complications noted in 45 ACL direct reattachments using the endoscopic staple (see Table 30–1).

It should be noted that these complication rates were compiled from a group of elite arthroscopic surgeons with extensive experience in arthroscopic surgery. It is the authors' belief that the incidence of complications among the general population of patients of orthopaedic surgeons performing arthroscopically assisted ACL surgery is higher than the numbers presented in this chapter indicate.

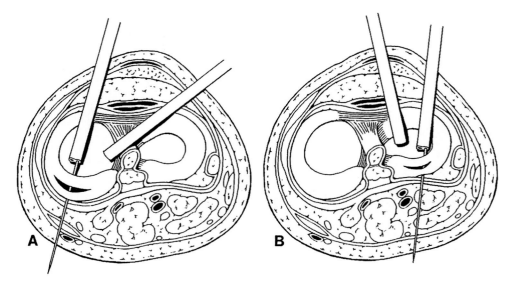

Figure 30–4 • *A,* When suturing through the ipsilateral portal, the saphenous nerve is at risk during medial meniscal repair. *B,* The popliteal neurovascular structures are at increased risk of injury when lateral meniscal posterior horn tears are repaired by suturing through the ipsilateral portal.

cific guidelines in sizing of the bone plug is necessary. Creation of any stress risers should be avoided.

Patellar Tendon Rupture

This complication occurs rarely and appears to be related to the width of the graft harvested from the tendon. Generally, one-third of the patellar tendon can be harvested without any risk of tendon rupture. The exact measurement for harvesting the tendon should be at the level of the tubercle attachment. At this location, the tendon is narrower than at the attachment to the patella.

Patellar Compression Syndrome

Tight closure of the patellar tendon defect may produce patellar compression, resulting in anterior knee pain syndrome. Studies are in progress to see whether leaving the defect open and closing just the paratenon may prevent this disabling complication.

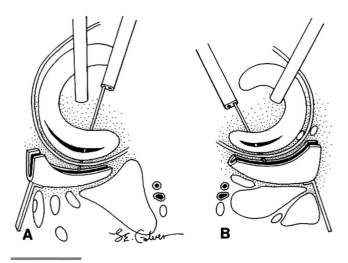

Figure 30–5 • Accessory posterior incisions are utilized in conjunction with deflecting retractors. Suturing is performed through the contralateral portal. The neurovascular structures are less likely to be injured during medial meniscal repair (*A*) or lateral meniscal repair (*B*) when these techniques are employed.

Patellofemoral Chondrosis/Chondromalacia

These complications appear to be caused by injury to the patella and extensor mechanism at the time of graft harvesting. Meticulous attention to recommended guidelines should prevent this complication from occurring.

COMPLICATIONS OF GRAFT HARVESTING FOR AUTOLOGOUS BONE-TENDON-BONE ONE-THIRD PATELLAR TENDON

Patellar Fracture

Patellar fractures secondary to graft harvesting have been reported. The incidence is seemingly low, although the exact incidence has not been tabulated. This complication can be avoided by following sound surgical principles in obtaining the bone plugs from the patella. Following spe-

Infrapatellar Contracture Syndrome

Paulos et al.[8] reported this complication following ACL reconstruction. Several causes of this complication have been postulated. These include quadriceps shut-down, the presence of bony and cartilaginous particles in the joint or the fat pad, and postoperative hemarthrosis.

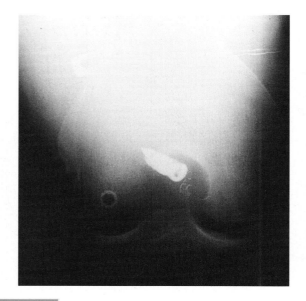

Figure 30–6 • Retracted LCR staple in semitendinous reconstruction (stapling).

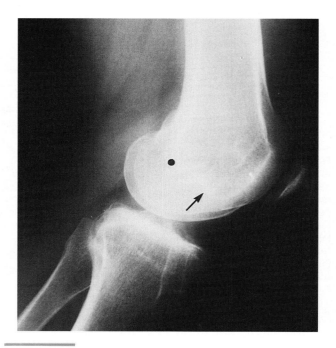

Figure 30–7 • Anterior placement of the femoral tunnel. Correct location (*bullet*). Incorrect location (*arrow*).

COMPLICATIONS OF OTHER TYPES OF ACL RECONSTRUCTION

Hamstring Tendon Grafts

There may be injury to the sartorius nerve or its branches as well as damage to the hamstring tendons themselves during harvesting. Fixation problems may occur (Fig. 30–6).

Iliotibial Band Grafts

In the case of harvesting the iliotibial band, there may be muscle herniation if the defect is not closed. If the iliotibial defect is closed too tightly, patellar compression syndrome may result.

COMPLICATIONS OF GRAFT POSITIONING

Placement of bony tunnels in such a fashion as to achieve isometricity is a critical step in ACL reconstruction. Tunnels placed too far anteriorly or posteriorly may lead to impingement and loss of motion in extension or flexion, respectively (Fig. 30–7). Placing the tibial tunnel too close to the articular surface results in loss of isometricity (Fig. 30–8). Tibial or femoral fracture may occur as a result of inappropriate tunnel placement.[9]

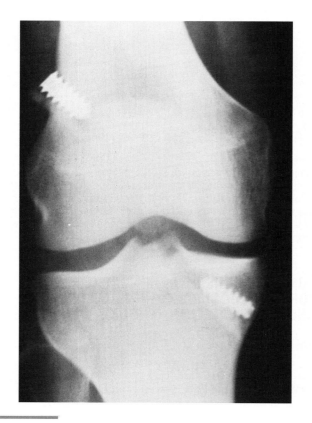

Figure 30–8 • Inappropriate placement of interference screws.

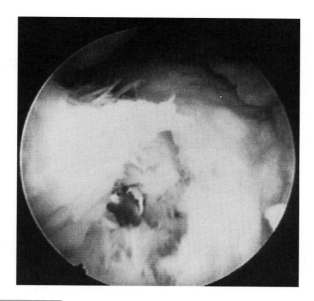

Figure 30–9 • Penetration of the interference screw in the joint. Arthroscopic view.

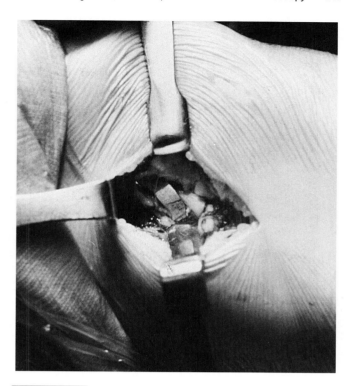

Figure 30–11 • Broken staple on the lateral aspect of the femur.

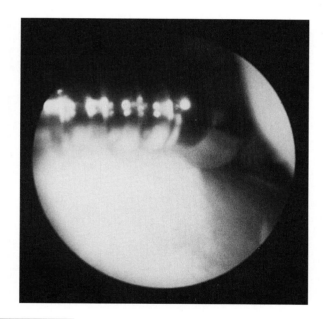

Figure 30–10 • Hardware loose in the joint. Retracted from the femoral tunnel.

COMPLICATIONS FROM THE USE OF HARDWARE

Placement of hardware in an incorrect position may lead to joint penetration and articular cartilage destruction inside the joint (Figs. 30–9 and 30–10). Other complications related to hardware use include staple pullout, loosening, and breakage (Fig. 30–11). Screw back-up and loosening can occur with interference screws and with suture-over-post fixation (Fig. 30–12).

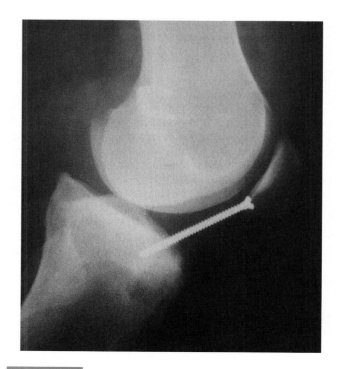

Figure 30–12 • Retraction of hardware in iliotibial band transfer for anterior cruciate ligament insufficiency.

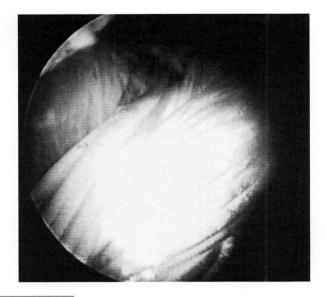

Figure 30–13 • Arthroscopic view of a normal Gore-Tex ligament.

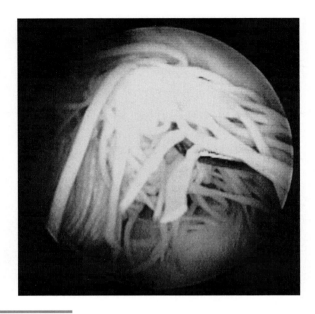

Figure 30–14 • Arthroscopic view of ruptured Gore-Tex fibers.

COMPLICATIONS OF ACL SUBSTITUTES

Synthetics

Synthetic materials are predisposed to complications such as synovitis, abrasions, breakage, and fractures (Figs. 30–13 and 30–14). In Small's report,[3] synthetic ACL reconstruction showed the highest complication rate (3.7%) when compared with autologous ACL reconstruction and allograft ACL reconstruction.

Allograft

Complications of allograft ACL reconstructions include graft nonviability, graft rejection, and graft disruption. A tibial bubble may occur as a result of ethylene oxide graft preservation (Fig. 30–15). Viral transmission can occur, although only one such incident has been documented. This incident occurred before 1985. An unprepared graft was used. Freeze-dried and irradiated allograft has significantly less potential for viral transmission. Tunnel widening and radiographic lucency are, occasionally, troublesome findings after allograft ACL reconstruction (Figs. 30–16 and 30–17). The exact significance of these findings is not known. Theories postulated include graft rejection and low-grade infection.

General Complications

For surgeons who have not yet developed the necessary psychomotor skills, there may be a higher complication rate with arthroscopically-assisted ACL surgery than with

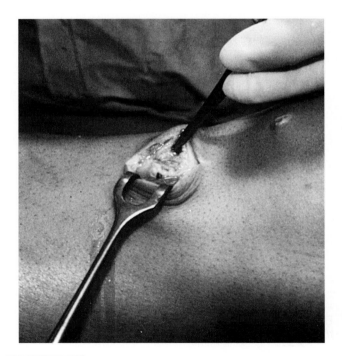

Figure 30–15 • Synovitis/granuloma formation on tibial tunnel entrance in an allograft sterilized with ethylene oxide.

conventional open reconstruction (Fig. 30–18). There should be fewer complications and less morbidity with arthroscopically assisted ACL reconstructions once the necessary psychomotor skills have been developed.

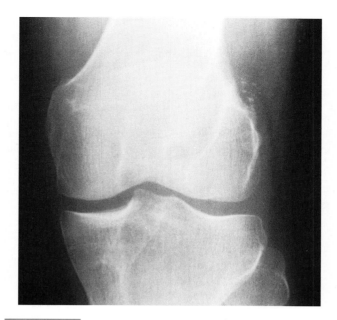

Figure 30–16 • Ballooning of anterior cruciate ligament tunnels with allograft—5 years postoperative.

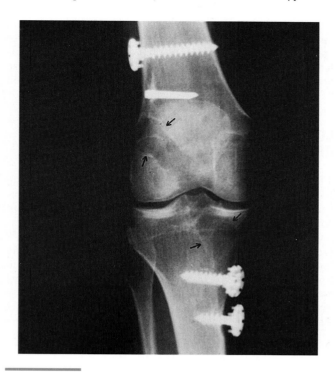

Figure 30–17 • Large cystic changes after anterior cruciate ligament allograft—8 months postoperative.

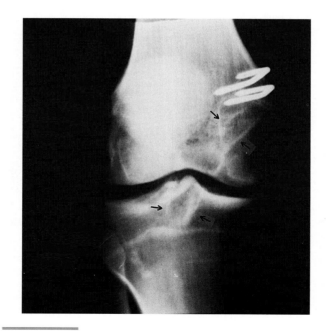

Figure 30–18 • Placement of the anterior cruciate ligament graft (*arrows*) in the wrong condyle (medial).

Adherence to the following principles should reduce the risk of complications in arthroscopically assisted ACL surgery:

1. Implementing careful patient selection, preoperative evaluation, and planning.
2. Following the fundamental surgical principles applicable to arthroscopic surgery.
3. Having a thorough knowledge of gross and arthroscopic anatomy of the knee.
4. Having a meticulous and systematic surgical approach.
5. Handling soft tissue carefully.
6. Using proper, inspected instruments and equipment.
7. Implementing supervised postoperative rehabilitation.

COMPLICATIONS OF ARTHROSCOPICALLY ASSISTED POSTERIOR CRUCIATE LIGAMENT RECONSTRUCTION

This procedure is not yet popular. It is less commonly done than arthroscopic ACL reconstruction, and no specific information is available in reference to its complication rate. Because of the complex anatomy of the popliteal area and posterior cruciate ligament, the structures at risk include the ACL, the articular cartilage, the popliteal artery, and the tibial nerve. A posteromedial accessory incision is recommended to palpate the site for the tibial pin penetration and drilling so that the popliteal structures are protected. Other complications that occur in arthroscopically assisted posterior cruciate ligament surgery are not different from those seen in arthroscopically assisted ACL surgery.

COMPLICATIONS OF LATERAL RETINACULAR RELEASE PROCEDURES

The procedure with the highest complication rate among arthroscopic procedures (7.2%) is arthroscopic lateral retinacular release (see Table 30–3). Several different types of complications have been identified. Among the more disabling complications is medial subluxation of the patella.[10] Hemarthrosis, however, has been found to be, by far, the most common complication.[11] Several factors have been found to correlate directly with the incidence of hemarthrosis. The use of a tourniquet is associated with a higher incidence of hemarthrosis. The hemarthrosis rate when a tourniquet was used was found to be 9.2%; when a tourniquet was not used, the hemarthrosis rate was 3.3%.

This difference is statistically significant (p = .037). Coupens and Yates[12] also found a higher complication rate when a tourniquet was used. The subcutaneous, arthroscopically controlled lateral retinacular release was found to have a higher complication rate than the lateral retinacular release performed as a purely endoscopic technique (10.2% versus 4.5%). The difference was statistically significant (p = .0057). The use of an electrocautery did not appear to lower the incidence of complications. The complication rate when an electrocautery was used was 8.6%. When an electrocautery was not used, the complication rate was 6.3%. The difference was not statistically significant (p = .05). There was found to be a significant correlation with the use of a postoperative suction drain for 24 hours or more. The complication rate when a postoperative suction drain was used for 24 hours or more was 13.4%. When a suction drain was used for less than 24

hours or not at all, the complication rate was 3.4%. This was found to be the most statistically significant factor when studying potential reasons for the high incidence of hemarthrosis following lateral retinacular release (p = >.001). A possible cause is the loss of the tamponade effect when a suction drain is used.

Suggestions, therefore, for minimizing complications in lateral retinacular release procedures include not using a tourniquet, performing a purely endoscopic procedure, and using a postoperative suction drain for less than 24 hours or not at all.

References

1. DeLee J: Complications of arthroscopy and arthroscopic surgery: result of a national survey. Arthroscopy 1:214–220, 1985.
2. Small NC: Complications in arthroscopy: the knee and other joints. Arthroscopy 4:253–258, 1986.
3. Small NC: Complications in arthroscopic surgery performed by experienced arthroscopists. Arthroscopy 3:215–221, 1988.
4. Henning CE, Clark JR, Lynch MA, et al. Arthroscopic meniscus repair with a posterior incision. Instr Course Lect 37:209–221, 1988.
5. Barber FA and Stone RG: Meniscal repair: an arthroscopic technique. J Bone Joint Surg Br 67:39–41, 1985.
6. Harner CD, Fu FW, Fu FH, et al.: Recognition and management of the stiff knee following arthroscopic anterior cruciate ligament reconstruction. Presented at the Annual Meeting of the American Academy of Orthopaedic Surgeons, Anaheim, Calif., 1991.
7. Malek MM: Complications of ACL surgery. Presented at the Summer Institute of the American Academy of Orthopaedic Surgeons, San Diego, Calif., 1988.
8. Paulos LE, Rosenberg TD, Drawbert J, et al.: Infrapatellar contracture syndrome. Am J Sports Med 15:331–341, 1987.
9. Berg EE: Lateral femoral condyle fracture after endoscopic anterior cruciate ligament reconstruction. Arthroscopy 10:693–695, 1994.
10. Hughston JC and Deese M: Medial subluxation of the patella as a complication of lateral retinacular release. Am J Sports Med 11:253–257, 1983.
11. Small NC: An analysis of complications in lateral retinacular release procedures. Arthroscopy 4:282–286, 1989.
12. Coupens SD and Yates CK: The effect of tourniquet use and Hemovac drainage of postoperative hemarthrosis. Arthroscopy 1:214–220, 1991.

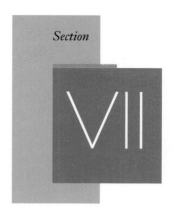

VII

The Ankle

Diagnostic Arthroscopy of the Ankle

James W. Stone • *James F. Guhl*

Burman performed the first reported attempts at diagnostic ankle arthroscopy on cadaveric specimens in 1931.[1] Using relatively primitive optics and large-diameter arthroscopes, he concluded that clinical applications for ankle arthroscopy were limited. The first significant technical advance that made ankle arthroscopy a practical surgical procedure was the development of high-quality fiberoptic arthroscopes of approximately 4–5 mm diameter. However, these arthroscopes were difficult to use in the ankle because of the tight ligament restraints and highly congruous curved articular surfaces. The development of mechanisms for joint distraction was the second significant technical advance that allowed improved arthroscopic inspection of the joint and the ability to perform surgical procedures arthroscopically. The third technical advance was the development of high-resolution, small-diameter, wide-angle arthroscopes of approximately 2.7 mm and smaller. These arthroscopes afford excellent visualization with decreased risk of iatrogenic articular cartilage damage. The fourth and most recent advance has been the development of noninvasive techniques for joint distraction. This technique utilizes sterile straps placed behind the heel and over the midfoot. Traction is applied to the strap, and sufficient joint opening is achieved to allow most arthroscopic procedures to be performed and decrease the risks inherent in the use of invasive joint distraction. This chapter discusses the indications and set-up for ankle arthroscopy and the technique for diagnostic ankle arthroscopy.

INDICATIONS FOR ANKLE ARTHROSCOPY

Historically, the presence of unexplained pain, swelling, instability, or mechanical symptoms such as locking or giving way has been the primary indication for ankle arthroscopy. As experience with the technique has increased and as the ability to diagnose various conditions using preoperative studies such as radiographs, bone scan, computed tomography, and magnetic resonance imaging

has improved, ankle arthroscopy without a specific preoperative diagnosis is less frequently performed. A diagnostic arthroscopy of the entire ankle joint is, however, the starting point for any arthroscopic ankle procedure. Several of the more common indications for ankle arthroscopy follow.

Soft-Tissue Indications

Soft-tissue impingement lesions are increasingly recognized as causes of mechanical joint symptoms, most commonly occurring after trauma to the joint. Wolin and colleagues[2] initially described the "meniscoid" lesion as a fibrocartilaginous mass in the lateral talomalleolar joint that generally formed after inversion ankle sprain. The lesion resembled the knee meniscus in consistency, and patients with persistent symptoms responded to surgical excision. The advent of ankle arthroscopy has kindled a renewed interest in these lesions and has helped to define their location, pathologic conditions, and causes.[3]

These lesions usually occur after inversion ankle sprain in patients who fail to respond to the usual conservative treatment. The patients continue to complain of anterolateral joint pain, clicking, and giving way, although they do not have objective evidence of joint laxity on stress radiographs. The most common arthroscopic finding is a mass of firm tissue arising from the area of the distal tibiofibular joint and protruding into the lateral talomalleolar joint (Fig. 31–1). The lesions can be removed by using mechanical instruments such as basket forceps, and the tibiofibular joint can be further cleaned by using a small curet.

Alternatively, the holmium:YAG laser removes these lesions efficiently, ablating the soft tissue while simultaneously achieving hemostasis.

Other types of soft-tissue indications for ankle arthroscopy include scar tissue bands or more generalized soft tissue adhesions or arthrofibrosis, which can cause severe limitation of joint motion after trauma. Adhesions

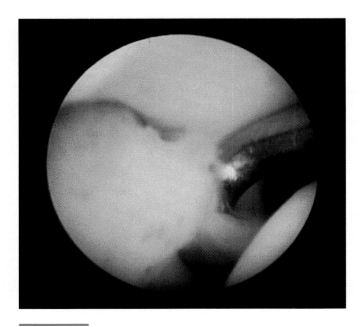

Figure 31–1 • Arthroscopic view of right ankle with arthroscope in the anterolateral portal looking laterally (tibia above, talus in foreground, and fibula left). A mass of synovium is noted arising from the distal tibiofibular joint and is palpated with a probe.

that cause mechanical symptoms such as clicking and locking are easily removed arthroscopically. Joints with dense arthrofibrosis can be quite challenging to débride arthroscopically. The most difficult challenge may be the achievement of initial visualization, which must be done carefully by using a small joint shaver to remove fibrotic material in the anterior joint compartment, exercising care not to injure normal articular cartilage. Again, the holmium:YAG laser may assist in removing dense scar tissue in this type of joint.

There are several types of specific synovitis that can affect the ankle joint and that may be amenable to arthroscopic treatment. Rheumatoid arthritis is usually treated successfully with medications. However, when medical management fails to relieve the joint inflammation and synovitis, a surgical synovectomy may provide symptomatic relief for these patients. This procedure can be performed arthroscopically by using a combination of mechanical instruments, shavers, and the holmium:YAG laser. The laser is a great advantage in this instance because the rheumatoid synovium is ablated and hemostatis is achieved simultaneously.

Pigmented villonodular synovitis can occur either as a generalized disorder of the ankle joint or as a localized form. The localized form may cause mechanical symptoms similar to those seen with loose bodies. Arthroscopic excision is appropriate in cases of localized lesions, and synovectomy can be performed in the generalized cases.

Synovial chondromatosis with multiple intra-articular cartilaginous or osteocartilaginous loose bodies is an excellent indication for ankle arthroscopy. The loose bodies cause pain and mechanical symptoms such as locking. They can also be responsible for significant articular carti-

lage damage. The loose bodies can be removed arthroscopically, but the procedure is a demanding one in which a diligent search for all loose bodies must be made, and the surgeon must be comfortable using the usual anterior operating portals in addition to accessory anterior and posterior portals. Small loose bodies can hide deep in the medial and lateral gutters or in the posterior joint compartment. If small cartilaginous buds are noted in the synovium, then a synovectomy can be performed.

Ankle arthroscopy is rarely indicated for crystalline synovitis such as gout or pseudogout.

Chondral and Osteochondral Lesions

Osteophytes

Osteophytes are commonly seen in the ankle, especially arising from the anterior tibia, and are usually associated with some amount of post-traumatic or arthritic joint degeneration. Anterior tibial osteophytes may coexist with osteophytes of the talar neck. They can cause symptoms, especially as the ankle is dorsiflexed and they come into contact with each other. Symptoms usually include anterior joint pain and limitation of dorsiflexion. Plain radiographs document the size of the lesion and assist the surgeon in planning the extent of resection. A bone scan demonstrates increased uptake in the area of the osteophytes in symptomatic patients. Anterior tibial osteophytes are easily approached arthroscopically and can be resected by using an osteotome, pituitary rongeur, or bur (Fig. 31–2). An intraoperative radiograph can be obtained to document adequate surgical resection of the osteophyte. The results of osteophyte excision are best when there is minimal generalized articular cartilage damage to the remainder of the joint.

The authors have seen several patients with "post-fracture" osteophytes on the distal fibula. These types of osteophytes occur when the distal fibula fracture heals with a degree of shortening and rotation so that a spike of bone projects from the proximal fragment anteriorly. When such a bony protrusion causes local symptoms, it can be removed arthroscopically.

Loose Bodies

Loose bodies in the ankle joint can arise from several sources, including osteochondritis dissecans, synovial chondromatosis, osteophytes, and acute chondral or osteochondral fractures. They can cause mechanical symptoms that include catching, locking, and swelling. Chondral loose bodies cannot be seen on routine radiographs, but computed arthrotomography (arthrogram/computed tomography scan) allows visualization of such lesions. Plain radiographs alone can be misleading. A lesion that appears to be an osseous loose body may actually be extra-articular or intracapsular and would not be amenable to arthroscopic excision. The procedure for arthroscopic removal of loose bodies is the same as for synovial chondromatosis. In addition to removing the loose bodies, a search for their

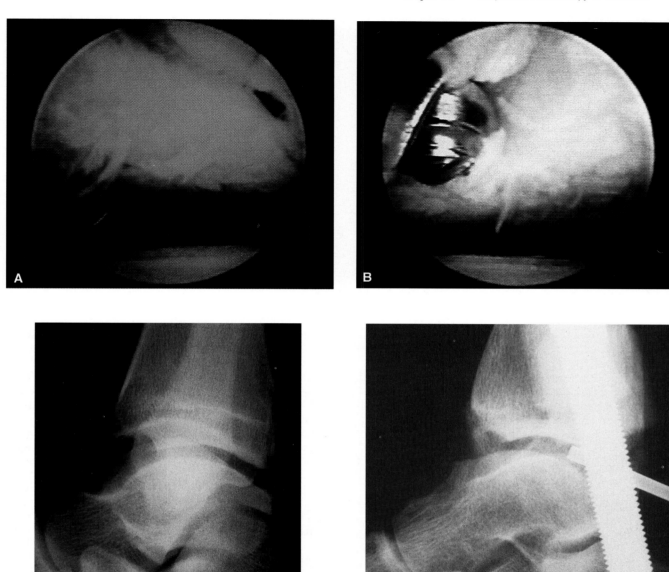

Figure 31–2 • *A,* Arthroscopic view of anterior tibial osteophyte (talus below, osteophyte above). *B,* Anterior tibial osteophyte being resected using a round bur. *C,* Preoperative lateral radiograph showing anterior tibial osteophyte. *D,* Postoperative lateral radiograph showing adequate surgical resection.

source must be performed so that more loose bodies can be prevented from forming.

Osteochondral Talar Dome Lesions

Osteochondral lesions of the talar dome, the general term for lesions including osteochondritis dissecans, can result in fragment separation and loose body formation. The goal of treatment of intact lesions is to prevent fragment separation and articular cartilage loss. Evaluation and treatment of these lesions are performed arthroscopically by drilling of the lesion, internal fixation, bone grafting,

or fragment excision.[4] These procedures are covered in Chapter 32.

Degenerative Joint Disease

The role of arthroscopy in degenerative joint disease is controversial. Patients are initially treated nonoperatively with measures such as nonsteroidal anti-inflammatory drugs, a cane, weight reduction, and judicious use of intra-articular corticosteroids. Arthroscopic débridement can be performed when symptoms persist despite aggressive non-operative management. Osteophytes are removed along with loose, flaking articular cartilage fragments and loose bodies. If significant full-thickness articular cartilage loss has occurred, then arthroscopic débridement can provide only limited and temporary relief. In this circumstance, arthrodesis may be the only alternative.

Arthroscopic ankle arthrodesis using crossed transmalleolar screw fixation has been performed with excellent results in patients who have severe arthritis but little or no deformity. The procedure has a high union rate and avoids many of the complications associated with open arthrodesis techniques.[5]

Ankle Instability

There are two techniques for arthroscopic treatment of lateral ligament laxity resulting in joint instability. The first technique utilizes a staple introduced laterally into the ligament complex, and the second technique utilizes suture anchors placed into the area of the insertion of the anterior talofibular ligament on the talus.

Infection

A septic ankle joint can be irrigated and débrided by using arthroscopic techniques, and drains may also be inserted. This technique may avoid some of the morbidity associated with open approaches to joint drainage.

INSTRUMENTATION FOR ANKLE ARTHROSCOPY

Arthroscopes

The authors routinely use the small-diameter arthroscopes for ankle arthroscopy. The 2.7 mm arthroscope is small enough to be easily maneuvered within the joint but strong and rigid enough to resist bending. It is beneficial to have both 30 degree and 70 degree angle-of-view arthroscopes available. The single-unit arthroscope/camera combination provides the smallest lever arm and most compact unit. An interchangeable cannula system allows switching of portals without having to reinsert the camera through the skin, thus decreasing soft-tissue trauma and potential injury to superficial nerves.

Fluid Inflow

Although an arthroscopic fluid pump may be utilized for inflow, the authors generally use gravity inflow through a dedicated inflow cannula placed posterolaterally. The fluid pump has the advantage of consistent inflow, but if pressure monitoring is not accurate, fluid can extravasate quickly into the soft tissues. Gravity inflow through a dedicated cannula provides excellent inflow. When the inflow cannula is placed posterolaterally, the arthroscope and instruments are manipulated by using the two anterior portals. The posterior inflow tends to force loose bodies toward the arthroscope anteriorly, decreasing the chance

for such loose bodies to be directed to the less accessible posterior joint recess. When posterior viewing is necessary, the arthroscope can be switched to the posterolateral position by using the interchangeable cannula system, with the inflow through the anterior portal.

Mechanical Instruments and Shavers

Standard arthroscopic instruments including basket forceps and an assortment of loose body forceps should be available in sizes smaller than those used for knee and shoulder arthroscopy. A selection of small cervical curets and straight and angled ring curets is useful for débridement of osteochondral lesions. Small joint motorized instruments such as synovial resectors and abraders are frequently required.

Laser

The holmium:YAG laser can be useful in a tightly constrained joint such as the ankle. This laser utilizes a small-diameter fiberoptic cable enclosed in a strong metal handpiece to transmit the laser energy. The handpieces are available in 0 degree, 15 degree, 30 degree, and side firing probes that can be maneuvered about the joint more easily than standard instruments of wider diameter. The laser is particularly useful for ablating abnormal soft tissues such as synovitis or synovial impingement lesions, and it provides the significant benefit of simultaneous hemostasis. Chondral lesions are also easily débrided and contoured with the laser.

OPTIONS FOR JOINT DISTRACTION IN ANKLE ARTHROSCOPY

Invasive Joint Distraction

The method for invasive ankle joint distraction for arthroscopic surgery was pioneered by Guhl.[6] He developed an external outrigger that applied distraction force via pins placed proximally and distally to the ankle joint. In the outrigger's most common application, 3/16 inch threaded Steinmann pins are placed into the tibia and calcaneus from the lateral side. Attention to detail is important when inserting these pins to avoid potential complications, the most important of which is nerve damage. The tibial pin is placed approximately 5 cm proximal to the ankle mortise. The skin alone is incised with a scalpel, and then blunt dissection is performed with a hemostat, pushing the anterior tibial musculature posteriorly so that the hemostat touches the lateral border of the tibia. The fibula is not used for invasive distraction because the risk of postoperative fracture is significant. The Steinmann pin is then inserted unicortically by using a tissue-protecting cannula approximately 1 cm posterior to the anterior tibial crest (Fig. 31–3). Penetration of the anterior tibial crest gives poor fixation and increases risk of fracture. The calcaneal pin is inserted posteriorly to the peroneal tendons laterally. The pin is angulated approximately 20 degrees distally and

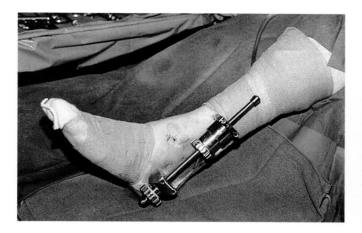

Figure 31–3 • Intraoperative photograph showing invasive ankle distractor in position.

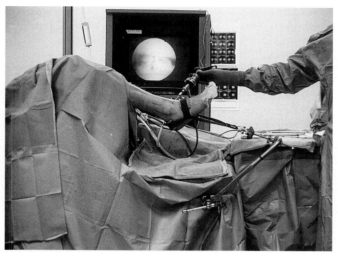

Figure 31–4 • The authors' current recommendation for non-invasive distraction. The hip and knee are supported in a flexed position by using a well-padded leg holder. The video equipment is placed on the side opposite the extremity operated on.

can be placed bicortically. The external outrigger is then applied, and an amount of distraction force sufficient to create an adequate joint opening is applied.

An alternative method is to place the pins from the medial aspect of the ankle joint into the tibia and the talus. The advantage of this method is that the distraction is applied across only the ankle joint rather than across the ankle and subtalar joints. A disadvantage is that medial placement can block medial transmalleolar approaches to the talar dome. The authors recommend that the talar pin be placed using fluoroscopic guidance to ensure that the pin enters the center of the talar neck rather than the proximal or distal articular surfaces.

Noninvasive Distraction

The occurrence of a small but significant number of complications related to the use of invasive distraction stimulated the development of noninvasive methods of joint distraction. The first reported method utilized a loop of Kerlix gauze wrapped around the heel and midfoot. The loop was then placed beneath the foot of the operating surgeon, and variable distraction force could be applied by pressing on the loop. This method, although effective, is somewhat clumsy and places additional, unnecessary demands on the operating surgeon.

New methods of joint distraction have been developed simultaneously but independently by Guhl, Ewing, and Glick. In Glick's technique, the patient is placed supine on the operating table, and the foot of the table is lowered so that the patient's leg hangs dependently. After the ankle is prepared and draped, a sterile strap is applied to the foot, and weights are attached to the strap through a hole in the drape. Ewing devised a method of noninvasive distraction that utilizes a bar attached to the operating table and extending past the foot. After preparing and draping the ankle, the sterile strap is applied to the foot and then attached to the bar, which includes a gauge to measure distraction force. This method is effective, but draping in a sterile fashion is somewhat cumbersome.

Guhl devised a method that uses a similar strap but utilizes a completely sterile system that can be converted to invasive distraction if necessary. The patient is positioned supine on the operating table, and the hip and knee are supported in a flexed position by a well-padded knee support (Fig. 31–4). The entire leg can be prepared into the field, and sterile drapes are placed. A sterile clamp is then attached to the operating table siderail, and a sterile bar is inserted into the clamp. The straps are then placed on the foot, and the strap is attached to the bar by using the distractor outrigger (Fig. 31–5). Gross distraction

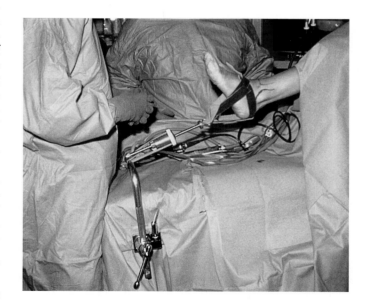

Figure 31–5 • Close-up view showing noninvasive straps applied to the foot and ankle and connected to a sterile bar.

adjustments are made by positioning the sterile bar, and fine adjustments are made by using the knurled knob on the distractor. This position places the foot and ankle in a comfortable plantigrade position that allows adequate exposure for placement of both anterior and posterior portals. The authors have had no complications related to the use of the noninvasive distractor apparatus. The combination of effective noninvasive distraction with high resolution small-diameter arthroscopes has made the use of invasive joint distraction a rare event.

Diagnostic Ankle Arthroscopy

After careful positioning of the patient, skin preparation, and sterile draping, the noninvasive ankle distractor is applied to the foot. Anatomic landmarks are marked on the skin by using a sterile marker. The border of the medial malleolus and anterior tibial plafond are marked, followed by marking of the fibular margins. The positions of the anterior tibial tendon and the peroneus tertius are marked anteriorly, along with the lateral border of the Achilles tendon. These tendons provide the anatomic landmarks for creation of the arthroscopic portals. An attempt should be made to visualize the subcutaneous course of the superficial peroneal nerve dorsal intermediate branch, which usually passes near the location of the anterolateral portal. The nerve can often be seen by inverting the foot and ankle and plantarflexing the lateral toes.

The appropriate portal position for the anteromedial portal is localized by using a hypodermic needle placed at the approximate level of the joint line adjacent to the medial border of the anterior tibial tendon. The surgeon should determine the proximal or distal position that allows the needle to pass most easily across the joint. A position too proximal causes the arthroscope and instruments to strike the talus, and a position too distal causes impingement on the tibia. To create the portal, the skin alone is incised, and then the subcutaneous tissues are bluntly dissected to the level of the capsule by using a fine hemostat. The portal is then created by using a blunt obturator. A sharp obturator can cause significant articular cartilage injury and is not necessary to penetrate the thin capsule of the ankle joint. After creating the anteromedial portal, the location for the posterolateral portal is determined by using a hypodermic needle placed adjacent to the lateral border of the peroneus tertius tendon. With the arthroscope in the anteromedial portal, transillumination of the anterolateral soft tissues can be used to confirm the location of the dorsal intermediate branch of the superficial peroneal nerve and any associated vessels so as to minimize the likelihood of iatrogenic neurovascular injury. In addition, the hypodermic needle can be seen to pass at an appropriate angle within the joint.

After the two anterior working portals are made, a posterolateral portal is created under direct visualization. The arthroscope is directed posteriorly so that the inferior slip is identified. A spinal needle is then introduced into the joint from a point adjacent to the lateral border of the Achilles tendon. This point is generally approximately 1–

2 cm distal to the anterior portals so that the cannula can accommodate the posterior curvature of the talus.

The authors place inflow through the posterolateral portal cannula. This dedicated portal allows excellent inflow and pressure. In addition, because flow is directed from a posterior to an anterior direction, loose bodies and other pieces of soft or hard tissue are directed anteriorly where they may be grasped with an instrument or removed with a shaver, rather than being directed into the posterior joint compartment where retrieval can be difficult. Another alternative to posterior inflow is the use of an arthroscopy fluid pump.

Diagnostic arthroscopy is initiated with the arthroscope in the anteromedial portal, the inflow placed posterolaterally and the probe placed anterolaterally. In general, it is easier to maneuver the arthroscope from anterior to posterior by using the anteromedial portal because of the presence of a slight indentation in the anteromedial tibia known as the notch of Harty (after the anatomist who described this consistent anatomic finding). The entire joint should be examined in a systematic manner so as not to miss any pathologic condition, starting anteromedially and then switching the arthroscope to the anterolateral portal and viewing posterolaterally. Depending on the pathologic condition in the joint, there may be a significant amount of synovitis obscuring visualization. The first step is to débride this hypertrophic synovium by using a synovial resector. Care must be taken to prevent iatrogenic articular cartilage injury or injury to the anterior neurovascular structures if initial joint visualization is difficult.

After obtaining initial visualization, the tip of the medial malleolus and deltoid ligament are inspected, and then the arthroscope is directed up the medial gutter to examine the medial talomalleolar joint (Fig. 31–6). The arthroscope is then brought over the convexity of the medial talar dome and gently passed from anterior to pos-

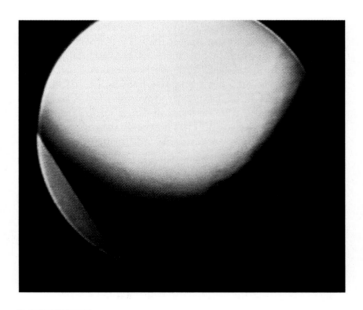

Figure 31–6 • Arthroscopic view of right ankle and tip of medial malleolus.

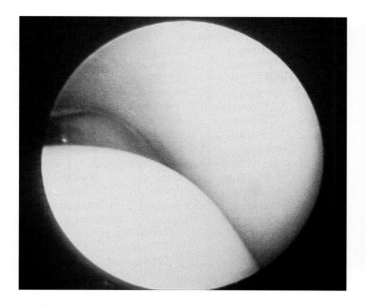

Figure 31–7 • Arthroscopic view of medial talar dome and tibial plafond.

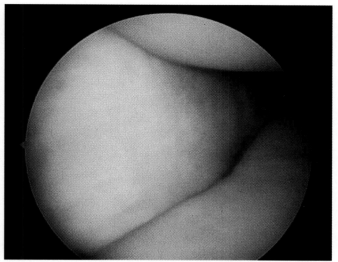

Figure 31–9 • Arthroscopic view of distal tibiofibular joint (tibia above right, talus below right, fibula left).

terior while simultaneously palpating the articular surfaces with a probe (Fig. 31–7). As the arthroscope is swept from medial to lateral, the inferior slip of the posterior tibiofibular ligament (transverse tibiofibular ligament) is visualized as a prominent structure (Fig. 31–8). Just superiorly, the inferior border of the main portion of the posterior tibiofibular ligament is seen. The distal tibiofibular joint is identified and inspected as the arthroscope is gently maneuvered from posterior to anterior. A variable quantity of synovium is present in this joint (Fig. 31–9).

Viewing with the arthroscope across the joint from medial to lateral, the inferior slip of the anterior tibiofibular ligament is noted to be a prominent, vertically oriented structure (Fig. 31–10). The lateral talomalleolar joint can usually be inspected from the medial portal with a 30 degree angled arthroscope, and then the arthroscope can be directed to the tip of the lateral malleolus and anterior talofibular ligament (Fig. 31–11). The arthroscope should then be brought anteriorly over the talar neck, and with the viewing angle directed proximally the anterior tibia is

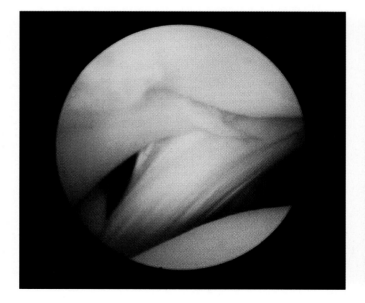

Figure 31–8 • Arthroscopic view of posterolateral structures (tibia above, talus below, transverse tibiofibular ligament [syndesmotic ligament] running obliquely).

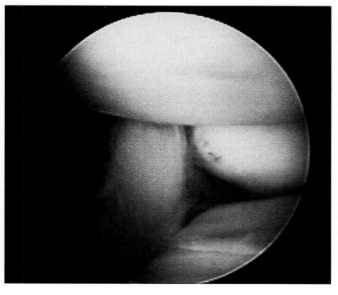

Figure 31–10 • Arthroscopic view of anterolateral structures (tibia above, talus below right, fibula central right, anterior tibiofibular ligament center left running vertically).

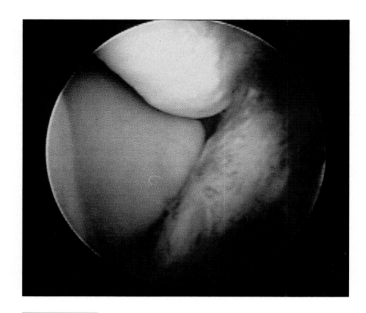

Figure 31–11 • Arthroscopic view of lateral gutter (fibula above, talus right, anterior talofibular ligament running obliquely left foreground).

inspected. This is a common location for osteophyte formation. Such an osteophyte may require débridement as the initial step in joint visualization when its size impairs arthroscope passage across the joint. The anterior talar neck is then inspected for osteophytes and loose bodies in the anterior recess.

After anteromedial inspection, the arthroscope is placed into the joint via the anterolateral portal, and the joint is inspected in reverse order. The tip of the fibula and the anterior talofibular ligament are inspected, and then the arthroscope is directed up the lateral gutter to view the lateral talomalleolar joint. The posterior talofibular ligament can sometimes be seen across this joint posteriorly.

The distal tibiofibular joint and then the dome of the talus and tibial plafond are inspected. Finally, the arthroscope is directed down the medial gutter to the tip of the medial malleolus and then over the anterior talar neck.

The authors believe that the complete ankle joint inspection should include posterolateral viewing. This can be accomplished easily by using an interchangeable cannula system or a switching stick to place the arthroscope into the portal previously used for inflow. This view gives an excellent perspective of the posterior talar dome and may allow the best visualization of a posteromedial osteochondral lesion. In addition, the deltoid ligament is inspected nicely from this approach.

The preceding technique describes a reproducible, step-by-step approach to diagnostic ankle arthroscopy. Even when the problem is known preoperatively, a thorough diagnostic joint inspection is mandatory before proceeding with the surgical portion of the procedure. By performing the diagnostic procedure in the same manner on every arthroscopy, the surgeon can be sure that pertinent pathologic processes will not be missed during ankle arthroscopy.

References

1. Burman MS: Arthroscopy or the direct visualization of joints: an experimental cadaver study. J Bone Joint Surg 13:660–695, 1931.
2. Wolin I, Glassman F, Sideman S, et al.: Internal derangement of the tibiofibular component of the ankle. Surg Gynecol Obstet 91:193–200, 1950.
3. Ferkel RD, Karzel RP, Del Pizzo W, et al.: Arthroscopic treatment of anterolateral impingement of the ankle. Am J Sports Med 19:440–446, 1991.
4. Stone JW and Guhl FJ: Ankle arthroscopy. In Pfeffer GB and Frey CC (eds.): Current Practice in Foot and Ankle Surgery, vol 1. New York, McGraw-Hill, 1993, pp 1–29.
5. Glick JM, Myerson MS, Morgan CD, et al: Arthroscopic ankle arthrodesis. Presented at the Ninth Annual Meeting of the Arthroscopy Association of North America, Orlando, Fla., April, 1990.
6. Guhl JF: New concepts (distraction) in ankle arthroscopy. Arthroscopy 4:160–167, 1988.

32 Operative Arthroscopy of the Ankle

Richard D. Ferkel • *Charles M. Ruland*

Arthroscopy of human cadaveric ankle joints was first reported by Burman in 1931.[1] Since its first description in human patients by Takagi[2] in 1939, ankle arthroscopy has become an important diagnostic and therapeutic procedure for the documentation and treatment of disorders of the ankle. Arthroscopic examination of the ankle joint allows direct visualization and probing of the intra-articular structures. Visualization of the ligament structures during intraoperative stress-testing maneuvers may determine laxity or instability. Numerous arthroscopic procedures of the ankle may be performed, including biopsy, débridement, synovectomy, loose body removal, chondroplasty, and arthrodesis. Many authors[3–18] have described their experience and techniques with ankle arthroscopy. These techniques have continued to progress via technological advances in video cameras, fiberoptic light sources, small-joint arthroscopes and instrumentation, and effective distraction of the ankle joint by invasive and noninvasive means. Studies with long-term follow-up have allowed a critical evaluation of the results of arthroscopic treatment of specific pathologic entities of the ankle joint.[19]

PATIENT SELECTION

Indications

There are numerous indications for ankle arthroscopy. However, surgical intervention should be reserved for those patients who have failed to respond to nonoperative methods of treatment. Diagnostic arthroscopy should be considered after a thorough history, physical examination, and appropriate diagnostic studies have failed to explain the pathologic process. Diagnostic indications for ankle arthroscopy include unexplained pain, swelling, stiffness, instability, hemarthrosis, locking, and abnormal snapping or popping. Operative indications for ankle arthroscopy include removal of loose bodies, excision of anterior tibiotalar spurs, débridement of meniscoid and other soft-tissue impingement lesions, evaluation and débridement

of osteochondral lesions of the talus, synovectomy for systemic inflammatory conditions such as rheumatoid arthritis and post-traumatic synovitis, evaluation of associated intra-articular problems and stabilization procedures for ankle instability, débridement of post-traumatic and degenerative arthritis, and ankle arthrodesis for patients with end-stage post-traumatic and degenerative arthritis with minimal deformity.[20] The use of ankle arthroscopy in the acute setting, such as evaluation of the articular injury in fractures of the ankle, has not been clearly defined.

Contraindications

Absolute contraindications for ankle arthroscopy include localized soft-tissue and systemic infection and severe degenerative joint disease. With severe degenerative joint disease, successful distraction of the joint is often unobtainable and range of motion is limited, resulting in inadequate visualization of the joint. Relative contraindications for ankle arthroscopy include moderate degenerative joint disease with restricted range of motion and reduced joint space, severe edema, and tenuous vascular status. A relative contraindication such as reflex sympathetic dystrophy must be considered individually for each patient.

Preoperative Evaluation

Proper selection of patients for operative ankle arthroscopy depends on meticulous preoperative assessment. Often, an accurate preoperative diagnosis facilitates an arthroscopic procedure. Patient evaluation includes a thorough history, physical examination, and radiologic evaluation.

A thorough history is essential. The nature of the patient's chief complaint—usually pain, swelling, stiffness, instability, snapping, popping, or locking—should be understood. The duration, severity, provocation, and timing of symptoms should be documented. Often, but not always, an accident or trauma may initiate an ankle problem. Therefore, the mechanism of injury and the exacerbating activities are documented. A general medical history should be obtained, with special care to reveal any symptoms suggestive of a systemic or rheumatologic disorder.

Physical examination of the joint should include inspection of localized areas or generalized swelling and ecchymosis. Palpation should be performed to pinpoint exact areas of tenderness. Range of motion should be tested, and any pain, locking, or abnormal crepitus, snapping, or popping should be recorded. The ankle joint should be tested for instability and compared with the normal side. Instability tests include the anterior drawer and the varus/valgus stress test. The subtalar joint should also be tested for instability. Often, local anesthetic agents can be injected into specific areas to aid in establishing a diagnosis.

Routine blood tests are obtained to check for systemic and rheumatologic conditions and infection. Aspiration of the ankle joint and analysis of joint fluid can be helpful in the differential diagnosis because inflammatory, noninflammatory, and septic processes can be distinguished by examination.

Routine radiographs (anteroposterior, lateral, and mortise views) should be obtained for all patients. Diagnostic capabilities have improved significantly with advances in computed tomography (CT) and magnetic resonance imaging (MRI). Three-phase bone scanning can also be helpful in differentiating soft tissue from bony involvement (such as osteomyelitis). Stress x-ray films of the ankle should be obtained if instability is suspected.

Conservative Treatment

Initial treatment for most disorders of the ankle depends on the problem. In general, nonoperative treatment may include rest, nonsteroidal anti-inflammatory drugs, corticosteroid injections, an orthosis or shoe modification, and physical therapy to maintain range of motion and strength. Immobilization with a brace, splint, or cast may be needed.

Patient Education

Preoperative preparation includes extensive discussions with the patient regarding the nature of the surgical procedure and the alternative modes of treatment. Office pamphlets, anatomic models, illustrations, and videotapes of the specific procedures can be used to inform the patient fully. The patient must be provided with realistic expectations about the possible results of the surgical procedures. Potential problems and complications of the surgery are also reviewed.

ARTHROSCOPIC SURGERY TECHNIQUE

Arthroscopic Equipment

Both the 4.0 mm and 2.7 mm arthroscopes with 30 degree and 70 degree obliquity can be used for ankle arthroscopy.

The 2.7 mm short video arthroscope is preferred for visualization throughout the ankle joint and particularly in the tighter spots in the medial and lateral gutters and the posterior aspect of the ankle. The shorter lever arm helps to prevent chondral injury and instrument breakage. In addition, the lightweight arthroscope is easier for the surgeon to handle with one hand. The 70 degree arthroscope is helpful for seeing over the medial and lateral domes of the talus to visualize the gutters and to evaluate certain osteochondral lesions of the talus. An interchangeable cannula system that allows the arthroscope to be switched from portal to portal without reinstrumentation may prevent nerve and wound damage. Small-joint arthroscopic instruments are preferred because they are easier to maneuver within the tight joint spaces. Instruments typically used include 3.5 mm, 2.9 mm, and 2.0 mm shavers; burs; 3.5 mm, 4.5 mm, and 7.0 mm ring curets; a 1.5 mm probe; 2.7 mm graspers and baskets; and small banana blades.

A high inflow and outflow system is critical and can often be accomplished with gravity drainage from the posterolateral portal. If the posterior portal is difficult to obtain or maintain, or where higher fluid pressure is desired, an arthroscopy pump can be used. A higher pressure and flow volume can assist with hemostasis and improve visualization. Extravasation of fluid in the foot and ankle must be monitored closely to prevent increased compartmental pressure.

Visualization of the ankle joint can improve significantly via an ankle distractor. Without the distractor, the central tibial plafond and talar dome, the posteroinferior tibiofibular ligament, and the transverse tibiofibular ligament are poorly seen. A noninvasive soft-tissue distraction set-up or an invasive mechanical distraction using tibial and calcaneal pins may be used. The decision to use noninvasive or invasive distraction is made at the time of surgery and depends on the tightness of the ankle joint and the location of the pathologic condition. Ferkel's technique for invasive distraction was described by Guhl[21] (Fig. 32–1). For noninvasive soft-tissue distraction, a device that grips around the posterior aspect of the heel and the dorsum of the foot is attached to a strain gauge (Fig. 32–2). The anterior neurovascular bundle may be compromised if excessive pressure is placed on the dorsum of the foot. Periodic relaxation of the device prevents complications. Presently, noninvasive distraction is used in almost all ankle arthroscopy cases.

Positioning

The patient is placed in a supine position. A tourniquet is placed around the upper thigh. The thigh is secured by an unsterile thigh holder and positioned with the hip flexed 45–50 degrees. The thigh holder is placed proximal to the popliteal fossa and is well padded to avoid injury to the sciatic nerve. The patient is then prepared and draped in a standard fashion. A sterile foot holder is then used to support the foot and ankle in the desired position. The foot holder is secured to the operating table with a sterile clamp that is placed over the drapes on the side of the table. Both the anterior and posterior portions of the ankle are accessible. Noninvasive distraction is usually attempted initially.

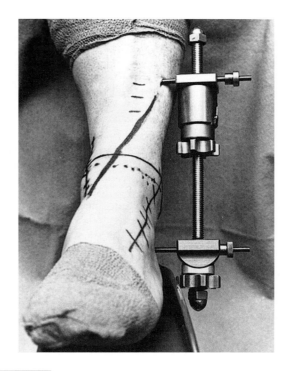

Figure 32–1 • The invasive distractor inserted with pins in the tibia and calcaneus on the lateral side. (From Ferkel RD and Fasulo GJ: Arthroscopic treatment of ankle injuries. Orthop Clin North Am 25:17–32, 1994.)

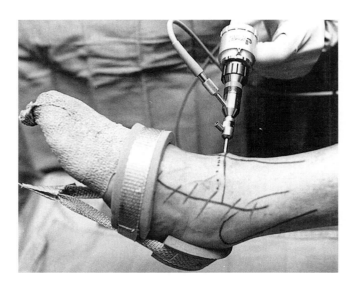

Figure 32–2 • Use of a noninvasive distraction strap. This strap can be attached to weights or to a distraction device that generates a constant force. (From Ferkel RD and Fasulo GJ: Arthroscopic treatment of ankle injuries. Orthop Clin North Am 25:17–32, 1994.)

If visualization is inadequate, pins can be inserted to use the invasive distractor.

Anatomic Landmarks

The dorsalis pedis artery, deep peroneal nerve, saphenous vein, tibialis anterior, peroneus tertius tendons, and superficial peroneal nerve and its branches should be identified and outlined with a marking pen over the surface of the ankle. Determining the location of the superficial peroneal nerve and its branches can be facilitated by holding the foot plantar flexed and inverted. The joint line is also identified and marked with dorsiflexion and plantar flexion of the ankle.

Arthroscopic Portals

The most common anterior portals are the anteromedial and anterolateral portals. An anterocentral portal has been described, but because of the risk to the dorsalis pedis artery and vein and to the deep branch of the peroneal nerve, the authors discourage use of this portal (Fig. 32–3).

The posterior portals are the posterolateral, trans-Achilles, and posteromedial portals. Because of the risk of serious injury to the Achilles tendon, the posterior tibial

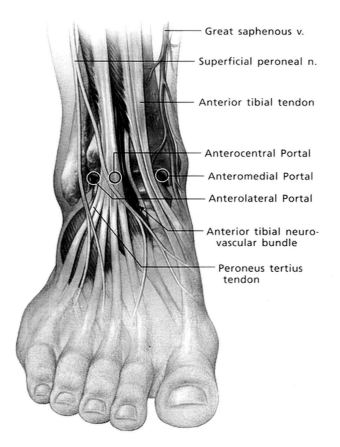

Figure 32–3 • Anterior portals. Use of the anterocentral portal is not recommended. (From Ferkel RD and Scranton PE: Current concepts review: arthroscopy of the ankle and foot. J Bone Joint Surg Am 75:1233–1242, 1993.)

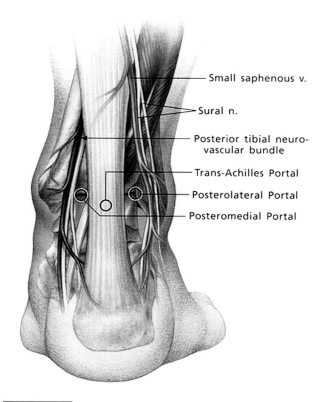

Small saphenous v.

Sural n.

Posterior tibial neuro-vascular bundle

Trans-Achilles Portal

Posterolateral Portal

Posteromedial Portal

Figure 32–4 • Posterior portals. The posterolateral portal is used most commonly; use of the posteromedial portal and the trans-Achilles portal is not recommended. (From Ferkel RD and Scranton PE: Current concepts review: arthroscopy of the ankle and foot. J Bone Joint Surg Am 75:1233–1242, 1993.)

artery and nerve, and the flexor tendons located medially, the posterolateral portal is regarded as the only safe portal (Fig. 32–4).

Establishment of Portals

Sterile Ringer lactate solution is infused into the ankle joint with an 18 gauge needle medial to the tibialis anterior tendon to establish the anteromedial portal (see Fig. 32–3). Backflow of fluid from the needle confirms entry into the joint. A No. 11 scalpel is then used to make a vertical skin incision while the tibialis anterior tendon is palpated. Blunt dissection using a mosquito clamp is performed through the subcutaneous tissue down to the capsule. A blunt trocar with an attached arthroscopic cannula is then placed carefully into the ankle joint. Additional Ringer lactate solution is infused into the joint through the arthroscopic cannula side port by a syringe, and the joint is viewed from the anteromedial portal.

With direct arthroscopic vision, a 25 gauge 1-1/2 inch needle is then inserted into the ankle joint to locate the position for the anterolateral portal (see Fig. 32–3). The anterolateral portal is established by using a technique similar to that in the preceding paragraph, and an inflow cannula is inserted into the ankle joint. Sequential examination of the ankle joint and structures is now performed

by using the eight-point anterior, three-point central, and three-point posterior sequence (see the following section).

Commonly, the posterolateral portal (see Fig. 32–4) is used for inflow or observation in the seven-point posterior examination. The key to establishing the posterolateral portal is adequate joint distention with constant distraction. The posterolateral portal is established under direct visualization by taking the arthroscope from the anteromedial portal and maneuvering it posteriorly through the notch of Harty. An 18 gauge spinal needle is then inserted through the posterior capsule medial to the posteroinferior tibiofibular and transverse tibiofibular ligaments. When the posterolateral portal is used, distraction often needs to be increased for an adequate view. The cannula should be inserted with care to avoid injury to the branches of the sural nerve and the short saphenous vein. The posterolateral portal is used initially as the primary inflow portal, and it may be used subsequently for visualization or instrumentation by means of an interchangeable system of cannulae. The posteromedial portal is almost never used because of the risk to the posterior neurovascular structures.

Arthroscopic Examination

A 21-point arthroscopic examination of the ankle has been recommended to ensure a systematic evaluation of the ankle.[10] The eight-point anterior examination includes the deltoid ligament; the medial gutter; the medial, central, and lateral aspects of the talus; the talofibular articulation; the lateral gutter; and the anterior gutter. The three-point central examination from the anterior portal includes the medial, central, and lateral portions of the tibiotalar joint. The three-point posterior examination from the anterior portal includes the posteroinferior tibiofibular ligament, the transverse tibiofibular ligament, the capsular reflection of the flexor hallucis longus tendon, and the medial and lateral synovial recesses. The seven-point posterior examination includes the medial gutter; the medial, central, and lateral aspects of the talus; the talofibular articulation; the lateral gutter; and the posterior gutter. Generally, the combination of the anteromedial, anterolateral, and posterolateral portals provides excellent visualization of the entire joint. With a three-portal system, adequate inflow can be maintained with gravity drainage. Often, there is no need for an arthroscopic pump.

Postoperative Management

The ankle joint is subjected to a markedly increased hydrostatic pressure compared with other joints that are commonly treated with arthroscopy. The wound sealing effect of the soft tissue, such as muscles and subcutaneous tissue, is absent at the ankle. Edema, intra-articular hemorrhage, and effusion of the joint pose greater postoperative problems, and careful attention to wound closure is important. After the arthroscopic examination is completed, all wounds are closed with a 4-0 nonabsorbable nylon suture. A bulky compressive dressing and a well-padded posterior splint are applied for 5–7 days. Postoperative rest with elevation of the limb and ankle immobilization is necessary. After 1 week, a short leg compression stocking is applied, and a brace or a movable short-leg walker is used for ambulation. Weight-bearing status depends on the operative procedure performed. Rehabilitation is started at 2 weeks postoperatively and is gradually advanced to include strengthening and increased range of motion.

ARTHROSCOPIC TREATMENT OF ANKLE PATHOLOGY

Loose Bodies

Chondral and osteochondral loose bodies of the ankle joint are often caused by trauma (ankle sprains and fractures of the ankle and talus), degenerative and posttraumatic arthritis, osteochondral lesion of the talus (osteochondritis dissecans), and synovial chondromatosis.

Loose bodies may cause locking, catching, swelling, pain, and decreased range of motion as they float freely within the joint. These symptoms can be intermittent because the loose bodies may become fixed to the synovium and, therefore, asymptomatic, only to recur when the chondral or osteochondral fragments come loose. Physical examination is usually unremarkable. Rarely is there any specific area of tenderness or a palpable loose body.

Standard radiographs and CT usually demonstrate osseous loose bodies; however, chondral loose bodies remain radiolucent on plain radiographs and may not be detected by CT. The arthrogram can be effective in demonstrating loose bodies, especially in synovial chondromatosis. MRI with an intra-articular injection of gadolinium may demonstrate the bony or cartilaginous lesion when other imaging studies are unsuccessful. Often, a combination of diagnostic tests must be used to diagnose loose bodies. To facilitate surgical approach and removal, it is important to determine preoperatively whether the loose bodies are intracapsular, extracapsular, or intra-articular.

Removal of chondral and osteochondral loose bodies can be accomplished arthroscopically.[22–24] Operative treatment begins with a careful examination to evaluate the entire ankle joint. Distraction can improve visualization and access to the loose bodies. Loose bodies in the anterior compartment are most easily removed from an anterior portal with a grasper while visualizing from the other anterior portal or from the posterolateral portal. Loose bodies in the posterior compartment are best removed while visualizing from an anterior portal and performing the removal with instrumentation placed through the posterolateral portal or by manipulating the loose bodies into the anterior compartment and proceeding with the removal with an anteriorly placed instrument. Following removal, another arthroscopic examination is performed to detect any remaining loose bodies and to determine the origin of the lesion. If a substantial chondral or osteochondral defect in the articular surface is found, then débridement, burring, and, possibly, drilling should be performed. Osteochondral loose bodies with sufficient bone attached to allow healing can be replaced and pinned in a manner similar to that for separated osteochondral lesions of the talus. Avoiding arthrotomy in these situations is desirable.[24–26]

The clinical results of arthroscopic loose body removal depend on the underlying cause of the loose bodies and the presence of degenerative or post-traumatic arthritis in the ankle joint. When significant degenerative or post-traumatic arthritis is present, the results are less predictable.

Tibiotalar Osteophytes

Tibiotalar osteophytes usually occur secondary to trauma or degenerative changes and are most commonly seen at the anterior lip of the distal tibia. Spurs may also occur anterolaterally between the talus and lateral malleolus,[27] on the anterior aspect of the medial malleolus, and in the posterior aspect of the ankle joint. With anterior spurs, the beak-like prominence of the distal tibia is often associated with a corresponding lesion on the anterior neck of the talus, which may be either a defect or an opposing osteophyte. This "kissing" lesion may be the result of direct trauma following a forced dorsiflex injury to the ankle or the result of forced plantar flexion causing capsular avulsion. These spurs are prevalent in dancers[28] and athletes.[29–31]

Tibiotalar spurs may cause bony impingement resulting in decreased range of motion, pain, catching, and joint swelling.[32] Clinically, a patient may have anterior ankle pain exacerbated by walking upstairs, squatting, or running. Tenderness is localized over the bony prominence of the anterior ankle joint and exacerbated by passive dorsiflexion of the ankle. Range of motion is limited, especially in dorsiflexion. Plain radiographic evaluation demonstrates the anterior osteophyte. Normally, the angle between the distal end of the tibia and the talus is greater than 60 degrees[8] (Fig. 32–5*A*). However, with osteophytic formation on the distal part of the tibia or the talar neck, this angle diminishes to less than 60 degrees[8] (Fig. 32–5*B*). A lateral-stress radiograph taken with the ankle in maximum dorsiflexion may demonstrate impingement of the osteophytes anteriorly. A bone scan usually shows increased uptake in the area of impingement in symptomatic lesions and may demonstrate a fracture through the osteophyte, if present.

Stoller, Hekmat, and Kleiger[28] reported that most spurs do not produce painful symptoms; therefore, patients who have persistent pain in the anterior aspect of the ankle and have an anterior tibiotalar spur evident on a lateral radiograph need additional diagnostic evaluation and management. Conservative treatment includes rest, nonsteroidal anti-inflammatory drugs, a heel lift, and intra-articular steroid injections with long-acting anesthetics. If pain persists despite nonoperative treatment, then the physician may consider using a bone scan to confirm that there is an abnormal increase in the uptake in the region of the spur. If there are persistent or progressive symptoms, pain and tenderness localized to the anterior aspect of the bony prominence, limited range of motion, or positive radiologic test results, arthroscopic or open

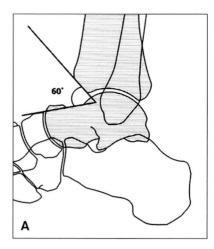 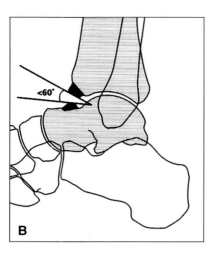

A

B

Figure 32–5 • *A*, The normal angle between the distal tibia and talus is 60 degrees or greater. *B*, Osteophytic formation on the distal tibia or talar neck, with the angle diminished to less than 60 degrees. (From Mann RA and Coughlin M (eds.): Surgery of the Foot and Ankle, 6th ed. St. Louis, C.V. Mosby, 1992.)

resection of the spur may be considered.[17, 27, 32–34] Often, surgical localization can be difficult so it is important to determine the precise anatomic location and medial and lateral extent of the osteophyte preoperatively. A CT scan may be helpful for this purpose.

A classification system for anterior spurs was developed by Scranton and McDermott[33] that consists of grades I–IV, based on the size of the spur and the extent of ankle arthritis (Fig. 32–6). Scranton and McDermott compared open resection with arthroscopic resection of painful anterior impingement spurs and showed that treatment and recovery correlated with the grade. Grades I, II, and III spurs were suitable for resection arthroscopically. However, the patients who were managed arthroscopically recovered in approximately half the time as those who were managed with arthrotomy. Grade IV spurs were initially thought to be inappropriate for arthroscopic resection; however, with increased experience the authors have successfully resected a number of grade IV spurs.

Arthroscopic resection of anterior tibiotalar osteophytes is associated with decreased morbidity as compared with open techniques.[33] Adequate visibility must be maintained and extreme caution must be exercised to prevent injury to the neurovascular structures. The shaver blades should never be directed dorsally into the soft tissues. Anterior osteophytes are often visualized without distraction; however, distraction may be necessary to "get around" the osteophyte during resection. Most osteophytes can be resected by using rongeurs, abraders, or small osteotomes placed through the anterior portals while visualizing through an anterior portal (Fig. 32–7). Occasionally, it is necessary to place the arthroscope through the posterolateral portal to remove an osteophyte (Fig. 32–8). Mechanical distraction of the ankle is frequently necessary to visualize the anterior osteophyte through the posterior portal. A partial synovectomy may be required when a large amount of synovitis is present. Intraoperatively, it is easy to become confused as to the extent of the anterior osteophyte. Therefore, the surgeon must expose both the superior and inferior surfaces of the osteophyte by using the shaver on the bone to elevate and remove the capsule. The normal articulation is then visualized and used to judge the amount of osteophyte to be

removed. An intraoperative lateral radiograph should always be obtained to verify satisfactory resection of the osteophyte.

Anterior Soft-Tissue Impingement

Persistent pain localized to the anterolateral corner of the ankle joint after an inversion ankle sprain is a common problem. In 1950 Wolin and colleagues[35] described an anterolateral (meniscoid) band of hyalinized connective tissue between the talus and the fibula. They thought that impingement of this meniscoid tissue led to pain and that its removal with an open procedure resulted in relief of the painful symptoms. In 1982 Waller[36] called the problem "anterolateral corner compression syndrome" and noted pain to be localized along the anteroinferior border of the fibula and the anterolateral talus. This lesion was thought to be caused by an inversion injury to the ankle. Others confirmed these findings and found that the lesion reflects a chronic synovitis and fibrosis.[37–40] Adjacent talar or fibular chondromalacia may be associated with this lesion.

The anterolateral impingement usually occurs in the superior portion of the anterior talofibular ligament but can also localize to the distal portion of the anteroinferior tibiofibular ligament (syndesmotic impingement) (Fig. 32–9). Bassett, Gates, and Billys[41] reported impingement from a separate fascicle of the anteroinferior tibiofibular ligament. Soft-tissue impingement can occur simultaneously along the entire lateral gutter and into the syndesmosis.

These patients with anterolateral impingement have persistent anterolateral pain despite prolonged conservative treatment, which includes rest, immobilization, nonsteroidal anti-inflammatory drugs, local steroid injections, and standard physical therapy. Plain radiographs show normal results for approximately half of the patients, and others may show mild spurring, calcification, and joint space narrowing.[38] Stress x-ray results are normal. MRI may be helpful in the diagnosis in 30–40% of patients.[38] If conservative treatment fails after a minimum of 3 months, the diagnosis of anterolateral impingement should be considered.

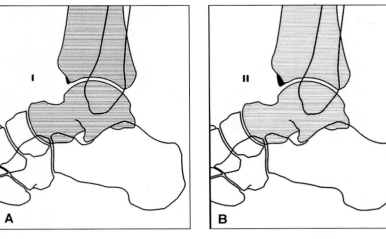

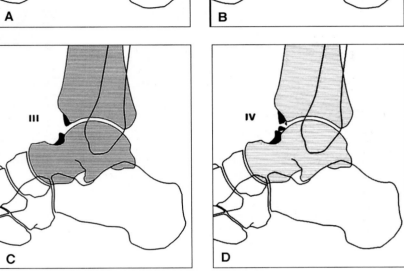

Figure 32–6 • The grades of ankle spurs as classified by Scranton and McDermott. *A*, Grade I: synovial impingement. Roentgenograms show an inflammatory reaction with spurs as large as 3 mm. *B*, Grade II: osteochondral reaction exostosis. Roentgenograms show spurs of more than 3 mm. No talar spur is seen. *C*, Grade III: severe exostosis with or without fragmentation. In addition, secondary spur formation is noted on the dorsum of the talus, often with fragmentation of the osteophytes. *D*, Grade IV: pantalocrural osteoarthrotic destruction. Roentgenograms suggest degenerative osteoarthrotic changes medially, laterally, or posteriorly. (From Ferkel RD and Scranton PE: Current concepts review: arthroscopy of the ankle and foot. J Bone Joint Surg Am 75:1233–1242, 1993.)

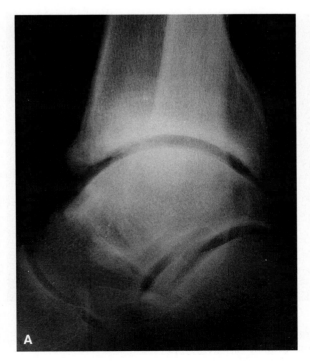

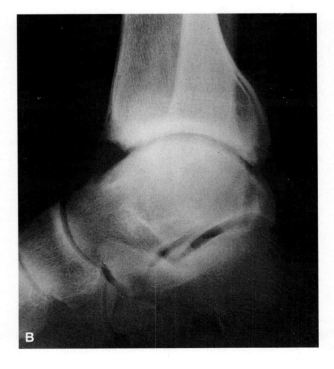

Figure 32–7 • Osteophyte removal. *A*, Large anterior distal tibial osteophyte. *B*, Postoperative radiograph demonstrates removal of the distal tibial osteophyte.

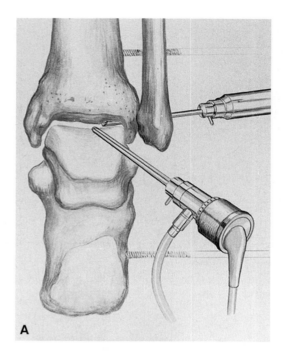

A

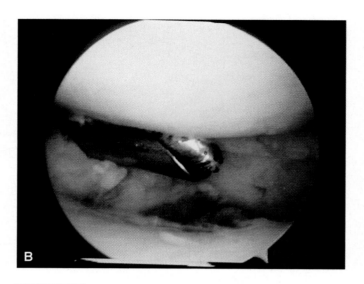

B

Figure 32–8 • *A* and *B*, Excision of the anterior osteophyte with a motorized bur through posterolateral visualization.

Arthroscopic treatment of anterolateral impingement includes débridement of the synovitis and fibrosis of the anterolateral gutter by using basket forceps or a motorized shaver. If present, the thickened band or meniscoid lesion is excised (Fig. 32–10). Care must be taken to preserve the anterior talofibular ligament. Treatment for syndesmotic impingement includes débridement of the anteroinferior tibiofibular ligament and distal tibiofibular joint. In addition, if a separate fascicle of the anteroinferior tibiofibular ligament is present, it should be excised.

Long-term results of arthroscopic synovectomy and débridement for anterolateral impingement demonstrate good-to-excellent results in approximately 75–90% of patients.[38, 39, 42–45]

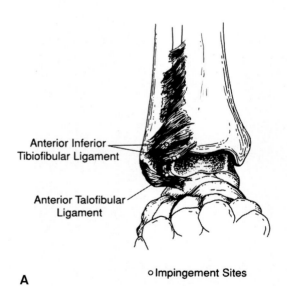

Anterior Inferior Tibiofibular Ligament

Anterior Talofibular Ligament

o Impingement Sites

A

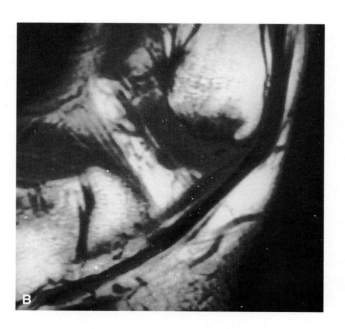

B

Figure 32–9 • Anterior impingement sites. *A*, Note that the anteroinferior tibiofibular ligament may have a separate fascicle that can impinge against the lateral dome of the talus. (From Mann RA and Coughlin M [eds.]: Surgery of the Foot and Ankle, 6th ed. St. Louis, C.V. Mosby, 1992.) *B*, T1-weighted sagittal view of the ankle with anterolateral impingement. Scar tissue appears as a decreased signal intensity between the talus and the fibula.

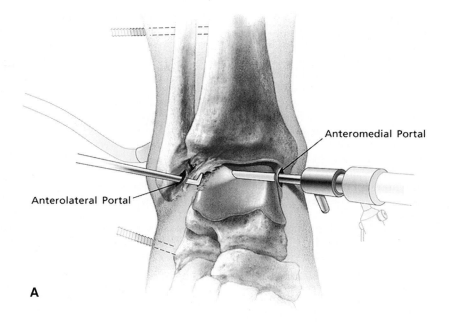

A

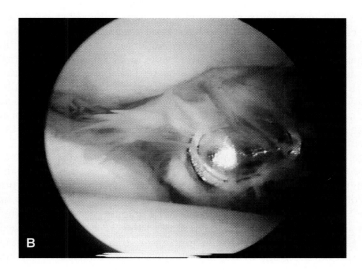

B

Figure 32–10 • Soft-tissue impingement lesion. *A*, At arthroscopy, synovitis of the lateral gutter with chondromalacia of the talus and fibula is seen, and occasional loose bodies are present. *B*, From the anterolateral portal a full-radius shaver is used to resect the fibrous bands and débride the talus and fibula.

Osteochondral Lesion of the Talus

The authors currently describe as osteochondral lesion of the talus the pathologic entity formerly called transchondral fracture, osteochondral fracture, osteochondritis dissecans, talar dome fracture, and talar flake fracture. This lesion may range from a small defect in the talar articular surface to a subchondral cyst or osteochondral fragment that is nondisplaced or displaced within the joint. The exact causes of osteochondral lesions of the talus remain controversial. Although trauma is believed to play a major role, idiopathic osteonecrosis may be another factor, supported by the fact that many patients have no history of trauma,[46] and approximately 10% of patients have bilateral involvement without a history of trauma.[47–49]

Medial lesions in this study are more common,[47] more posterior,[47] more cup-shaped, and deeper than lateral lesions, and they are usually nondisplaced. Lateral lesions are more commonly induced by trauma and are more anterior than medial lesions,[47] and they are usually shallow, wafer-shaped, and frequently displaced from their subchondral bed. Diagnosis may be difficult, given a high incidence of misdiagnosis or delayed diagnosis of osteochondral lesion of the talus with unexplained chronic ankle pain reported.[50] Patients frequently have chronic ankle pain, particularly following an associated trauma such as an inversion injury. In some cases, no such mechanism of injury is documented. Other presenting symptoms include recurrent swelling, stiffness, weakness or giving way, and occasional locking or catching.

The diagnosis of osteochondral lesion of the talus has traditionally been made by plain radiograph. However, a plain radiograph frequently does not demonstrate the lesion. Alexander and Barrack[51] reported that mortise and anteroposterior views can be taken in various degrees of plantar flexion and dorsiflexion to demonstrate the lesion. In a study by Zinman, Wolfson, and Reis,[52] CT scans have been found to be superior to x-ray films for both the diagnosis and follow-up of osteochondral lesions of the talus.

Currently, the single best test for osteochondral lesions of the talus is bilateral hindfoot CT scans with or without contrast medium in the coronal and transverse planes.

MRI has been advocated as being comparable to CT in its diagnostic capabilities.[53] Anderson et al.[53] compared CT with MRI in 24 cases, and in most of them CT was comparable to MRI; however, CT failed to diagnose stage 1 lesions in four patients. Cheng, Ferkel, and Applegate[54] reviewed x-ray films, CT scans, MRI scans, and intraoperative videotapes in 80 cases; they concluded that CT is the method of choice if there is a known diagnosis of osteochondral lesions of the talus. However, if the x-ray film and clinical findings are nondiagnostic, then MRI may be more valuable because of its ability to image soft tissue and bone.

A radiographic staging of osteochondral lesions of the talus was described by Berndt and Harty.[47] Four stages were proposed to describe the amount of destruction and displacement of the fragment (Table 32–1). Ferkel and Sgaglione[50] proposed a CT staging system that corresponds to the stages described by Berndt and Harty but that also takes into account the extent of osteonecrosis, the subchondral cyst formation, and the separation of fragments that are not seen radiographically (see Table 32–1 and Fig. 32–11). MRI has also been used to stage osteochondral lesions of the talus.[55, 56] Anderson and colleagues[53] compared CT with MRI results in 24 cases and also developed an MRI classification system (Table 32–2).

In 1986 Pritsch, Horoshovski, and Farine[26] developed a staging system based on the arthroscopic appearance of the overlying cartilage. They classified osteochondral lesions of the talus into three grades: intact, firm, shiny articular cartilage; intact but soft cartilage; and frayed cartilage. They also noted a poor correlation between the x-ray film appearance and the arthroscopic findings; they thought the arthroscopic appearance was the most important determinant for treatment. Cheng, Ferkel, and Applegate[54] correlated the CT scan and MRI staging systems with a new arthroscopic staging system (Table 32–3).

Controversy exists as to the appropriate treatment for osteochondral lesions of the talus. Conservative management of nondisplaced osteochondral lesions has been the traditional treatment, with arthrotomy or arthroscopy reserved for displaced fragments or failed conservative treatment.[47, 57, 58] Ferkel currently recommends conservative treatment in both the acute and chronic situations for CT scan stages 1 and 2 lesions. This conservative treatment includes 6–12 weeks of casting, with the length determined by the size of the lesion. At the present, there is no good evidence to support that non–weight-bearing in a cast is any better than weight-bearing, and therefore non–weight-bearing is not advocated. If the patient remains symptomatic after the proposed conservative treatment, then arthroscopic evaluation and treatment are suggested. Arthroscopy is advocated for all symptomatic CT scan stages 3 and 4 lesions. The only exception to the rule is for children whose growth plates remain open at the distal, tibial, and fibular epiphysis. For them, conservative treatment with casting before surgical intervention is recommended.

Open treatment for osteochondral lesions of the talus usually requires extensive arthrotomy and transmalleolar osteotomies to perform excision of loose bodies, drilling of the defect, fixation of the fragments, or bone grafting.[22, 23, 26, 57, 59–69] These approaches may be associated with malleolar nonunion and malunion and joint stiffness. Arthroscopy has eliminated many of these problems and has significant advantages in evaluating the condition of the articular surfaces when diagnosis of early, radiologically silent lesions, such as subchondral compression, and differentiation of partially detached and completely detached lesions are possible. With arthroscopy, removal of loose bodies and small osteochondral fragments, débridement of lesions, drilling of partially separated fragments and defects, pinning of reducible fragments, transmalleolar drilling, and bone grafting can be performed. The use of distraction improves access, especially to posterior lesions, allowing adequate débridement and curettage of the bed.[21, 70, 71]

Arthroscopic treatment of osteochondral lesions of the talus begins with inspection, identification, and staging of all lesions. Any loose body or osteochondral fragment is removed. Probing of the talar articular surface is essential for appreciating the extent of the overlying cartilaginous softening and blistering and for staging the lesion adequately. The authors do not advocate removing softened but intact cartilage but recommend drilling of these intact symptomatic lesions. If the lesion is loose, it should be removed. Débridement of the lesion is performed by using the full-radius resector, high-speed bur, mini-section punch, minicurets, grasper, and arthroscopic scalpel. Following débridement, a scalpel may then be used to excise loose chondral fragments and areas of surface blistering. There is controversy about whether drilling or abrasion of

---

Table 32–1   **Radiographic Staging of Osteochondral Lesions of the Talus**

Stage	Berndt and Harty System	Stage	CT System
I	Compressed	I	Cystic lesion with an intact roof
II	Disrupted	IIA	Cystic lesion with communication to talar dome surface
		IIB	Open articular surface lesion with overlying nondisplaced fragment
III	Partially displaced	III	Undisplaced lesion with lucency
IV	Displaced	IV	Displaced fragment

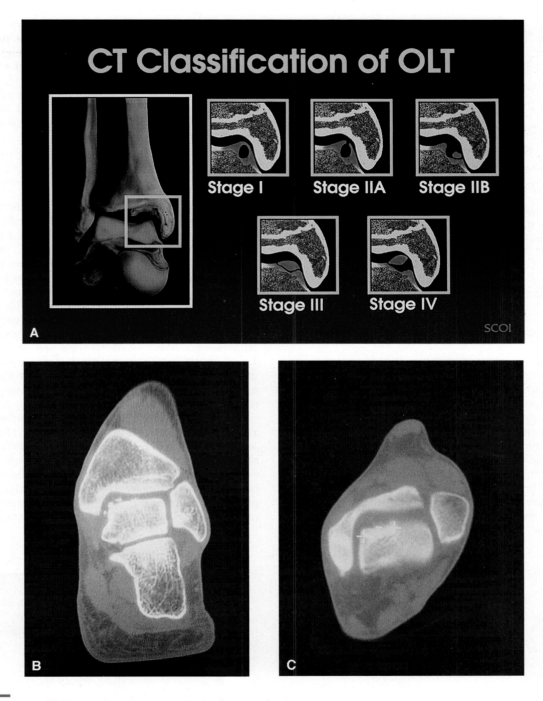

Figure 32–11 • Computed tomography (CT) staging. *A,* Classification of stages. *B,* Stage IV CT scan, coronal view. *C,* Stage IV CT scan, axial view.

the subchondral surface is the treatment of choice. Generally, drilling techniques are recommended for lesions larger than 1 cm, whereas abrasion may be adequate for smaller lesions. Drilling is performed through the three basic arthroscopic portals or with a transmalleolar technique in a superior-to-inferior fashion (Fig. 32–12). Transmalleolar drilling is performed by using a 0.062 inch K-wire at approximately 3–5 mm intervals to a depth of approximately 10 mm.[62] A small joint ankle guide may be used with the transmalleolar drilling of the lesion. Occasionally, fluoroscopy may be used to assist with drilling. Fluoroscopy is not frequently required since the advent of mechanical distraction techniques. Distraction of the ankle allows dorsiflexion and plantar flexion of the ankle so that drilling may be performed throughout the entire lesion. Occasionally, a lesion may be secured in place by

Table 32–2	**MRI Classification**
Stage I	Subchondral trabecular compression
	Plain x-ray film normal, abnormal bone scan
	Marrow edema on MRI
Stage IIA	Formation of subchondral cyst
Stage II	Incomplete separation of fragment
Stage III	Unattached, undisplaced fragment with presence of synovial fluid around fragment
Stage IV	Displaced fragment

Table 32–3	**Surgical Grade Based on Articular Cartilage**
Grade A	Smooth, intact but soft or ballottable
Grade B	Rough surface
Grade C	Fibrillations/fissures
Grade D	Flap present or bone exposed
Grade E	Loose, undisplaced fragment
Grade F	Displaced fragment

absorbable pins, screws, or K-wires (Fig. 32–13). This is especially important when the lesion is large and anatomic reduction is possible. Lateral lesions, especially anterior ones, may be more amenable to pinning than medial ones. Absorbable pins allow accurate fixation with early motion and avoid additional surgery for pin removal. Following drilling, the tourniquet is deflated and the fluid flow turned off. This allows visualization of the pathologic area and evaluation of whether adequate vascular access was created over the pathologic site.

Postoperatively, a bulky compression dressing is applied with a posterior splint in the neutral position. Range-of-motion exercises are begun at approximately 1 week, but weight-bearing is avoided for 4–8 weeks, depending on the size of the lesion.

The results of arthroscopic treatment are as good or better than those of open treatment and are associated with lower morbidity and shorter recovery time.[17, 19–22, 24–26, 50, 59, 64, 67, 68, 72–79]

Synovitis

The synovium of the ankle joint may become inflamed and hypertrophied secondary to various arthritides, infections, degenerative or neuropathic changes, and trauma (Table 32–4). An adequate work-up should be performed to determine the causes of the synovitis. Often, patients with undiagnosed and persistent synovitis, who have failed to respond to conservative treatment, can benefit from diagnostic arthroscopy and synovial biopsy.[80] Rheumatoid and other inflammatory arthritides, pigmented villonodular synovitis, and infectious arthritis can be diagnosed with arthroscopy. Many synovial diseases for which open synovectomy has been recommended can be treated arthroscopically. Nonspecific generalized or localized post-traumatic synovitis often responds well to arthroscopic treatment.[39, 81]

The patient is placed in a supine position, and thigh and ankle holders are used. This allows the foot to be secured in place and permits easy simultaneous access to the anteromedial, anterolateral, and posterolateral portals. For localized anterior synovitis, distraction is not always necessary. However, distraction is helpful to permit complete visualization, especially in cases of generalized synovitis. The 2.9 or 3.5 mm full-radius blade is preferred for

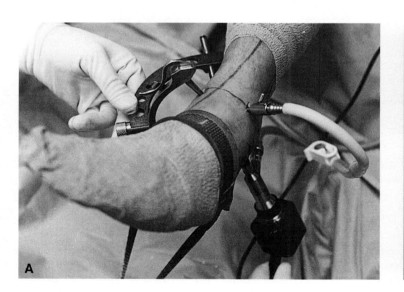

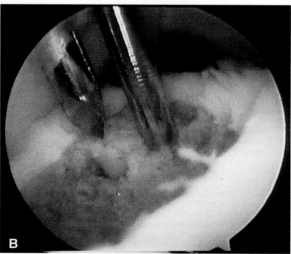

Figure 32–12 • Transmalleolar drilling of posteromedial lesion. *A,* The arthroscope is inserted through the posterolateral portal, and a small joint drill guide is inserted through the anteromedial portal. *B,* While viewing from a posterolateral portal, drill holes are made through the medial malleolus into the talus, utilizing the guide.

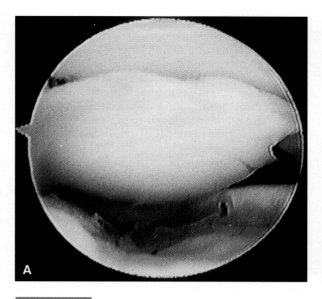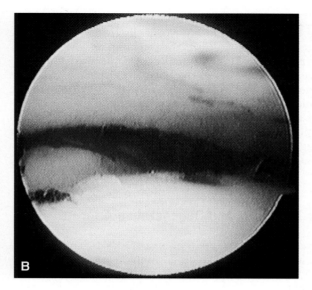

Figure 32–13 • Internal fixation of an osteochondral lesion of the lateral dome of the talus, left ankle. *A*, Osteochondral fracture visualized from the anteromedial portal, with inflow posteriorly and anterolateral portal used for probing and instrumentation. The fragment has rotated 180 degrees. *B*, Internal fixation of the acute osteochondral fracture with absorbable pin.

ankle synovectomy. The synovectomy and débridement should be performed sequentially and thoroughly. The entire joint should be débrided and freed from scar, fibrotic material, and synovitis. Débridement of associated chondromalacia and removal of loose bodies may be performed after improvement of visualization. Because patients with rheumatoid arthritis or other synovial disease have thin, friable capsules, a "whisker" shaver tip is preferred for débriding anteriorly or posteromedially under the neurovascular structures to avoid injury to these structures. Following complete synovectomy, the tourniquet should be released and drains inserted if extensive bleeding is noted.

Table 32–4	**Sources of Synovial Irritation**
Congenital	Plicae
	Congenital bands within the ankle
Trumatic	Sprains
	Fractures
	Previous surgeries
Rheumatic	Rheumatoid arthritis
	Pigmented villonodular synovitis
	Crystal synovitis
	Hemphilia
Infectious	Bacterial
	Fungal
Degenerative	Primary
	Secondary
Neuropathic	Charcot joints
Miscellaneous	Ganglions
	Arthrofibrosis

A compressive dressing with a short leg splint should be applied. The postoperative regimen should include early range-of-motion exercises and protected weight-bearing, depending on the extent of resection.

Ankle Instability

Lateral ankle sprains resulting from an inversion injury are common. Rarely do these injuries lead to instability, and therefore nonoperative treatment is indicated. However, recurrent lateral ankle sprains may result in chronic instability that does not respond to conservative treatment. Patients with lateral instability often complain of pain and swelling following each episode of injury. Often, symptoms include looseness, weakness, and giving way. In these cases, surgical repair may be necessary to correct the instability.

Arthroscopy can be useful in the evaluation and treatment of chronic lateral ankle instability. The amount of subluxation within the ankle mortis can be evaluated, thereby providing dynamic information not available from simple stress films.[80] Often, chronic lateral ankle instability is associated with intra-articular pathologic conditions, especially chondral injuries and even a meniscoid lesion.[6] Failure to recognize these associated lesions can compromise results; therefore, arthroscopic evaluation of the joint before a stabilization procedure has been advocated to prevent missing significant intra-articular pathologic conditions.[78, 82] Arthroscopic ligament stabilization has been described by Lundeen and Hawkins[83, 84]; however, these techniques are investigative, and no long-term results have been reported.

The technique for arthroscopic stabilization of the ankle for lateral instability is not discussed here because the authors do not utilize this technique. The reader is referred to Hawkins.[84] Initially, a staple was utilized to secure the soft tissues to the bone after the talus had been abraded. Because of problems with the staples, a suture technique using suture anchors was developed. The anchors are placed percutaneously through the lateral portal and planted parallel to the tibiotalar joint. Postoperative management includes a weight-bearing cast for 6 weeks and subsequent rehabilitation.

Post-Traumatic and Degenerative Arthritis

Conservative management of post-traumatic and degenerative arthritis of the ankle is often successful with non-steroidal anti-inflammatory drugs, intra-articular steroid injections, and bracing, preferably with a rigid ankle-foot orthosis. If a trial of conservative management has failed, the symptoms of early degenerative or post-traumatic arthritis are often amenable to arthroscopic débridement.[9, 17, 80, 81] Synovectomy, removal of loose bodies, débridement of loose chondral fragments, débridement of soft-tissue impingement, lavage, and osteophyte removal appear beneficial. Abrasion and drilling of exposed subchondral bone may promote fibrocartilage regeneration. Severely arthritic joints with extensive deformity, fibrosis, or significant instability are not candidates for arthroscopic débridement.

Ankle arthrodesis is the preferred operative procedure for the treatment of end-stage degenerative or post-traumatic arthritis in most patients. A variety of open techniques have been described for performing an ankle arthrodesis. An arthroscopic approach to ankle arthrodesis has been developed and is indicated for patients with end-stage degeneration of the ankle joint with minimal deformity.[85, 86] The goal of arthroscopic ankle arthrodesis is to allow preparation of the joint surfaces for successful arthrodesis without extensive arthrotomy, soft-tissue dissection, devascularization of the bony tissue, and unsightly scars. The principles of arthroscopic arthrodesis of the ankle are similar to those associated with open arthrodesis: débridement of all hyaline cartilage and underlying necrotic bone, reduction in an appropriate position for fusion (ideally, neutral to 5 degrees of dorsiflexion with 5 degrees valgus), and rigid internal fixation. Distraction of the ankle facilitates maximum exposure of the joint during the procedure. The use of sharp-cup and ring curets, shavers, and burs is essential. Fixation is usually accomplished by insertion of percutaneous cannulated screws through the medial and lateral malleoli (Fig. 32–14).

Early clinical functional results with arthroscopic ankle arthrodesis were good to excellent in 92% of patients.[85] More recent series demonstrate good-to-excellent results in approximately 85% of patients,[87, 88] with a rapid time to fusion, a low rate of nonunion, and few complications. In a comparison of an open and arthroscopic technique, Myerson and Quill[89] reported that the mean time to arthrodesis was faster and recovery time quicker in the arthroscopic group.

However, the two groups were not similar because the patients selected for open arthrotomy and arthrodesis, as a group, had many more complex problems, both in the overall alignment of the ankle and quality of the bone. Patient selection may have accounted for the difference between the two groups in the time to fusion. The extent of deformity, quality of local circulation, presence of prior infection, and vascularity of the talus and distal tibia had some bearing on patient selection and decision-making regarding surgery.

Arthroscopic ankle arthrodesis appears to result in similar or better results in selected patients. The technique is particularly appealing for elderly patients and those with rheumatoid arthritis who are unable to tolerate prolonged non–weight-bearing postoperatively.[16] However, a prospective, randomized study comparing open and arthroscopic fusion in similar groups is needed to compare the two techniques adequately.

For an arthroscopic ankle arthrodesis, the patient is placed in a supine position on the operating table with a fluoroscopic attachment. The leg to be operated on should be placed so that the ankle is easily accessible to fluoroscopy and use of the image intensifier. Ankle distraction should be performed for maximum visualization and access to the entire ankle joint. The standard anterolateral, anteromedial, and posterolateral portals are used. The arthroscope is first inserted in the anteromedial portal to assess the amount of distraction. Once adequate visualization is achieved, the posterolateral portal is established for fluid flow and eventual instrumentation to the posterior compartment.

The entire articular surface of the tibial plafond, talar dome, and the medial and lateral talomalleolar surfaces should be systematically removed with ring curets supplemented by a motorized abrader and shaver placed through the anterolateral portal. All remaining hyaline cartilage and sclerotic subchondral bone should be removed until underlying viable cancellous bone is exposed. Care should be taken to maintain the anatomic bony contour of the talar dome and the tibial plafond. Previously existing varus or valgus deformity may be corrected at this time, although advanced deformities should be treated by open techniques. Avoid resecting too much bone or squaring off the surfaces so as to prevent the creation of a varus or valgus deformity that may result in a delayed union or malunion. In general, the posterior compartment may be abraded from the anterior portals. If the motorized bur does not reach adequately into the posterior compartment, a 15 degree angled curet may be used. Occasionally, it may be easier to reach the posterior compartment by abrading through the posterolateral portal while viewing through the anterolateral portal. In general, the medial portion of the débridement process is performed with the arthroscope placed anterolaterally and the abrader placed anteromedially. Conversely, the lateral half of the débridement process is generally accomplished with the arthroscope placed anteromedially and the abrader placed anterolaterally.

Anterior lip osteophytes should be removed so that they do not block reduction of the talar dome convexity into the tibial plafond cavity. This may be achieved by abrading and viewing through the anterior portals. If the

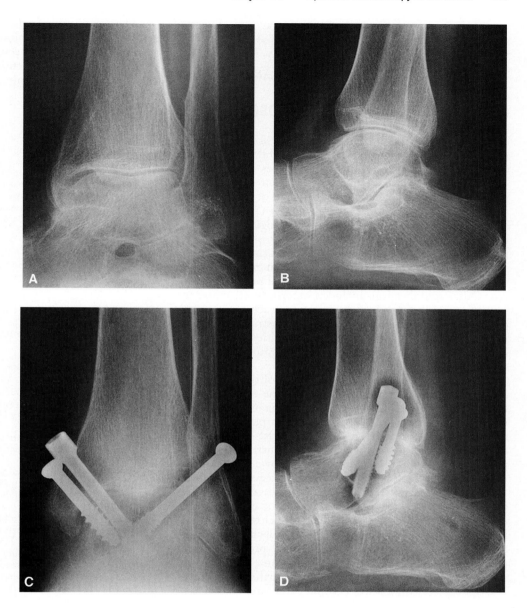

Figure 32–14 • Arthroscopic ankle arthrodesis. *A* and *B*, Preoperative anteroposterior and lateral radiographs demonstrate joint space narrowing. *C* and *D*, Anteroposterior and lateral radiographs show insertion of cannulated screws through the medial malleolus and fibula into the talus.

anterior capsule is adherent to the anterior osteophyte, visualization through the posterolateral portal makes it possible to assess the amount of bone required to be removed. A small osteotome is placed through a 1/2 inch incision made directly over the osteophyte to facilitate its rapid removal.

Once cancellous bone with viable vascularity is established over the entire fusion area, two guide pins are drilled percutaneously into the medial and lateral malleoli under direct vision by using a small joint drill guide. Small stab incisions are used to insert the screws. The first pin is drilled from the proximal part of medial malleolus just above the joint line. The second pin is drilled laterally through the lateral malleolus and the posterior aspect of the joint line. The medial pin is directed slightly posteriorly, and the lateral pin is directed anteriorly. The tips of the pins should penetrate the tibial plafond and lateral malleolus and may be viewed directly by using the arthro-

scope. Distraction is then released and the arthroscopic instruments are removed. The ankle surfaces are then compressed.

Fluoroscopy should be used at this time to confirm a satisfactory position of fusion. Fusion surfaces should be in intimate contact, and the foot should be in the desired position. While maintaining this position, the guide pins should be advanced back into the talus. The depth of the pins may be determined by using the image intensifier. A 6.5 mm self-drilling, self-tapping cannulated screw is then placed over the guide pin and advanced through the malleoli and into the talus. The position of the fusion is confirmed during and after insertion of the hardware by using fluoroscopy.

Postoperatively, the ankle is immobilized in a posterior splint. After 1 week a short leg non–weight-bearing cast is applied for an additional 3 weeks. At the end of that time, a short leg weight-bearing cast is applied. The cast is removed when fusion is verified by an x-ray film. A movable short-leg walker can be used at 3–4 weeks with weight-bearing, depending on bone quality, rigid fixation, and good patient compliance.

COMPLICATIONS OF ANKLE ARTHROSCOPY

There are many potential complications associated with ankle arthroscopy. Ferkel, Heath, and Guhl[90] reported an overall complication rate of 9% in a series of 612 cases. The most common complication was neurologic (49%), primarily involving the superficial branch of the peroneal nerve (15/27 or 56%), the saphenous nerve (5/27 or 18%), and the sural nerve (6/27 or 22%). Neurologic damage can be caused by placement of the distraction pins or placement of the operative instruments through the portal sites. Neurologic and arterial damage has been reported with use of the anterocentral and posteromedial portals.

Other complications included superficial infections in six patients, adhesions in three patients, fractures in three patients, deep infection in two patients, instrument failure in two patients, ligament injury in two patients, and incisional pain in two patients. Several other minor complications were seen in one patient each.

Invasive distraction was used in 317 of the 612 cases. Distraction pins were associated with some transient pin-track pain. Two stress fractures of the tibia occurred early in the series because of inappropriate pin placement (too anterior or too posterior) or a too-rapid rate of rehabilitation. One stress fracture of the fibula occurred due to pin placement in the fibula. Statistically, the overall complication rate was not affected by the use of invasive distraction. Superficial wound infection appeared to be related to the closeness of portal placement, the type of cannula used, early mobilization, and the use of tapes to close the portals. Deep wound infection correlated with a lack of administration of preoperative antibiotics. No problems have occurred since the use of skin sutures and preoperative antibiotics. Increased experience of the arthroscopist was also associated with a lower complication rate.

AVOIDANCE OF COMPLICATIONS

Careful preoperative planning, a knowledge of surface anatomy, and use of appropriate distraction and instrumentation techniques help to avoid complications. The skin is incised by using a scalpel blade, with blunt dissection performed to the capsule by using a mosquito clamp. This minimizes risk to the neurovascular structures and tendons. Use of the posteromedial and anterocentral portals is discouraged because of their proximity to neurovascular structures and tendons. Arthroscopic cannulae should be used to minimize soft-tissue trauma around the portals. The portals should be sutured to minimize wound problems, and antibiotics should be administered for 24 hours. It is imperative to avoid multiple portals in proximity. Invasive distraction pins should be inserted through cannulae with blunt dissection from skin to the bony surface and placed unicortically only one thumb-breadth below the anterior cortex.

The majority of complications reported with ankle arthroscopy have been minor and transient; however, serious complications do occur. The surgeon must exhibit exceptional care and attention to detail when performing ankle arthroscopy to minimize potential complications.

References

1. Burman MS: Arthroscopy of direct visualization of joints: an experimental cadaver study. J Bone Joint Surg 13:669, 1931.
2. Takagi K: The arthroscope. J Jpn Orthop Assoc 14:359, 1939.
3. Andrews JR, Previte WJ, and Carson WG: Arthroscopy of the ankle: technique and normal anatomy. Foot Ankle 6:29, 1985.
4. Chen YC: Clinical and cadaver studies on the ankle joint arthroscopy. J Jpn Orthop Assoc 50:631, 1976.
5. Chen Y: Arthroscopy of the ankle joint. In Watanabe M (ed.): Arthroscopy of Small Joints. New York, Igaku-Shoin, 1985, pp 104–127.
6. Drez D Jr, Guhl JF, and Gollehon DL: Ankle arthroscopy: technique and indications. Foot Ankle 2:138, 1981.
7. Drez D Jr, Guhl JF, and Gollehon DL: Ankle arthroscopy: technique and indications. Clin Sports Med 1:35, 1982.
8. Ferkel RD: Arthroscopy of the ankle and foot. In Mann RA and Coughlin M (eds.): Surgery of the Foot and Ankle, 6th ed. St. Louis, C.V. Mosby, 1993, pp 1277–1310.
9. Ferkel RD and Fischer SP: Progress in ankle arthroscopy. Clin Orthop 240:210, 1989.
10. Ferkel RD: Arthroscopic Surgery: The Foot and Ankle. Philadelphia, Lippincott-Raven, 1996.
11. Gollehon DL and Drez D: Ankle arthroscopy: approaches and technique. Orthopedics 6:1150, 1983.
12. Gollehon DL and Drez D: Arthroscopy of the ankle. In McGinty J (ed.): Arthroscopy Surgery Update. Rockville, Md., Aspen, 1985, p 161.
13. Harrington KD: Degenerative arthritis of the ankle secondary to longstanding lateral ligament instability. J Bone Joint Surg Am 61:354, 1979.
14. Johnson LL: Diagnostic and Surgical Arthroscopy, 2nd ed. St. Louis, C.V. Mosby, 1981, p 412.
15. Parisien JS: Arthroscopy of the ankle: state of the art. Contemp Orthop 5:21, 1982.
16. Parisien JS and Shereff MJ: The role of arthroscopy in the diagnosis and treatment of disorders of the ankle. Foot Ankle 2:144, 1981.
17. Parisien JS and Vangsness T: Operative arthroscopy of the ankle: three years' experience. Clin Orthop 199:46, 1985.
18. Watanabe M: Selfoc-Arthroscope (Watanabe No. 24 Arthroscope). Monograph. Tokyo, Teishin Hospital, 1972.
19. Martin DF, Baker DL, Curl WW, et al.: Operative ankle arthroscopy: long-term follow-up. Am J Sports Med 17:16, 1989.
20. Ferkel RD and Scranton PE: Current concepts review: arthroscopy of the ankle and foot. J Bone Joint Surg Am 75:1233, 1993.
21. Guhl JF: New techniques for arthroscopic surgery of the ankle: preliminary report. Orthopedics 9:261, 1986.
22. Baker CL, Andrews JR, and Ryan JB: Arthroscopic treatment of transchondral talar dome fractures. Arthroscopy 2:82, 1986.
23. McCullough CJ and Venugopal V: Osteochondritis dissecans of the talus: the natural history. Clin Orthop 144:264, 1979.
24. McGinty JB: Arthroscopic removal of loose bodies. Orthop Clin North Am 13:313, 1982.
25. Parisien JS: Arthroscopic treatment of osteochondral lesions of the talus. Am J Sports Med 14:211, 1986.
26. Pritsch M, Horoshovski H, and Farine I: Arthroscopic treatment of osteochondral lesions of the talus. J Bone Joint Surg Am 68:862, 1986.
27. St Pierre RK, Velazco A, and Flemming LL: Impingement exostoses of the talus and fibula secondary to an inversion sprain. Foot Ankle Int 3:282, 1983.
28. Stoller SM, Hekmat F, and Kleiger B: A comparative study of the frequency of anterior impingement exostoses of the ankle in dancers and nondancers. Foot Ankle 4:201, 1984.
29. McMurray TP: Footballer's ankle. J Bone Joint Surg Br 32:68, 1950.
30. O'Donoghue DH: Impingement exostoses of the talus and tibia. J Bone Joint Surg Am 39:835, 1957.

31. O'Donoghue DH: Chondral and osteochondral fractures. J Trauma 6:469, 1966.
32. Hawkins RB: Arthroscopic treatment of sports-related anterior osteophytes in the ankle. Foot Ankle 9:87, 1988.
33. Scranton PE Jr and McDermott JE: Anterior or tibiotalar spurs: a comparison of open versus arthroscopic debridement. Foot Ankle 13:125, 1992.
34. Ogilvie-Harris DJ, Mahomed N, and Demaziere A: Anterior impingement of the ankle treated by arthroscopic removal of bony spurs. J Bone Joint Surg Br 75:437, 1993.
35. Wolin I, Glassman F, Sideman F, et al.: Internal derangement of the talofibular component of the ankle. Surg Gynecol Obstet 91:193, 1950.
36. Waller JF: Hindfoot and midfoot problems of the runner in symposium on the foot and leg. In Mack RP (ed.): Running Sports. St. Louis, Mosby-Year Book, 1982, pp 64–71.
37. Ewing JW: Arthroscopic management of transchondral talar-dome fractures (osteochondritis dissecans) and anterior impingement lesions of the ankle joint. Clin Sports Med 10:677–687, 1991.
38. Ferkel RD, Karzel RP, Del Pizzo W, et al.: Arthroscopic treatment of anterolateral impingement of the ankle. Am J Sports Med 19:440–446, 1991.
39. Martin DF, Curl WW, Baker CL: Arthroscopic treatment of chronic synovitis of the ankle. Arthroscopy 5:110, 1989.
40. Thein R and Eichenblat M: Arthroscopic treatment of sports-related synovitis of the ankle. Am J Sports Med 20:496, 1992.
41. Bassett FH III, Gates HS III, and Billys JE: Talar impingement by anteroinferior tibiofibular ligament. J Bone Joint Surg Am 72:55, 1990.
42. McCarroll JR, Schrader JW, Shelbourne KD, et al.: Meniscoid lesions of the ankle in soccer players. Am J Sports Med 15:255, 1987.
43. Ferkel RD: Soft tissue pathology of the ankle. In McGinty JB (ed.): Operative Arthroscopy. New York, Raven Press, 1991, pp 713–725.
44. Liu SH, Raskin A, Osti L, et al.: Arthroscopic treatment of anterolateral ankle impingement. Arthroscopy 10:215, 1994.
45. Meislin RJ, Rose DJ, Parisien JS, et al.: Arthroscopic treatment of synovial impingement of the ankle. Am J Sports Med 21:186, 1993.
46. Campbell CJ and Ranawat CS: Osteochondritis dissecans: the question of etiology. J Trauma 6:201, 1966.
47. Berndt AL and Harty M: Transchondral fractures (osteochondritis dissecans) of the talus. J Bone Joint Surg Am 41:988, 1959.
48. Blom JM and Strijk SP: Lesions of the trochlea tali: osteochondral fractures and osteochondritis dissecans of the trochlea tali. Radiol Clin North Am 44:387, 1975.
49. Guhl JF: Ankle arthroscopy. Presented at the Biennial Meeting of the International Arthroscopy Association, Rome, 1989.
50. Ferkel RD and Sgaglione NA: Arthroscopic treatment of osteochondral lesions of the talus: long term results. Orthop Trans 14:172, 1990.
51. Alexander AH and Barrack RL: Arthroscopic technique in talar dome fractures. Surgical Rounds for Orthopedics January 1990:27.
52. Zinman C, Wolfson N, and Reis ND: Osteochondritis dissecans of the dome of the talus. J Bone Joint Surg Am 70:1017, 1988.
53. Anderson IF, Chrichton KJ, Grattan-Smith T, et al.: Osteochondral fractures of the dome of the talus. J Bone Joint Surg Am 71:1143, 1989.
54. Cheng MS, Ferkel RD, and Applegate GR: Osteochondral lesions of the talus: a radiologic and surgical comparison. Presented at the Annual Meeting of the Academy of Orthopaedic Surgeons, New Orleans, Feb., 1995.
55. Dipaola JD, Nelson DW, and Colville MR: Characterizing osteochondral lesions by magnetic resonance imaging. Arthroscopy 7:101, 1991.
56. Nelson DW, Dipaola J, Colville M, et al.: Osteochondritis dissecans of the talus and knee: prospective comparison of MR and arthroscopic classifications. J Comput Assist Tomogr 14:804, 1990.
57. Canale ST and Belding RH: Osteochondral lesions of the talus. J Bone Joint Surg Am 62:97, 1980.
58. Roden S, Tillegard P, and Unnander-Scharin L: Osteochondritis dissecans and similar lesions of the talus. Acta Orthop Scand 23:51, 1953.
59. Alexander AH and Lichtman DM: Surgical treatment of transchondral talar dome fractures (osteochondritis dissecans). J Bone Joint Surg Am 62:646, 1980.
60. Bauer M, Jonsson K, and Linden B: Osteochondritis dissecans of the ankle: a 20-year follow-up study. J Bone Joint Surg Br 69:93, 1987.
61. Flick AB and Gould N: Osteochondritis dissecans of the talus (transchondral fractures of the talus): review of the literature and new surgical approach for medial dome lesions. Foot Ankle 5:165, 1985.
62. Gebstein R, Conforty B, Weiss RE, et al.: Closed percutaneous drilling for osteochondritis dissecans of the talus. Clin Orthop 213:197, 1986.
63. Gould N: Technique tips. Foot Ankle 3:184, 1982.
64. Mukherjee SK and Young AB: Dome fractures of the talus: a report of ten cases. J Bone Joint Surg Br 55:319, 1973.
65. O'Donoghue DH: Chondral and osteochondral fractures. J Trauma 6:469, 1966.
66. O'Farrell TA and Costello BG: Osteochondritis dissecans of the talus: the late results of surgical treatment. J Bone Joint Surg Br 64:494, 1982.
67. Ove PN, Bosse MJ, and Reinert CM: Excision of posterolateral talar dome lesions through a medical transmalleolar approach. Foot Ankle 9:171, 1989.
68. Pettine KA and Morrey BF: Osteochondral fractures of the talus: a long term follow-up. J Bone Joint Surg Br 69:89, 1987.
69. Thompson JP and Loomer RL: Osteochondral lesions of the talus in a sports medicine clinic. Am J Sports Med 12:460, 1984.
70. Trager S, Frederick LD, and Sengson D: Ankle arthroscopy: a method of distraction. Orthopedics 12:1317, 1989.
71. Yates CK and Grana WA: A simple distraction technique for ankle arthroscopy. Arthroscopy 4:103, 1988.
72. Ferkel RD and Orwin JF: Ankle arthroscopy: a new tool for treating acute and chronic ankle fractures. Arthroscopy 9:352, 1993.
73. Ferkel RD: Ankle arthroscopy. In An illustrated Guide to Small Joint Arthroscopy. Andover, Mass., Dyonics, 1989.
74. Guhl JF: New concepts (distraction) in ankle arthroscopy. Arthroscopy 4:160, 1988.
75. Guhl JF (ed.): Ankle Arthroscopy: Pathology and Surgical Techniques. Thorofare, N.J., Slack, 1988.
76. Lee CK and Mercurio C: Operative treatment of osteochondritis dissecans in situ by retrograde drilling and cancellous bone graft: a preliminary report. Clin Orthop 158:129, 1981.
77. Loomer R, Fisher C, Lloyd-Smith R, et al.: Osteochondral lesions of the talus. Am J Sports Med 21:13, 1993.
78. Lundeen RO: Arthroscopic evaluation of traumatic injuries to the ankle and foot. Part I: acute injuries. J Foot Ankle Surg 28:499, 1989.
79. Naumetz VA and Schweigel JF: Osteocartilaginous lesions of the talar dome. J Trauma 20:924, 1980.
80. Heller AJ and Vogler HW: Ankle joint arthroscopy. J Foot Ankle Surg 21:23, 1982.
81. Lundeen RO: Arthroscopic evaluation of traumatic injuries to the ankle and foot. Part II: chronic posttraumatic pain. J Foot Ankle Surg 29:59, 1990.
82. Chen YD: Arthroscopy of the ankle joint. Arthroscopy 1:16, 1976.
83. Lundeen RO and Hawkins RB: Arthroscopic lateral ankle stabilization. J Am Podiatr Med Assoc 75:372, 1985.
84. Hawkins RB: Ankle instability surgery from an arthroscopist's perspective. In McGinty JB (ed.): Operative Arthroscopy. New York, Raven Press, 1991, pp 747–752.
85. Morgan CP: Arthroscopic tibiotalar arthrodesis. In McGinty JB (ed.): Operative Arthroscopy. New York, Raven Press, 1991, pp 695–701.
86. Myerson MS and Allon SM: Arthroscopic ankle arthrodesis. Contemp Orthop 19:21, 1989.
87. Ogilvie-Harris DJ, Lieberman I, and Fitsialos D: Arthroscopically assisted arthrodesis for osteoarthritic ankles. J Bone Joint Surg Am 75:1167, 1993.
88. Mann JA, Glick JM, Morgan CT, et al.: Arthroscopic ankle arthrodesis: experience with 75 cases. Presented at the Annual Meeting of the American Academy of Orthopaedic Surgeons, Orlando, Fla., Feb., 1995.
89. Myerson MS and Quill G: Ankle arthrodesis: a comparison of an arthroscopic and an open method of treatment. Clin Orthop 268:84–95, 1991.
90. Ferkel RD, Heath DD, and Guhl JF: Neurological complications of ankle arthroscopy: a review of 612 cases. Arthroscopy 10:352, 1994.

Subtalar Arthroscopy: Diagnostic and Operative Techniques

Mark M. Williams • *Richard D. Ferkel*

Refinements in instrumentation and techniques used for the large joints allow these instruments and methods to be used for the smaller joints, creating useful surgical alternatives to traditional open procedures. Small-joint arthroscopy has been documented to be effective in treating disorders of the ankle, wrist, and elbow, as well as of the great toe metatarsophalangeal joint.[1] The posterior subtalar joint has become yet another structure amenable to arthroscopic evaluation and treatment.

There are only four published reports regarding arthroscopy of the subtalar joint. Parisien was the principal investigator on two of them, the first of which was published in 1985.[2] He presented the feasibility of subtalar arthroscopy with a cadaveric study and followed this up in 1986 with three case reports.[3] In 1994 Williams and Ferkel[4] presented the only series of subtalar arthroscopy to date. The authors presented results on 50 subtalar arthroscopies performed during a 3-year period, with 32-month average follow-up. All patients underwent ankle arthroscopy followed by subtalar arthroscopy. Of the patients, 42% underwent diagnostic subtalar arthroscopy only. The other 58% of the patients underwent operative subtalar arthroscopy for various diagnoses. For these latter 29 patients, 86% of the results were good to excellent, with 12 month–minimum follow-up. Patient results were affected by associated ankle disorders, degenerative joint disease, age, and activity level. The report by Frey, Gasser, and Feder[5] was an anatomic cadaveric study that further defined the position and safety of arthroscopic portals in relation to neurovascular structures and tendons.

Subtalar arthroscopy usually refers to arthroscopy of the posterior subtalar joint or the posterior talocalcaneal joint. The sinus tarsi anterior and middle facets are not as easily accessible to arthroscopy. Pertinent anatomy is discussed as part of the general technique described later. This chapter reviews patient selection, operating room set-up, diagnostic and operative subtalar arthroscopy, and postoperative management.

PATIENT SELECTION

Indications

The diagnostic indications for posterior subtalar arthroscopy include persistent subtalar pain, swelling, locking, or catching that has been refractory to conservative management.

The therapeutic indications for subtalar arthroscopy include the treatment of various stages of degenerative joint disease, such as synovitis, loose bodies, and chondromalacia. Other indications include post-traumatic arthrofibrosis, sinus tarsi syndrome, painful os trigonum, and osteochondritis dissecans. Severe degenerative arthritis may require subtalar arthrodesis; Tasto[6] described his technique of arthroscopic subtalar arthrodesis, with apparently excellent fusion rates. Future indications may include fracture assessment and reduction. Other indications will undoubtedly occur as operative experience with the technique increases.

Contraindications

Absolute contraindications to subtalar arthroscopy include localized infection and advanced degenerative joint disease with deformity. Severe deformity may logistically prevent an adequate diagnostic or operative arthroscopy from being completed.

Relative contraindications include severe edema, poor vascularity, and severe arthrofibrosis, which may preclude visualization of anatomy.

In the authors' experience, when patients present with chronic sprain pain with discomfort in both the lateral subtalar region and the lateral gutter of the ankle and soft-tissue impingement findings are noted at ankle arthroscopy, subtalar joint arthroscopy is not indicated unless there are preoperative findings to suggest otherwise.[7]

Conservative Treatment and Preoperative Evaluation

Subtalar evaluation begins with a detailed history followed by a careful physical examination. Radiographs of the weight-bearing patient must be obtained and should include oblique views to allow visualization of the ankle and the subtalar joints. Occasionally, special views are necessary to understand the problem further. These include Broden, Cobey, and Isherwood views and stress x-ray films.

Before surgery, all patients are treated with conservative measures such as nonsteroidal anti-inflammatory drugs, ice, bracing, casting, and physical therapy. Physical therapy should emphasize modalities to control inflammation (such as phonophoresis and iontophoresis), stretching and strengthening of the foot and ankle, and proprioceptive training. Shoe modification and orthotic inserts should be considered. A trial of immobilization using a removable short-leg orthosis may be of some benefit in selected cases of chronic subtalar pain and swelling. Occasionally, subtalar lidocaine (Xylocaine) injection, with or without cortisone, may be of diagnostic and therapeutic benefit.

In patients with persistent symptoms, further diagnostic testing is indicated. Computed tomography scan, in both coronal and axial planes, is helpful for detecting degenerative joint disease, loose bodies, osteochondral lesions, nonunions of the os trigonum, and other abnormalities. A three-phase technetium bone scan can identify and localize occult disorders and evaluate nonunions. Magnetic resonance imaging is more beneficial in evaluating soft-tissue disease, including that of the surrounding tendons and ligaments, as well as osteochondral lesions and marrow edema. In addition, diagnostic studies such as computed tomography, magnetic resonance imaging, and bone scanning can be particularly helpful for surgical planning.

Patient Education

Patient education is a key component for a successful procedure. It is important that, before surgery, patients have a rudimentary understanding of the anatomy of the ankle and subtalar joint and what is planned on being accomplished or performed at surgery. At the Southern California Orthopaedic Institute, an education tape is shown to all patients at their preoperative visit. The tape also includes instructions on postoperative care. An instruction sheet is given to all patients at this time so they can have it available for reference after surgery.

OPERATING ROOM SET-UP

Anesthesia

Subtalar arthroscopy is typically performed using a general or regional anesthetic. Local anesthetic is not recommended because muscular relaxation is required to allow good joint distraction and intra-articular visualization of the ankle and subtalar joints. Also, should an invasive distractor be required, a local anesthetic is not ideal.

Patient Positioning

Subtalar arthroscopy is performed with the patient in a position similar to that for ankle arthroscopy (see Chapters 31 and 32). Depending on the surgeon's preference, the patient may be positioned in either a supine position or lateral decubitus position or with the knee flexed at 90 degrees, with the leg over the table or supported by a leg holder.

Equipment

Operative equipment includes a tourniquet, thigh holder, and small-joint instrumentation similar to that used for the ankle. Small arthroscopes of 2.7 and 1.9 mm diameter are required with the use of a small shaver and blades of similar sizes. Generally, a short 2.7 mm, 30 degree oblique arthroscope is used. A 2.7 mm, 70 degree oblique arthroscope is helpful in certain situations to allow visualization (Fig. 33–1). A short 1.9 mm, 30 degree oblique arthroscope is sometimes required in particularly tight joints. A "videoarthroscope" is recommended for avoiding a long lever arm and increased weight. For most cases, a 2.9 mm

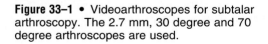

Figure 33–1 • Videoarthroscopes for subtalar arthroscopy. The 2.7 mm, 30 degree and 70 degree arthroscopes are used.

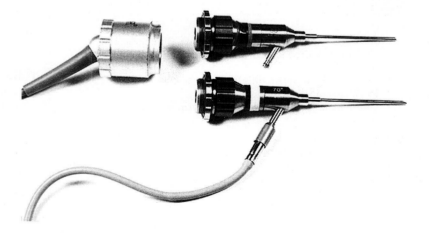

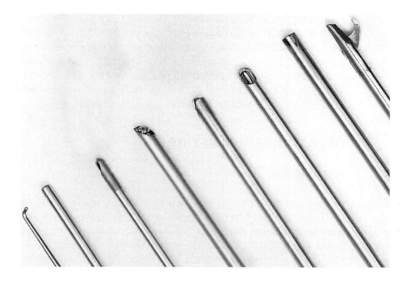

Figure 33–2 • Small-joint basket, shavers, burs, and probes are utilized with subtalar arthroscopy.

full-radius synovial resector and 2.9 mm bur are adequate, but smaller 1.9 and 2.0 mm blades should be available as needed. Appropriate small-joint hand instruments are necessary to facilitate débridement, loose body removal, and drilling. These instruments include probes, baskets, knives, graspers, and curets (Fig. 33–2). See Table 33–1 for a complete list of recommended instruments.

Soft-tissue and invasive distraction instrumentation should also be available and used as needed for visualization. Specific distraction techniques are presented in Chapter 31.

GENERAL TECHNIQUE

Regional Anatomy

The posterior subtalar joint, or the posterior talocalcaneal joint, includes the posterior talar and calcaneal facets. The posterior subtalar joint is separated from the anterior subtalar joint (talocalcaneonavicular joint) by the tarsal canal and sinus tarsi. The tarsal canal is formed by the inferior

Table 33–1	Instruments for Subtalar Arthroscopy

Needed
- 1.9 and 2.7 mm, 30 degree and 2.7 mm, 30 degree and 70 degree short videoarthroscopes with lightweight chip cameras
- 2.0 and 2.9 mm full-radius blades, whiskers, and burs
- 18 gauge spinal needle
- Two 19 gauge needles and 55 mL syringe with intravenous tubing

Otherwise include
   Small joint probe, small joint grasper
   Ring curets, pituitary
   K-wires
   Drill

talar sulcus and the superior calcaneal sulcus. The canal is bordered anteriorly and posteriorly by the respective joint capsules of the anterior and posterior subtalar joints. The tarsal canal's long axis is oriented obliquely in a 45 degree fashion, from posteromedial to anterolateral.

The ligamentous support of the ankle and subtalar joints has been extensively documented. Some controversy remains regarding the subtalar joint's ligamentous anatomy. Dissections performed by Ferkel have found three distinct layers of ligaments supporting the subtalar joint. These findings support work performed by Harper[8] in 1991. These layers are divided into superficial, intermediate, and deep layers. The superficial layer includes the talocalcaneal ligaments (lateral, posterior, and middle), the lateral root of the inferior extensor retinaculum, and the calcaneofibular ligament. Reflections of the lateral talocalcaneal and calcaneofibular ligaments are readily observed during subtalar arthroscopy. The intermediate layer includes the intermediate root of the inferior extensor retinaculum and the cervical ligament. The cervical ligament arises from the floor of the sinus tarsi and is thought to limit inversion. The deep layer of ligaments includes the medial root of the inferior extensor retinaculum and the interosseous talocalcaneal ligament (also known as the ligament of the tarsal canal). This ligament is the most important structure uniting the talus and calcaneus and prevents eversion, heel valgus, and longitudinal arch depression. This structure is readily visualized with diagnostic subtalar arthroscopy.

Portals

Primary Portals

Arthroscopy of the posterior subtalar joint is performed on the lateral side of the hindfoot by using two primary and two accessory portals (Fig. 33–3). It is imperative to outline pertinent bony and soft-tissue anatomy before subtalar arthroscopy. This is a concept similar to those of glenohumeral arthroscopy preceding subacromial bur-

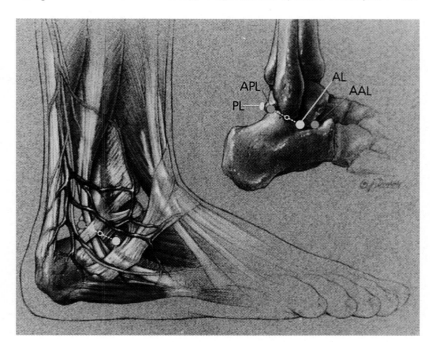

Figure 33–3 • Subtalar portals. The anterolateral (AL) and the posterolateral (PL) are the primary portals. The accessory anterolateral (AAL) portal and the accessory posterolateral (APL) portal are frequently used with operative procedures. (Copyright, Dr. Richard D. Ferkel.)

soscopy and anatomic outlines being made before soft-tissue extravasation.

Careful attention should be given to outlining the bony ankle joint with a marking pen. The superficial peroneal nerve and the dorsalis pedis neurovascular bundle should also be identified when possible and outlined. The tip of the fibula and the Achilles tendon serve as the anatomic landmarks for the subtalar portals. Note that the sural nerve is at risk when the posterolateral portal is established. Two studies have evaluated the neurovascular structures surrounding the subtalar portals.[5, 9]

Once bony anatomy and soft-tissue anatomy have been outlined, the posterolateral subtalar portal is identified and is marked at the fibular tip and just lateral to the Achilles tendon. Exact portal placement depends on the amount of distraction applied. The anterolateral portal is marked approximately 1 cm distal to the fibular tip and 2 cm anterior to it.

Accessory Portals

Accessory anterolateral and posterolateral portals are useful for instrumentation. The accessory posterolateral portal is established lateral to the posterolateral portal, with extreme care given to avoiding injury to the sural nerve, the lesser saphenous vein, and the peroneal tendons. These structures are also at risk, of course, when the posterolateral portal is established. The accessory anterolateral portal is normally placed slightly superior and anterior to the anterolateral portal. The accessory portal is established with a needle localization technique under direct visualization from either the posterolateral or anterolateral portal. It is important to keep enough separation between the primary portal and the accessory portal to allow triangulation and to prevent instrument crowding.

Normal Arthroscopic Examination

Authors' Preferred Technique

The authors' preferred technique is similar to that described for ankle arthroscopy in Chapter 32. Briefly, the patient is placed in the supine position, and a thigh holder is utilized to maintain hip flexion of 45 degrees. The thigh is well padded, and a tourniquet is applied but inflated only at the surgeon's discretion. A noninvasive distraction strap is placed on the ankle, keeping it low enough to allow subtalar portal placement. The strap is attached to a distraction device, as previously described in Chapter 32. This positioning allows 360 degree access to the foot and ankle (Fig. 33–4). It is critical that enough room be available posteriorly to work from the posterolateral portal. On a rare occasion, invasive distraction may be necessary. In that case, a sterile foot holder and clamp are attached to the table over the sterile drapes, and the invasive distractor is applied.

The joint is distended by inserting a 19 gauge needle into the posterolateral portal. Care is taken to avoid puncture of the lesser saphenous vein or sural nerve. When locating this portal it is important to avoid placing it too proximally, or the arthroscopist will inadvertently enter the posterior ankle joint instead. Exact posterolateral portal placement varies, depending on the amount of distraction. As in arthroscopy of other joints, bony landmarks are used as a guide only. Once the needle is positioned in the posterolateral portal, the joint is distended with fluid, and free backflow through the needle is confirmed. With the joint distended, the anterolateral portal is established in the position as previously outlined. Using another 19 gauge needle to verify correct portal placement, free flow of fluid must be confirmed through the anterior needle before making the portal incisions. When placing the

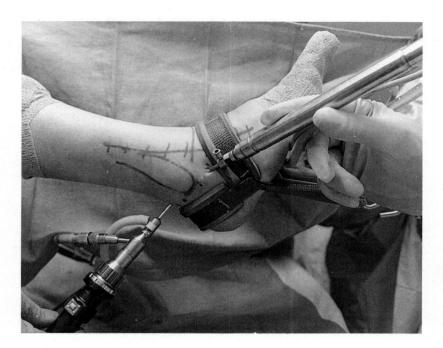

Figure 33–4 • Typical set-up for subtalar arthroscopy using soft-tissue noninvasive distraction. Note that the arthroscope is placed through the posterolateral portal while shaving is done through the anterolateral portal.

anterolateral needle, it should be positioned so that it is angled away from the sinus tarsi and placed with care to avoid abrading the articular surface.

After proper needle localization of portals, incisions are made with care to avoid injury to subcutaneous neurovascular structures. The anterolateral portal is established first and is used as the initial viewing portal. The skin is carefully incised, and the subcutaneous tissues are separated bluntly with a clamp. Branches of the superficial peroneal nerve are at risk particularly with anterolateral portal development. A short 2.7 mm, 30 degree oblique arthroscope is then inserted through an interchangeable cannula in the anterolateral portal. Inflow may be used through the arthroscopic cannula, and the posterolateral portal may be used for instrumentation. If visualization is obscured by lack of distraction, further noninvasive distraction is applied. If this is unsuccessful, then invasive distraction is applied. Once the anterolateral inspection is complete, the arthroscope is switched to the posterolateral portal to complete the diagnostic examination (see Fig. 33–4). Accessory anterolateral and posterolateral portals are utilized as needed to address disorders and facilitate inflow. Occasionally, the short 2.7 mm, 70 degree oblique videoscope is used for areas that are hard to see.

On occasion, it may be necessary to combine subtalar and ankle arthroscopy at the same sitting. In this instance, subtalar arthroscopy should be done first because, after ankle arthroscopy, fluid extravasation can make it difficult to locate the subtalar portals properly and perform subtalar arthroscopy.

13-Point Diagnostic Examination

As with diagnostic arthroscopy of all joints, it is important to have a reproducible, systematic method of anatomic review. Whenever the authors perform diagnostic subtalar arthroscopy, they employ a 13-point arthroscopic evaluation starting from anterior to posterior. It is critical that the examination be done the same way every time to avoid missing any disorder. After the anterolateral portal is used, the arthroscope is switched to the posterolateral portal. Inflow may be used through the arthroscope or the other portal. At the surgeon's preference, a gravity inflow or fluid management system may be used. The authors routinely do not use an arthroscopic pump.

The diagnostic examination begins anteriorly with the arthroscope in the anterolateral portal (Fig. 33–5*A*). The interosseous talocalcaneal ligament is readily observed. Both the deep (1) and the superficial (2) portions of the interosseous ligament are noted (Fig. 33–5*B*). As the arthroscopic lens is rotated from medial to lateral, the anterior aspect of the saddle-shaped posterior talocalcaneal joint (3) is visualized. Further laterally, the anterolateral corner (4) is examined, and the ligamentous reflections of the lateral talocalcaneal ligament (5) and the calcaneofibular ligament (6) are seen. The relationship of the calcaneofibular ligament is posterior to the lateral talocalcaneal ligament. As the arthroscopic lens is rotated medially, the central articulation (7) and the posterolateral gutter (8) are seen.

The arthroscope is then switched to the posterolateral portal, and the inflow may be placed in the anterolateral

Figure 33–5 • Thirteen-point subtalar examination. *A*, Diagnostic examination of the right posterior subtalar joint from the lateral view. This joint is separated from the tarsal canal by the interosseous talocalcaneal ligament. (From Ferkel RD: Arthroscopic Surgery: The Ankle and Foot. Philadelphia, Lippincott-Raven, 1996.) *B*, Arthroscopic view showing a right subtalar joint with the interosseous talocalcaneal ligament well demonstrated.

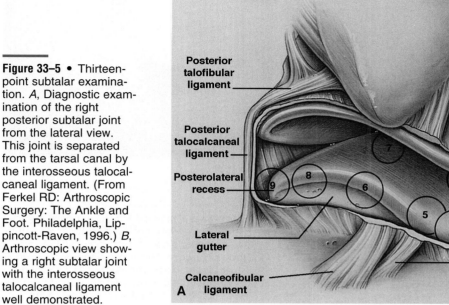

Lateral view

Posterior talofibular ligament

Posterior talocalcaneal ligament

Posterolateral recess

Lateral gutter

Calcaneofibular ligament

A

Medial roots of inferior extensor retinaculum

Tarsal canal

Cervical ligament

Interosseous talocalcaneal ligament

Anterior capsular ligament

Lateral talocalcaneal ligament

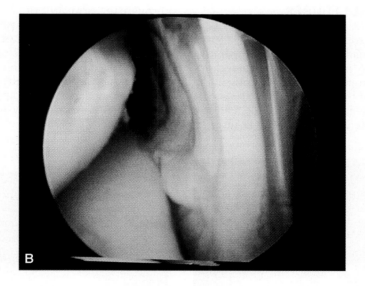

B

Illustration continued on following page

portal or through the arthroscope (Fig. 33–5*C*). The joint is once again examined from front to back, or anteriorly to posteriorly. Anteriorly, the interosseous ligament may be seen through the bony articulation. The lateral talocalcaneal ligament (5) and the calcaneofibular ligament (6) reflections are observed from the posterior view (Fig. 33–5*D*). As the arthroscope is withdrawn posteriorly, the posterolateral recess (9) and the posterior gutter (10) are identified. The arthroscopic lens is then rotated medially to observe the posteromedial recess (11) and the postero-

medial corner (12). The final structure seen is the posterior aspect of the talocalcaneal articulation (13). The posterior arthroscopic portal usually provides the best view of abnormalities of the os trigonum and of the Stieda process.

After the diagnostic portion of the procedure is complete, the disease observed is treated as needed. Afterward, the portals are closed with simple nylon ligatures, and the limb is immobilized in a soft, bulky, short-leg compressive dressing supported by a posterior plaster splint. Further postoperative care is discussed later.

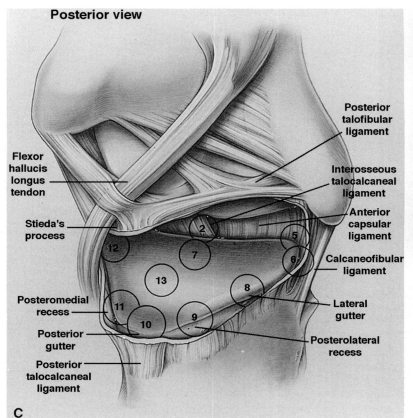

Posterior view

Flexor
hallucis
longus
tendon

Stieda's
process

Posteromedial
recess

Posterior
gutter

Posterior
talocalcaneal
ligament

Posterior
talofibular
ligament

Interosseous
talocalcaneal
ligament

Anterior
capsular
ligament

Calcaneofibular
ligament

Lateral
gutter

Posterolateral
recess

C

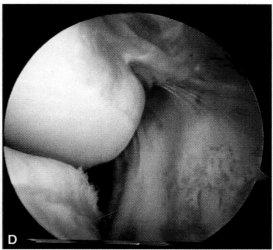

D

Figure 33–5 *Continued* • *C,* Diagnostic examination of the right posterior subtalar joint from
the posterior view. (From Ferkel RD: Arthroscopic Surgery: The Ankle and Foot. Philadelphia, Lippincott-Raven, 1996.) *D,* Lateral gutter of the right posterior subtalar joint from the
posterior view. Note the reflections of the
lateral talocalcaneal and calcaneofibular
ligaments.

SPECIFIC OPERATIVE PROCEDURES

In the authors' series,[4] the treatment of various stages of degenerative joint disease made up 34% of the operative procedures. It is possible to perform an adequate chondroplasty and abrasion arthroplasty arthroscopically in the subtalar joint with the use of the 2.9 mm synovial resector and bur. Portal selection for instrumentation depends on the site of the lesion. Generally, the shaver is inserted through the primary portal closest to the lesion and the arthroscope through the primary portal farthest away to allow better triangulation and to prevent instrument crowding. However, an accessory portal may be required because it can be difficult to see across the central talocalcaneal articulation, especially if there is poor distraction. These general principles apply also to operative techniques such as synovectomy and loose body removal (Figs. 33–6 and 33–7).

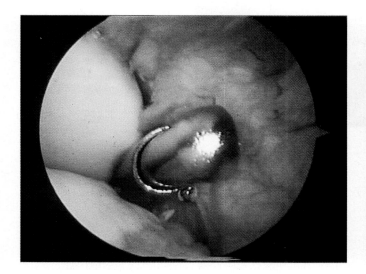

Figure 33–6 • Synovitis surrounding the lateral gutter of the right posterior subtalar joint. Visualization is through the posterolateral portal, and the shaver is coming in through the anterolateral portal.

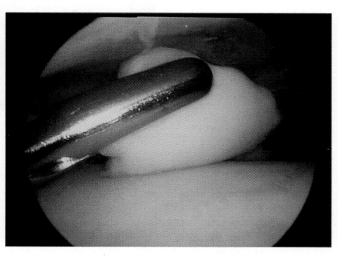

Figure 33–7 • Removal of osteochondral loose body. With visualization from the anterolateral portal, the grasper is inserted through the posterolateral portal to remove the loose body.

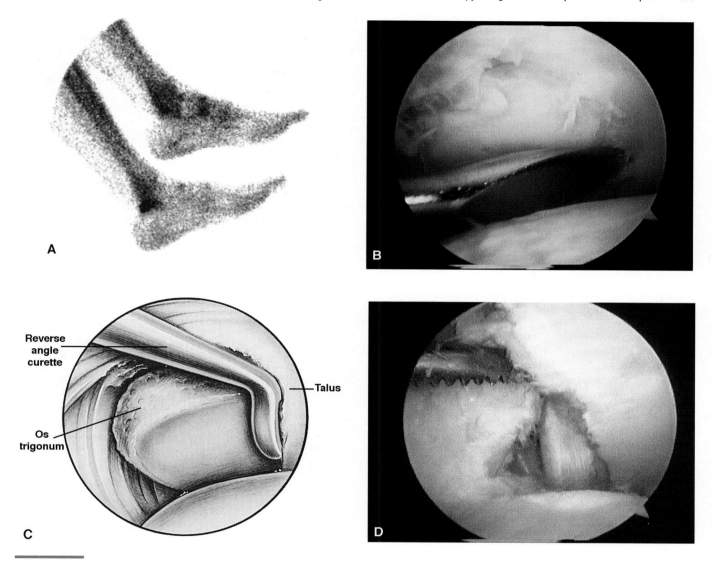

Figure 33–8 • Removal of os trigonum. *A*, Bone scan of a professional dancer with 1-year history of pain in the posterior right ankle. Note the well localized "hot" spot along the os trigonum. *B*, Insertion of a banana knife to free the os trigonum from the posterior talus. *C*, Use of a reverse-angle curet to assist in peeling the os trigonum away from the talus. (From Ferkel RD: Arthroscopic Surgery: The Ankle and Foot. Philadelphia, Lippincott-Raven, 1996.) *D*, Removal of the loose os trigonum with a grasper through the postero-lateral portal. Notice the flexor hallucis longus is preserved.

Another specific indication for operative subtalar arthroscopy is a painful os trigonum. The work-up should include plain radiographs, a three-phase technetium bone scan, and occasionally a computed tomography scan. A patient with a symptomatic nonunion of the os trigonum may demonstrate a "hot" bone scan, and a computed axial tomography scan can show the site of the fibrous union or nonunion, especially on the axillary views (Fig. 33–8*A*). In the authors' series,[4] 14% of the patients treated with oper-ative subtalar arthroscopy underwent an arthroscopic exci-sion of the os trigonum. In performing the excision, the os trigonum is usually visualized from the anterolateral por-tal, the inflow is through an accessory anterolateral portal, and the posterolateral portal is utilized to instrument the lesion. Occasionally, two posterior portals may be required. Arthroscopic banana knives, curets (reverse-

angle), and graspers facilitate excision of this lesion (Figs. 33–8*B* and 33–8*C*). Care must be taken to remove the os trigonum without injuring the flexor hallucis longus tendon and posteromedial neurovascular bundle (Fig. 33–8*D*).

POSTOPERATIVE CARE

Postoperatively, the patient is evaluated at 1 week, and the splint and sutures are removed. The patient then uses a compressive stocking and an ankle support shoe. The shoe preferred by the authors has a dual bladder that generates compression through small air cells and reduces swelling by circulating cold water around these air cells. At this first visit, weight-bearing is initiated, and crutches are discontinued as dictated by the type of procedure and patient comfort. An early rehabilitation program is encouraged, and patients undergo physical therapy emphasizing range-of-motion, strengthening, and proprioceptive exercises. Patients may return to their usual activities, such as sports, once they have maximized their range of motion and strength and have normal proprioception and no pain.

COMPLICATIONS

Complications from subtalar arthroscopy similar to those from ankle arthroscopy may be expected. In the authors' series,[4] there were no major complications, and there was only one minor complication of postoperative ecchymosis that resolved uneventfully. This is the only published series of cases and is not large enough to provide any statistically significant data regarding complication rates for relatively rare problems such as infection or neurovascular injury. Nevertheless, these problems should be expected to occur in frequency similar to that documented for the ankle.[9]

Certainly, the specific concern with subtalar arthroscopy is iatrogenic injury to underlying neurovascular structures that are especially at risk when establishing portals. The sural and superficial peroneal nerves and the lesser saphenous vein are particularly vulnerable with arthroscopic procedures on the lateral hindfoot. Careful attention should be given to trying to palpate any underlying nerves when outlining anatomy. Also, special care should be taken when establishing portals. The skin should not be incised below the dermis, and the subcutaneous tissues should be dissected bluntly with a small hemostat when placing arthroscopic cannulas. Attention to these details when establishing portals minimizes complications. The reader is referred to excellent anatomic studies regarding the sural nerve.[5, 10]

References

1. Ferkel RD and Van Buecken K: Great toe arthroscopy: indications, technique, and results. Presented at Arthroscopy Association of North America, San Diego, Calif., April, 1991.
2. Parisien JS and Vangsness CT: Arthroscopy of the subtalar joint: an experimental approach. Arthroscopy 1:53–57, 1985.
3. Parisien JS: Arthroscopy of the posterior subtalar joint: a preliminary report. Foot Ankle Int 6:219–224, 1986.
4. Williams MM and Ferkel RD: Subtalar arthroscopy: indications, technique, and results. Arthroscopy 10:345, 1994.
5. Frey C, Gasser S, and Feder K: Arthroscopy of the subtalar joint. Foot Ankle Int 15:425, 1994.
6. Tasto J: Subtalar arthrodesis. Presented at Specialty Day of the Arthroscopy Association of North America, Orlando, Fla., Feb., 1995.
7. Ferkel RD, Karzel RP, Del Pizzo W, et al.: Arthroscopic treatment of anterolateral impingement of the ankle. Am J Sports Med 19:440–446, 1991.
8. Harper MC: The lateral ligamentous support of the ankle. Foot Ankle Int 12:354–358, 1991.
9. Ferkel RD, Guhl J, Van Buecken K, et al.: Complications in 518 ankle arthroscopies. Orthop Trans 16:726, 1993.
10. Lawrence SJ and Botte MJ: The sural nerve in the foot and ankle: an anatomic study with clinical and surgical implications. Foot Ankle Int 15:490, 1994.

Index

Note: Page numbers in *italics* refer to illustrations; page numbers followed by (t) refer to tables.